A WORLD OF YOGA

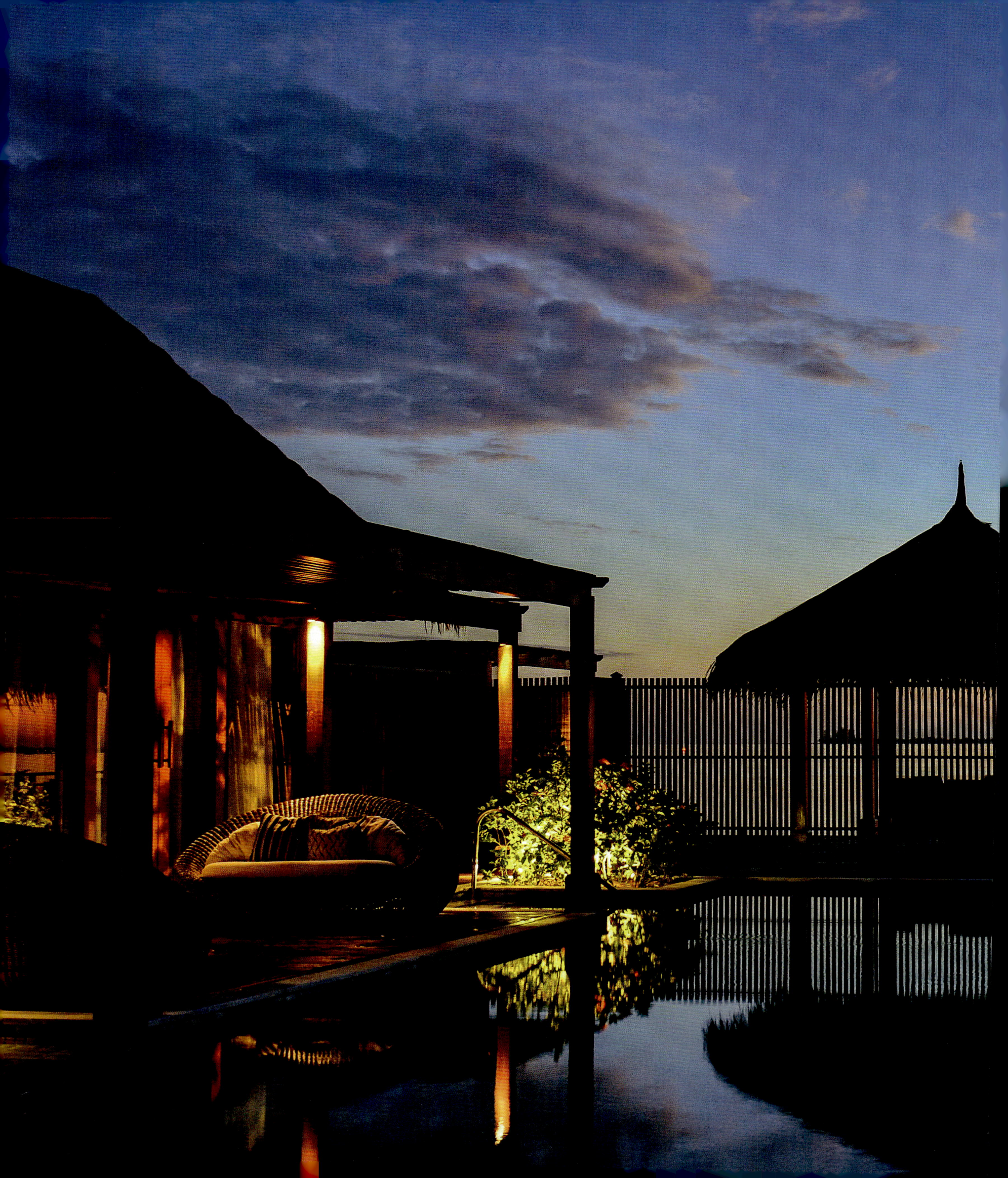

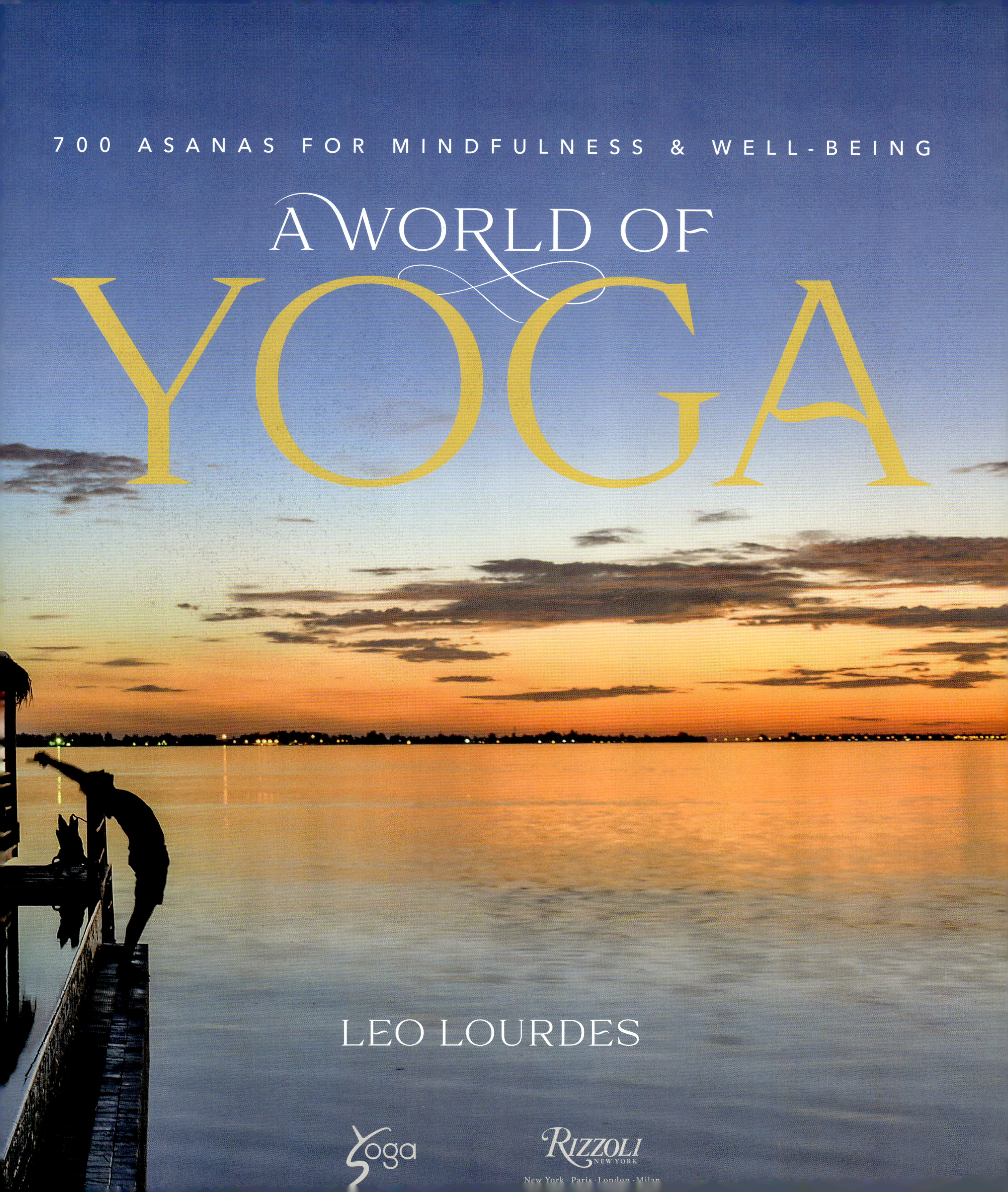

700 ASANAS FOR MINDFULNESS & WELL-BEING

A WORLD OF YOGA

LEO LOURDES

Yoga

RIZZOLI NEW YORK

New York · Paris · London · Milan

CONTENTS

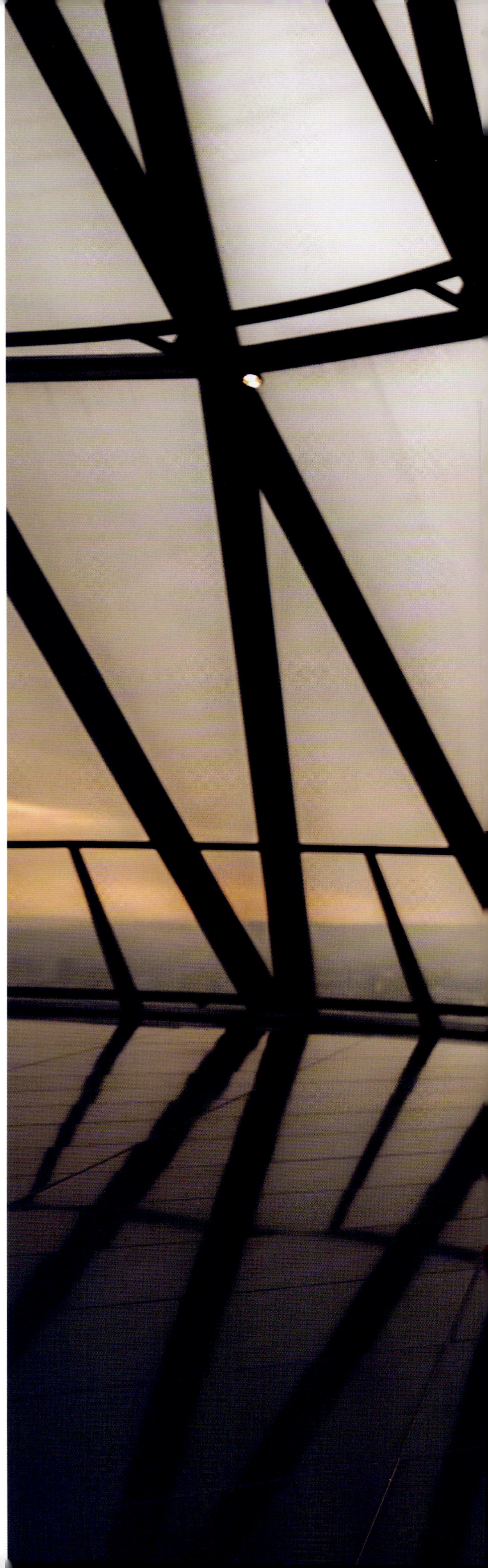

SAMDHI ANJANEYASANA · Horizon Crescent Lunge

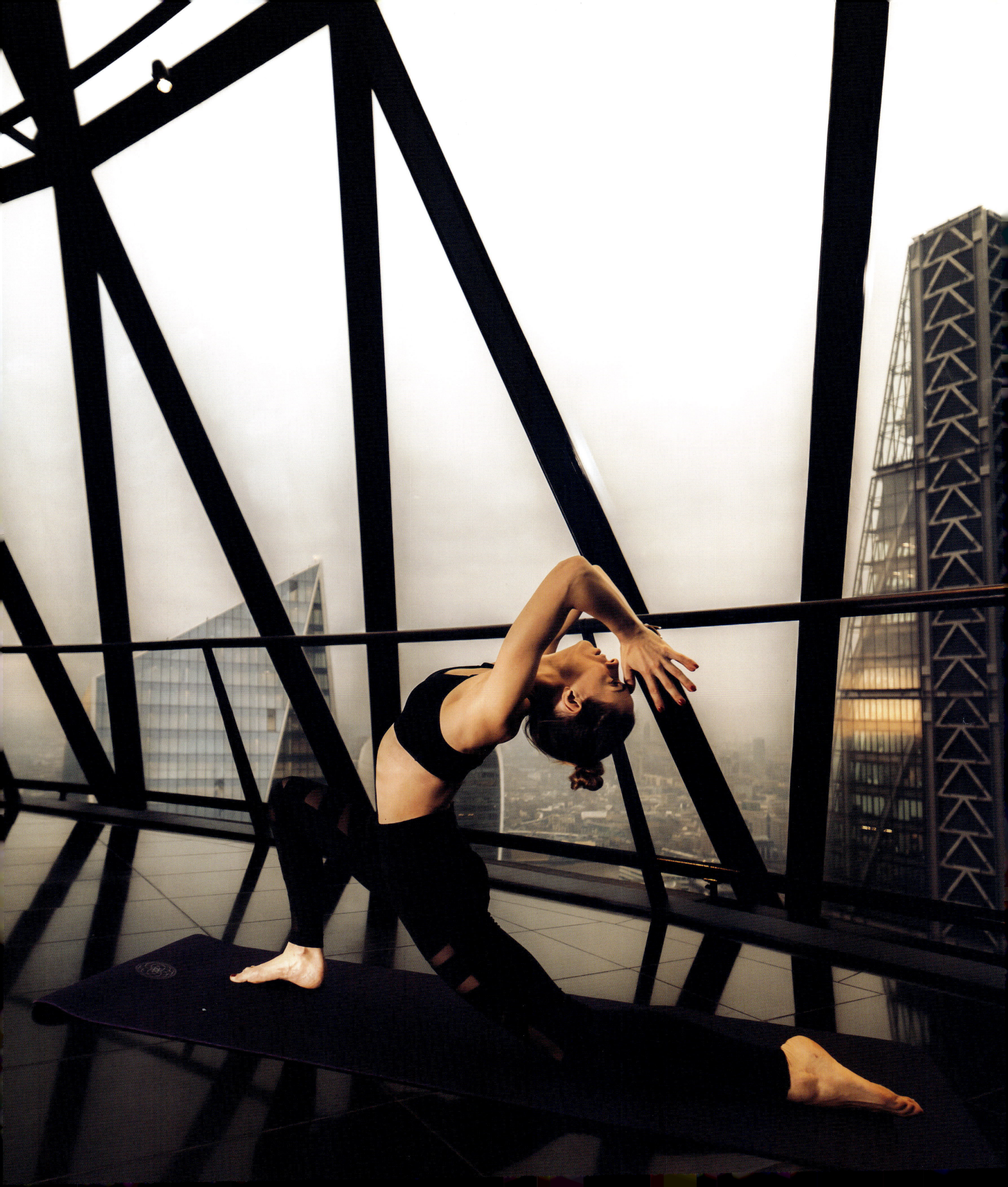

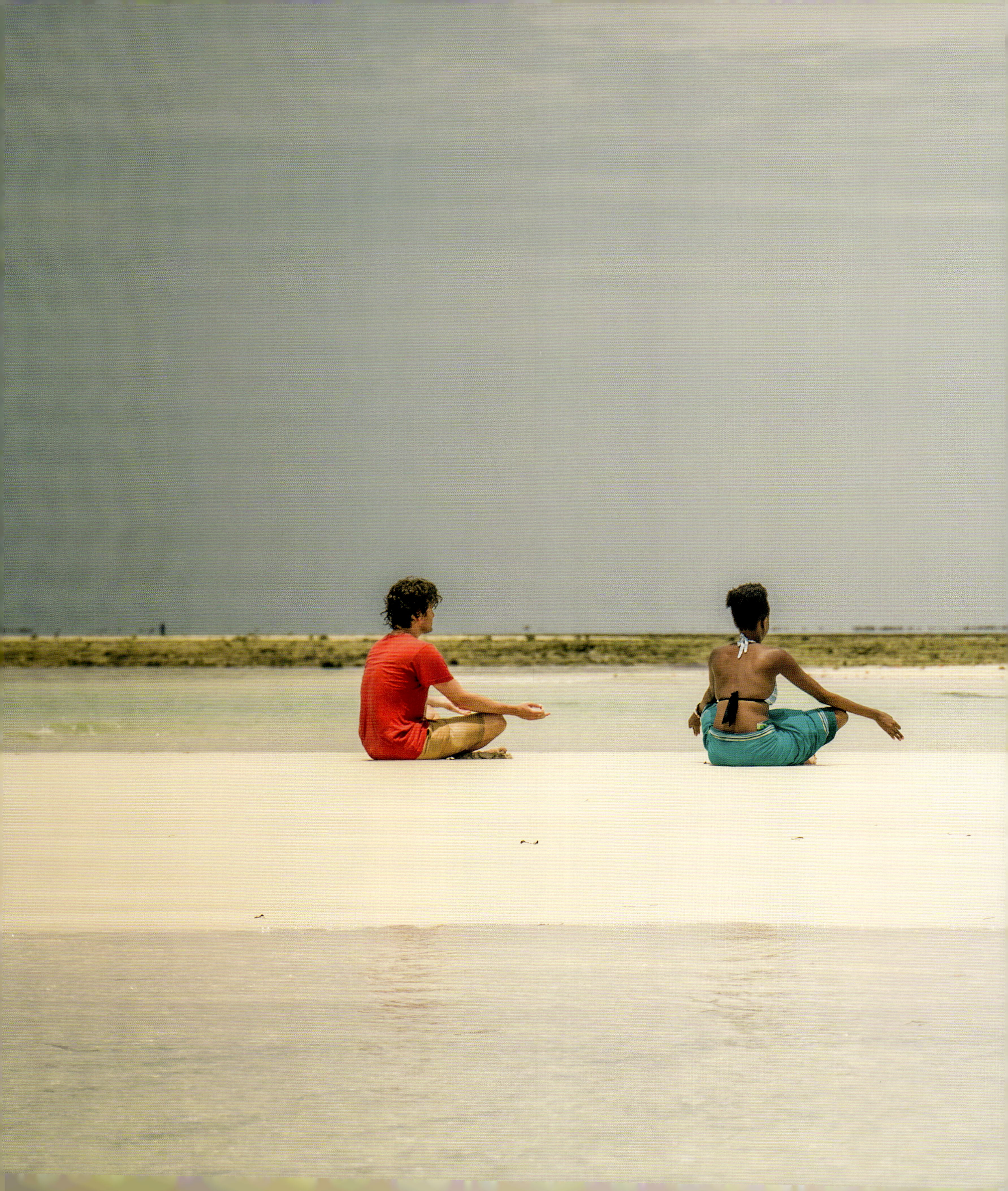

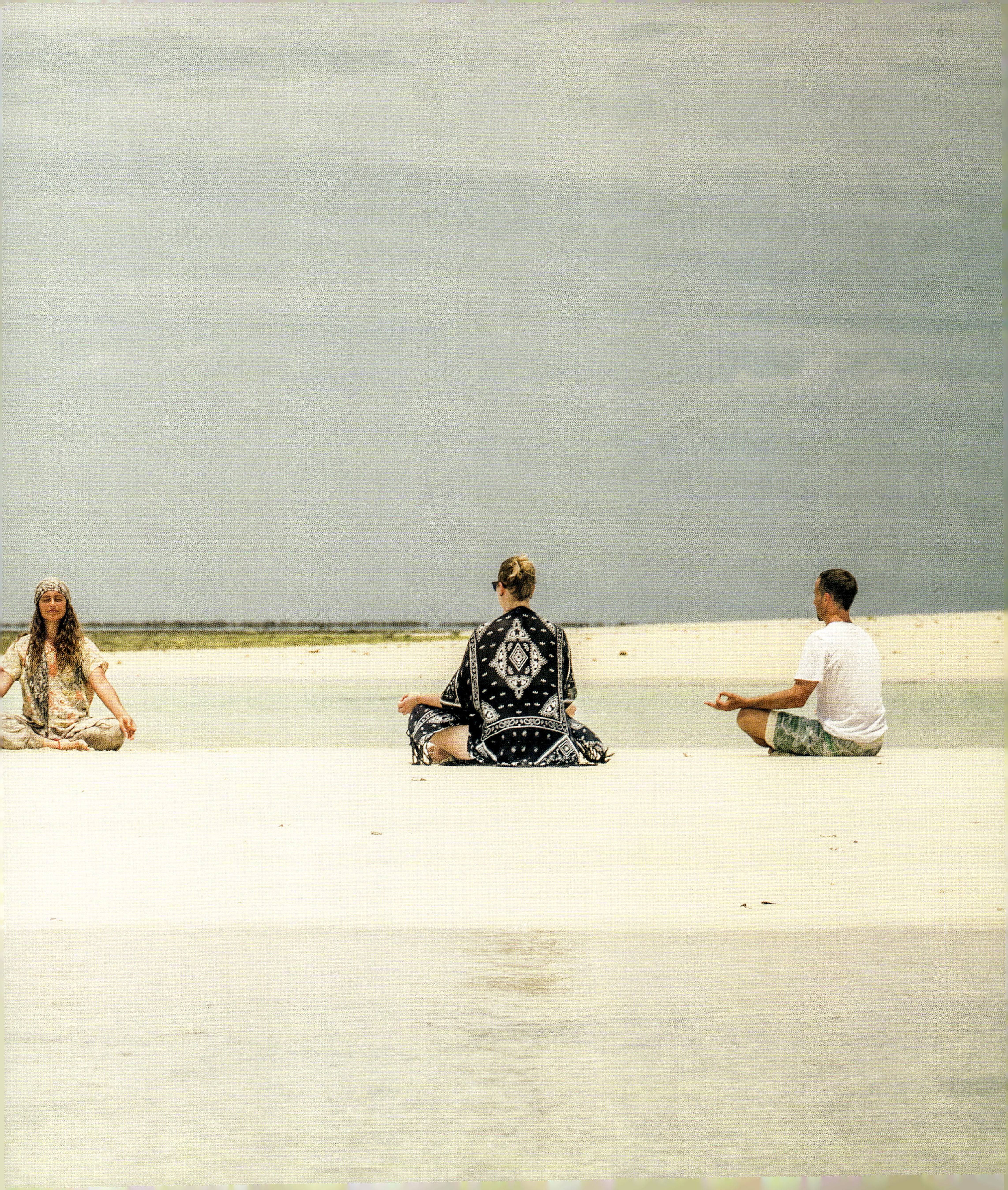

INTRODUCTION

I would not be here if not for yoga. I do not come from a viewpoint of trying to be your guru. Instead, I am here as your guide and friend. When people describe me as a guru, it makes me uncomfortable because people look to a guru for all kinds of answers. A guru is a spiritual teacher and a source of wisdom and knowledge—which my creation, Brahma Yoga, offers you—but I am not here to give you a premade perspective on life.

I am interested in *your* story. You are unique. You had a one in four trillion chance to be born. I will gladly listen to the life events that have contributed to who you are and the fiction of fear that, at times, has become all too real for you. It may be your circumstance, but it is not your truth. What I seek is the nascent part of you that is brimming with possibility. I will help you realize that possibility in yourself. That is my promise to you, and I will be by your side. Give yourself this opportunity to grow and develop a lifelong love of yoga.

In this book, you will experience six dedicated chapters based on the benefits you are drawn to by practicing Brahma Yoga. Each chapter includes affirmations I have created to inspire you. These reflections encourage a way to connect to the essence of each chapter and can be experienced as a guided visualization. I have also created Brahma Yoga sequences of poses and mudras based on your sun signs that will help you release the wisdom that resides within you.

My own love of yoga initially began as a quest. My great-grandfather came from Pondicherry, a former French colony in India, and yoga gave me a way to understand my roots while feeling a sense of connection to the diaspora that led my family to be uprooted through circumstance, or perhaps synchronicity. From direct experience, I know yoga is revolutionary, as it can change the way we treat the world and the life force within it. I understand the suffering life can bring and the challenges we face both individually and existentially with our planet and its ecology. I am no stranger to hardship myself. Imagine the worst, and you would be close to understanding what has happened to me throughout my life. Statistically, I should not be here, but to be here now is a gift, and I choose to be present and stay focused on my purpose.

Through principles of Tantra Yoga and chakra work, I healed my body from the abuses inflicted on me as a child. Through yoga asanas, I learned to love and reclaim my body with confidence beyond its history. Through pranayama breath work and visualization, I overcame complex post-traumatic stress disorder. Through Ayurveda, I explored naturopathic ways to listen to my body. Through yoga philosophy, I honed the intelligence of my mind. Through Raja Yoga, I developed extraordinary memory skills. Through chanting mantras, I released my voice and wrote, composed, produced, and performed songs using the science of sentics that evoked love and inspired emotional states. Through Kathak and Bharatanatyam dancing, I freed my spirit in ecstatic movement and storytelling. Through Vedic cosmology, I was able to connect all the dots and understand the occurrence of meaningful coincidences in my life. So my accumulated life experiences truly have been a grand experiment to becoming worthy of being your guide. I honor that with devotion and the utmost reverence.

I have always had a love of personal development driven as a quest to heal my life. I created a company called Futuremind and was the youngest consultant on London's prestigious Harley Street when I was 22 years old. I created Yogasphere, YS Yoga, and Brahma Yoga, and I launched my first yoga studio in The Shard in London and the second in Grosvenor Square in Mayfair. I have taught, shared wisdom with, and coached more than 40,000 people globally, including Oprah Winfrey in the Himalayas, Donna Karan at her home in the Hamptons, Dua Lipa and Helena Bonham Carter in London, and Elle Macpherson on a private island in the Maldives. I have been a stress-management consultant for Bank of America Merrill Lynch, ran Unilever's creative problem-solving program, and served as yoga master for Blackstone, an investment company. And even when the world unraveled due to the global pandemic and studios were forced to close, I continued to teach yoga online.

Based on these facts, you might have the impression that I have been successful in my life, but I have learned something important along the way. Life has taught me that I am still the same person whether I am living in luxury or in abject poverty. I am the same

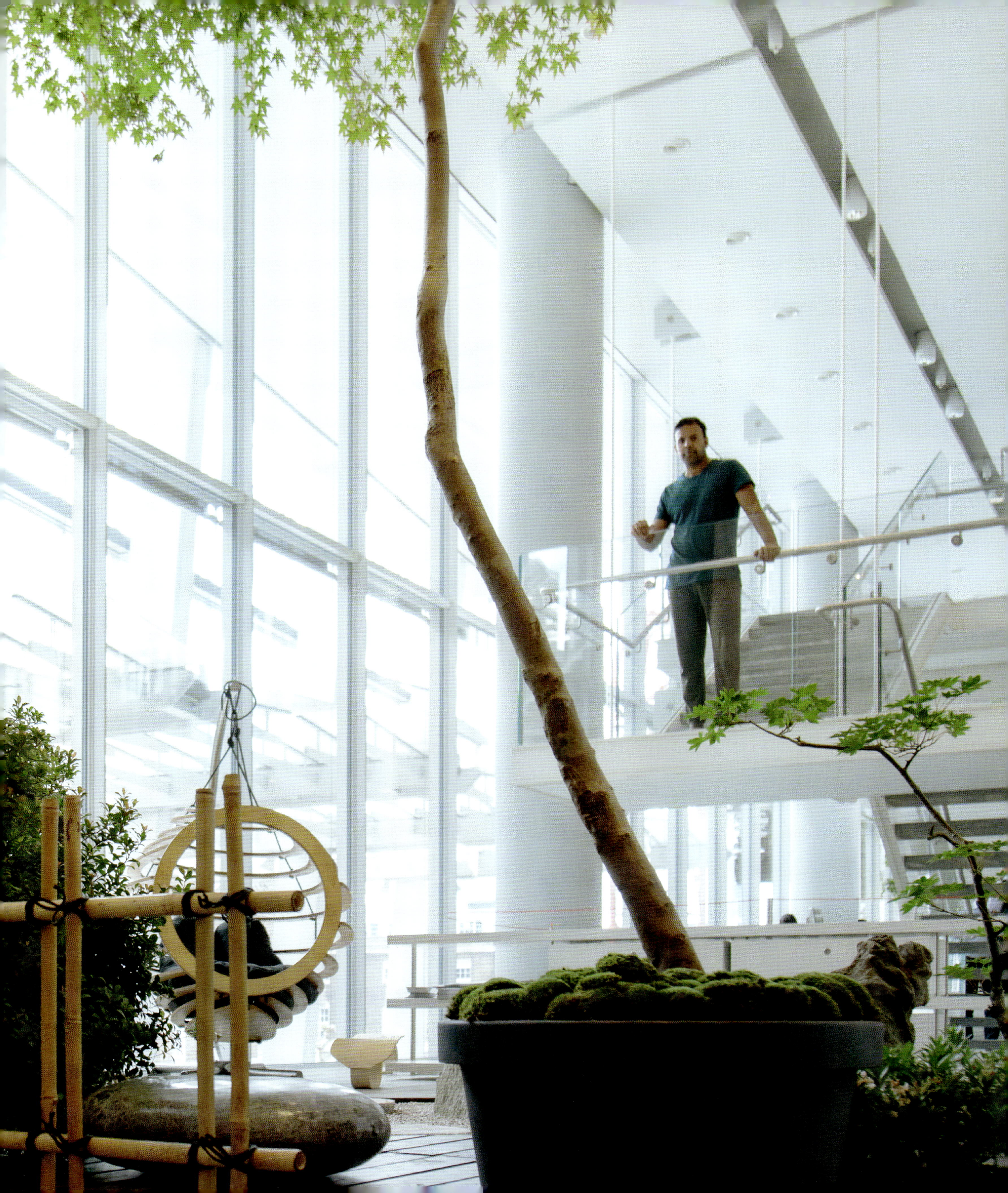

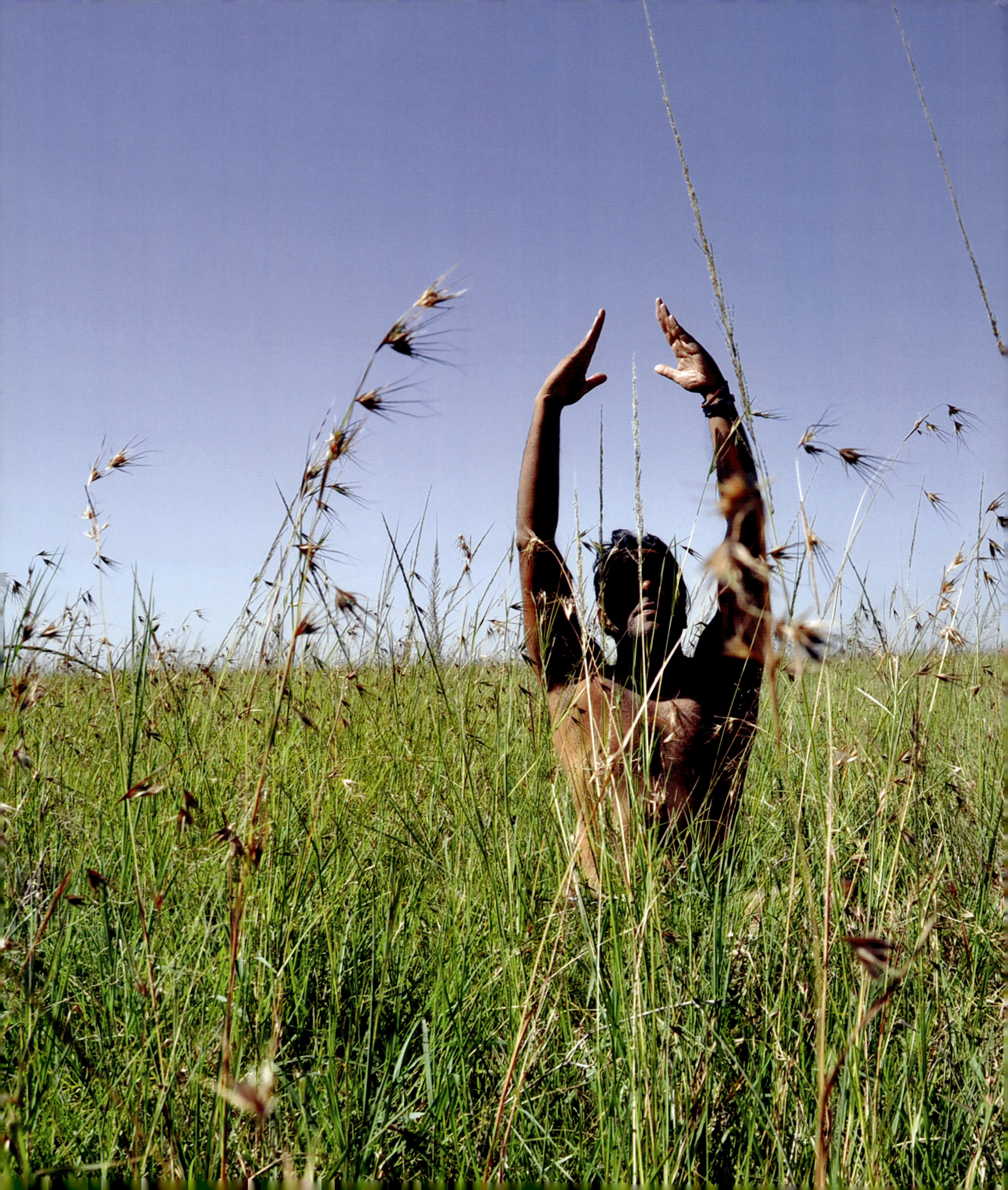

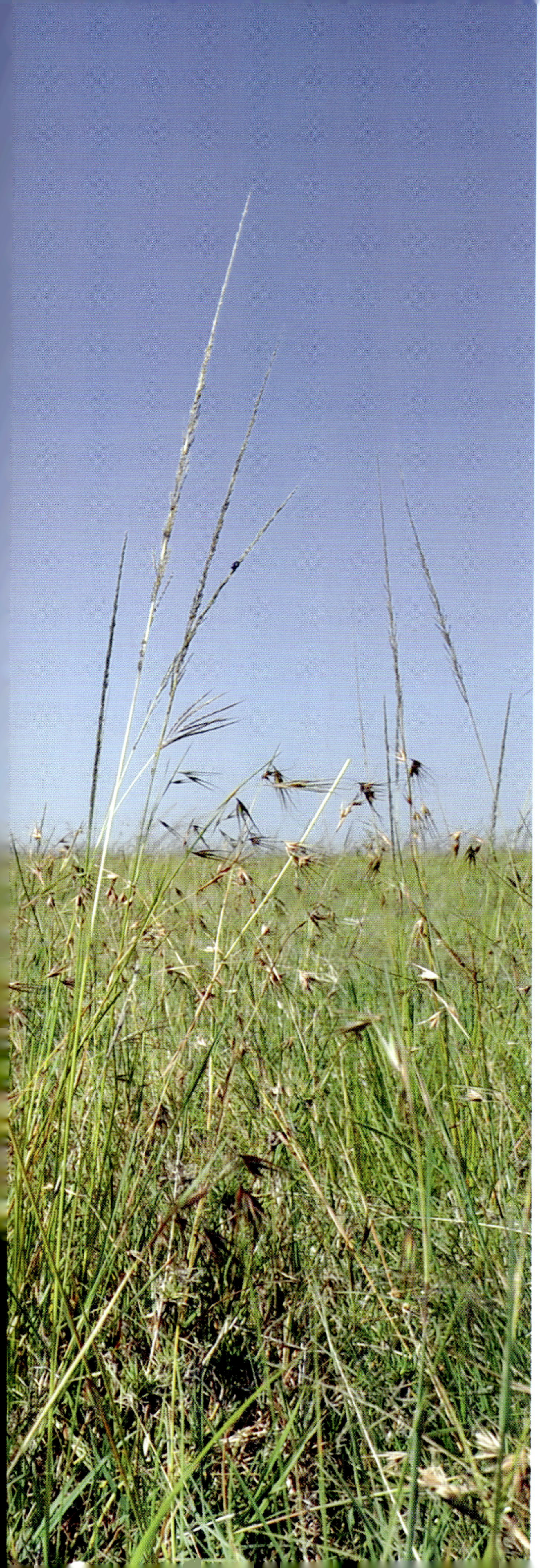

person now that I was when my fridge at home was bare. In fact, I was often the most creative when I had nothing. Then all I had was the joy in my heart to share, which made me feel like the richest person on Earth. Although I struggle with trusting others due to my personal history, I trust the universe, light, and spirituality with absolute certainty. I am empowered by creating joy for others through yoga, music, travel, and wellness.

When we stop feeling, we lose our humanity, so I am excited about the new range of feelings and realizations you will experience by practicing Brahma Yoga. I wish nothing more for you than to be loved fully down to every cell, across all ancestral lines and all incarnations, until love is radiating through your body. Brahma Yoga is my gift to you. Remember to always travel light.

ORIGINS OF BRAHMA YOGA

Yoga has the power to radically transform your life. Originating in ancient India more than 5,000 years ago, yoga is a practice that combines physical asana postures, breathing relaxation techniques, and meditation. It has been studied for its various health benefits, including reducing stress, improving flexibility and balance, and promoting overall well-being and strength. It has also been used as a complementary therapy for a variety of health conditions, including heart disease, chronic pain, and depression. More than a billion people worldwide currently practice yoga and meditation.

However, as yoga has gained global recognition, it has somewhat lost its way. Its growing popularity has led to its commodification, which has led to a homogeneity that does not clearly acknowledge its spiritual context, cultural diversity, and unique history. Indian teachers were initially brought to the West by wealthy patrons and colonial authorities. These teachers were pressured to modify the practice to fit Western expectations, curiosities, and ideals, and yoga was presented as a physical and mental discipline rather than as a spiritual practice.

This is one of the reasons I was inspired to create Brahma Yoga. I was worried about this trajectory that further detached from yoga's spirituality. Furthermore, I was concerned that the yoga methodologies of the 20th century were too patriarchal in their approach. There was too much regimental masculinity in the sequencing and not enough expression of femininity in the asanas. Virtually all of the early teachers who received recognition were men. When we dig deeper into the history of India, though, we find that there were greater sanctity and sacred reverence for females represented through its deities. Brahma Yoga connects us to both the divine masculine and sacred feminine.

Brahma Yoga seeks to reunite us through our practice to our place, presence, and purpose in this cosmos. It seeks to use the body as an elemental portal to align with the absolute transcendental reality of the universe. Brahma Yoga activates the vitality that thrives through the flow of energy, asanas, movement, mantras, and mudras. It reminds and awakens in each of us the yogic quest of enlightenment that leads to bliss, balance, creativity, love, acceptance, and freedom.

Consider Brahma Yoga not as a collection of traditions, but as a framework to offer inclusive spirituality without the separatism, compartmentalization, and complexity of ideology that religion brings. Through the practice of Brahma Yoga, you are not required to be part of a lineage, nor to be a devotee of any human, sage, saint, or guru. Be inspired, but be nonattached as you acknowledge the impermanence of everything and the beauty of that simple truth. Rather than approaching an altar held by a righteous priest or anyone purporting to help you grow in order to further their own commercial interests, let your body be the crucible of the offering and rituals of your practice. The forests, oceans, rivers, mountains, caves, and stars are the only temples you will need.

Brahma Yoga brings insight to your higher mind through intricate awareness of the body. The 700 asanas offered in Brahma Yoga are ways of arranging the body into different shapes for the sole purpose of a moving meditation, a radiant reflection of the main two shapes that other shapes are formed from—triangles and circles. As you bind, yoke, and unite the body, yoga becomes an irrigation system that moves the flow of oxygenated blood through the nervous, endocrine, respiratory, cardiovascular, digestive, urinary, and musculoskeletal systems of the human body. All of these systems work together to maintain homeostasis and allow the body to function properly. Brahma Yoga moves you through them with elegance rather than rehashing the usual sequence patterns. It helps you explore the mysteries of life through the portal of the body and offers freedom from all forms of attachment in order to help you experience your state of bliss.

In Indian Hindu mythology, Brahma was considered the creating force of the universe. Often depicted holding a lotus flower and a scripture, Brahma (the creator) is considered a part of the Trimurti (trinity) along with Vishnu (the preserver) and Shiva (the destroyer). The universe is cyclical, with a process of creation, preservation, and destruction. If we consider the cycles of birth and death, we can see that this process of creation and destruction is the very pulse of the way the universe functions.

Our focus when we practice Brahma Yoga is to sync with the divine pulsation of the universe through the concept of Pratyabhijna. Associated with the nondual Shaiva

SUPTA USTRASANA · Resting Camel

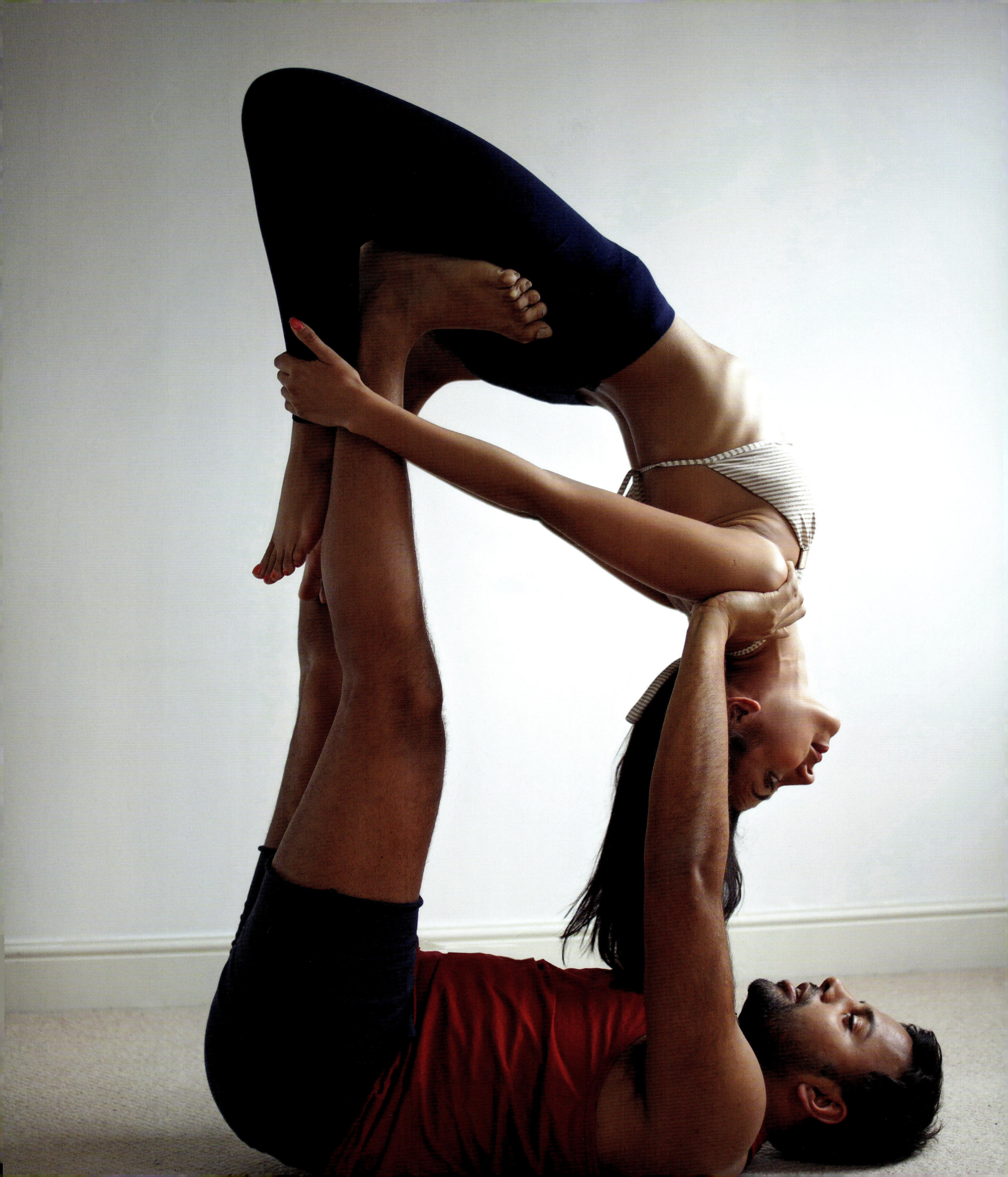

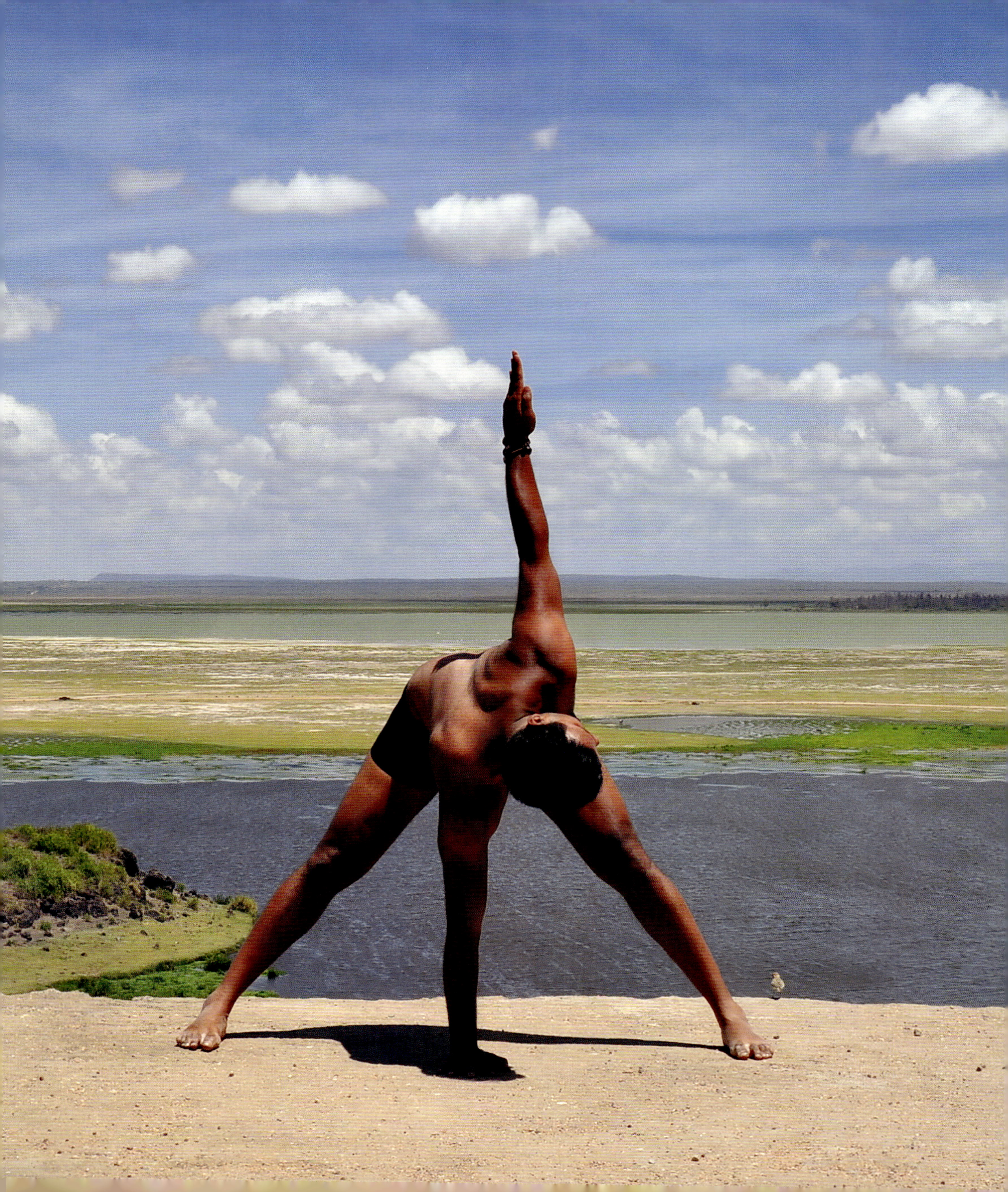

tradition, Pratyabhijna means "recognition" or "re-cognition" and refers to recognizing one's true nature as eternal and paying attention to all the signs, symbols, and intuitions that lead you. The goal of the Pratyabhijna path is to realize that the world and the individual self are not separate, but rather manifestations of the same ultimate reality.

Brahma Yoga helps us unravel the misguided mind through its interpretations, representations, opinions, beliefs, and classifications. From the abstractions of the mind, we can manifest our awareness to adjust to the vibration and pulse of the universe. We assist this process in Brahma Yoga through a deeper appreciation of prakriti, which is referred to as the primordial nature. Prakriti is seen as the foundation of an individual's physical, mental, and emotional constitution, but it is not limited to the individual; it is also the creative source of the physical world. It is one of the fundamental concepts of Samkhya philosophy. The ultimate goal is to transcend prakriti, or to see through the illusion of separation between the individual self and the ultimate reality. Prakriti is made up of three basic gunas, or qualities: sattva (purity and balance), rajas (activity and passion), and tamas (inertia and darkness). These gunas are in a constant state of change and interaction, and their balance in an individual's prakriti is important.

Purusha, on the other hand, is considered to be the ultimate reality, the observer and subject of all experiences. Purusha is eternal, perpetual, and conscious. It is not affected by the changes of the material world and is beyond the realms of time and space. The goal in Samkhya philosophy is to realize the distinction between purusha and prakriti and to achieve liberation from the cycle of rebirth. The goal in Brahma Yoga differs, as we are choosing to increase the longevity of our lives and then come back in different forms.

Vedic cosmology's goal is also to achieve liberation from the cycle of rebirth and merge with the ultimate reality, known as Brahman. From the perspective of Brahma Yoga, it is a pathway and route to understand and map out the origin and structure of the universe. Both Vedic astrology and Brahma Yoga are rooted in the same Indian spiritual tradition and share some common principles, such as the belief in the interconnectedness of all things and the importance of self-awareness and self-realization. Brahma Yoga differs in its approach, however, as it encourages any dedicated aspirant to take a spiritual sabbatical to delay this merging with ultimate reality and to do so by consciously prolonging your life through yoga.

In terms of longevity, biological age refers to the functional state of an organism, which is determined by various factors, such as genetics, lifestyle, and environment. It is different from chronological age, which is simply the number of years that have passed since birth. By practicing healthy lifestyle habits, such as regular yoga, eating a primarily plant-based diet, getting enough sleep, and managing stress, you can help slow down the aging process and maintain a lower biological age.

Brahma Yoga uses kriyas as a way to navigate. Kriyas are powerful tools for spiritual growth and self-transformation and include various types of practices, such as pranayama (breathing exercises), asanas (yoga postures), mudras (hand gestures), bandhas (energy locks), mantras (sacred sounds), yantras (visualization), and dhyana (meditation).

Brahma Yoga also incorporates kundalini energy. Sushumna nadi is a subtle energy channel in the body that is believed in yoga philosophy to run along the spinal column. It is the central channel through which prana (life-force energy) flows and is associated with spiritual awakening and enlightenment. The sushumna nadi is surrounded by two other energy channels, the ida and pingala, which are associated with the left and right channels of the body respectively. The balance of energy among these three channels is thought to be important for physical and mental well-being and can be achieved through practices such as pranayama and meditation.

A mudra is a hand gesture or position that is used in spiritual practices, yoga, and meditation and has healing properties that help direct energy flow in the body. The thumb represents the element of fire, the index finger the element of air, the middle finger the element of space/ether, the ring finger the element of earth, and the little finger the element of water. There are 72 mudras in the Brahma Yoga system, and each one activates a state of realization or symbolism. Brahma Yoga gleaned some of its precious mudras from Kathak and Bharatanatyam, which are classical dance forms that originated in India and are known for their intricate footwork, expressive hand gestures, and dynamic movements. Brahma Yoga treats yoga as a moving meditation with fluid dancelike motions, as dancing offers a home for a spirit that at times struggles to be contained in its body. The largest challenge in life is trying to fit the enormity of your spirit inside your body.

To make the most of this book, begin by reviewing the two sequences that follow this essay. In the Brahma Surya / The Sun evocations (pages 18–21), you will evoke 21 nourishing emotions through 21 postures. To evoke something is to bring it to mind or reflect on a memory. In the Brahma Chandra / The Moon invocations (pages 22–24), you will invoke 16 symbolic animal guides through 16 postures. To invoke is to call upon something for support and guidance. The oldest civilizations in the world, across all spectrums of beliefs, have worshipped or used the sun and moon in their symbology.

After choosing to prepare the body by either warming up with the sun evocations or energizing with the moon invocations, you can then choose one of the 12 set sequences, which I call constellations, that are included in this book. You could choose to do a combination of two sequences based on your sun sign and moon sign. A sun sign, also known as a star or zodiac sign, is the astrological position that the sun was in at the time of a person's birth. It is associated with certain characteristics and personality traits, and the sun sign is said to be the expression of a person's identity and individuality. Though lesser known, a moon sign is determined by the position of the moon in the zodiac at the time of a person's birth. The moon is associated with emotions, feelings, and intuition, and the moon sign is said to indicate a person's emotional nature and inner self. While we often chase the solar power of the sun as the panacea for all our problems, we are underestimating the enormous power and potential of the moon.

Each of the six chapters in this book contains two sequences coordinating with these signs. In Toning and Flexibility, the featured sequences are Brahma Mesha / Aries (pages 76–79) and Brahma Vrishabha / Taurus (pages 80–83); in Rest and Rejuvenate, Brahma Mithuna / Gemini (pages 116–119) and Brahma Karkata / Cancer (pages 120–123); in Boost Vitality, Brahma Simha / Leo (pages 168–171) and Brahma Kanya / Virgo (pages 172–175); in Increase Energy, Brahma Tula / Libra (pages 220–223) and Brahma Vrishchika / Scorpio (pages 224–227); in Mindfulness and Realization, Brahma Dhanus / Sagittarius (pages 264–267) and Brahma Makara / Capricorn (pages 268–271); and in Inner Alignment, Brahma Kumbha / Aquarius (pages 316–319) and Brahma Meena / Pisces (pages 320–323). Alternatively, you could choose sequences based on the benefit or focus point contained in the title of each chapter.

To correspond with the sacred number of mala beads, there are also 108 sutras in the Brahma Yoga system, which are included with their corresponding signs throughout this book. The number of beads is significant—if you were to place 108 Earths side by side in a row, it would reach exactly from Earth to the sun.

This book is meant to awaken the mystery of life through Brahma Yoga. It is a portal for you to transform your mind, body, and spirit and enrich your life in wondrous ways beyond what you can even imagine. Explore and celebrate your journey in spirituality, wellness, yoga, and ecology. Live love and love light.

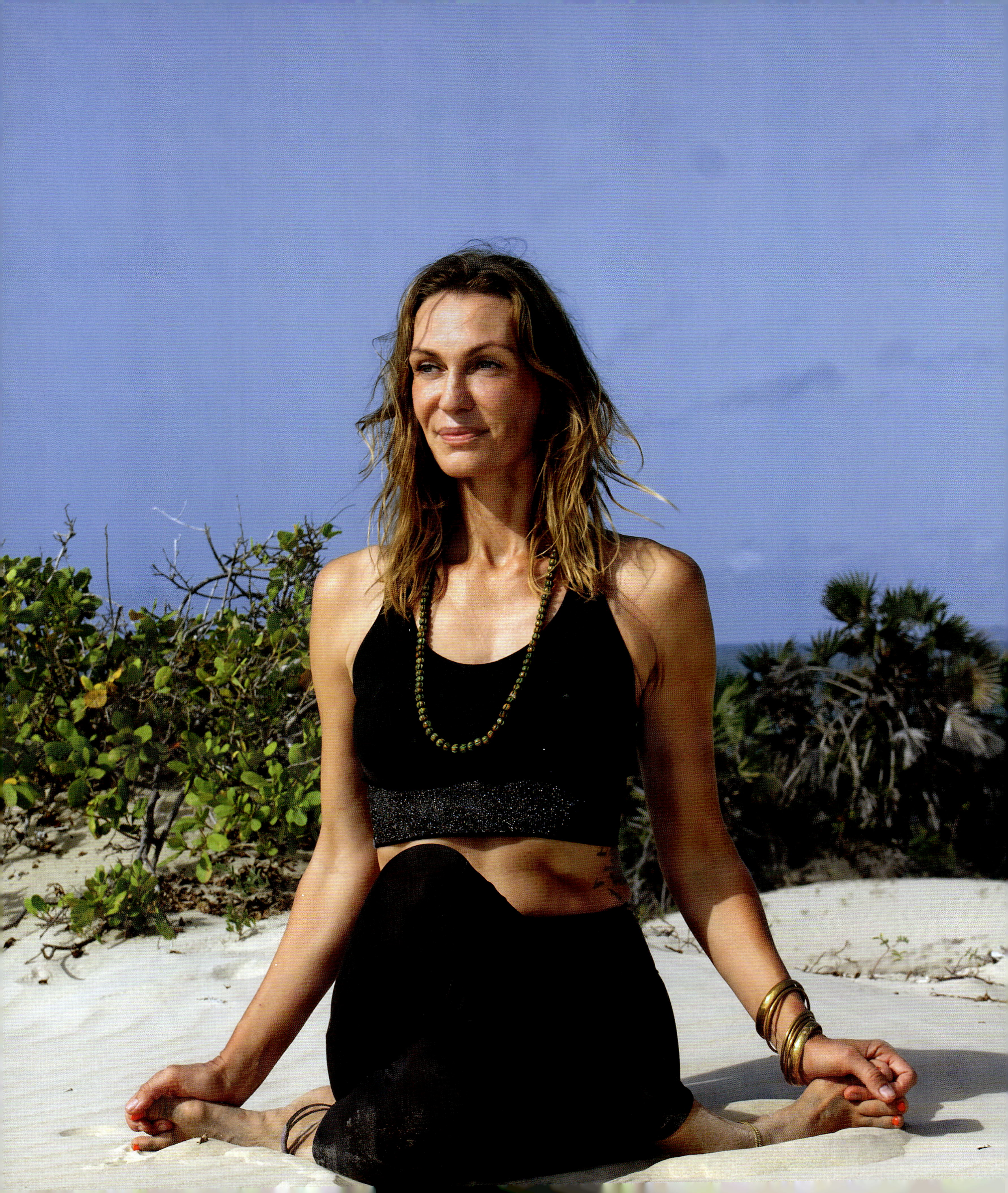

BRAHMA SURYA · The Sun

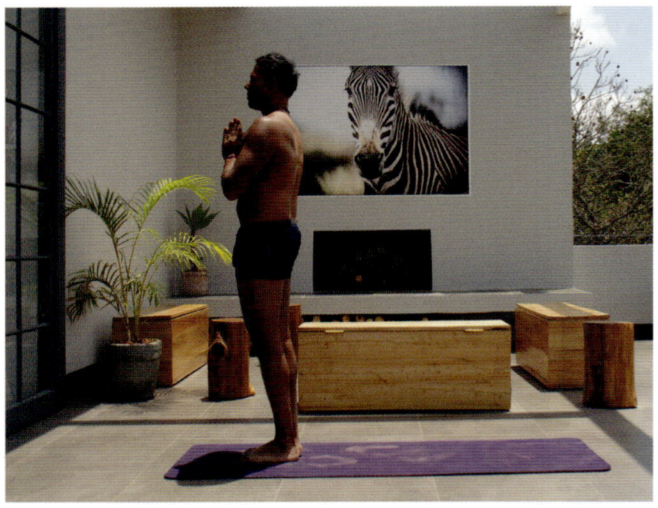

Appreciation
TADASANA & ANJALIMUDRA
Mountain & Love

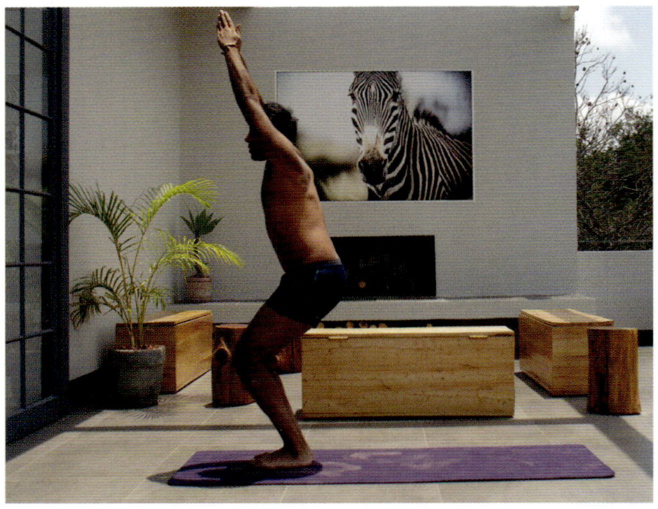

Courage
UTKATASANA
Chair

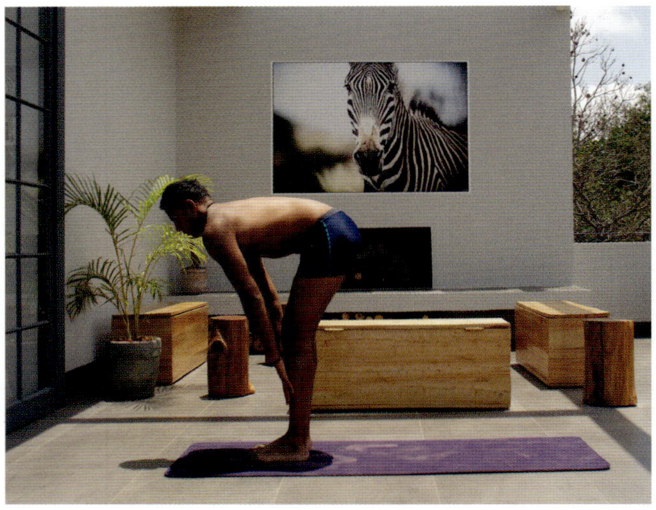

Curiosity
ARDHA UTTANASANA
Half Standing Forward Fold

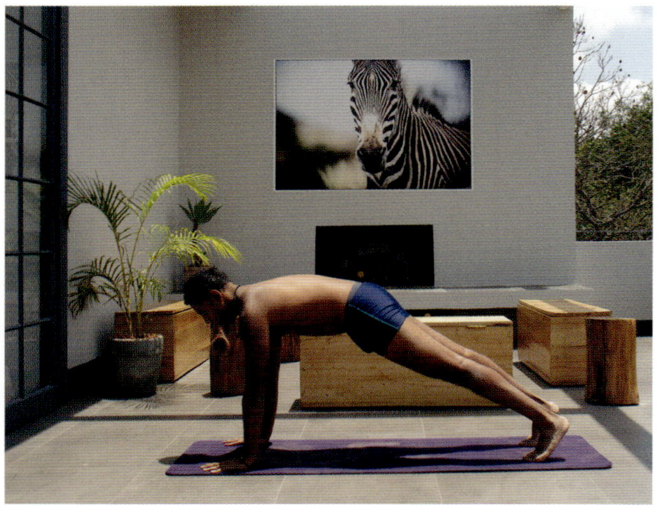

Enthusiasm
KUMBHAKASANA
Plank

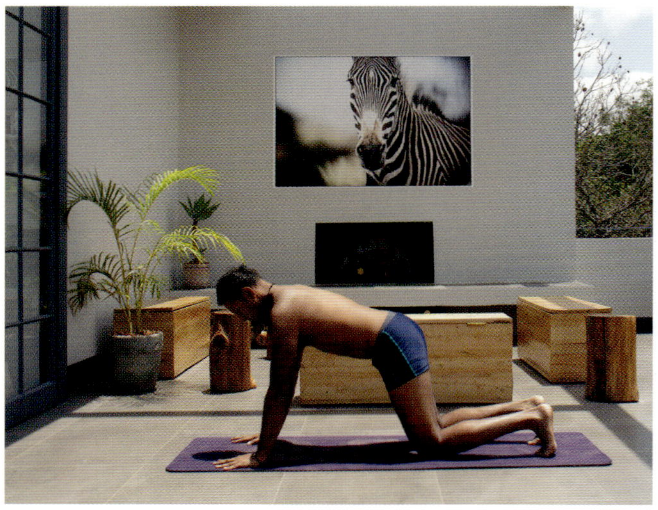

Relief
BHARMANASANA
Tabletop

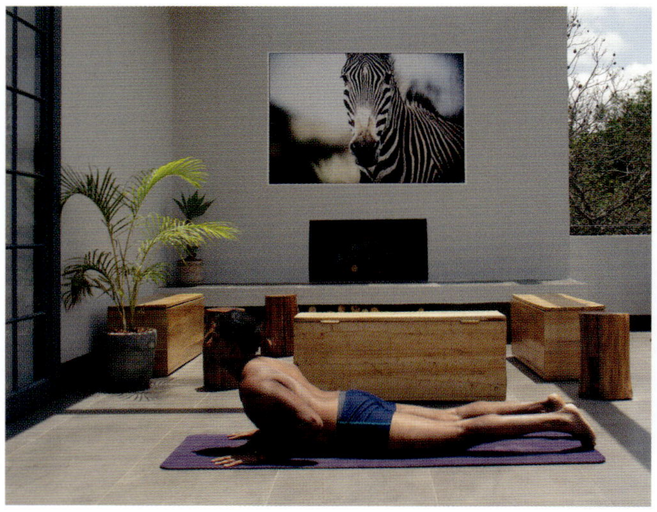

Optimism
BHUJANGASANA
Cobra

Under the power of the divine masculine of the sun, we have 21 asanas to evoke, warm up, and commence our yoga practice. Using Brahma Yoga's 21 positive states of being, we can instantly raise our consciousness and awaken the yogic quest of enlightenment that leads to bliss, balance, creativity, love, acceptance, and freedom. The 21 positive states are appreciation, courage, curiosity, enthusiasm, relief, optimism, contentment, joy, excitement, desire, surprise, delight, affection, passion, awe, bliss, enchantment, calmness, devotion, equanimity, and love.

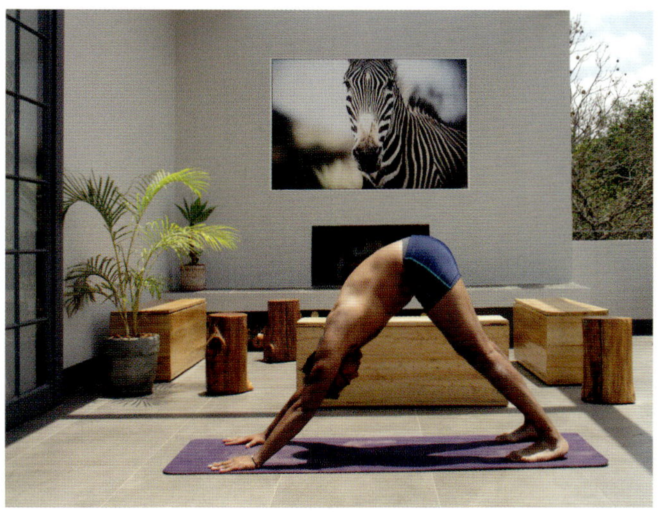

Contentment
ADHO MUKHA SVANASANA
Downward-Facing Dog

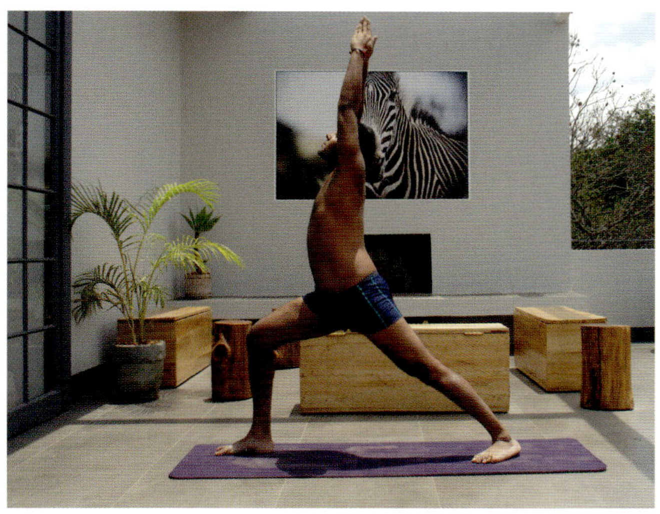

Joy
VIRABHADRASANA EKAM
Warrior I

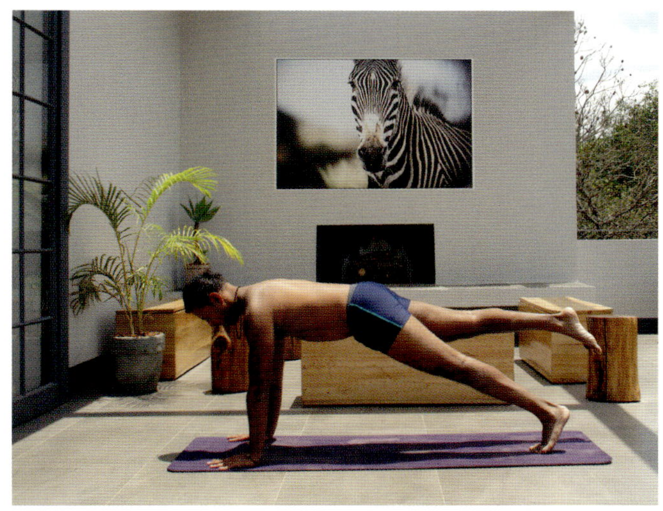

Excitement
EKA PADA KUMBHAKASANA
Leg-Lifted Plank

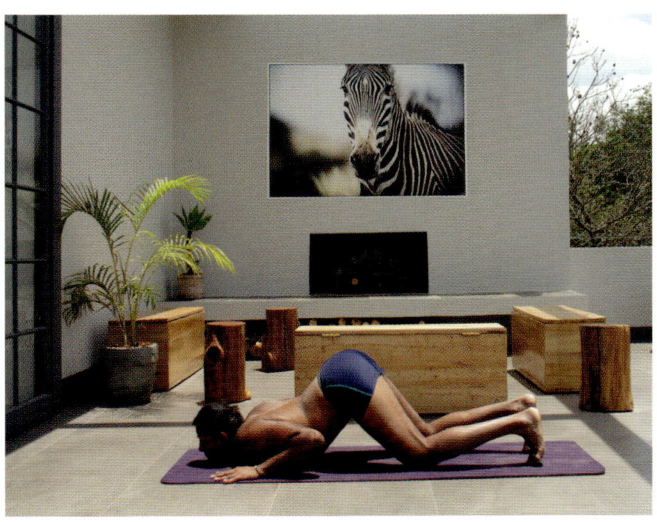

Desire
AJAGARASANA
Python

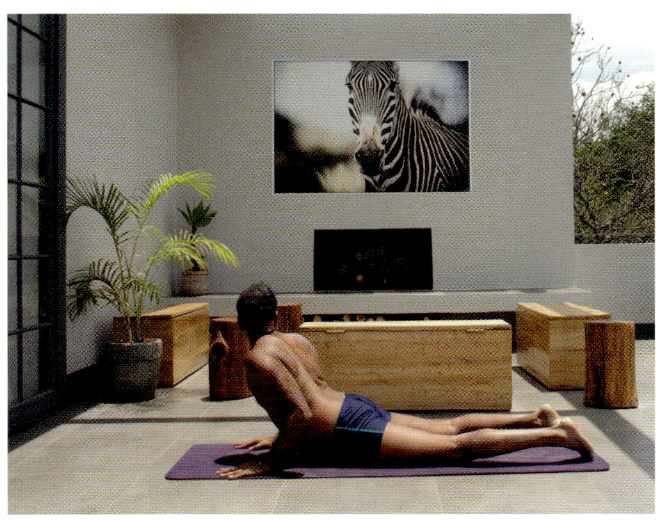

Surprise
UTTHITA NIRAVALASANA
Seal

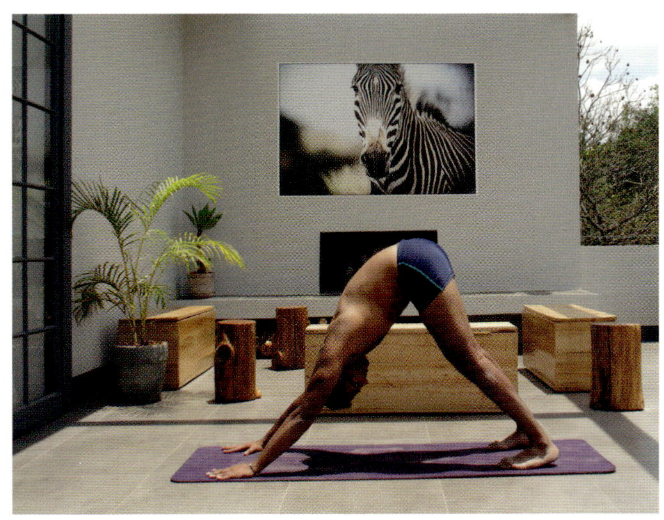

Delight
ADHO MUKHA SVANASANA
Downward-Facing Dog

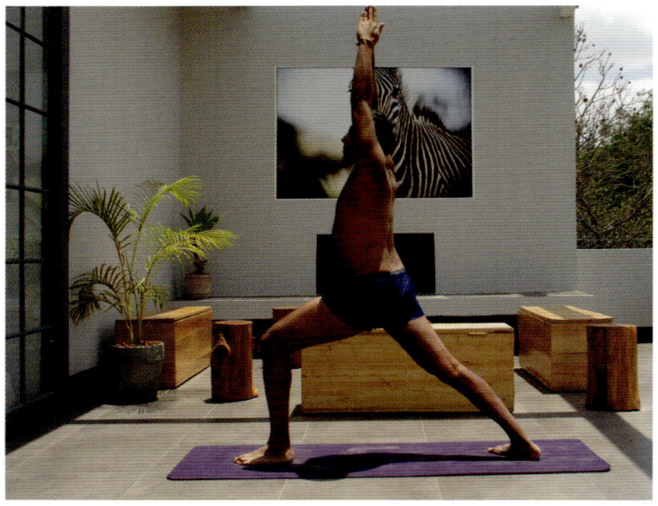

Affection
VIRABHADRASANA EKAM
Warrior I

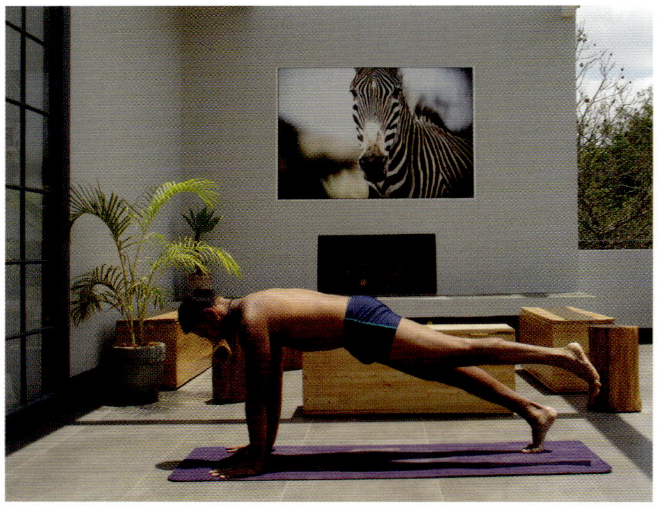

Passion
EKA PADA KUMBHAKASANA
Leg-Lifted Plank

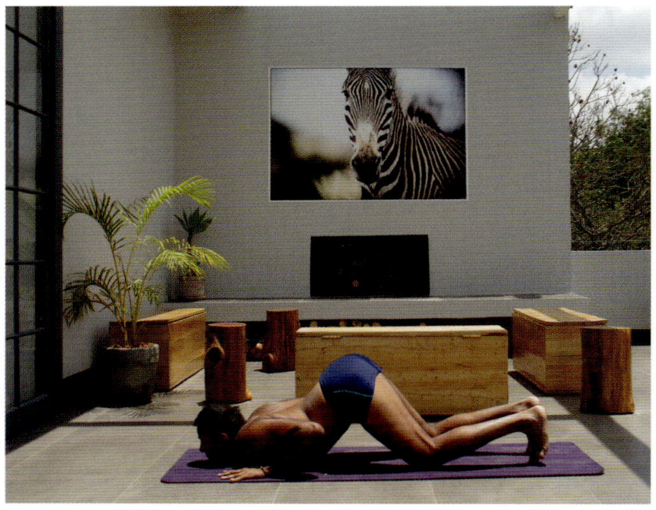

Awe
AJAGARASANA
Python

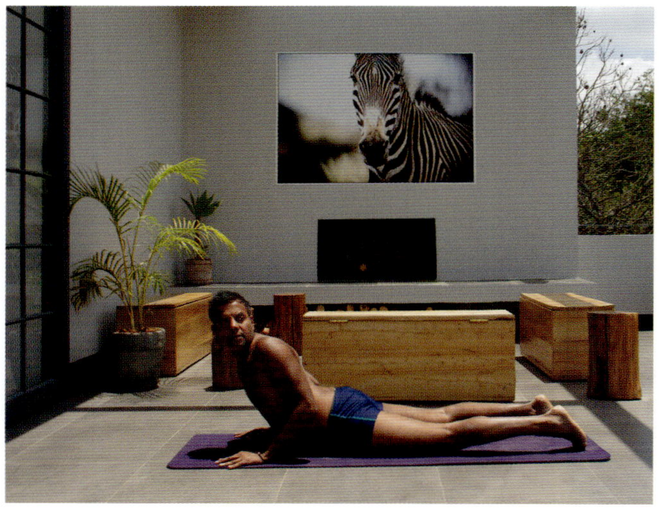

Bliss
UTTHITA NIRAVALASANA
Seal

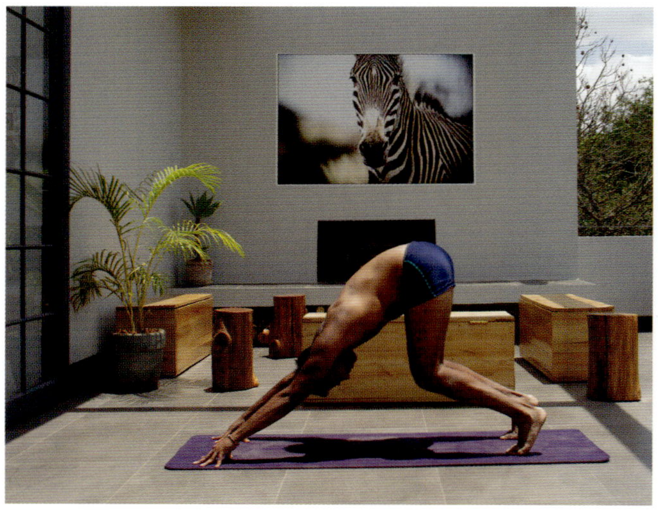

Enchantment
PANKHASANA
Feather

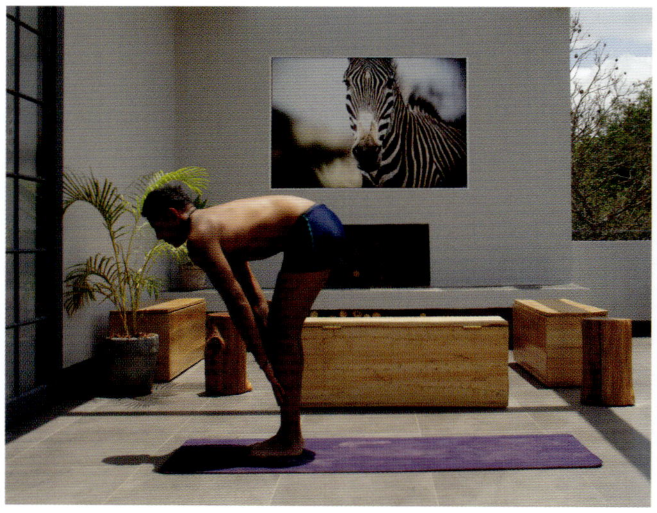

Calmness
ARDHA UTTANASANA
Half Standing Forward Fold

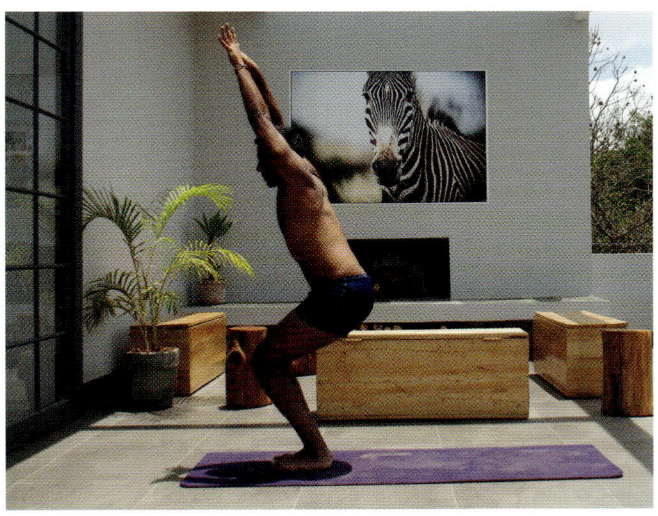

Devotion
UTKATASANA
Chair

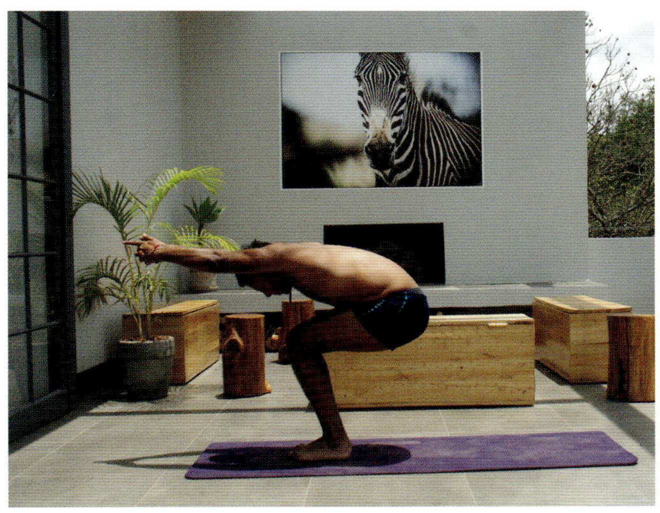

Equanimity
SAMDHIASANA
Horizon

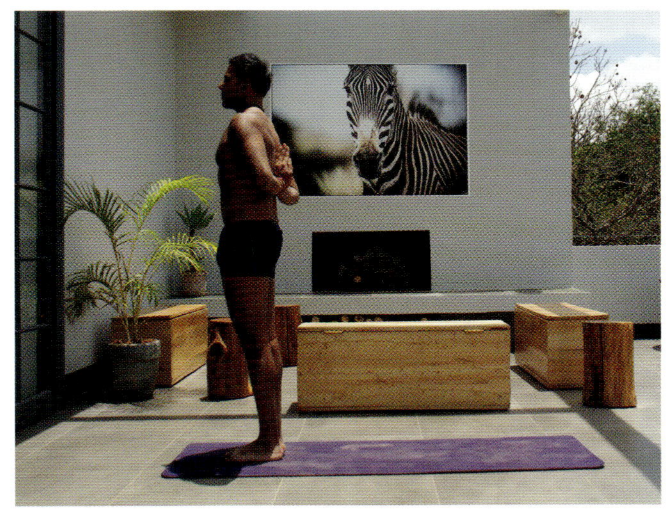

Love
TADASANA & VIPARITA ANJALIMUDRA
Mountain & Unconditional Love

Every inhale is a welcomed greeting
and every exhale a farewell,
a gentle inward hug for my organs.

BRAHMA CHANDRA • The Moon

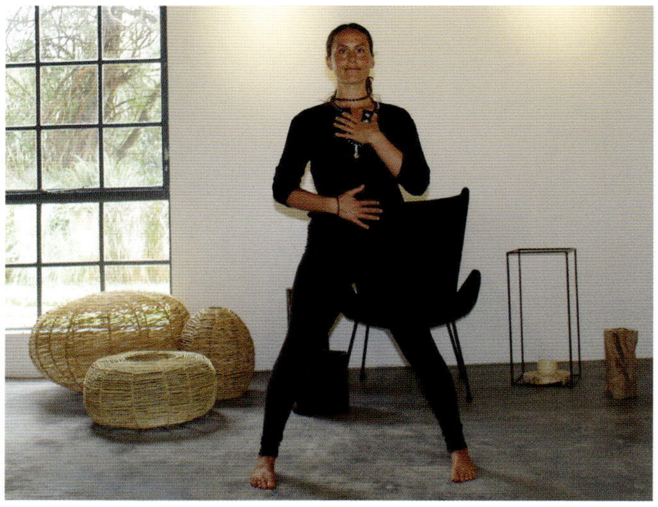

Ox
MONDIALASANA
Moondial

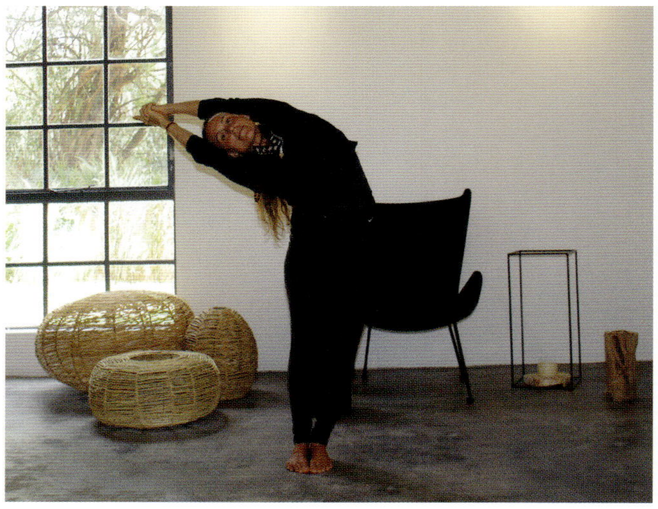

Deer
PINGALA PARSVA URDHVA HASTASANA
Moon-Charging Half Moon

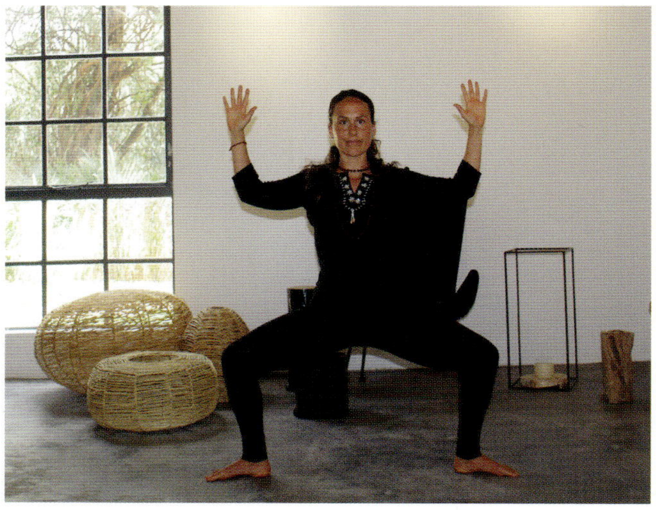

Giraffe
UTKATA KONASANA
Goddess

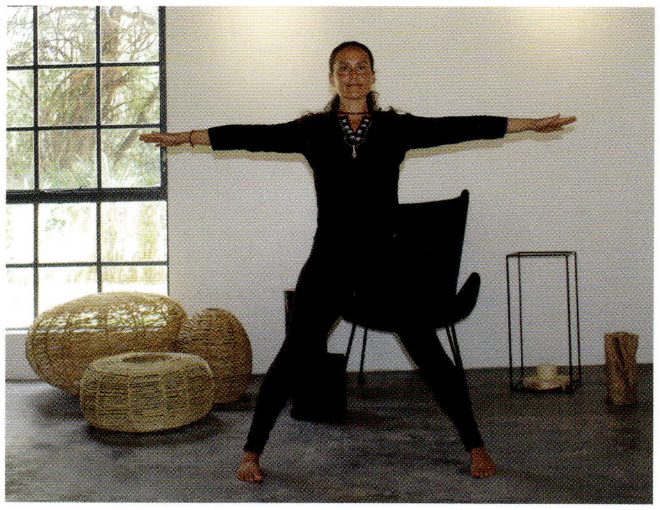

Tiger
CHANDRA DEVASANA
Moon Angel

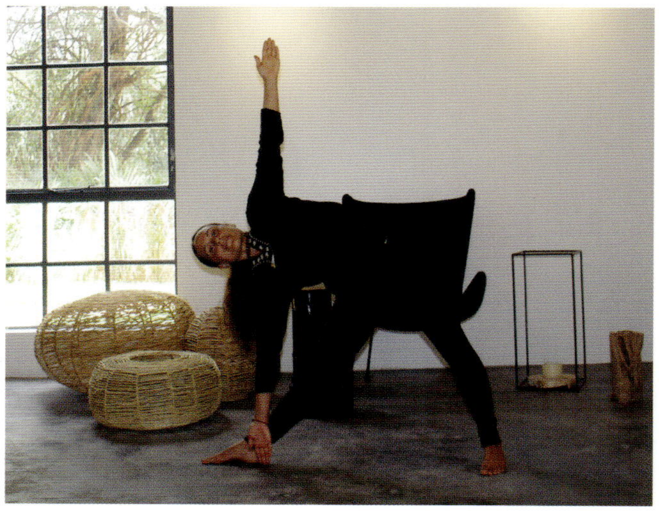

Panther
TRIKONASANA
Triangle

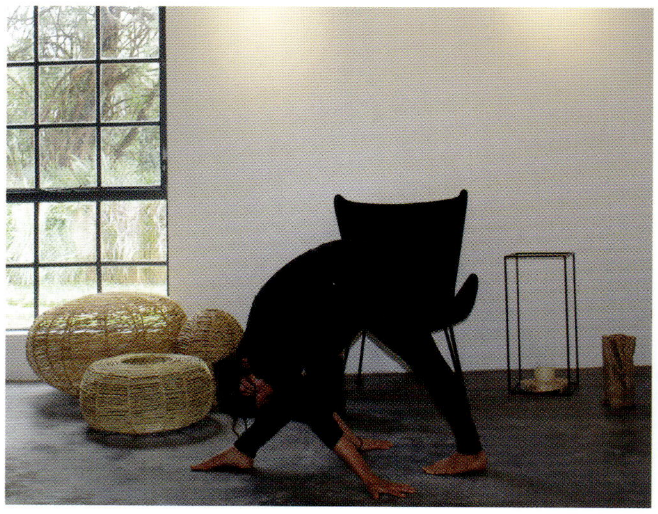

Goat
PARSVOTTANASANA
Pyramid

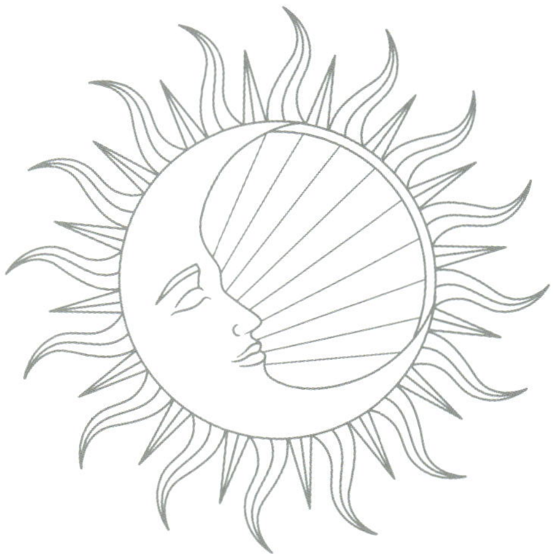

Under the wonder of the sacred feminine of the moon, we have 16 asanas to energize and invoke our yoga practice. We can connect with our symbolic animal guides: ox, deer, giraffe, tiger, panther, goat, rabbit, owl, zebra, penguin, elephant, dolphin, bear, horse, dog, or lion. We will have an enchanting experience of balancing our personality traits by identifying our levels of extroversion, agreeableness, openness, conscientiousness, and neuroticism.

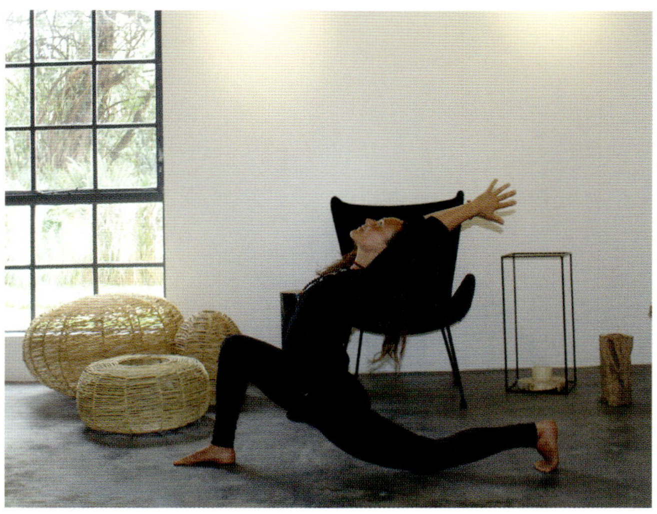

Rabbit
ANJANEYASANA
Crescent Lunge

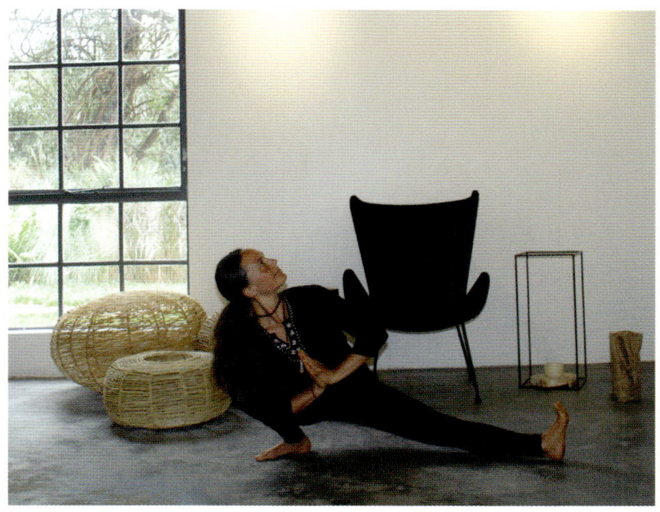

Owl
EKA PADA MALASANA
Extended Garland

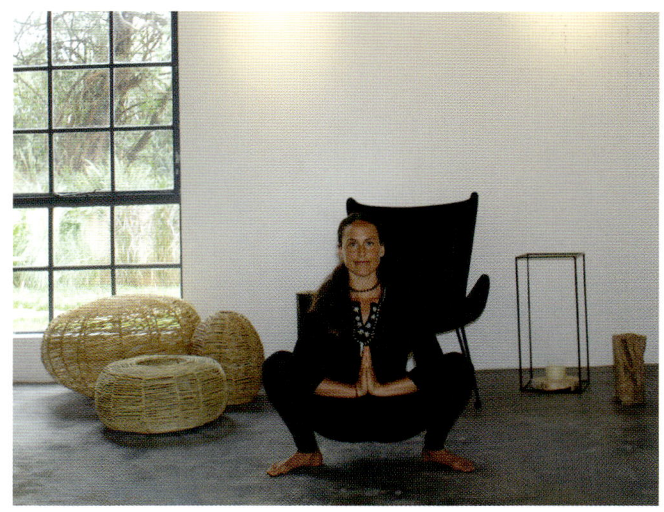

Zebra
MALASANA
Garland Squat

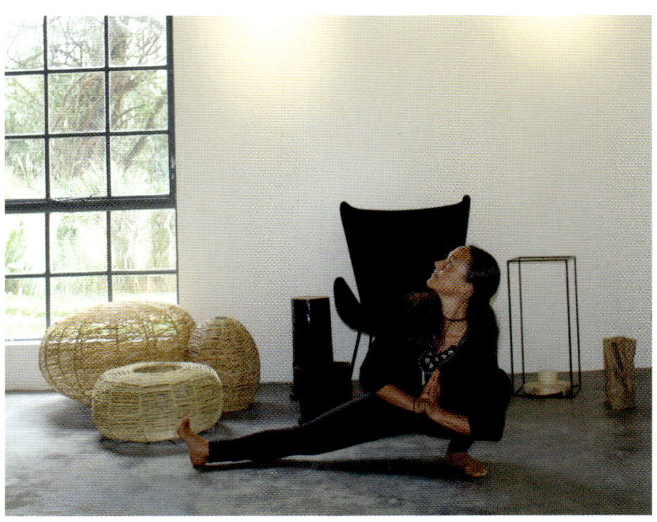

Penguin
EKA PADA MALASANA
Extended Garland

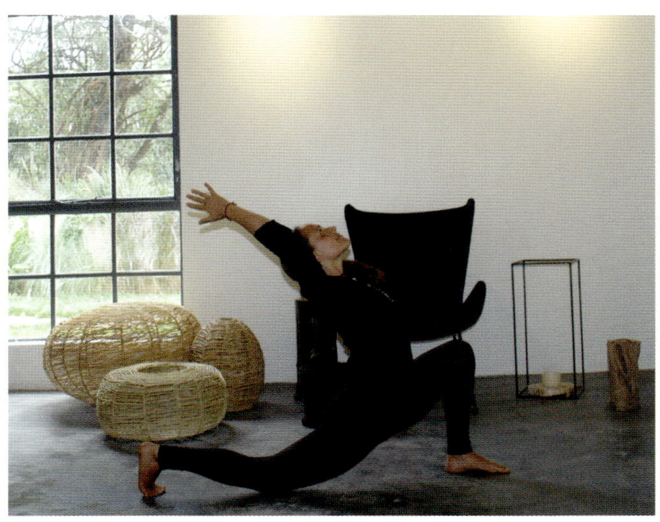

Elephant
ANJANEYASANA
Crescent Lunge

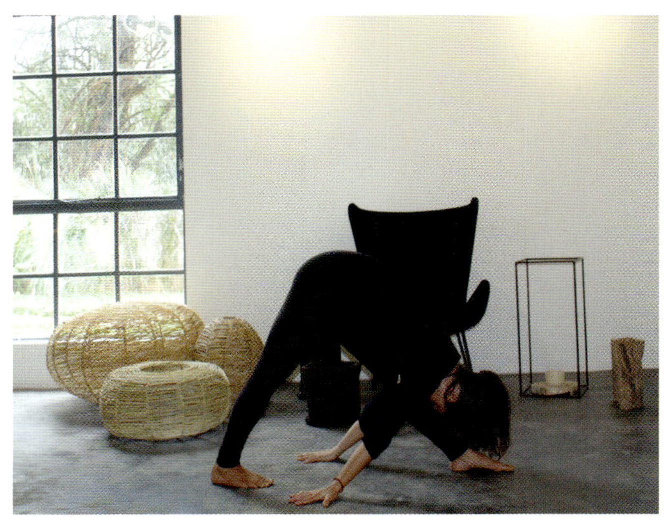

Dolphin
PARSVOTTANASANA
Pyramid

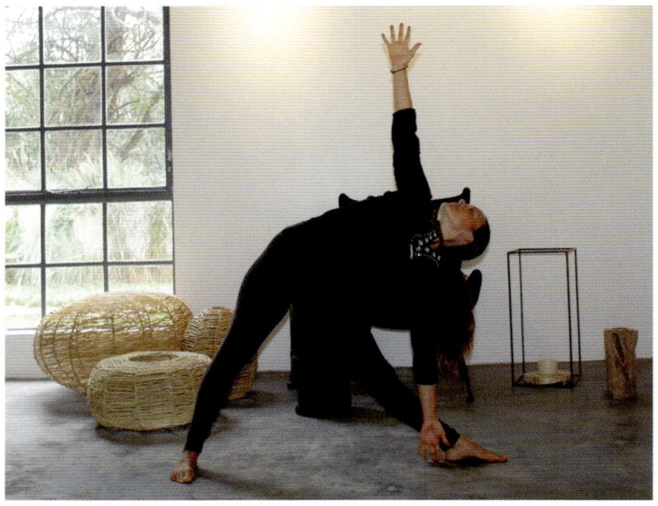

Bear
TRIKONASANA
Triangle

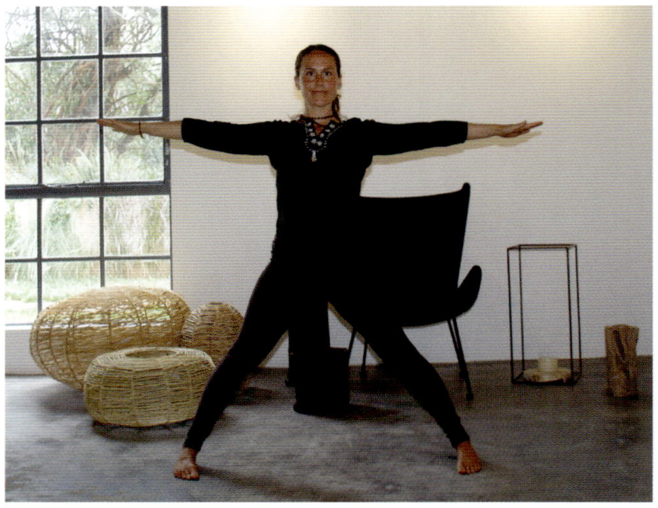

Horse
CHANDRA DEVASANA
Moon Angel

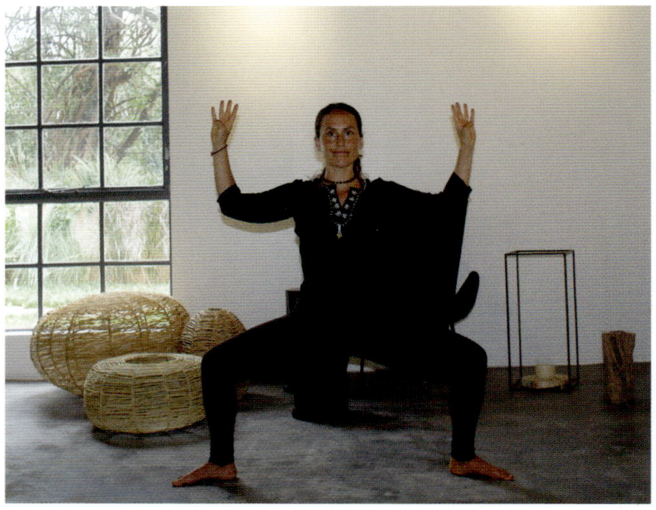

Dog
UTKATA KONASANA
Goddess

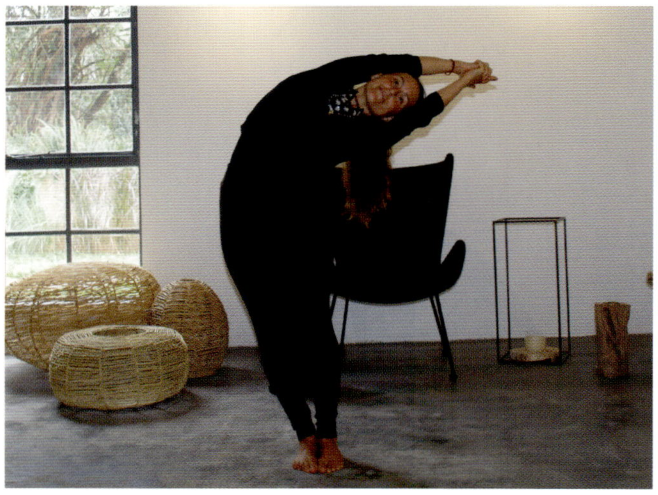

Lion
IDA PARSVA URDHVA HASTASANA
Sun-Rising Half Moon

The sun made me see it.
The moon made me do it.

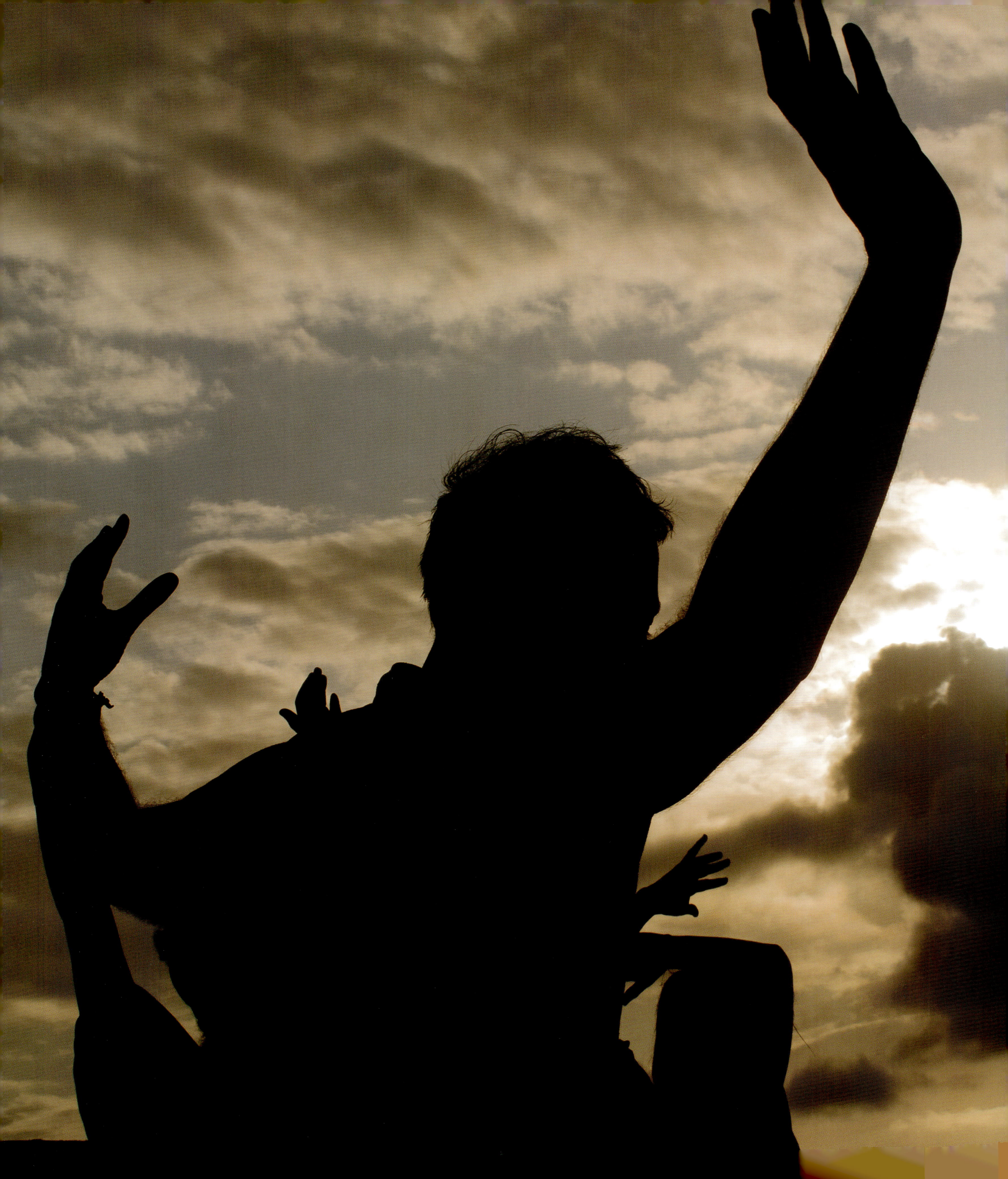

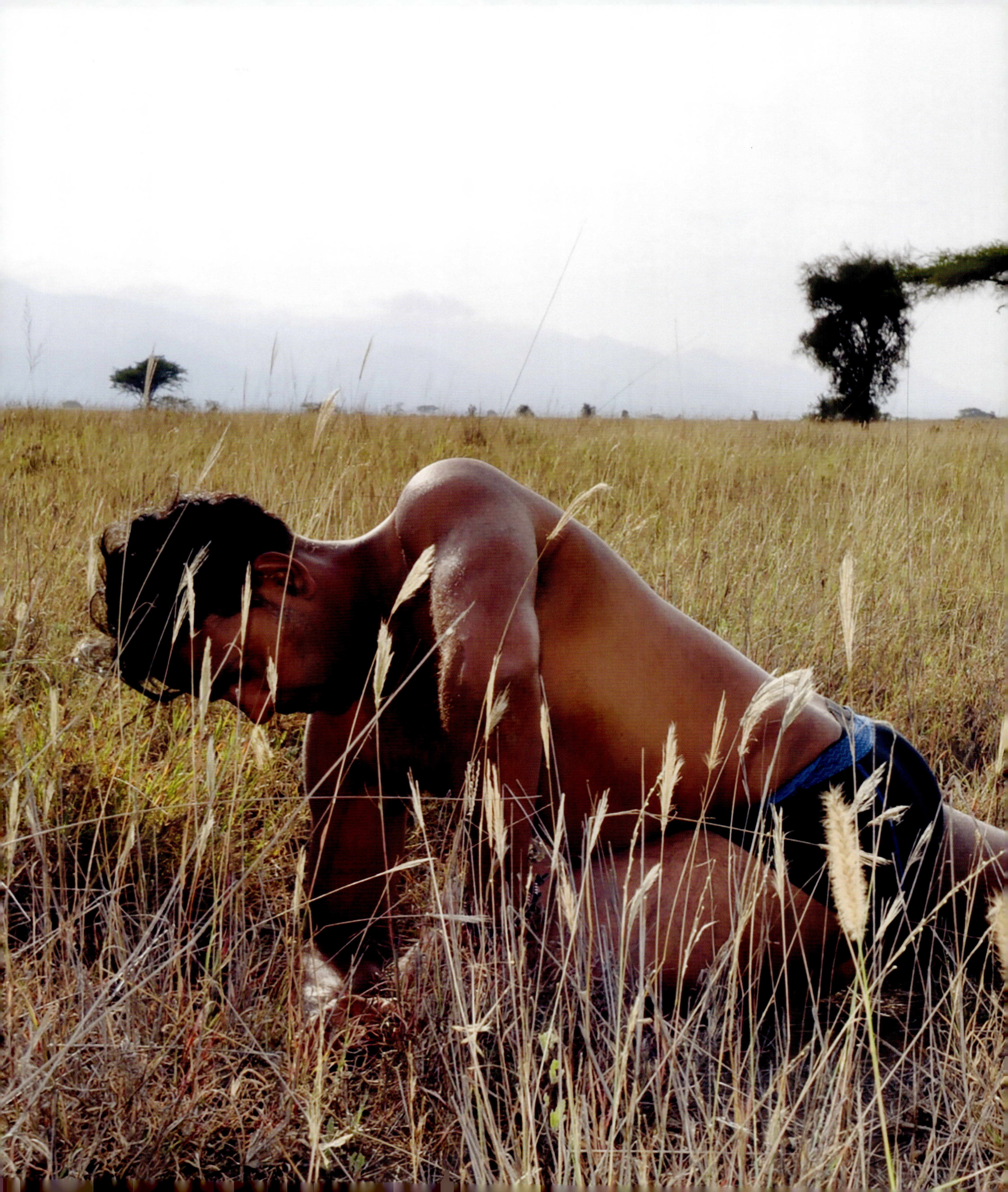

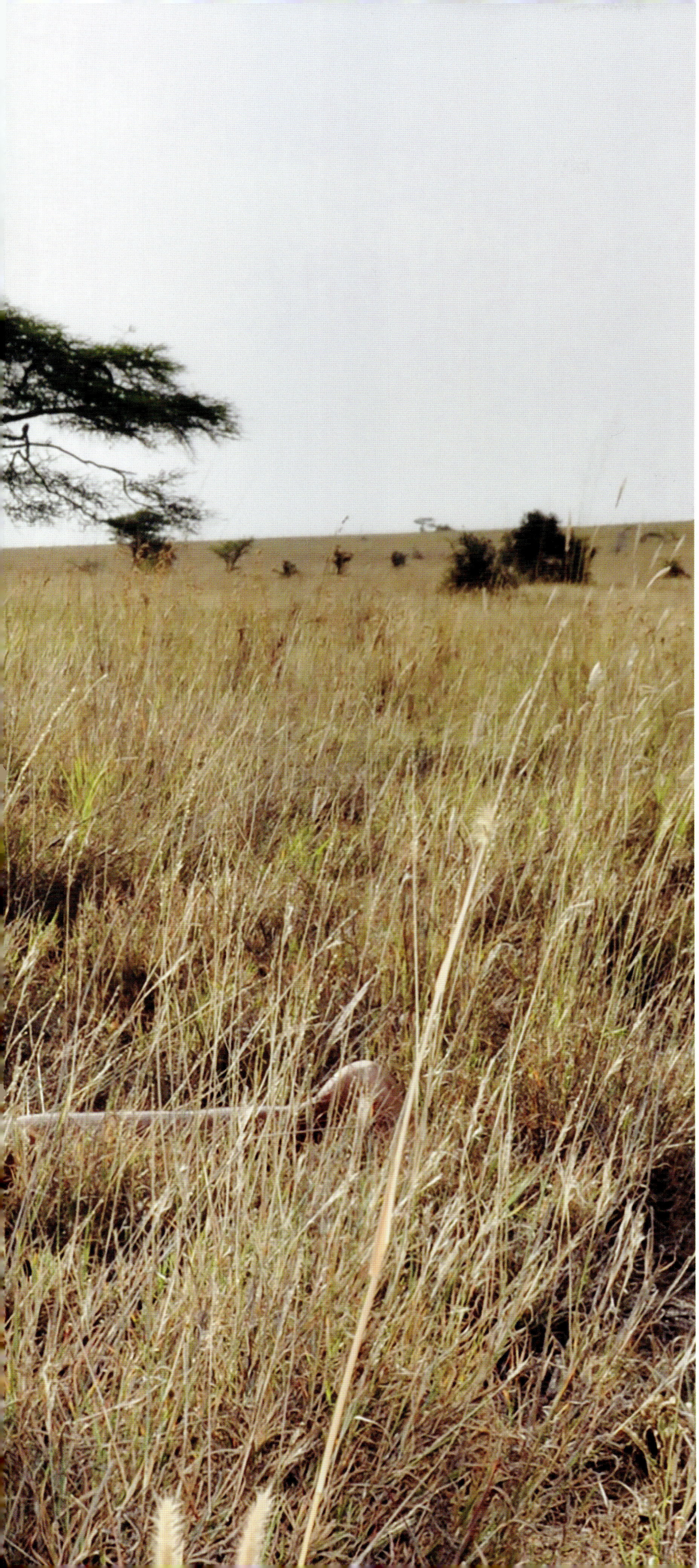

GEMS

We never really arrived here
We just pretended all these years
It felt so real
We convinced ourselves
To persuade others that we too belong
But our shield soon became our mask
It weighed heavier as we hid in our stories
Etching our truths deeper
Into the sanctuary of our skin
Leaving remnants to hide from sight
Discovered by uninvited hands
Like precious gems discarded as stones
The soil feels our longing to love
And loves us back
The acceptance of eternal rest as a seed
The gentle haunting lull of our spirits call
We are in stillness
While stains are concealed vigorously
Hoping to find atonement from time itself
Or from ancient gods like distant stars already dead
Beyond the hollows of history
We continue to remain present with Nature
Sharing the same divine fate

—Leo Lourdes

TONING & FLEXIBILITY

In Brahma Mesha / Aries, we are initiating the fire within. Brahma Vrishabha / Taurus, which is the settled season of earth, is the manifest state of our cultivation. Just like we toil and turn the land, through Brahma Yoga we can also transform our body. The sequences of poses across these two Vedic signs make the body stronger, increasing endurance without forsaking flexibility. I have found that many students, at least initially, excel in one area at the cost of the other.

In our yoga practice, we must first appreciate that toning of the muscles increases heat in the body. As you move through the sequences, your muscles will naturally contract and relax, generating heat. The more muscle fibers used, the greater the heat that is produced. When muscles are more toned, they are able to perform their functions more efficiently, not only in yoga but also in wider functional movements in your life. This leads to an increase in metabolism and energy-producing heat.

Our body composition refers to the proportion of water, bone, fat, and muscle we have. This should not be confused with the body constituents in Ayurveda called the doshas, which are vata, pitta, and kapha. I touched on this idea in the essay about the origins of Brahma Yoga when talking about the gunas. Your bodily composition is constantly changing based on the cycles of nature, your hormones, your health, and how you feed your body. When you do the two Brahma Yoga sequences in this chapter, you will build tone and explore positions that safely stretch and improve your flexibility.

I arranged the Brahma Mesha and Brahma Vrishabha sequences in this particular order because I know flexibility is essential to your health. It helps improve joint range of motion, thereby reducing the risk of injury. It improves posture, enhances your physical performance, and increases your body positivity, confidence, and self-esteem. It can bring a delightful, well-earned relaxation that comes from the hard work and commitment you put into your practice. A lack of flexibility can lead to muscle imbalances and joint stiffness. Those who don't practice Brahma Yoga are often blaming their body—its lack of function, its shape, its inflexibility, and so on—because they are disassociated. We should not do this; we should know that mind, body, and spirit are one in different expressions. We are not a noun; we are a process. These sequences challenge you in a way that keeps you wanting to learn more, not only to improve but also as a delicious process of self-discovery.

The slow, controlled movements and deep breathing bring relaxation, reduce muscle tension, increase blood flow to the muscles, strengthen our bones, and improve flexibility. We also do a range of isometric-based poses, where we hold a muscle in a static position for a period of time. This is followed by plyometric-based transitions between the postures, in which muscle contractions are followed by stretching. Brahma Yoga is a very effective way to improve flexibility because it involves a variety of stretches that target different muscle groups in the way the asanas are put together. It allows for adequate rest for some muscle groups while firing off others, all while keeping the heart simmering.

BRAHMA YOGA SUTRAS

BRAHMA MESHA • Aries

- Brahma Yoga honors that we are all one sharing this unique moment called life.
- I strengthen my indestructibility as I find things that I appreciate in myself.
- Preparation teaches me that we bend so we do not break, and that gravity is a field, not a force. I am vibration.
- I have perspective, and I am guided by following the signs of an illuminated path.
- I have stability and know that where there is stillness, there is great strength.
- History makes myths while living makes legends, so integration makes me the best that I can be.
- The identity I describe as "self" is simply an aspect, as I am consciousness experiencing itself in manifest form.
- I can unleash my subconscious primal wildness to unravel any negative conditioning.
- My actions affect others, so having an open heart makes the connection available to others.

BRAHMA VRISHABHA • Taurus

- I prioritize the coordination of my thoughts and behaviors, as I know I become what I most think about.
- I can control the restraint of my senses, and I can detach from anyone who hurts me with absolute ease.
- I find spirituality transcends the illusion of separation, dissolving the threshold of boundaries that divide us all.
- I am soaring, boundless, and free, and I know living my dreams is never a question of time but one of purpose.
- I feel loyalty when I am protective of others, especially with sensitivity and care.
- Brahma Yoga reveals that I am occurring naturally and play a crucial part amid the interdependent and outwardly opposing forces of the universe.
- Consolidation of my mind, body, and spirit occurs when I learn to surrender to the present moment.
- I am joyful, and I am devoted to merging my inner nature with Nature itself.
- A day at a time is all I need, and I thank the universe for who I am even if I am not exactly where I want to be.

Unwind today. Find some part of
the mind to release, some tension
in the body to undo like a knot.

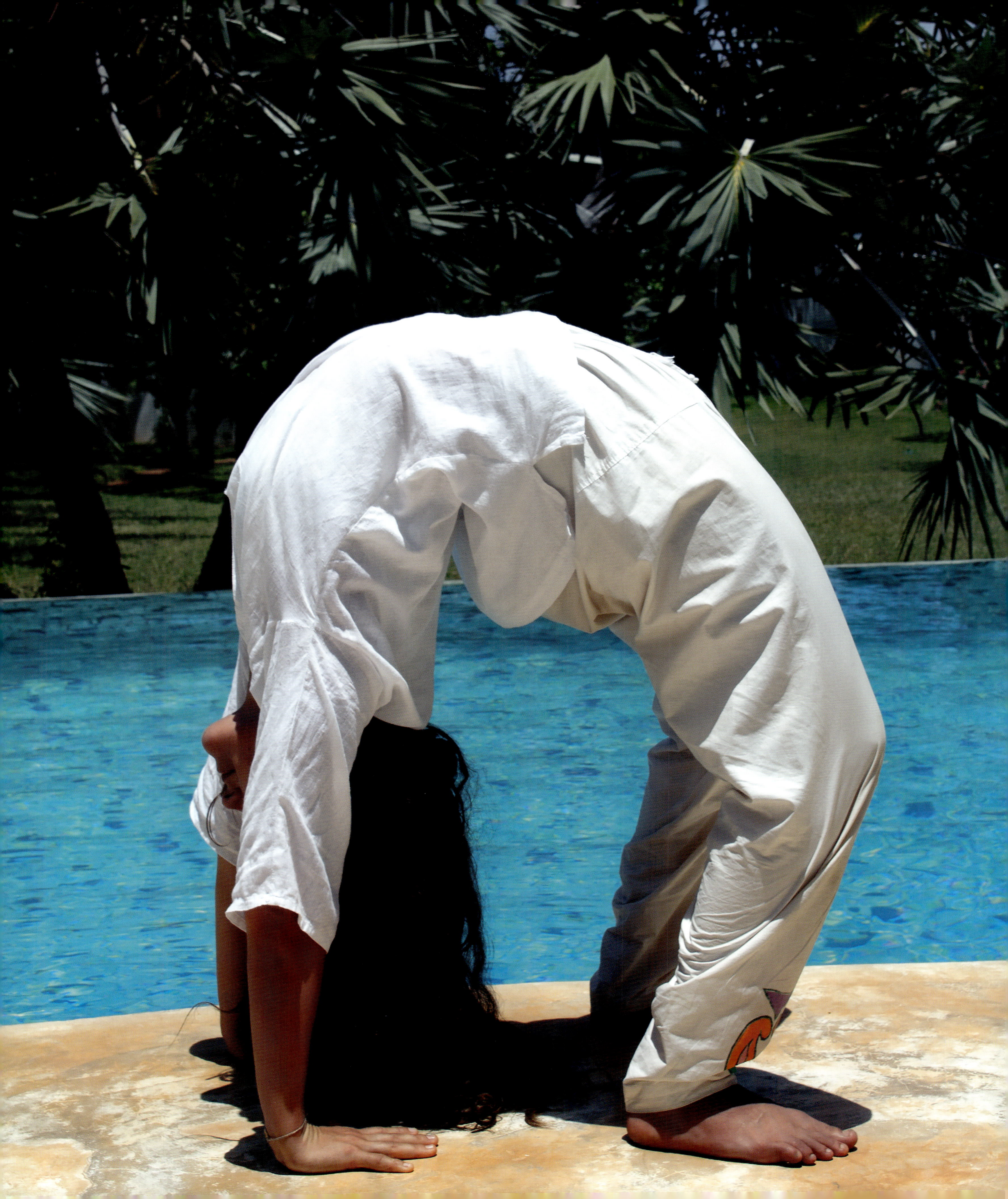

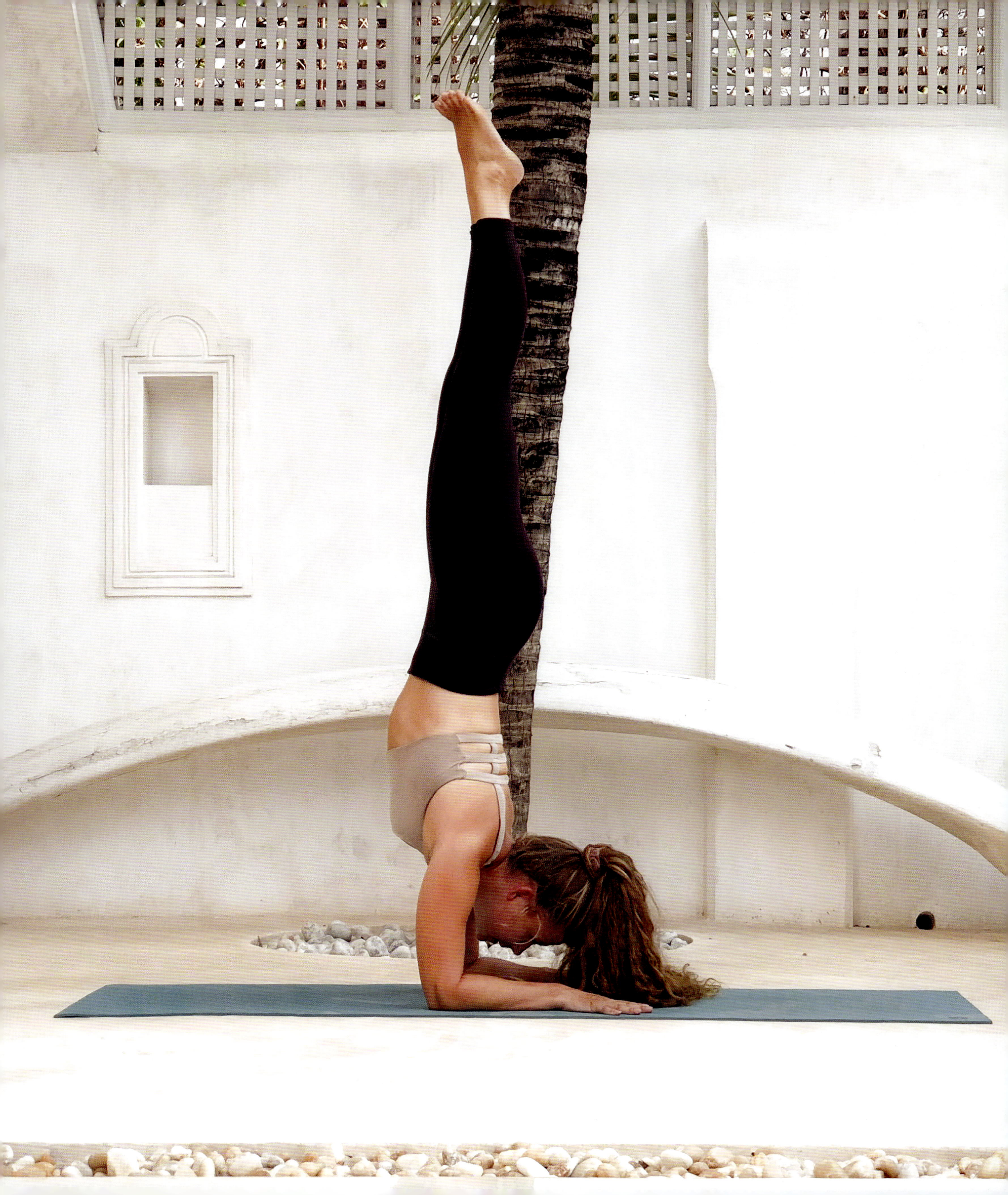

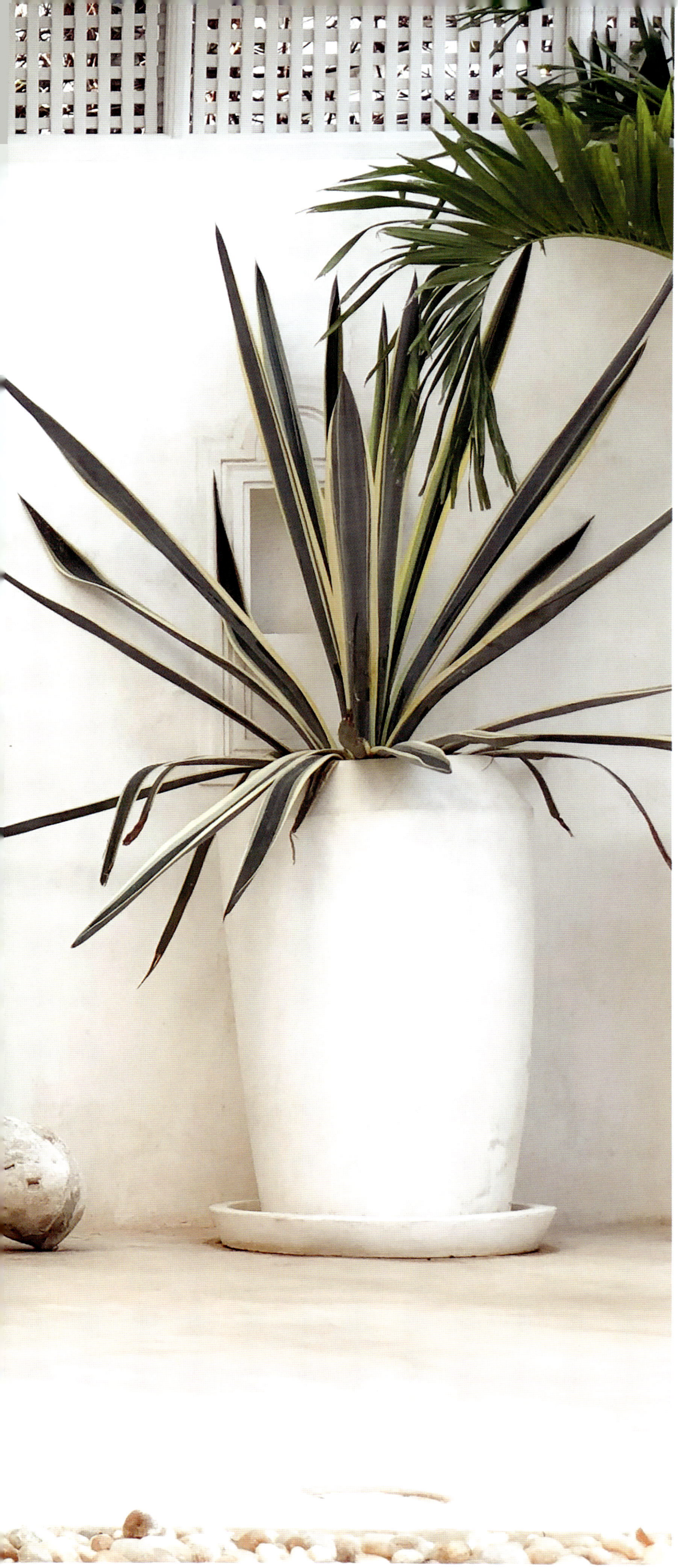

Through grounding,
we find growth.

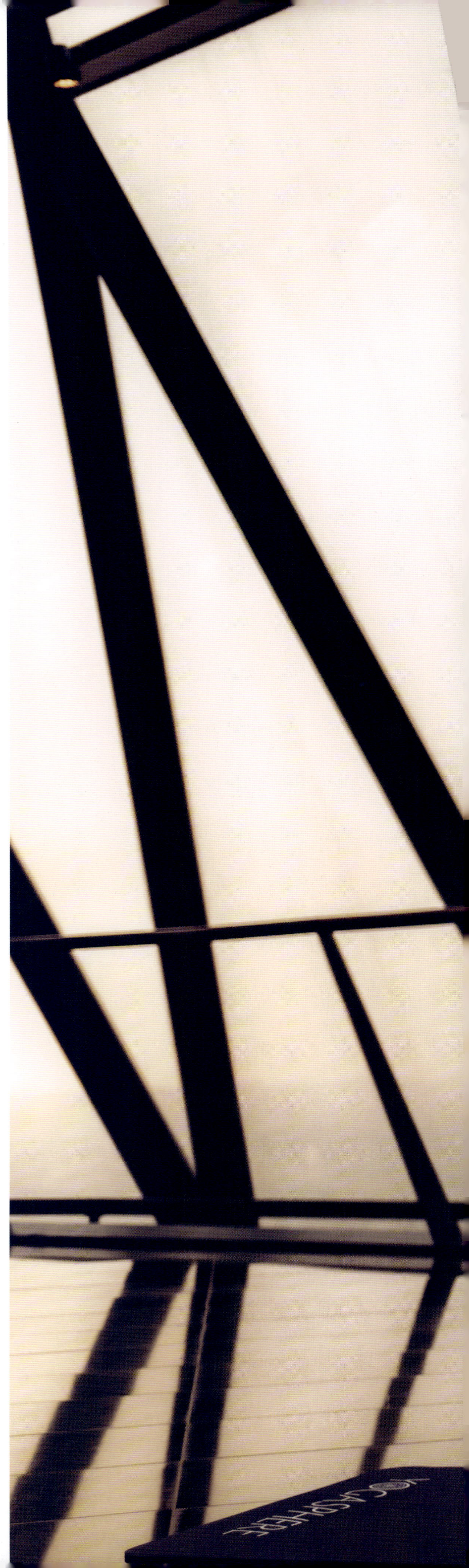

ARDHA SIRSASANA · Half Headstand

▼ **ADHO MUKHA VRKSASANA** · Downward-Facing Tree

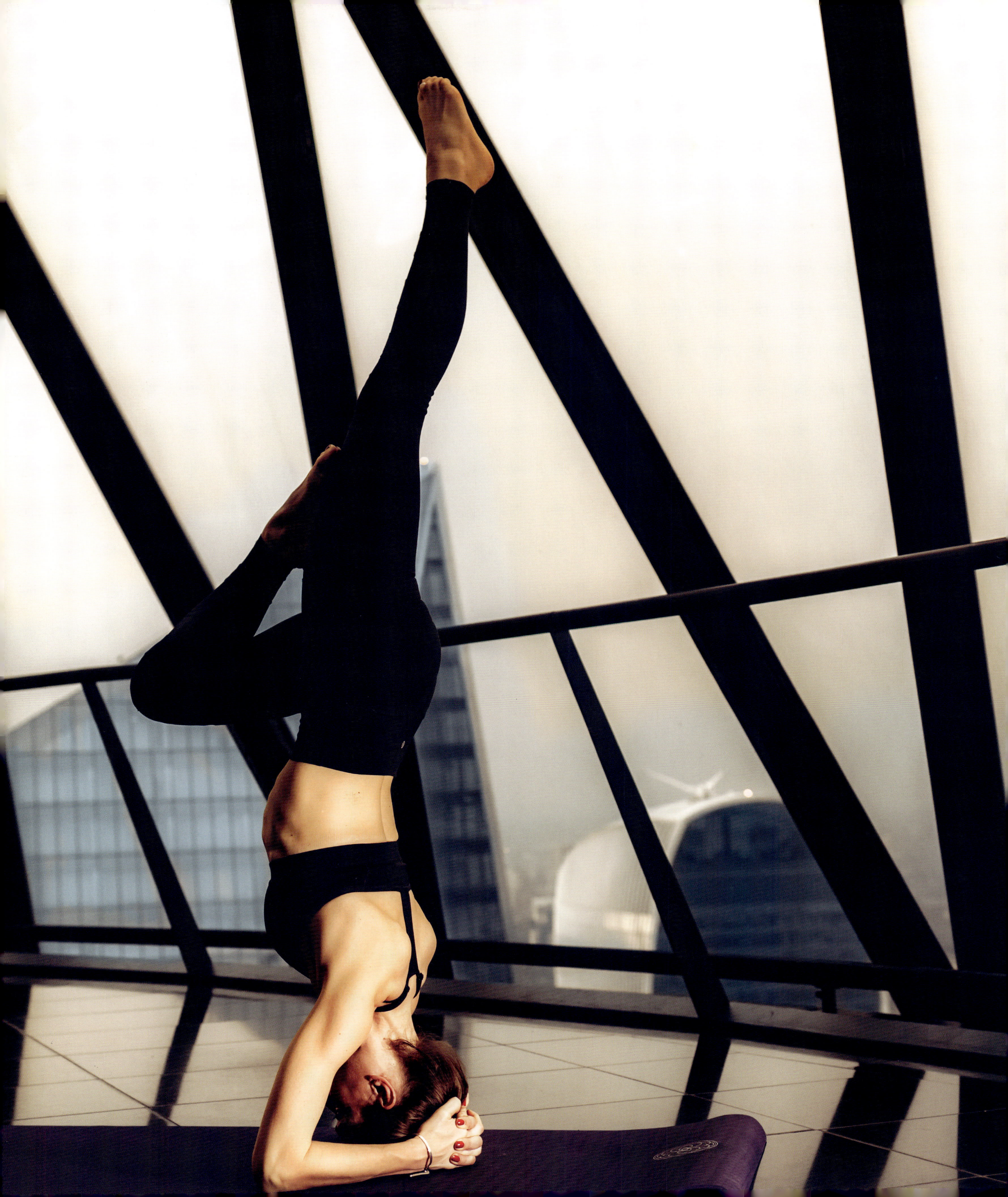

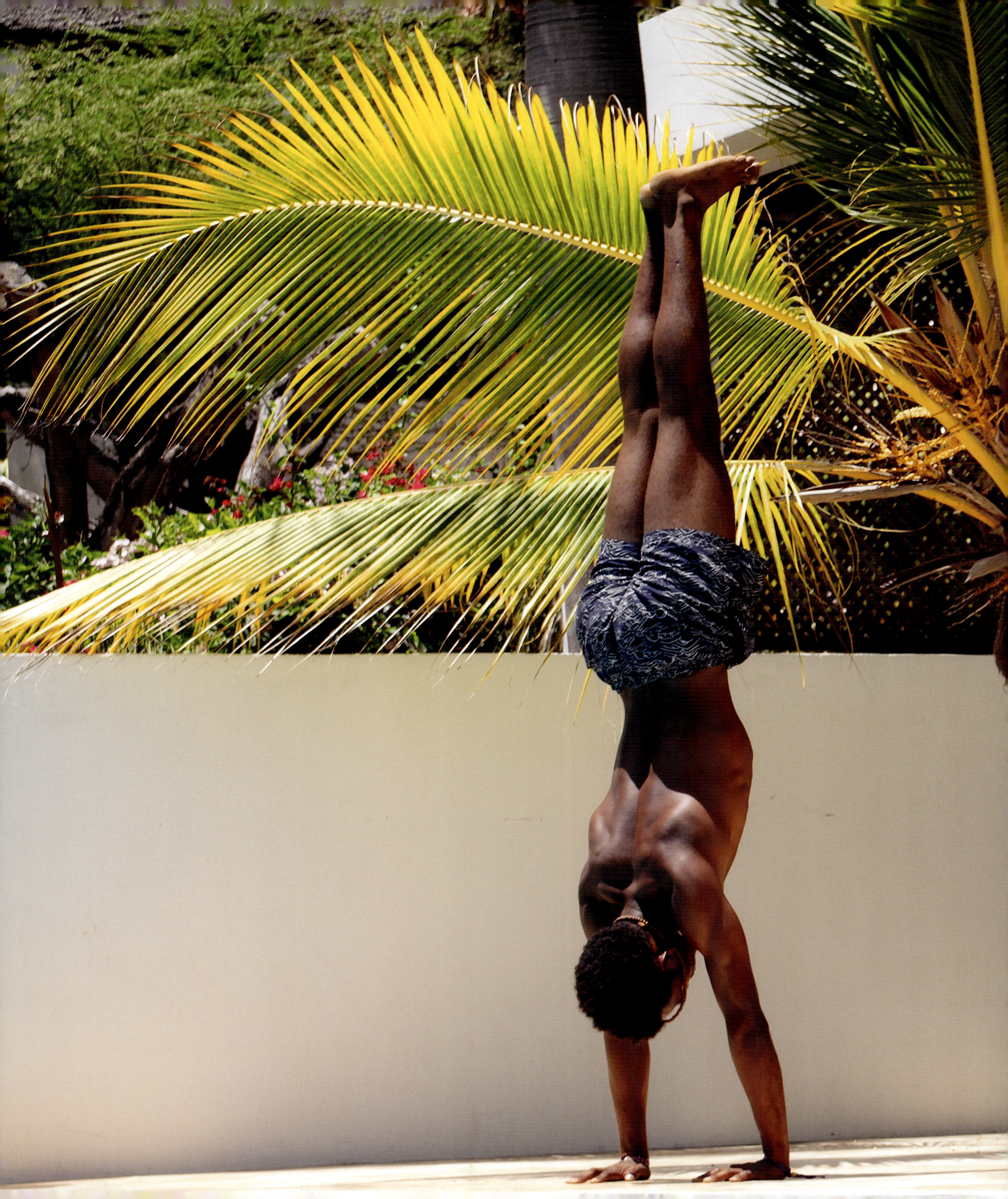

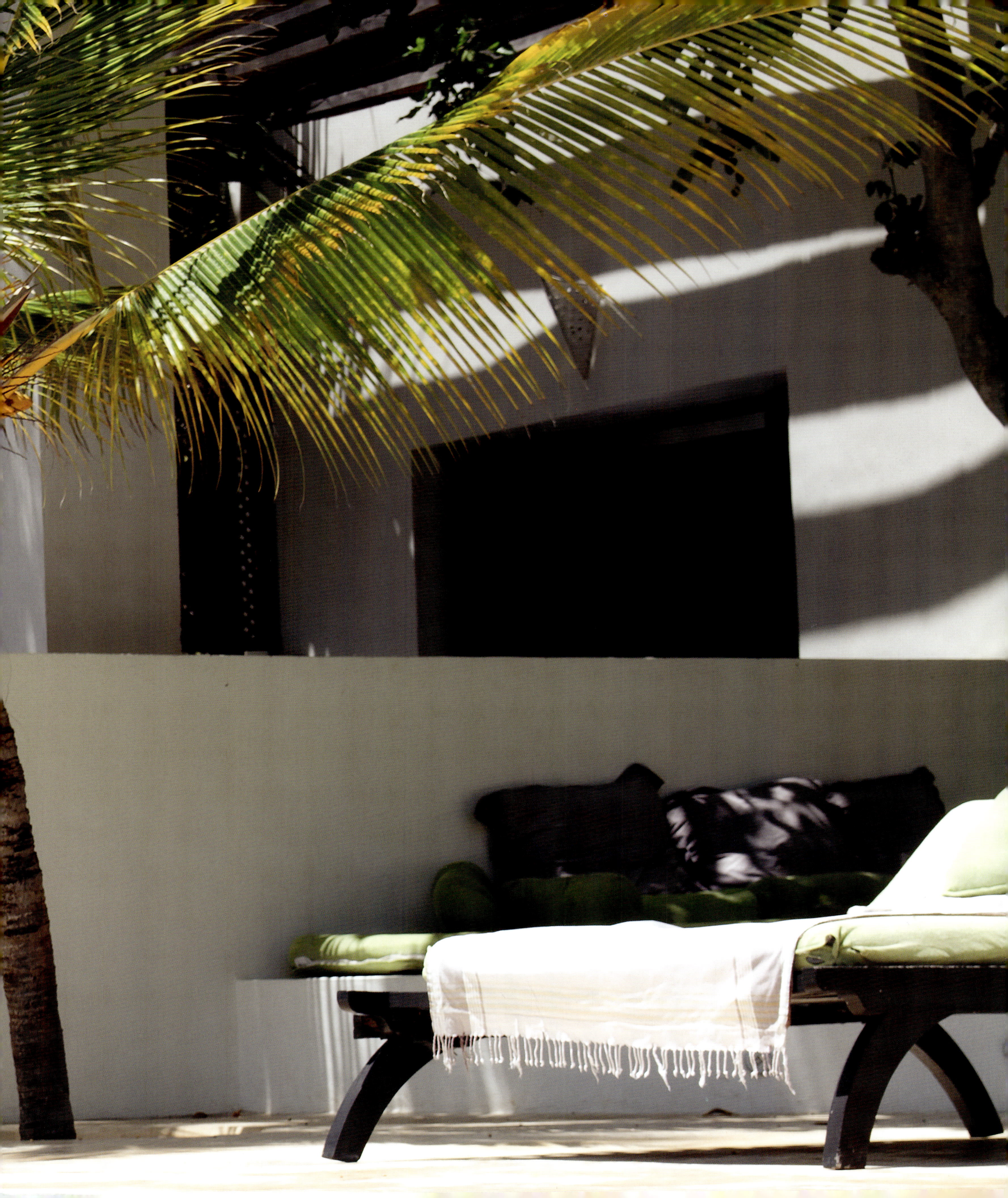

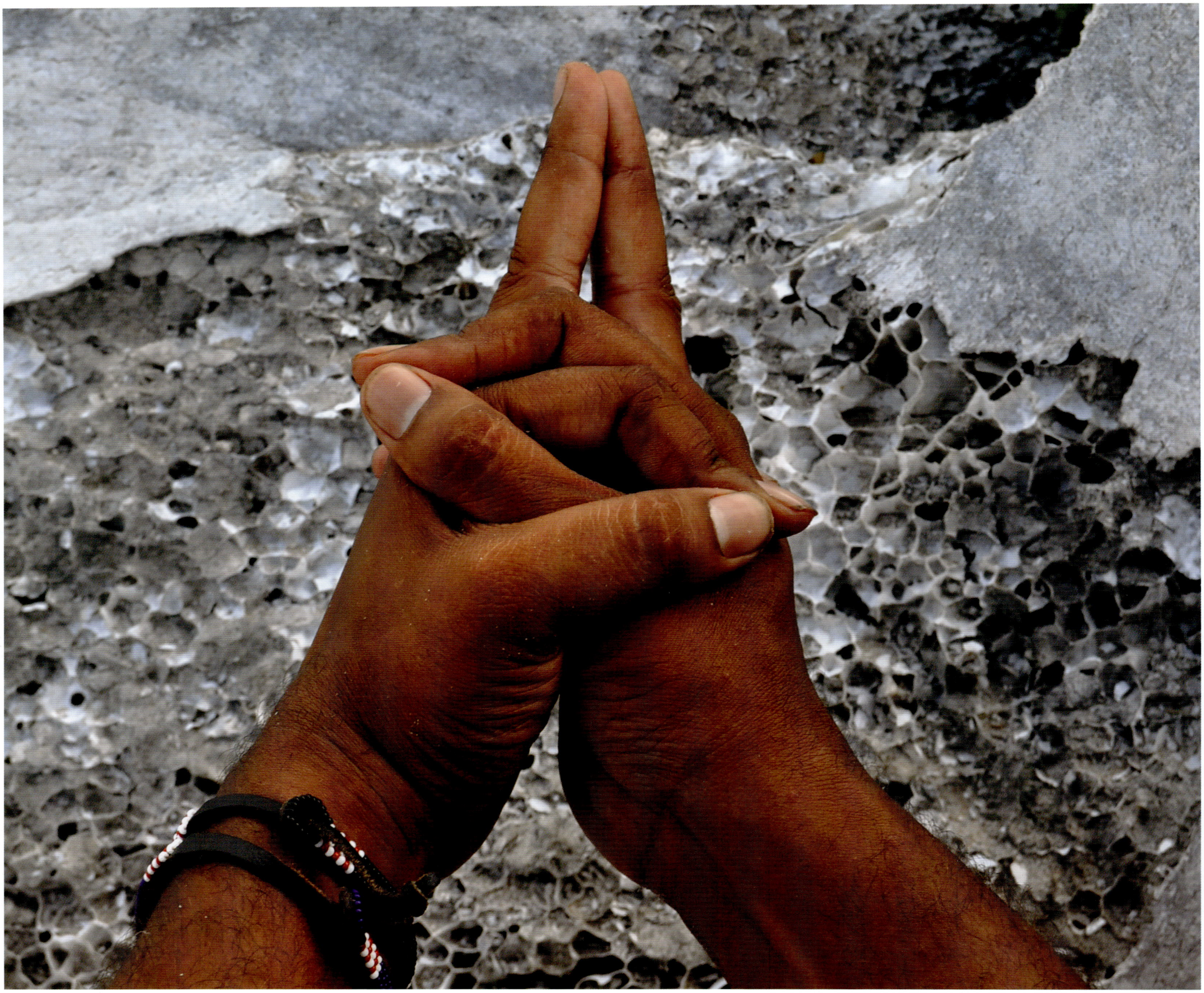

▲ **CHAKRAMUDRA** · Consolidation

UTTHITA HASTA PADANGUSTHASANA · Extended Hand-to-Toe

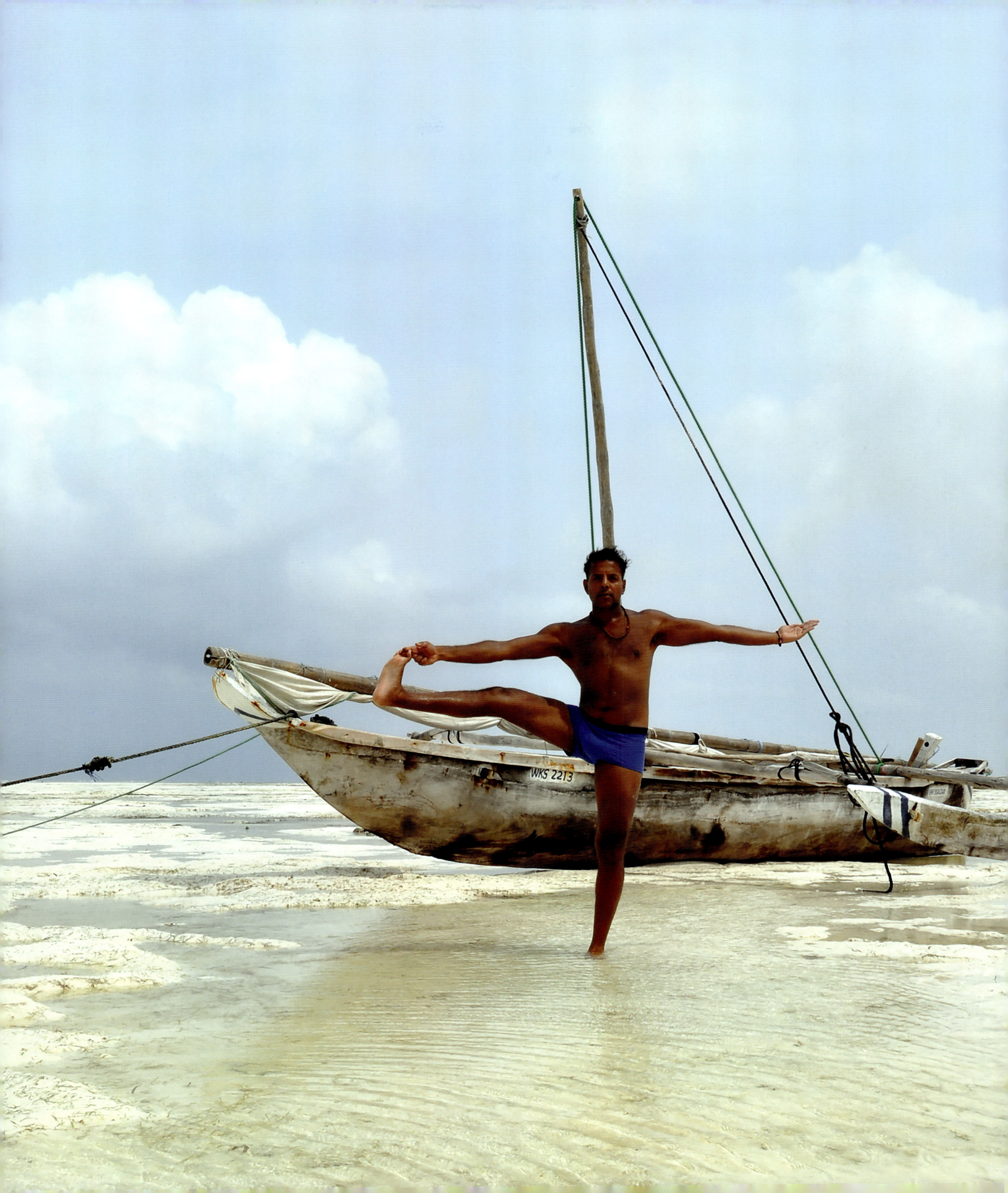
WKS 2213

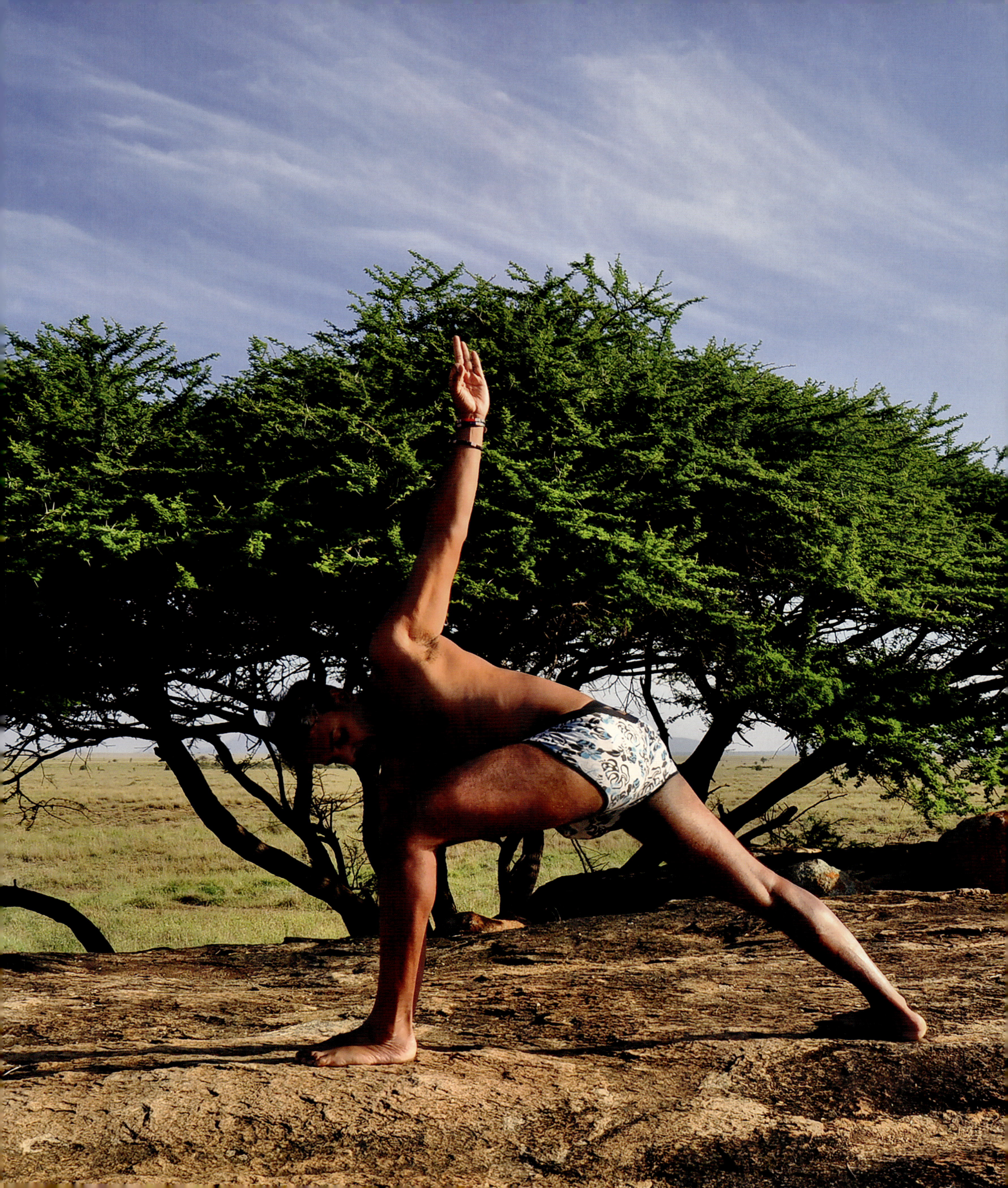

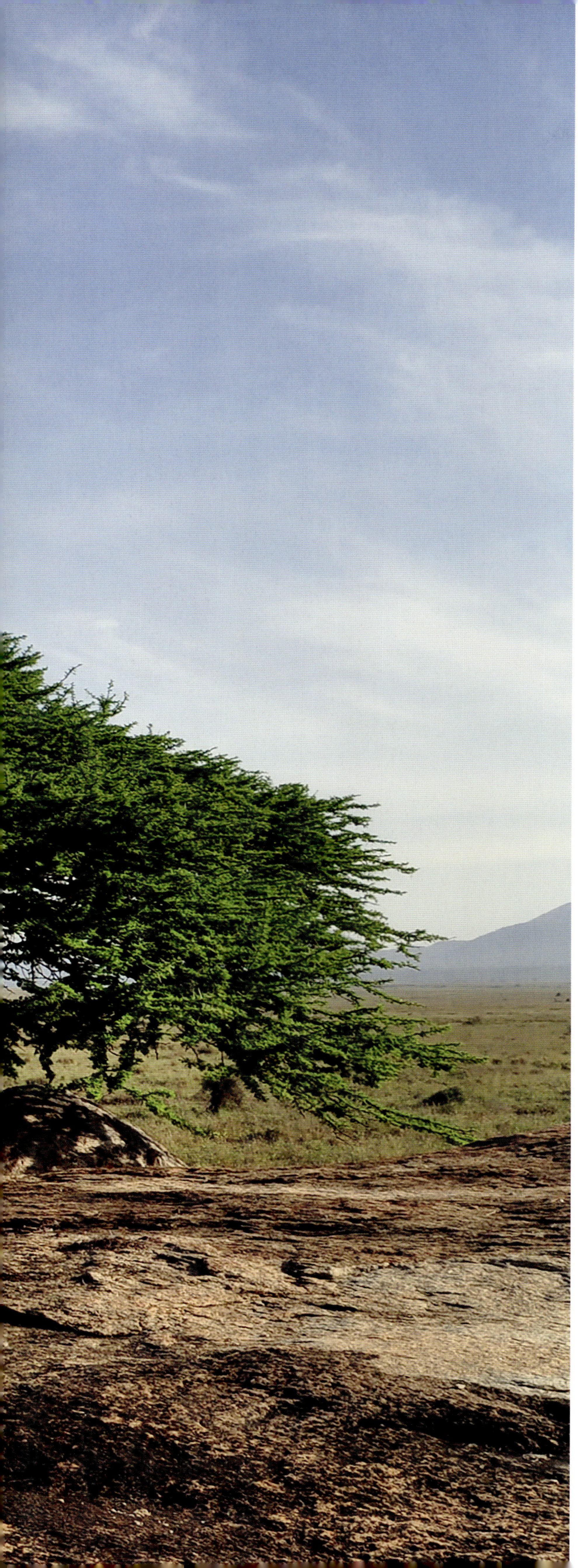

To know the depths
of your own heart
is the greatest
love affair you
will ever have.

PARIVRTTA PARSVAKONASANA · Twisted Side Angle

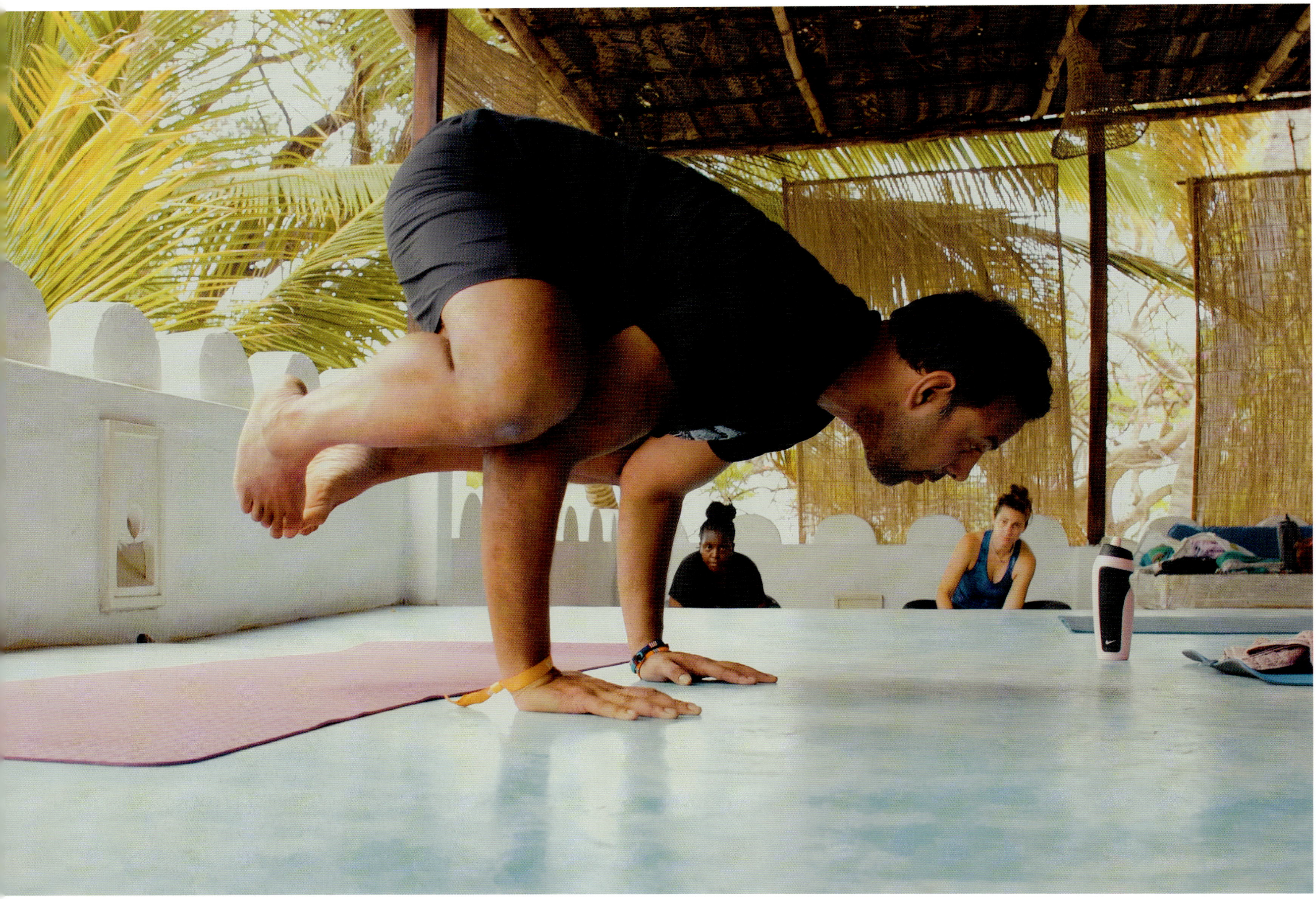

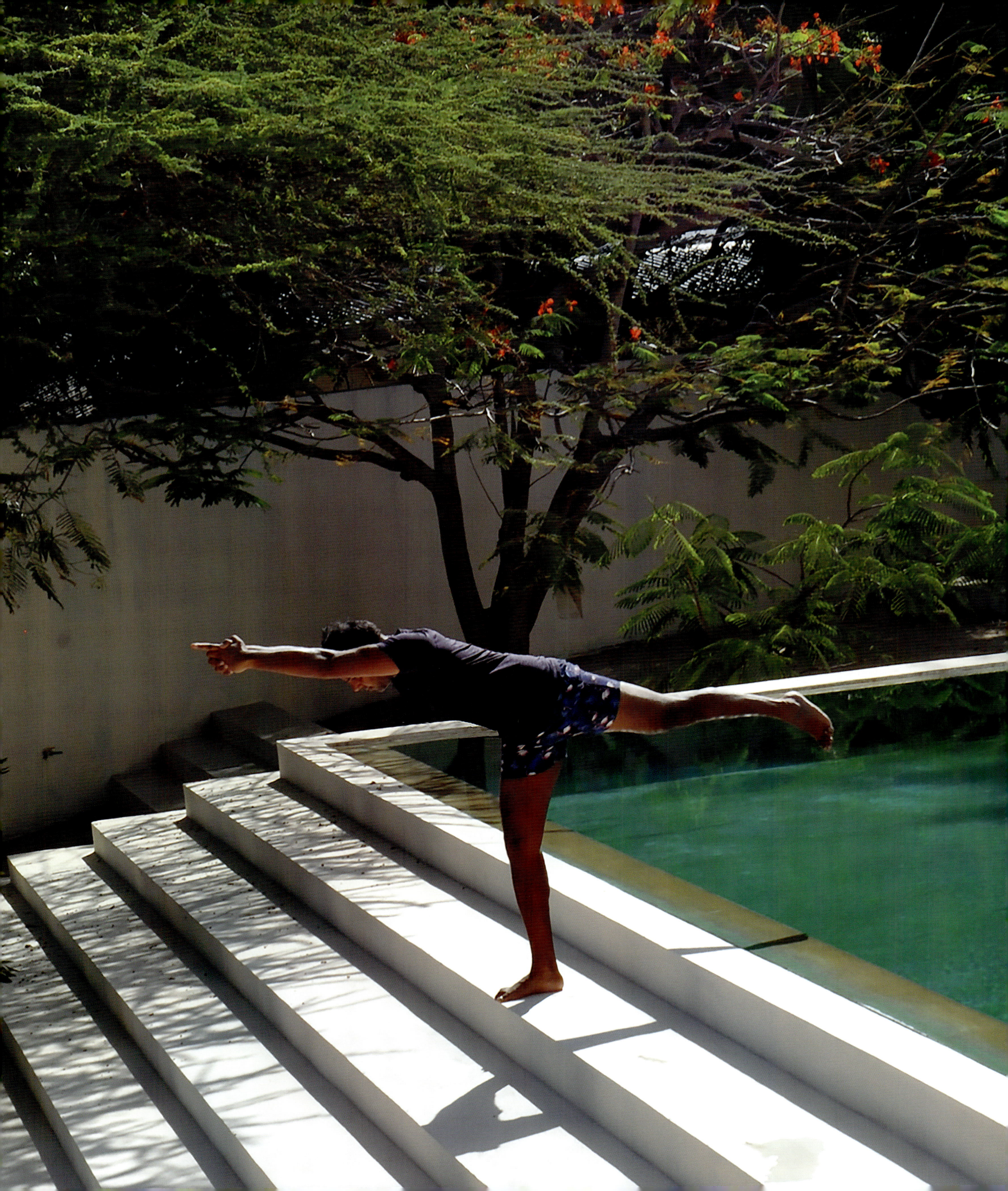

Navigate toward
what you want
rather than
fixating on the past.

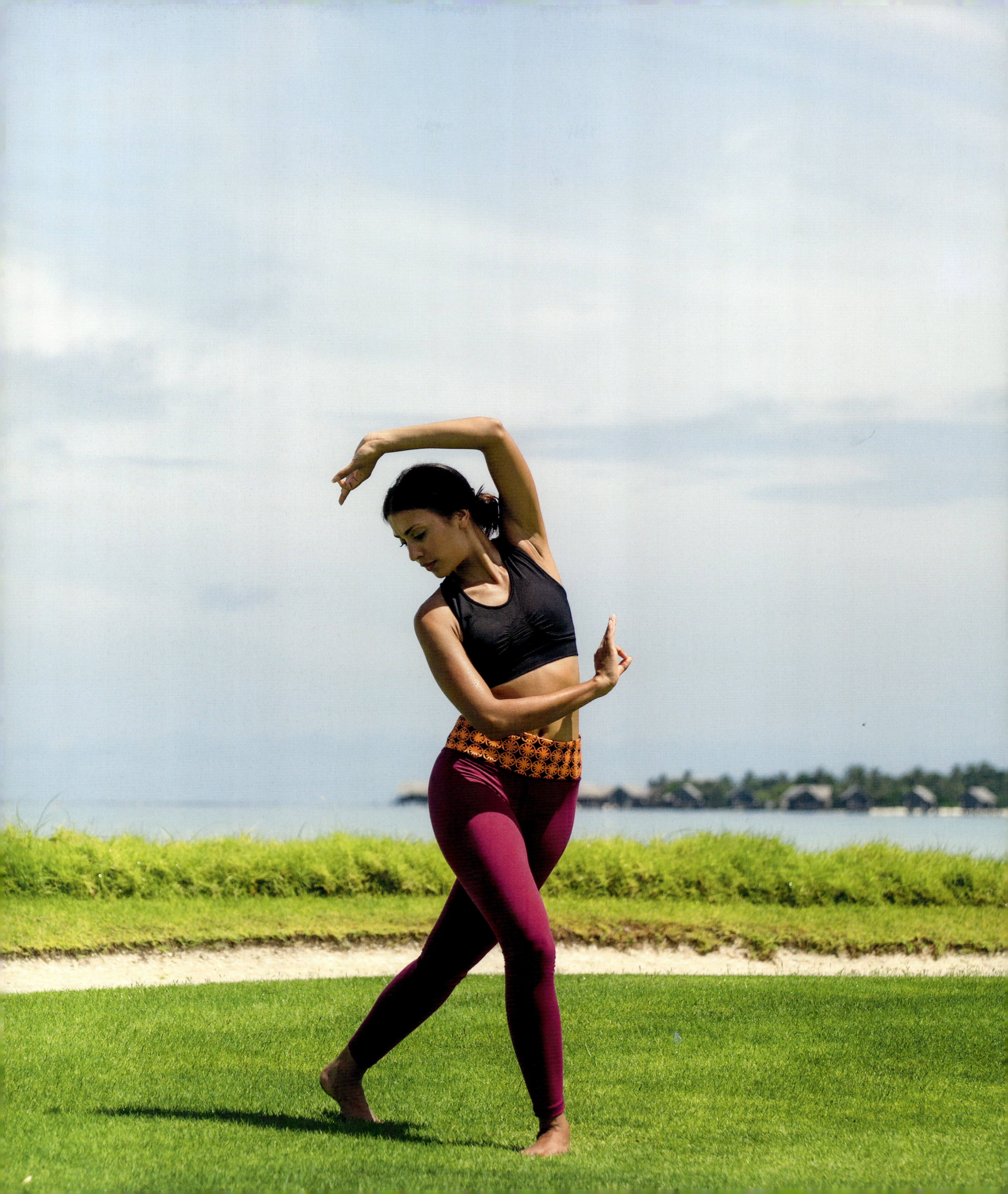

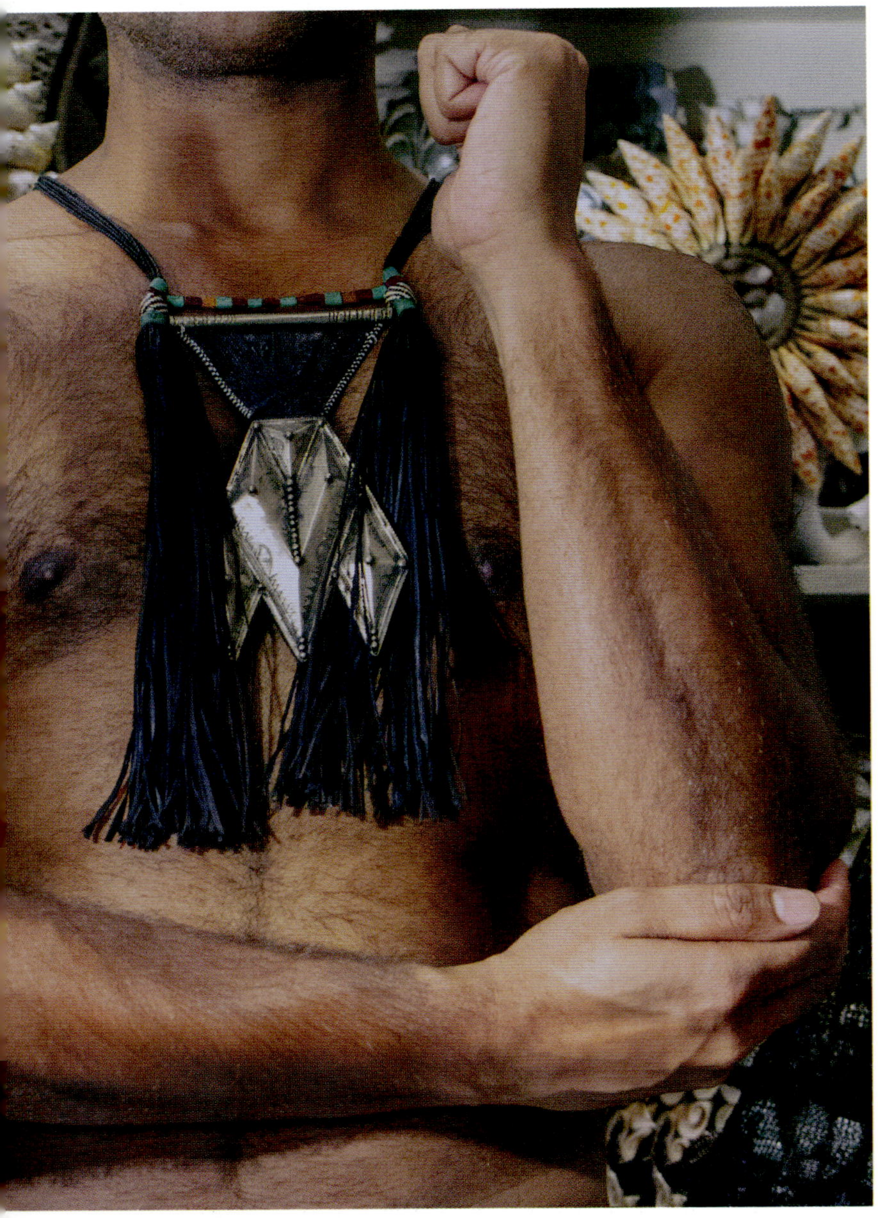

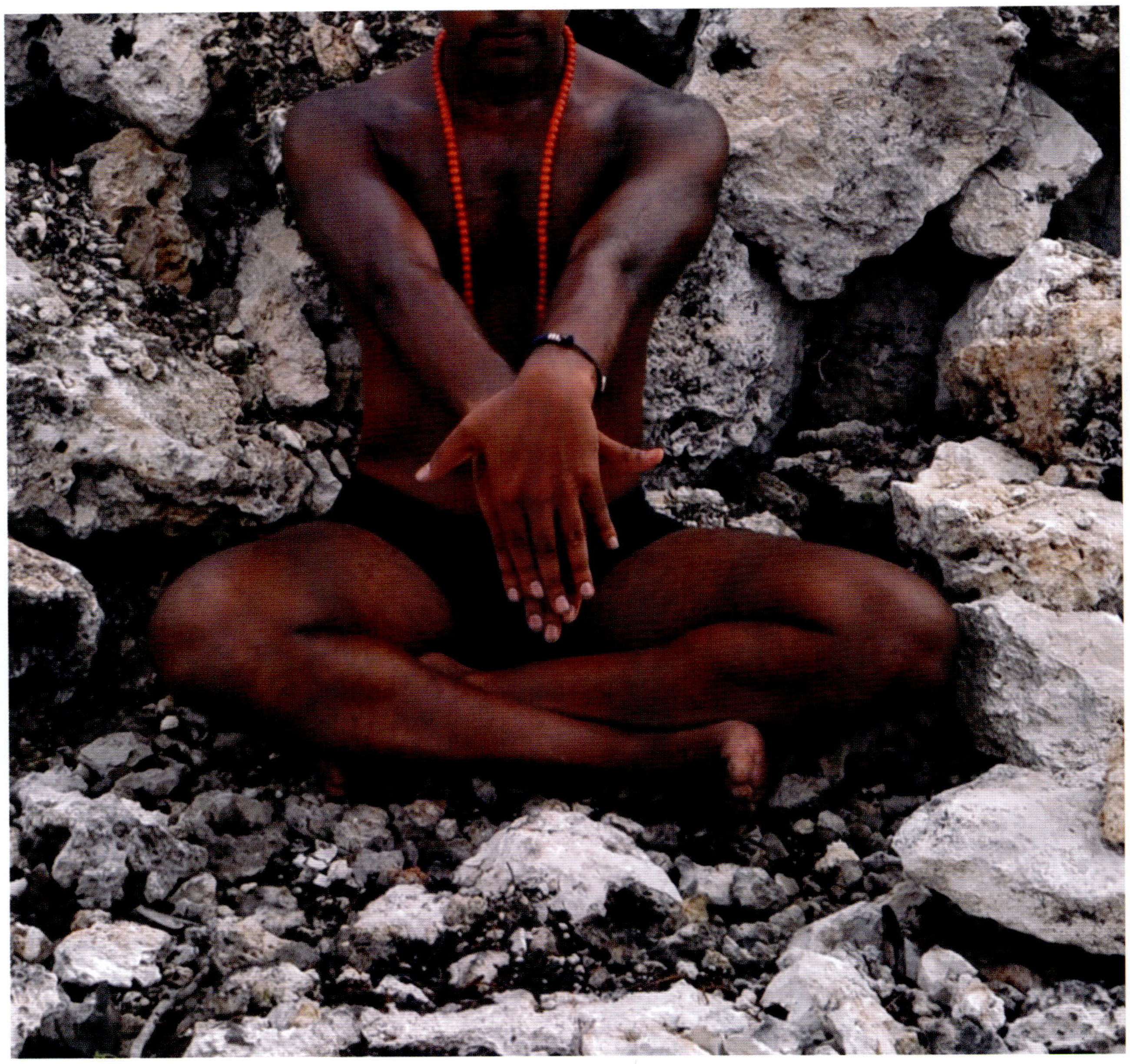

▲ **MUDGARAMUDRA** · Loyalty *(left)* **MATSYAMUDRA** · Integration *(right)*

UDAYA UTTHITA HASTA PADANGUSTHASANA · Rising Extended Hand-to-Toe

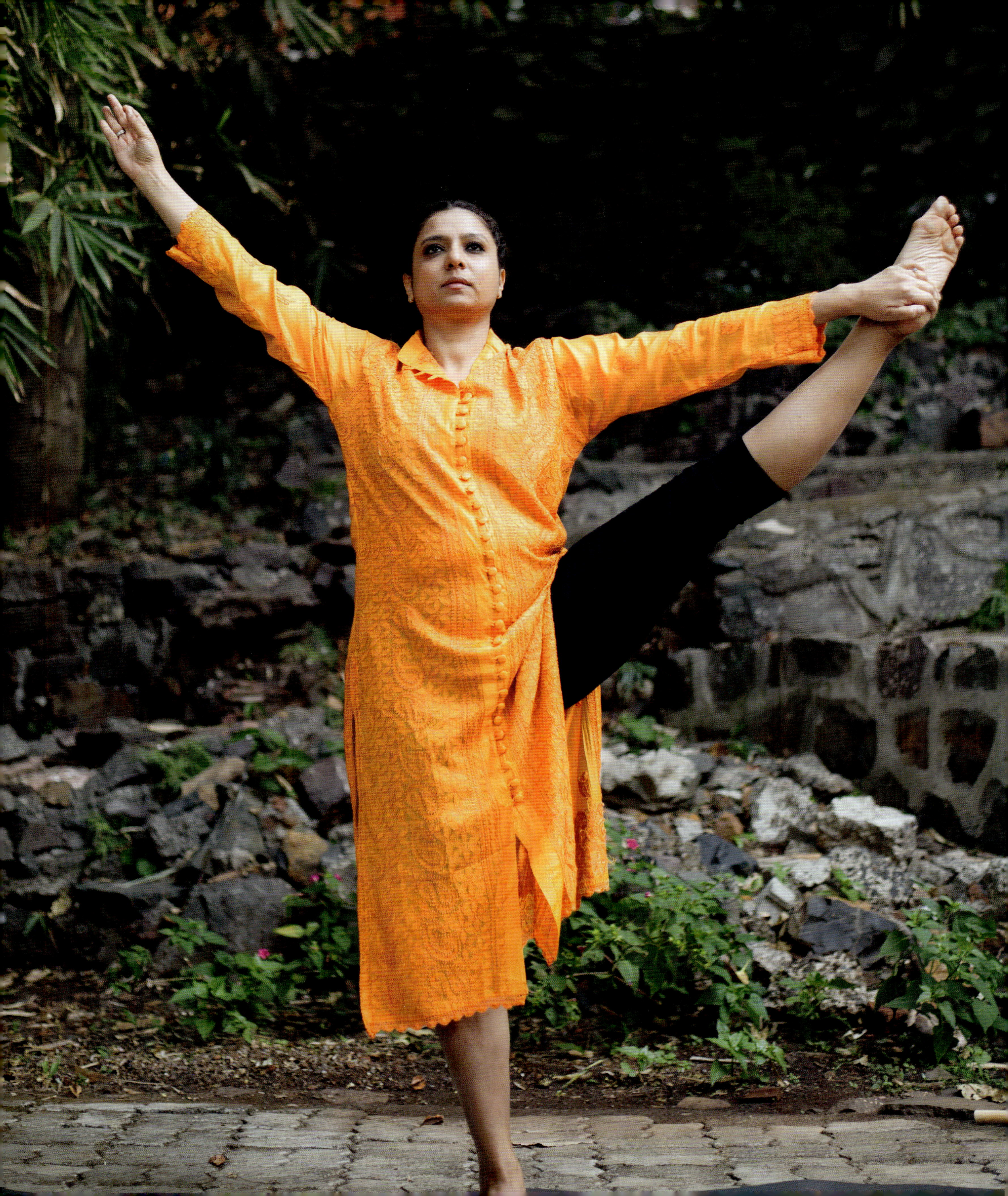

Yoga poses are living sculptures.
A sculpture is made beautiful as much from the knocks it receives as from the creative vision of its creator. You are no different.

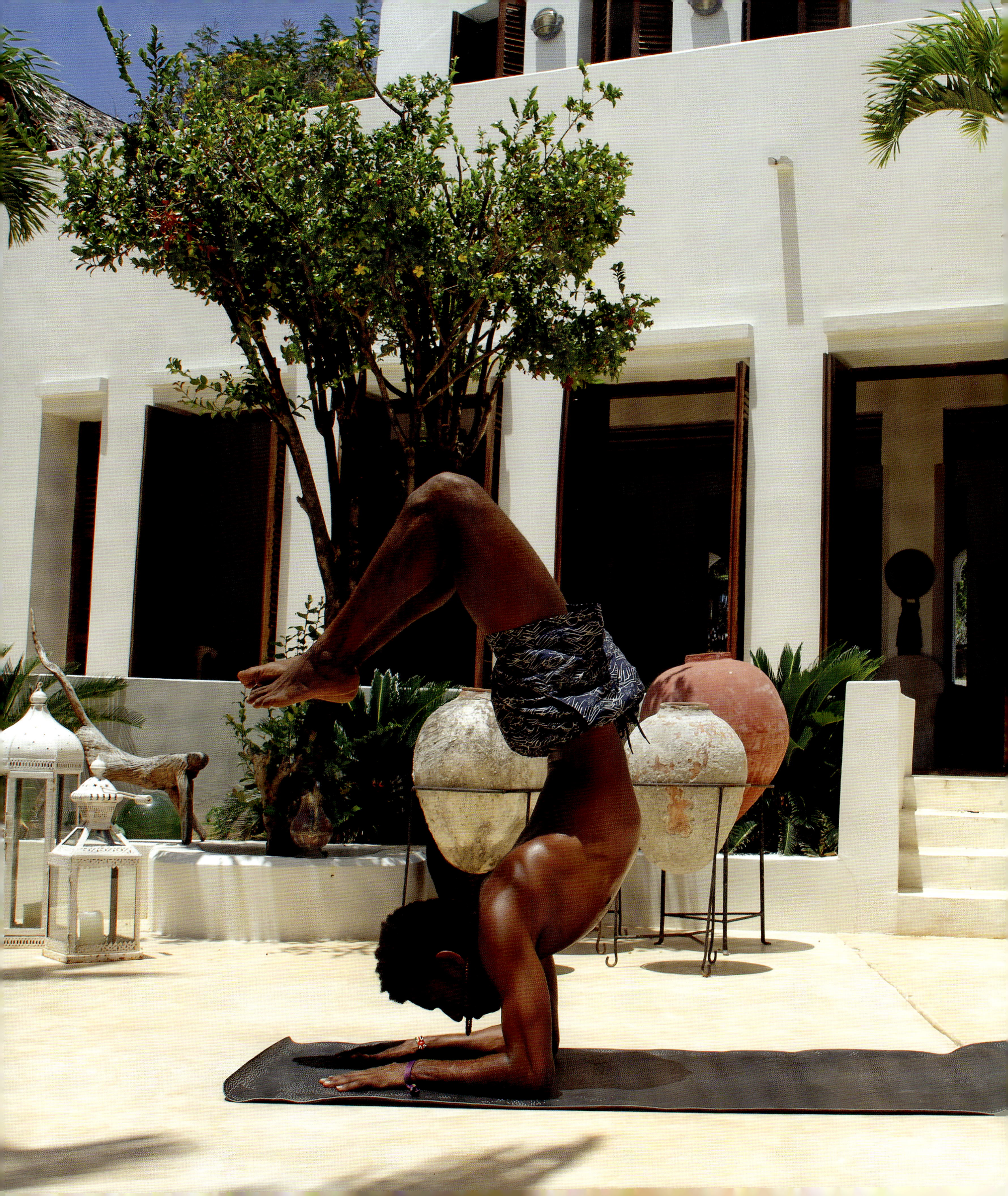

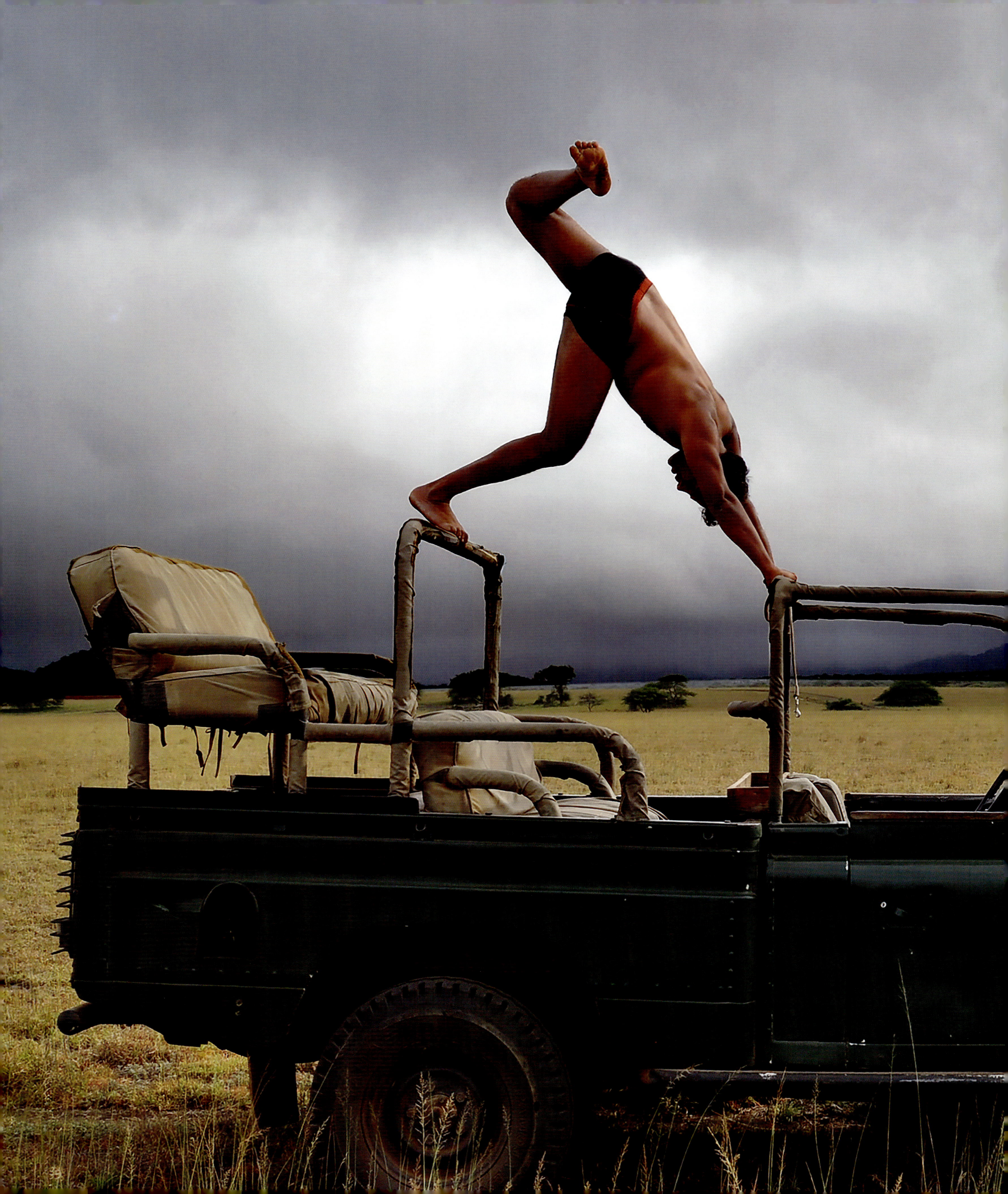

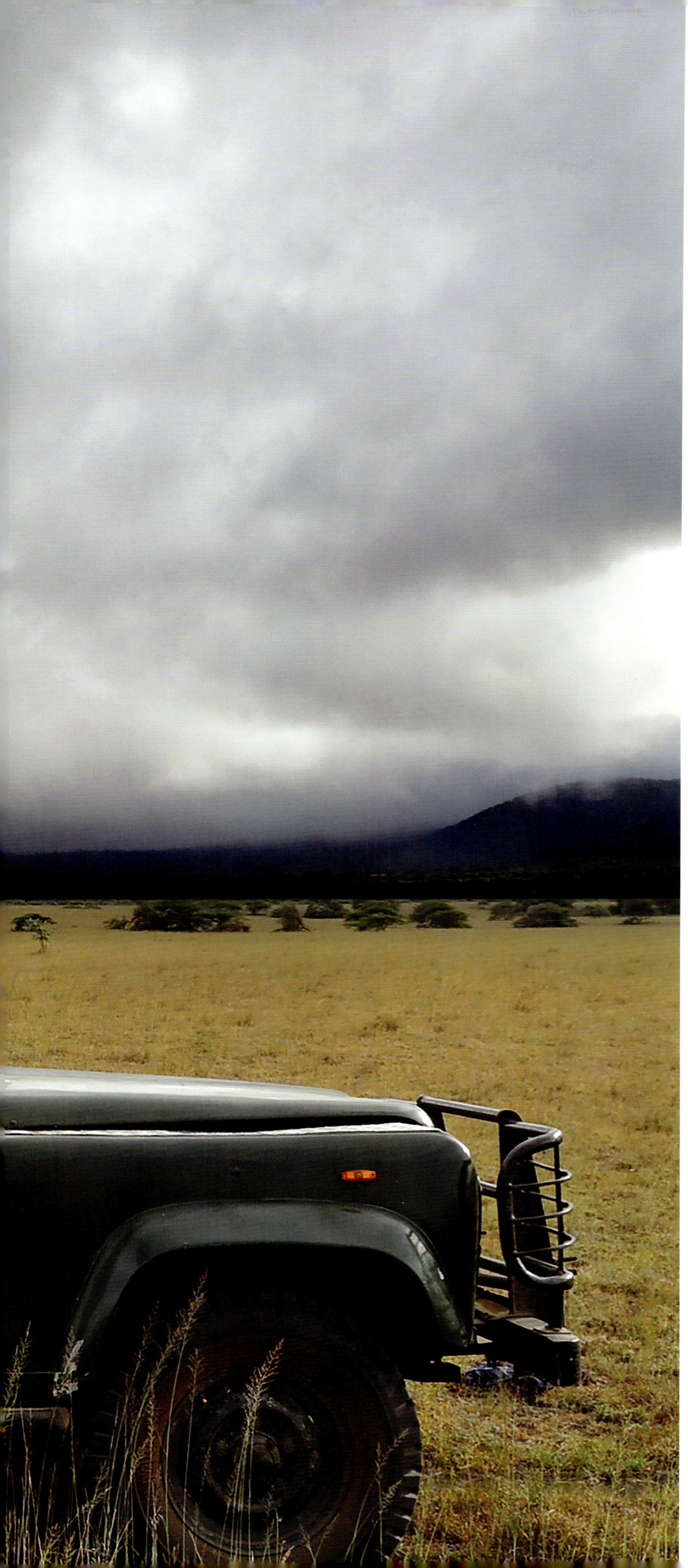

TRI PADA ADHO MUKHA SVANASANA • Three-Legged Downward-Facing Dog

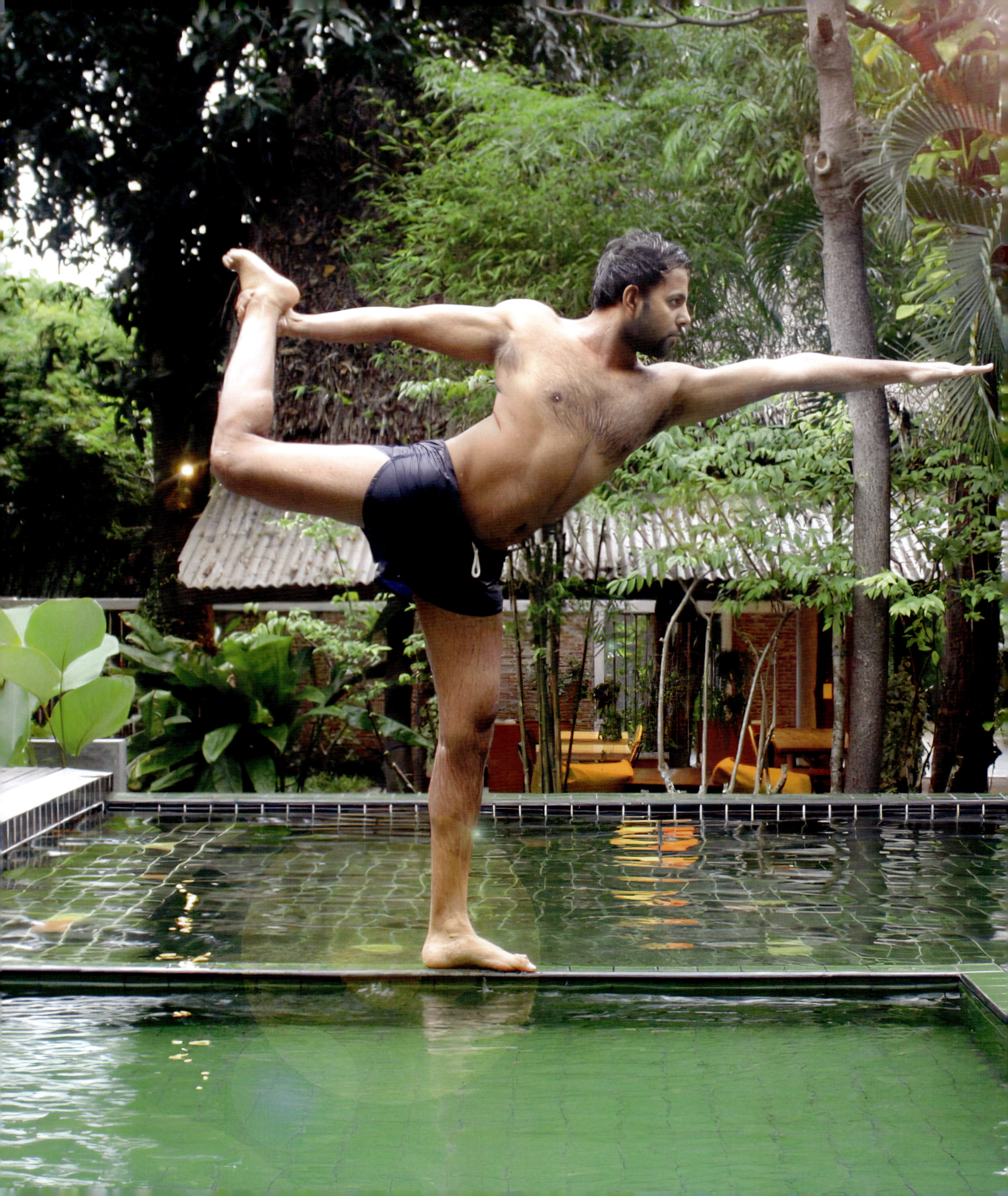

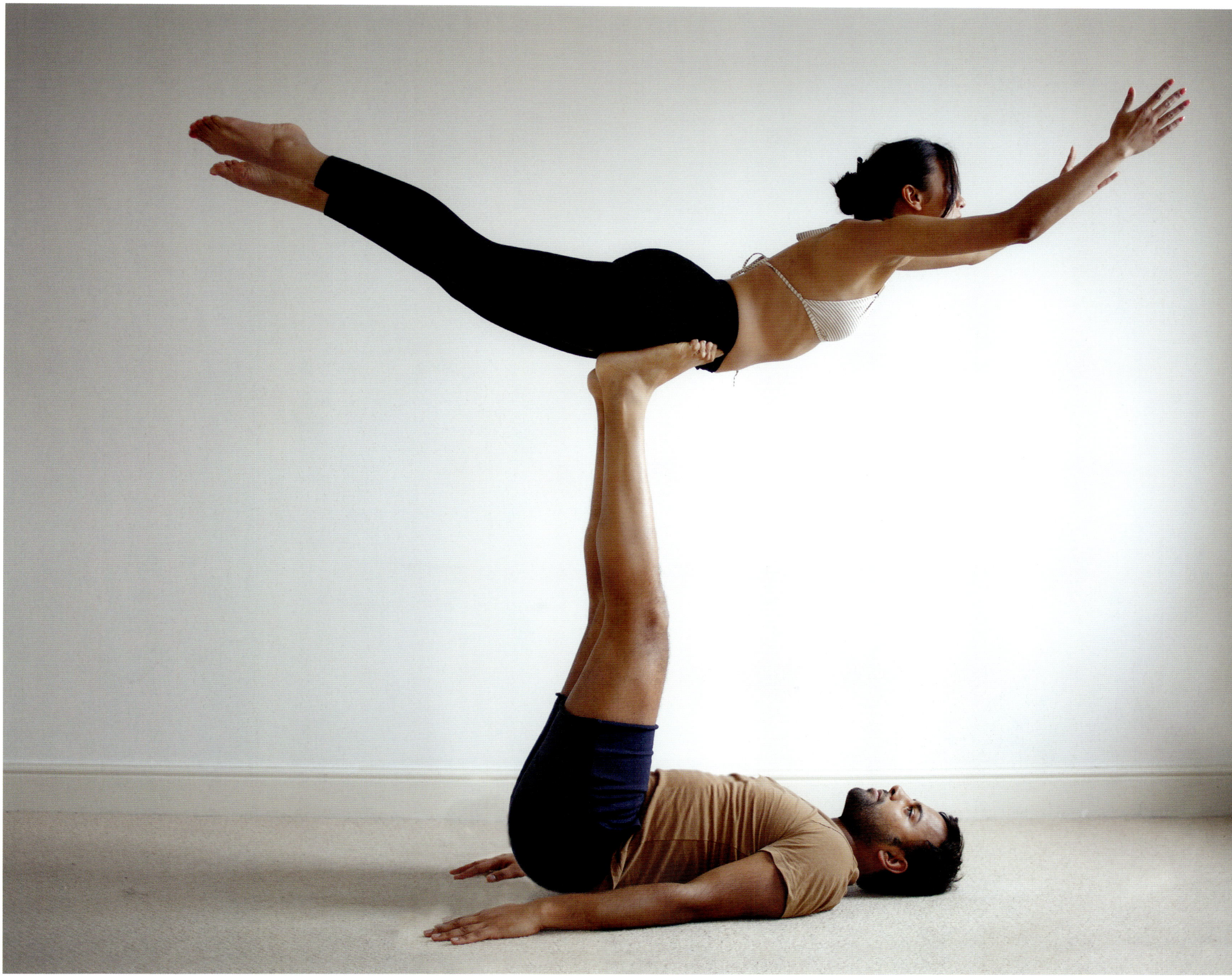

▲ **UTTHAN SALABHASANA** · Flying Locust

There is no need

to compete or compare

when you follow

an illuminated path.

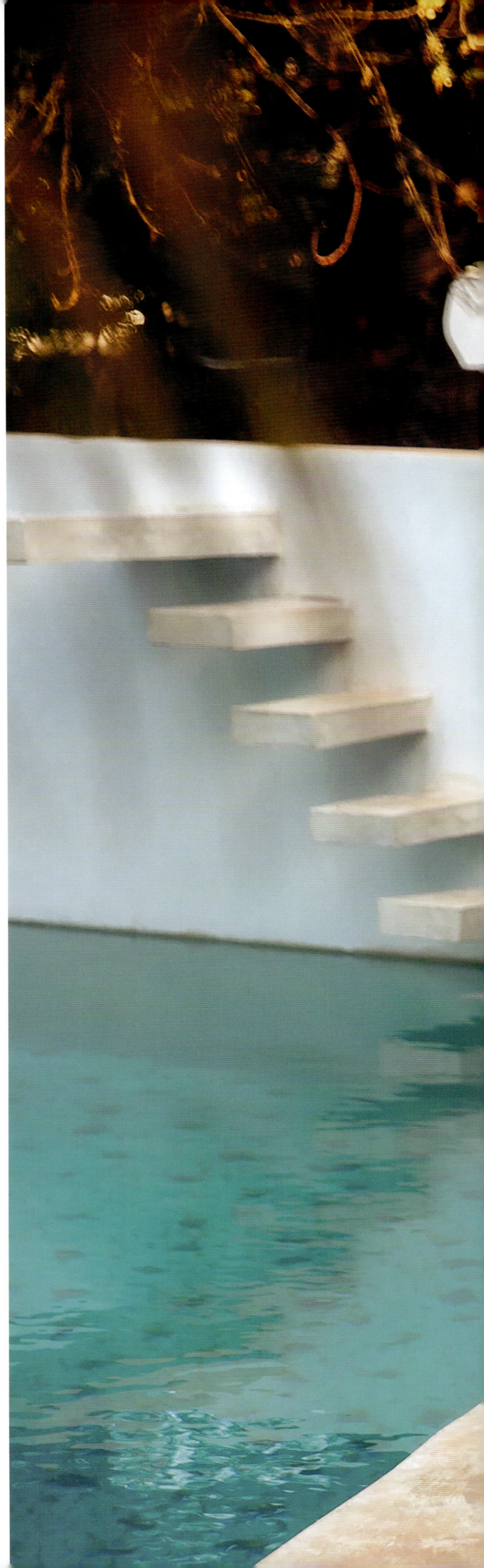

SIRSASANA · Headstand

▼ SAMDHI HANUMANASANA · Horizon Splits

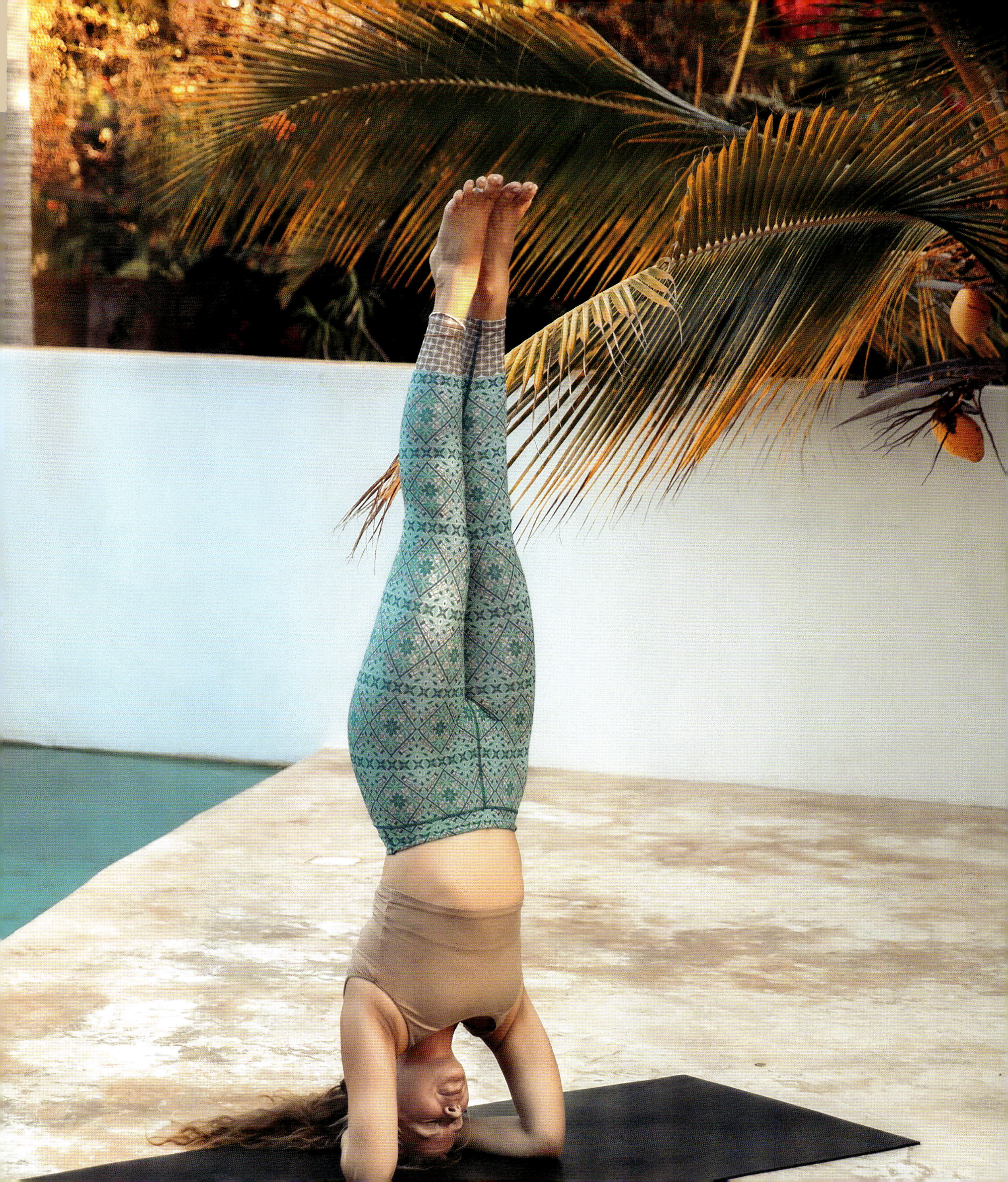

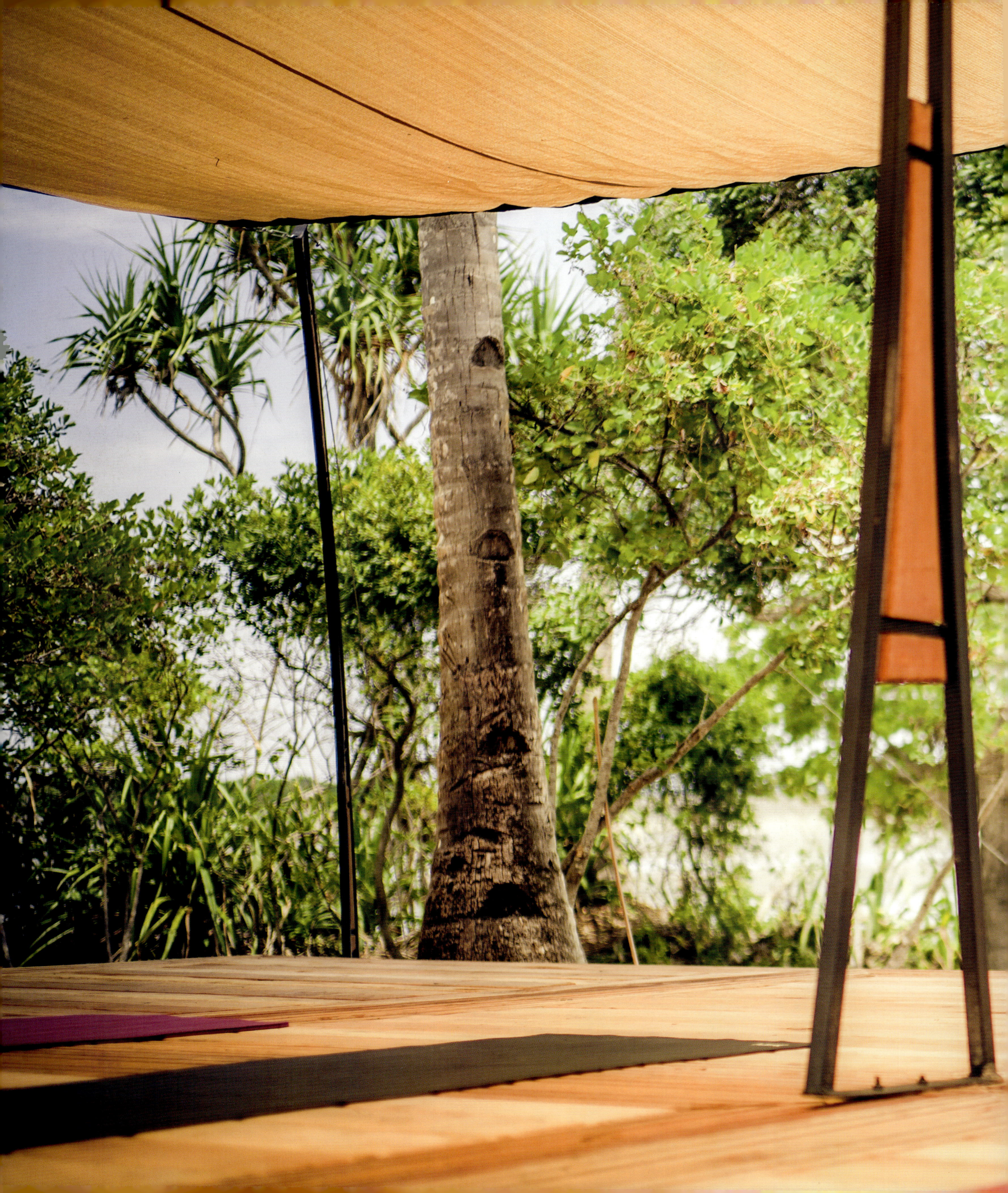

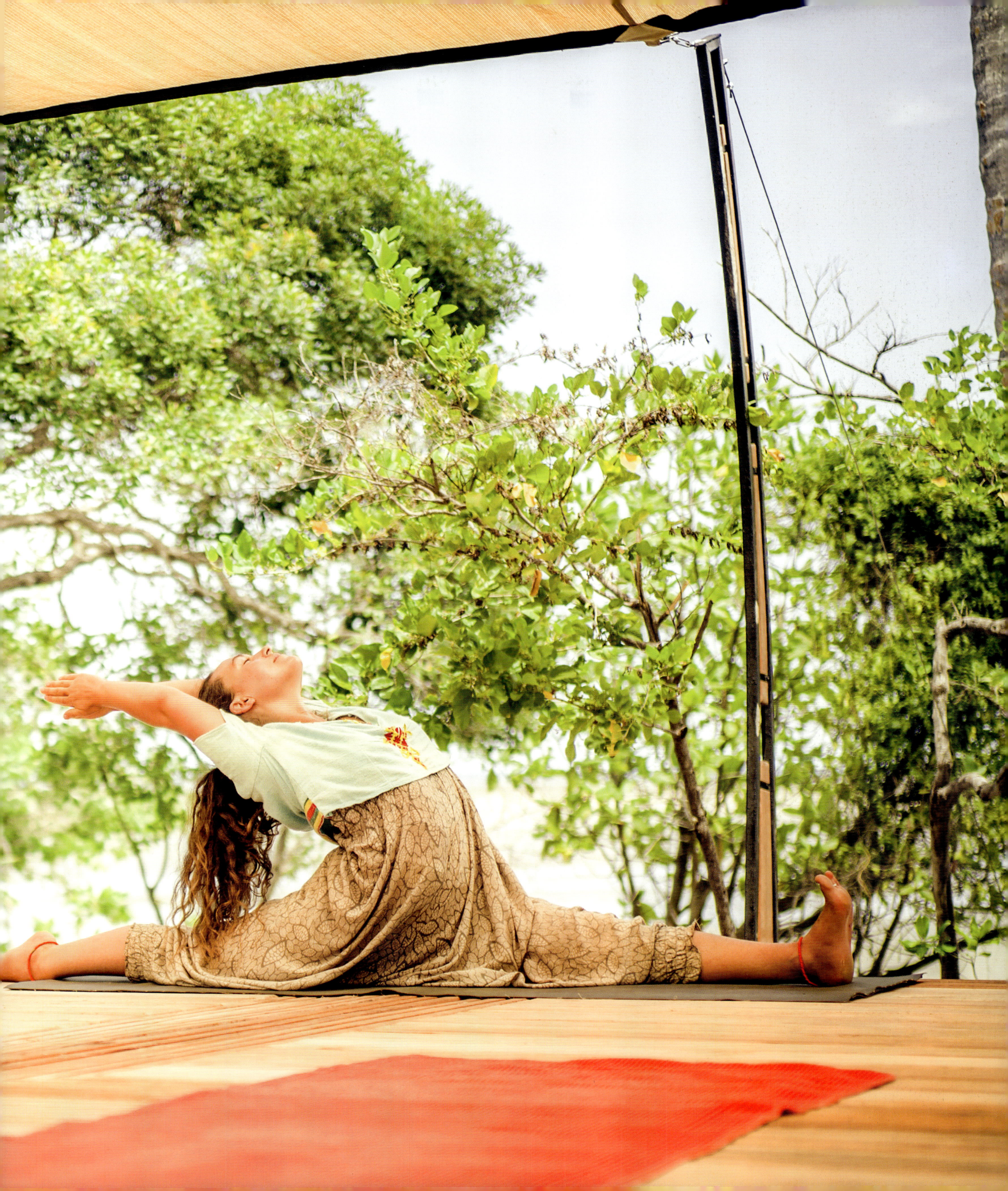

A spiral seems more complicated and longer than a line. To see things from all viewpoints is an advantage.

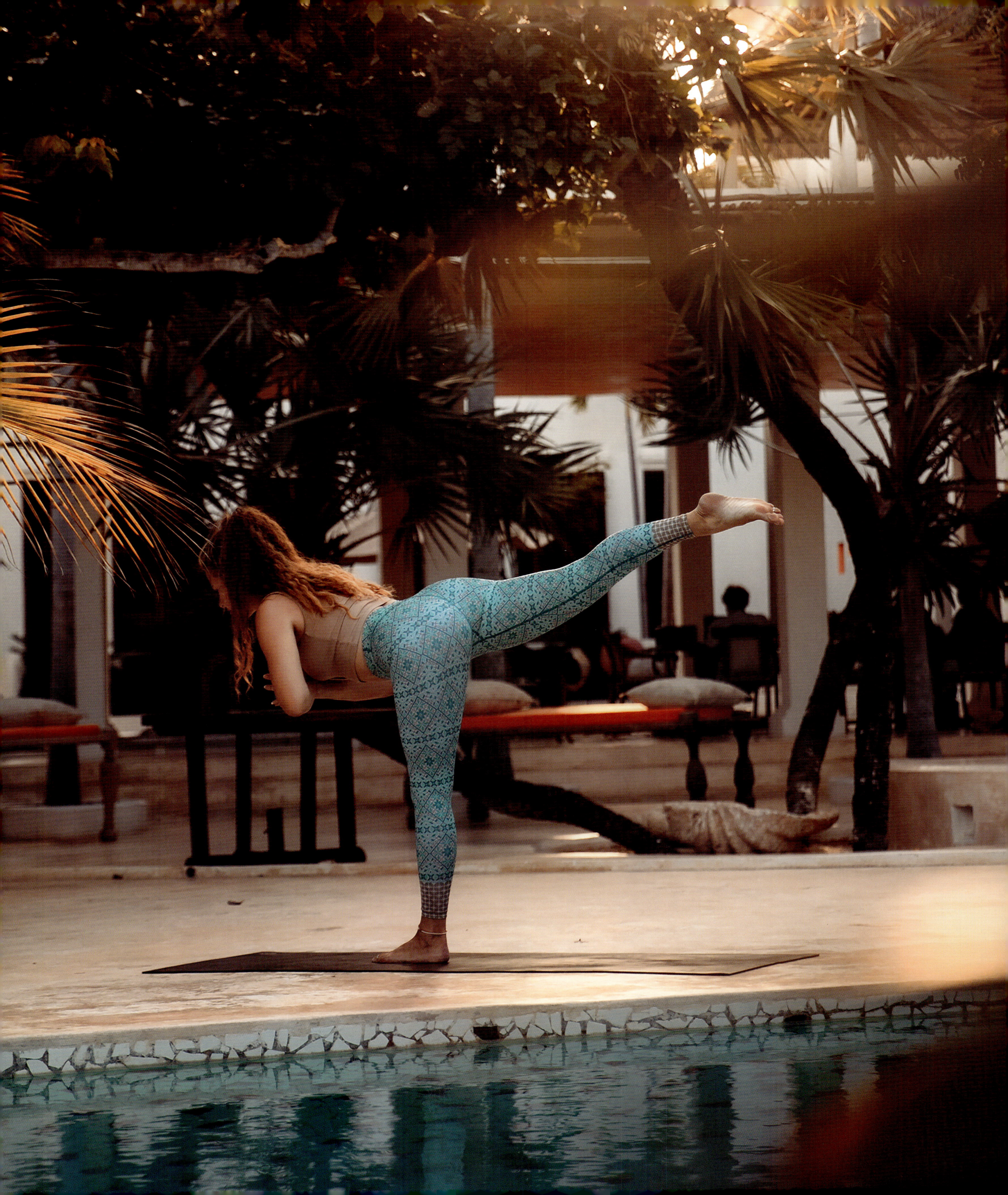

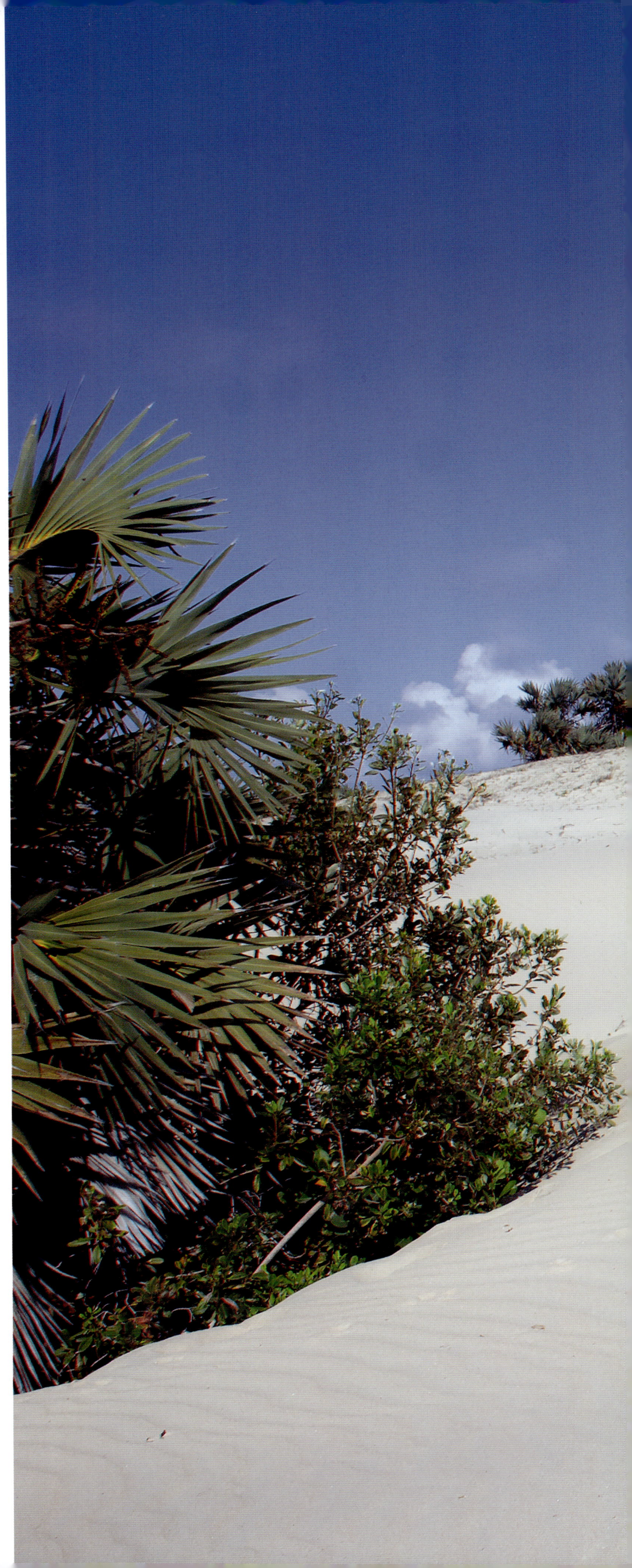

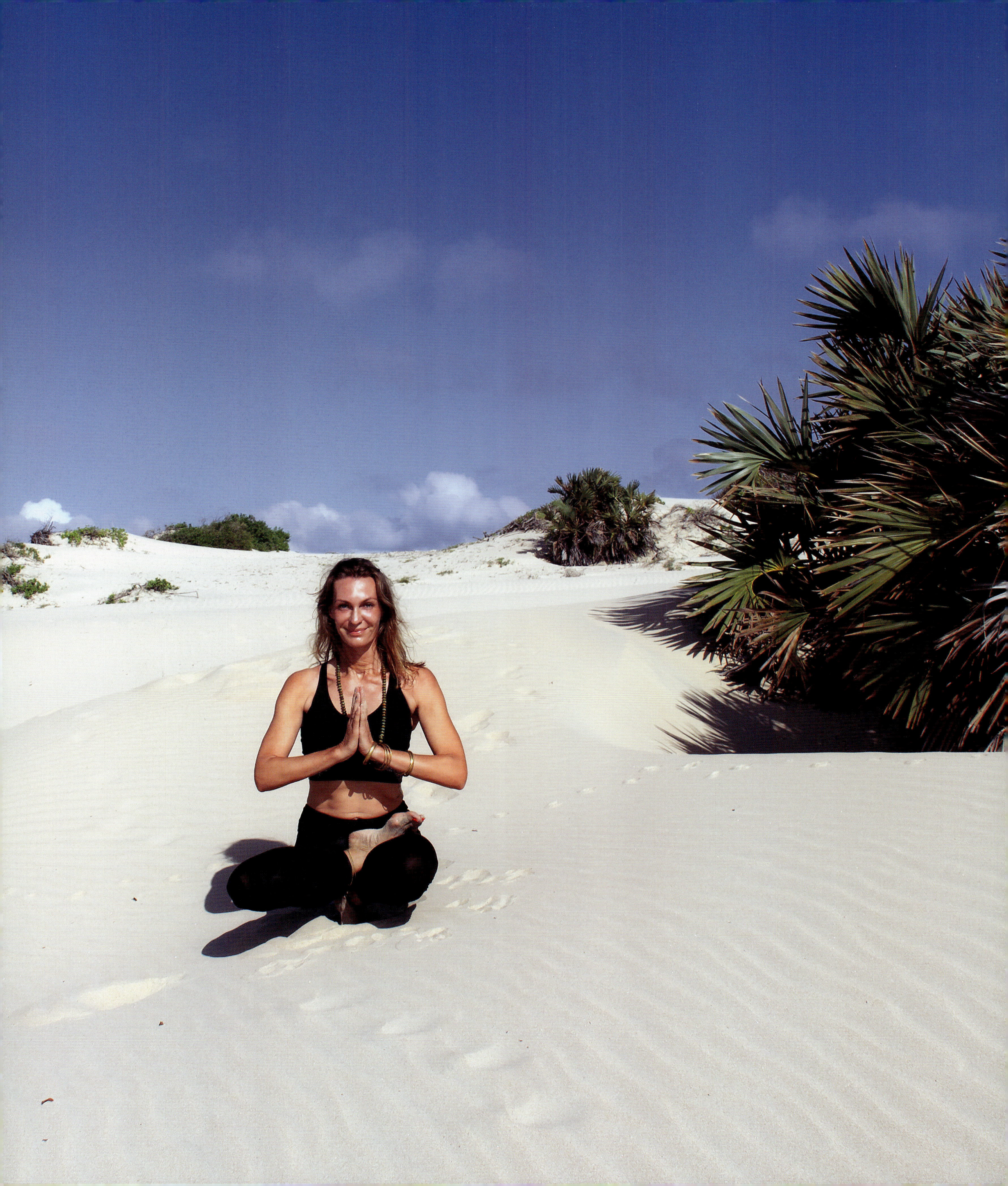

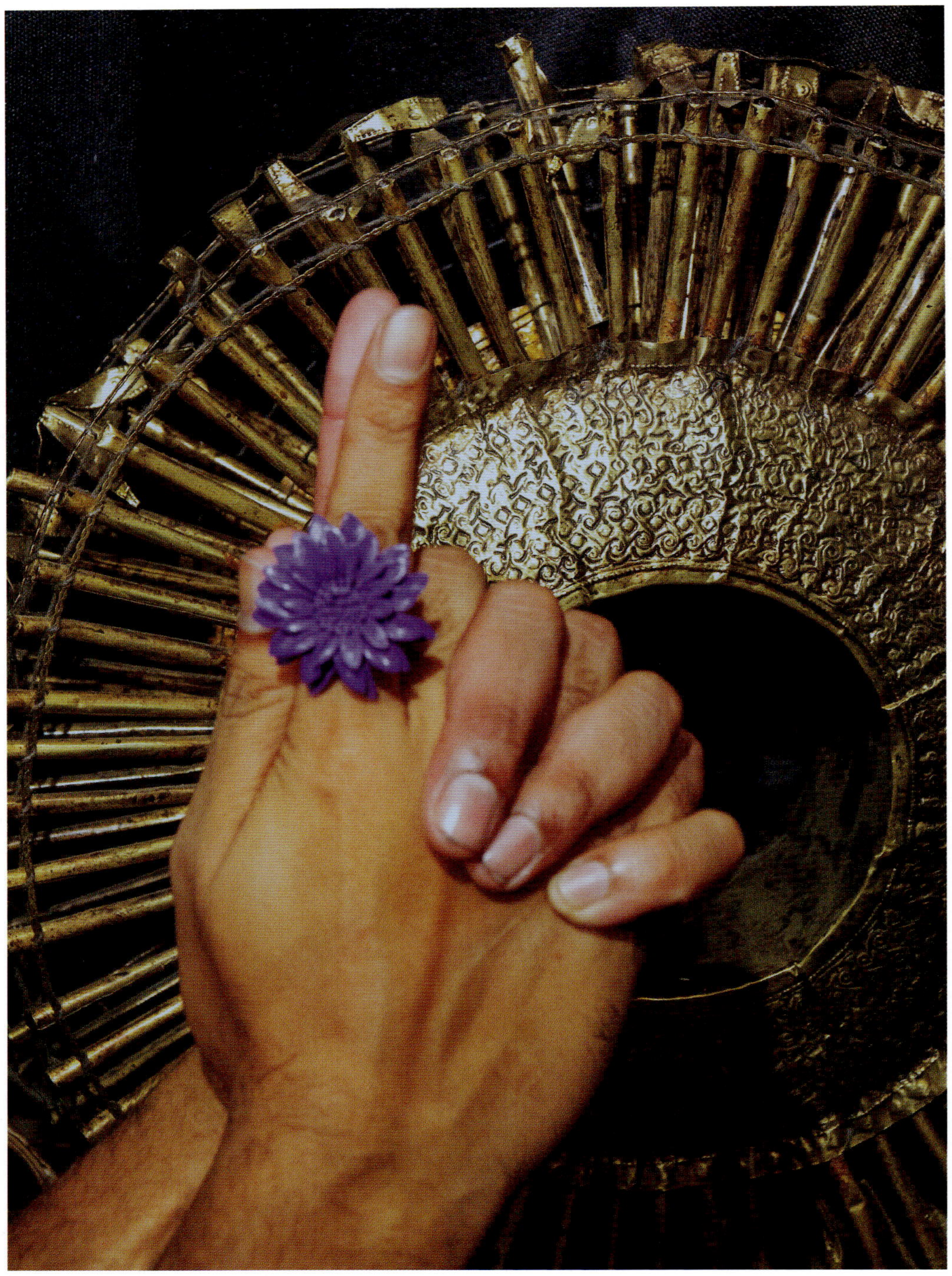

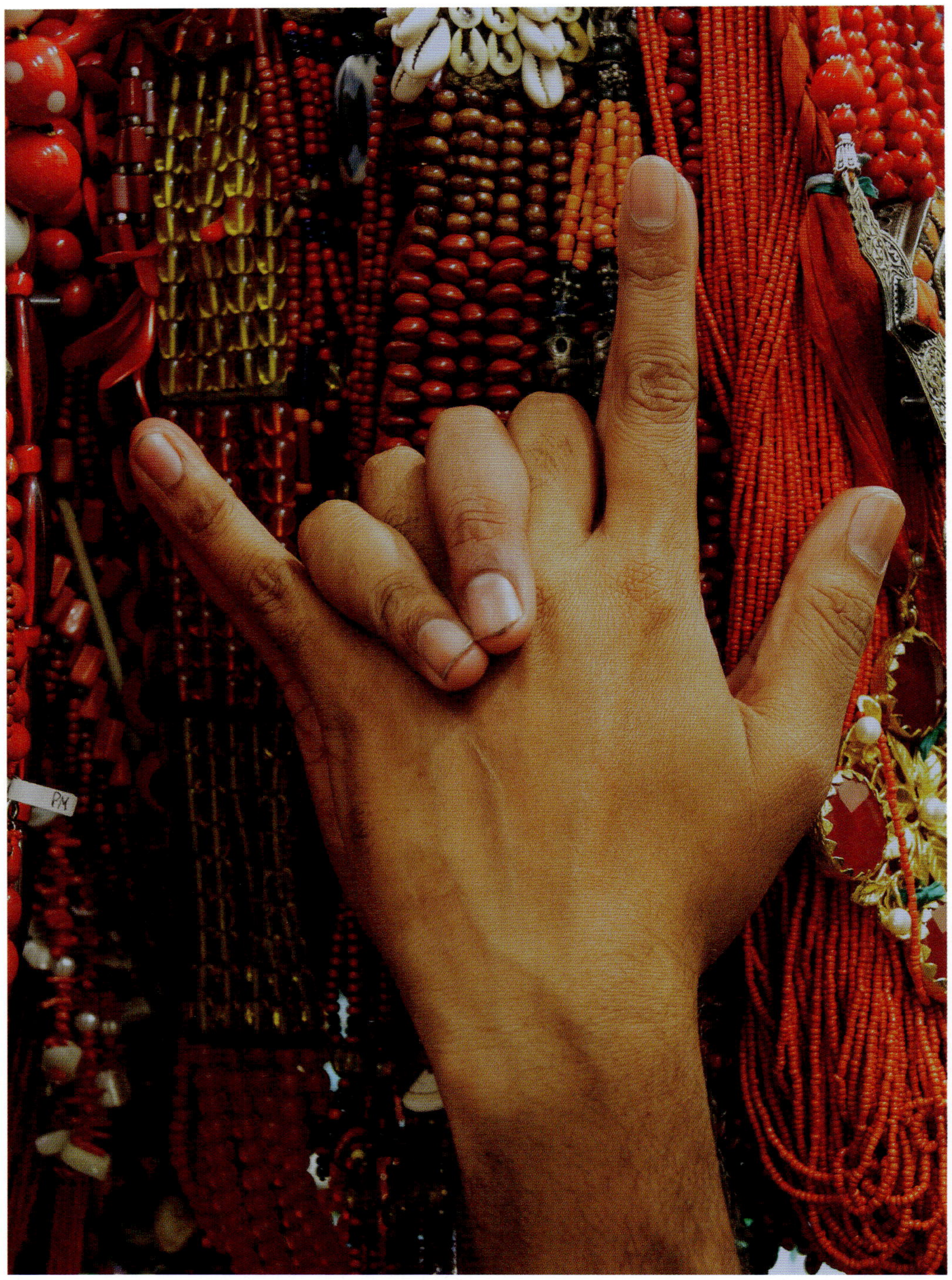

▲ **VAJRAMUDRA** • Indestructability *(left)* **ASHVARATNAMUDRA** • Perspective *(right)*

ARDHA PINCHA MAYURASANA • Half Feathered Peacock

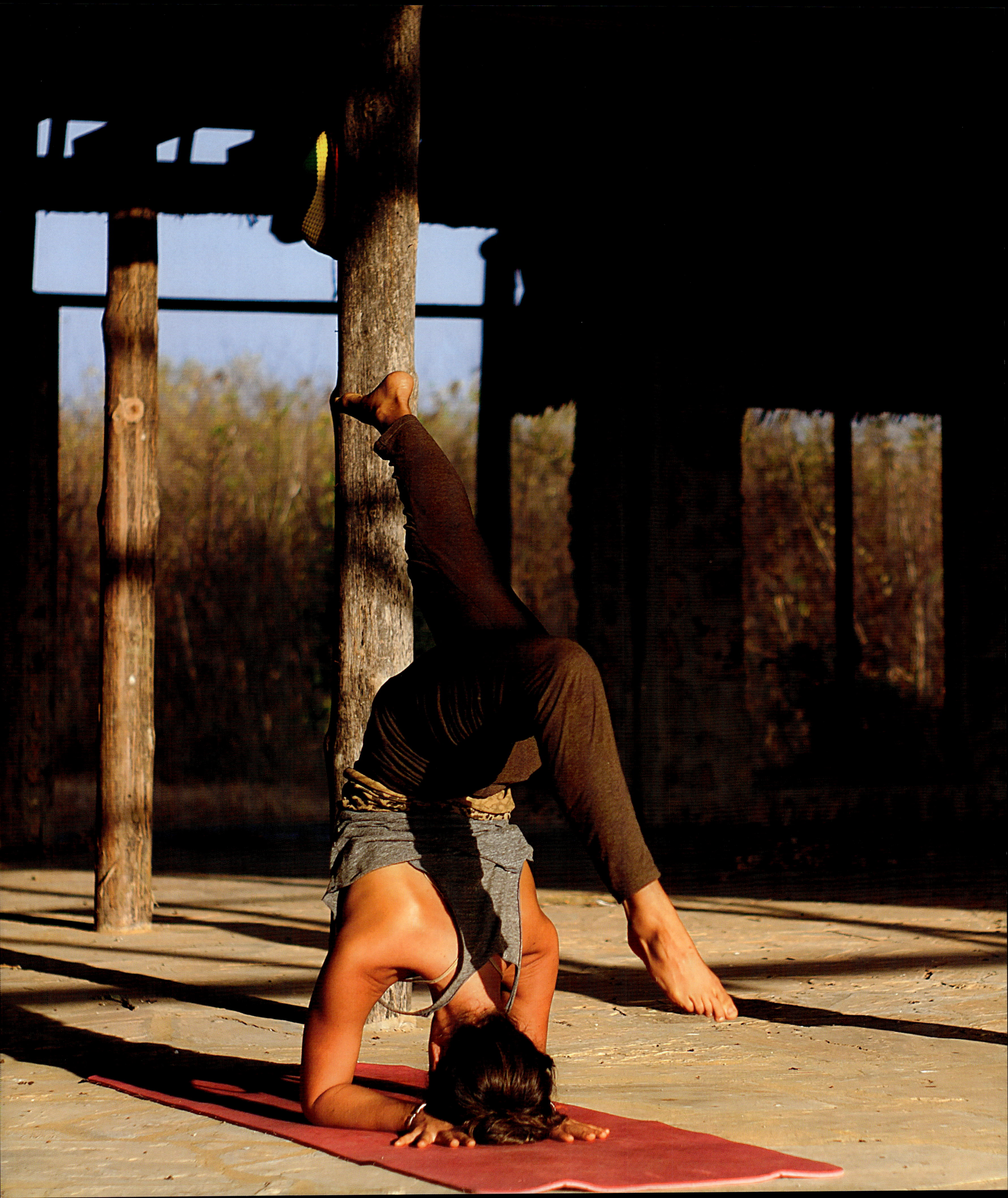

Be motivated by
igniting thought
into action.

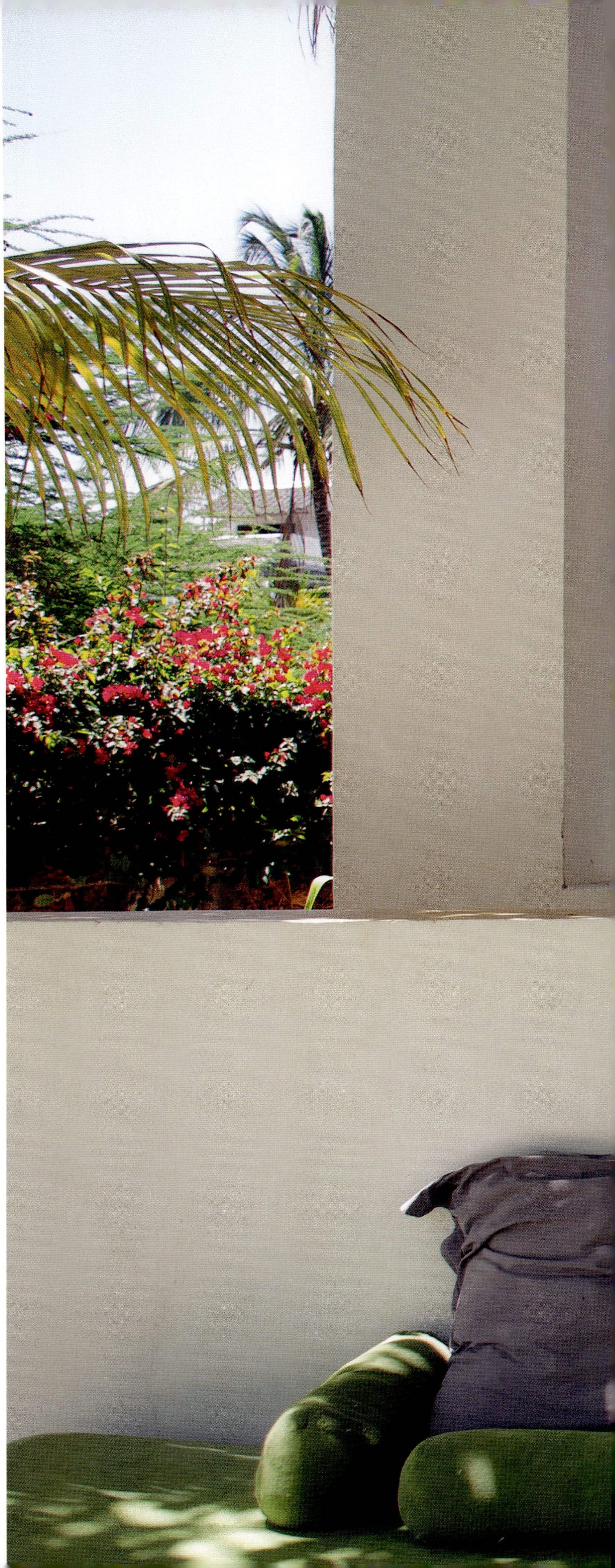

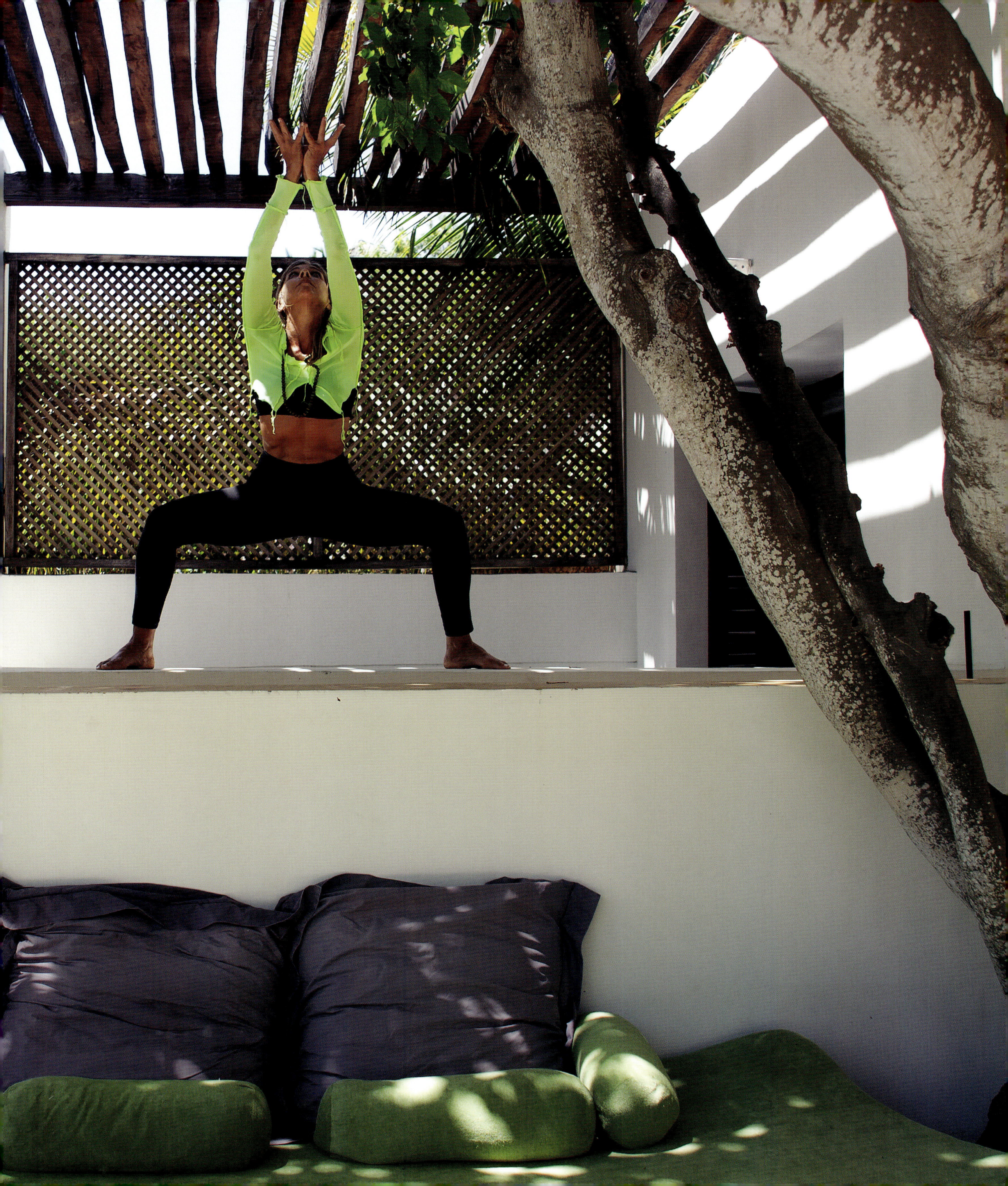

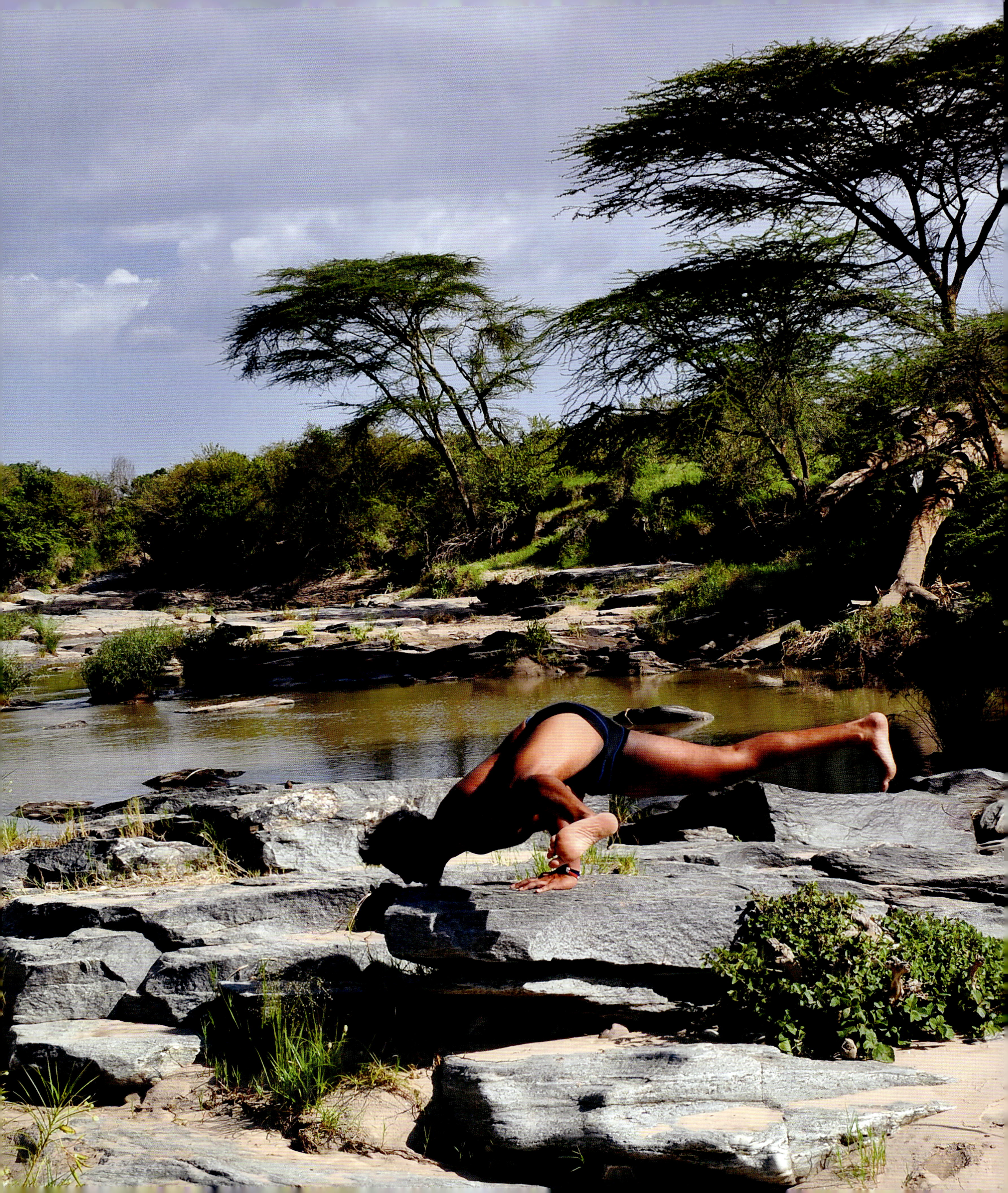

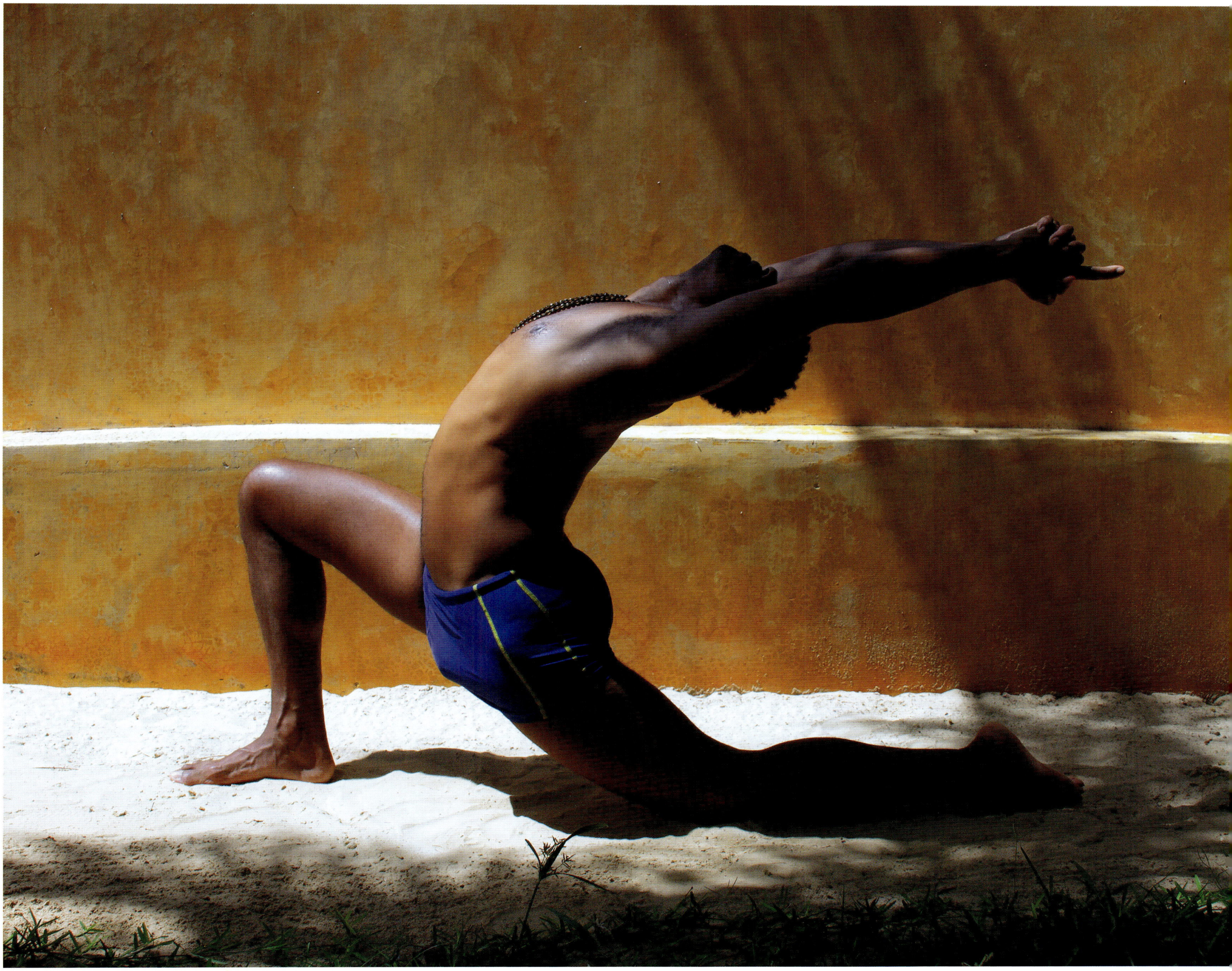

EKA PADA CHAUDA KOUNDINYASANA • Wide Flying Splits

▲ SAMDHI ANJANEYASANA • Horizon Crescent Lunge

Keep beginning, re-creating every day,

and the rest will fall into place.

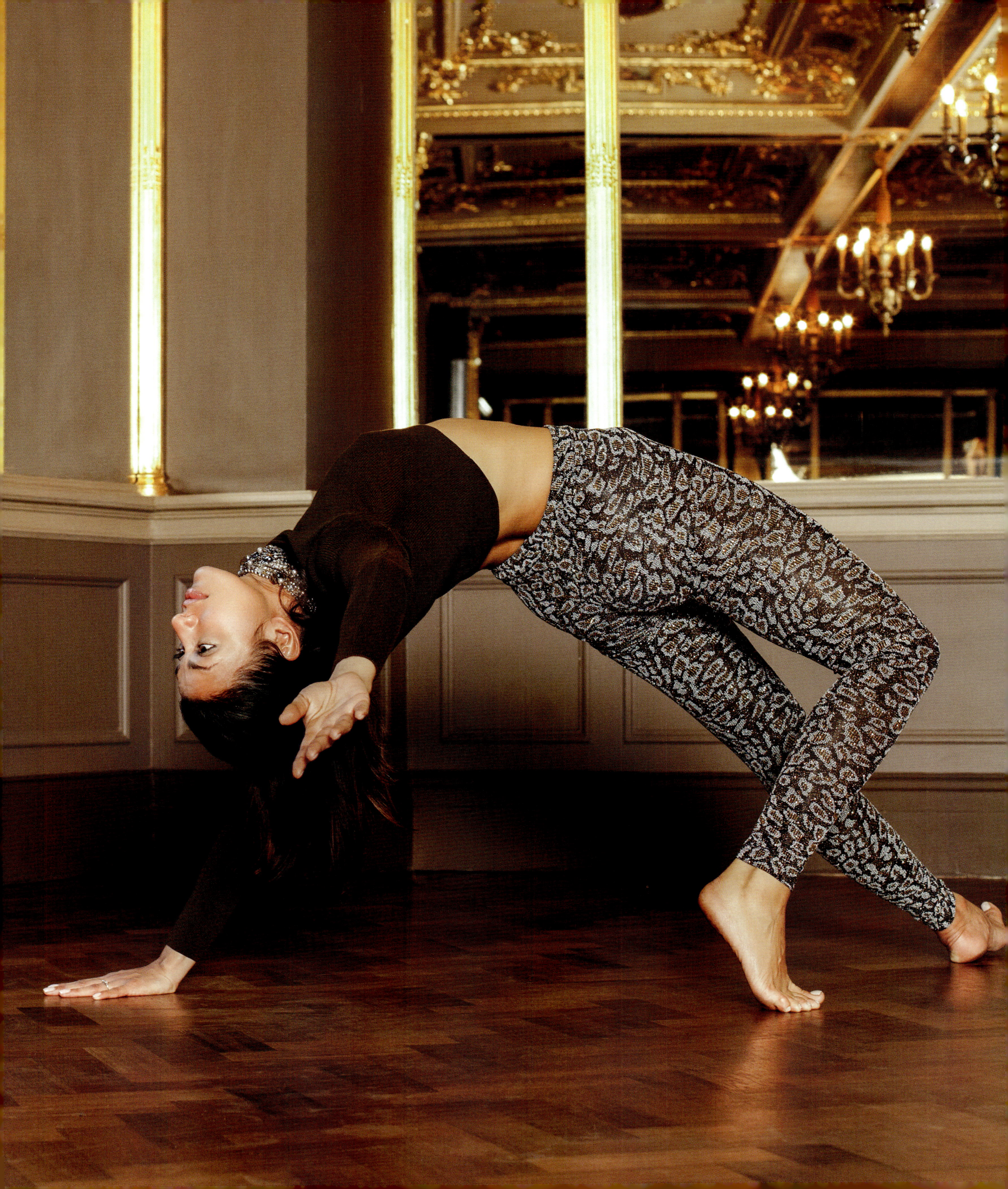

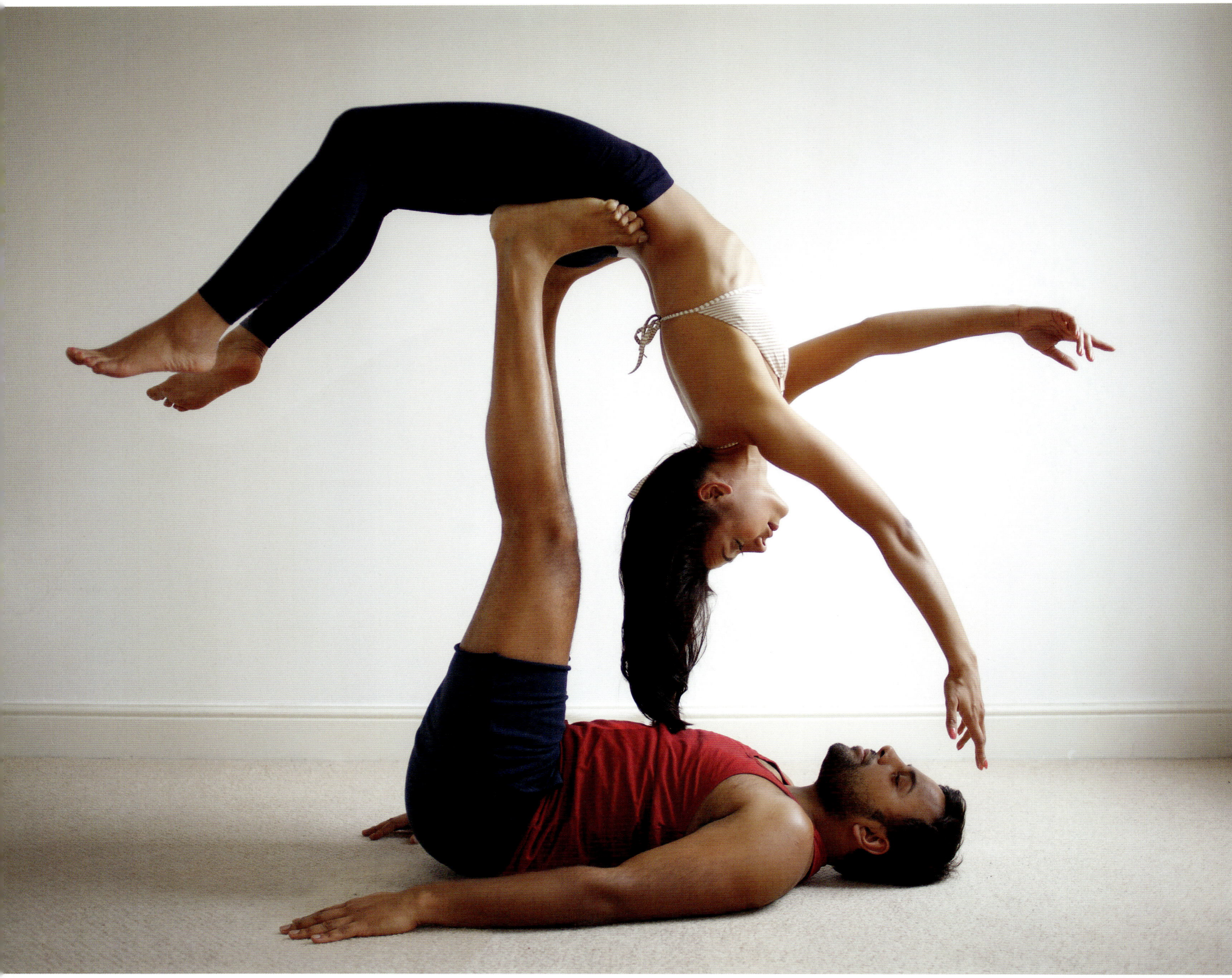

▲ **CHAKRAVHELASANA** · Whale Chakra

PARIVRTTA SURYA YANTRASANA · Compass

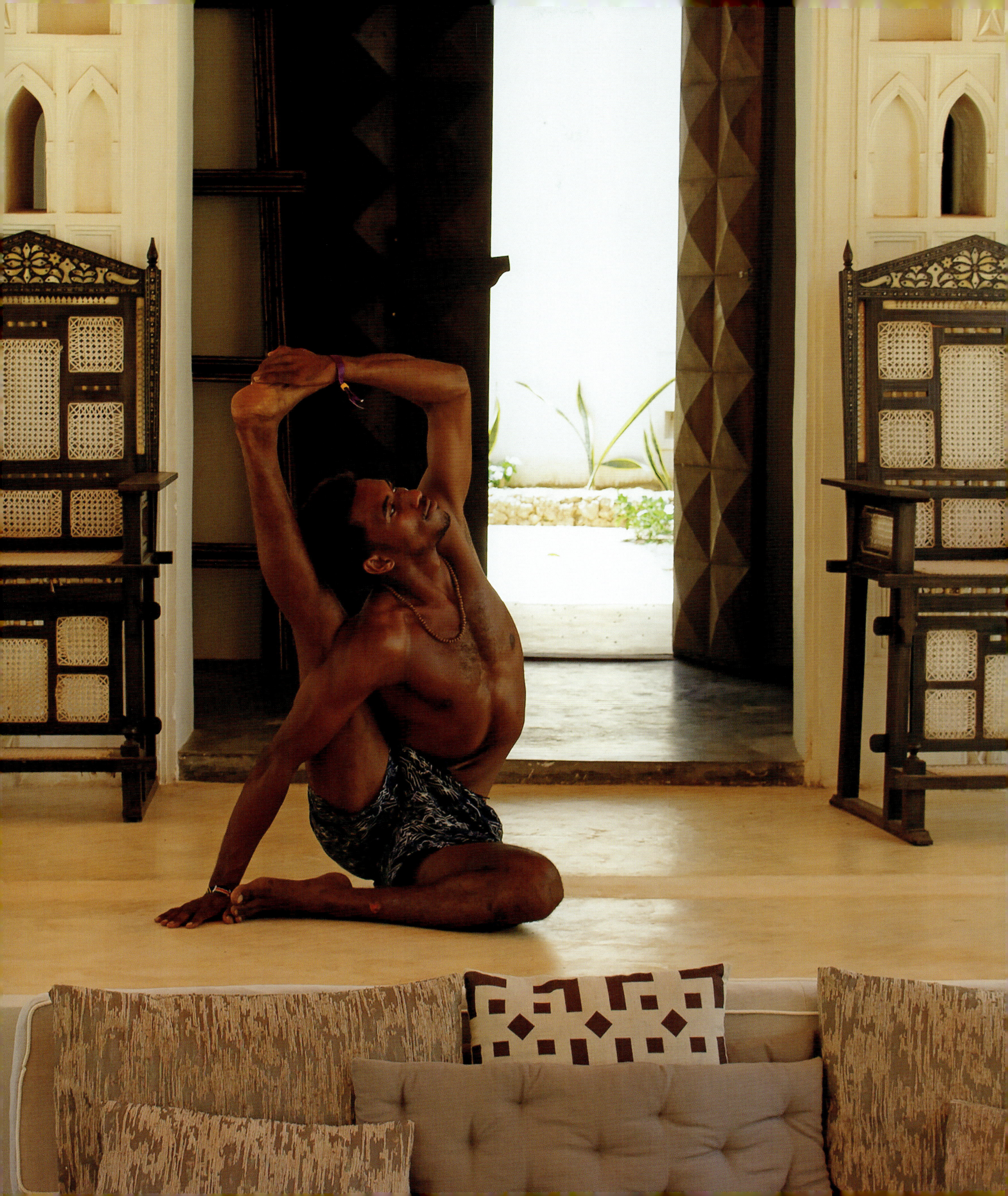

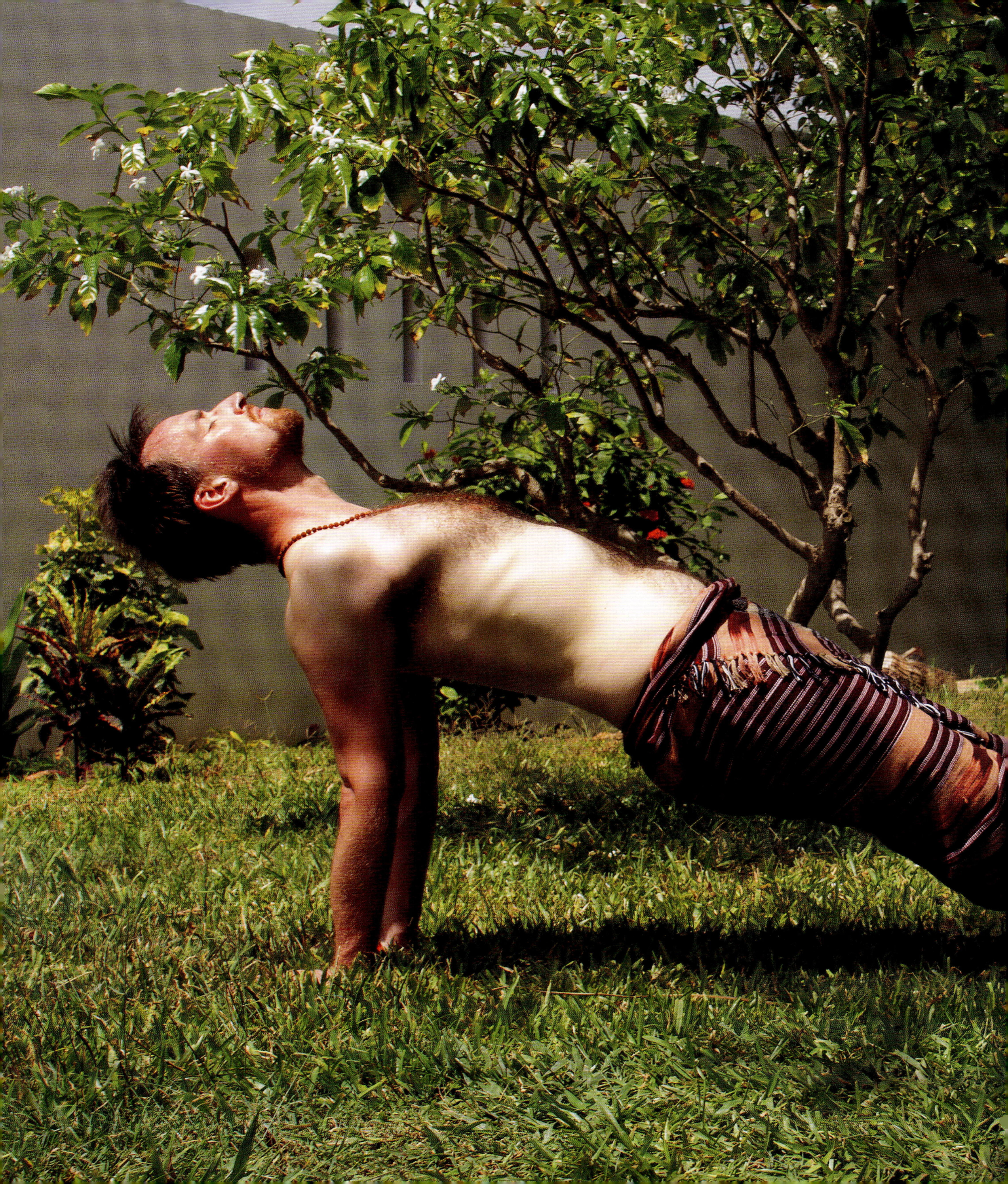

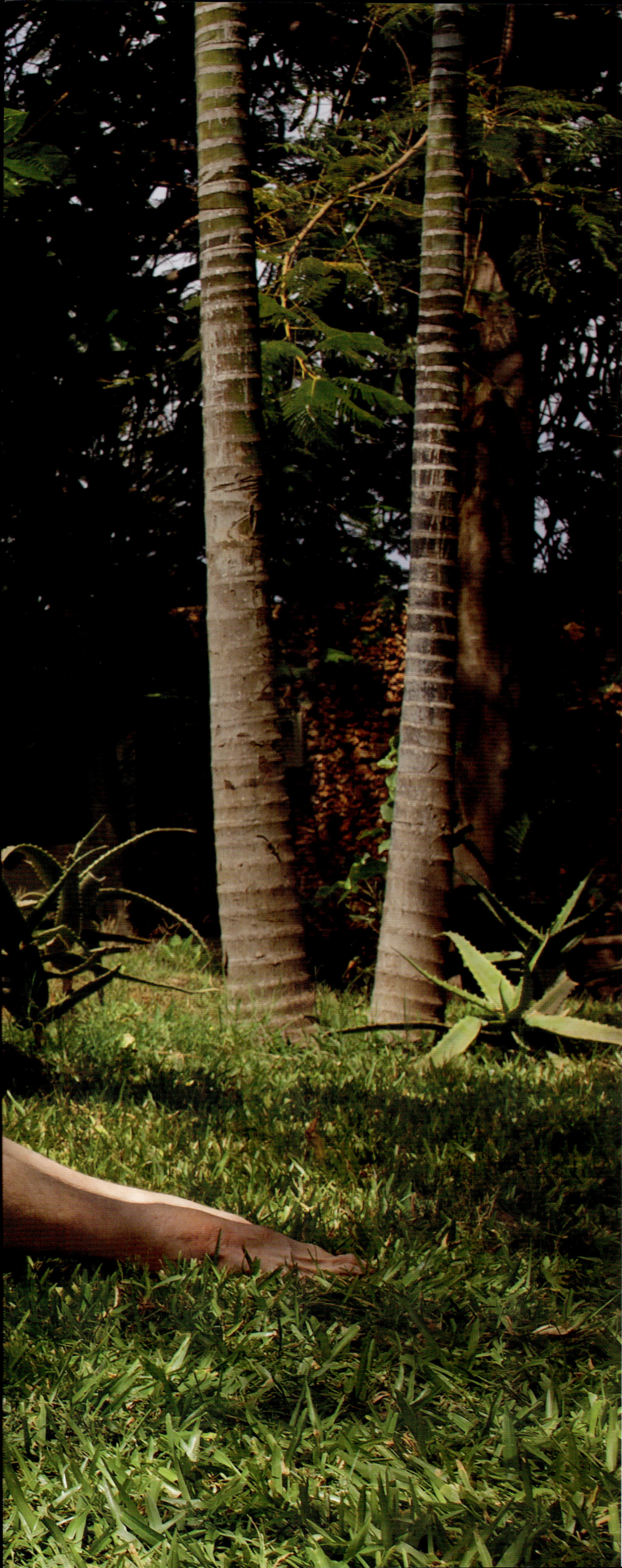

Every inhale
prepares you for
an outward quest,
and every exhale
is a journey
back home.

BRAHMA MESHA · Aries

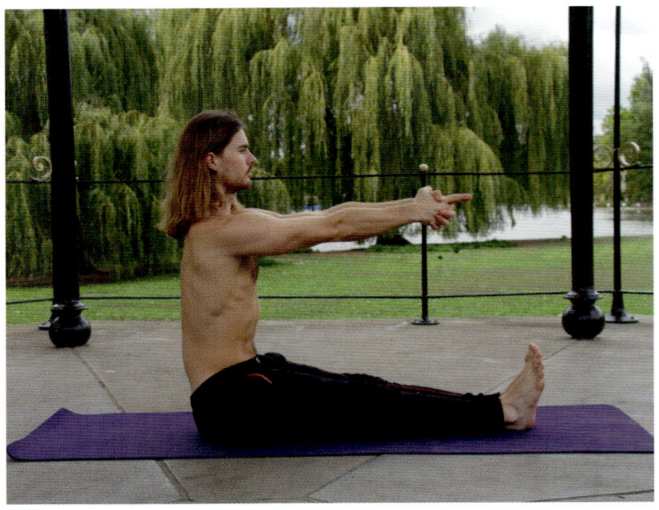

DANDASANA & VAJRAMUDRA
Staff & Indestructibility

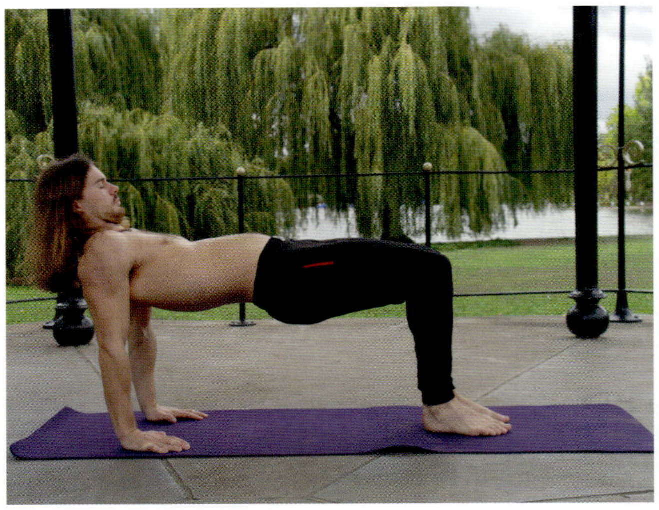

ARDHA PURVOTTANASANA
Half-Inclined Plane

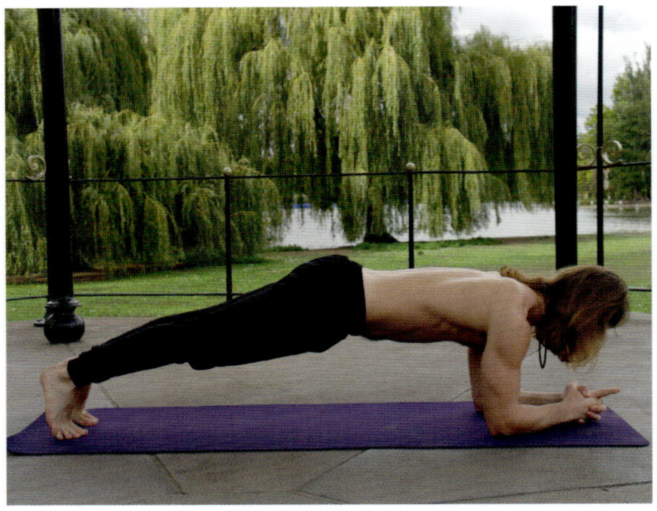

KUMBHAKASANA
Plank

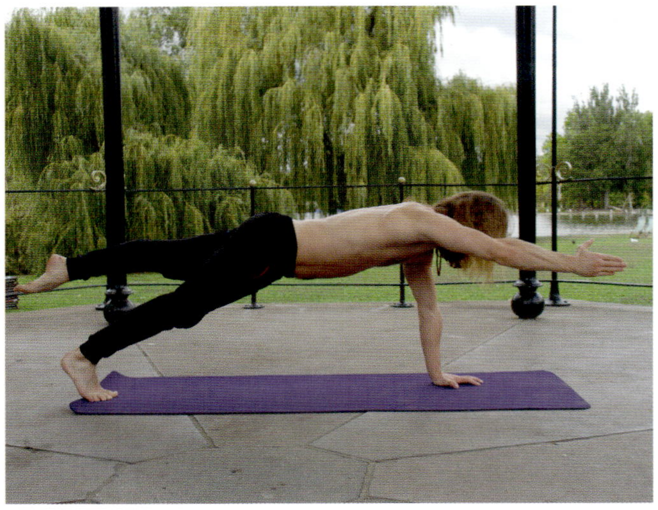

UTTHAN KUMBHAKASANA
Flying Plank

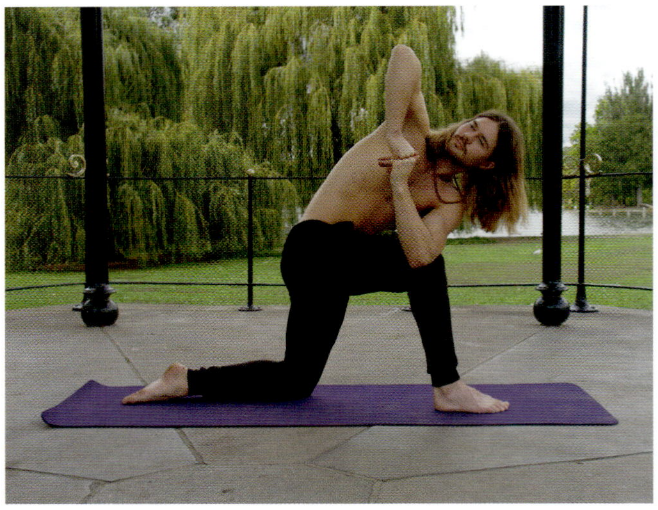

PARIVRTTA ANJANEYASANA & ADHOMUKHAMUDRA
Twisted Crescent Lunge & Preparation

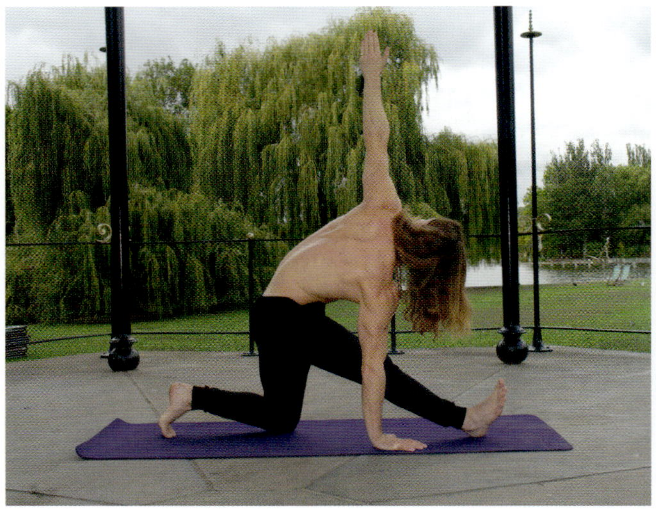

PARIVRTTA UTTANASANA
Twisted Forward Fold

In Brahma Mesha, we are initiating the season of elemental fire. This constellation of asanas, such as inversions, leads us to playfully explore exciting new edges of personal discovery. The balance poses build more focus in our practice, helping us develop confidence and one-pointedness. The held postures stoke our inner heat, galvanizing our interest while building our strength. The mudras release a passionate experience that involves indestructibility of our stamina, preparation to work within the field of gravity in new ways, perspective of a progressive mindset, integration of applied anatomical knowledge, stability in our body formations, and wildness of spirit.

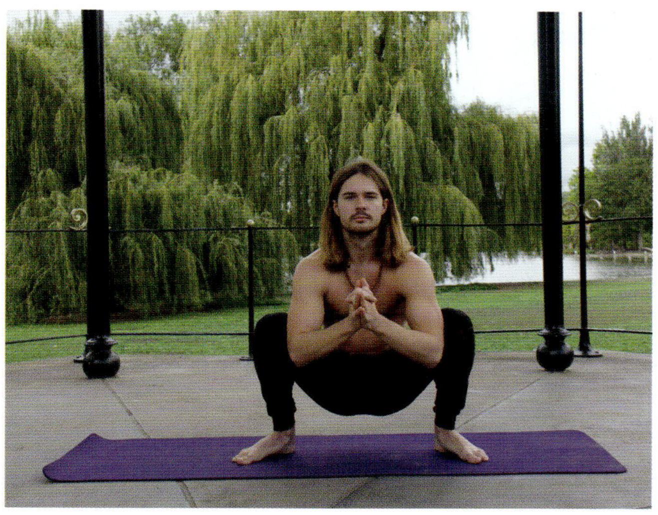

MALASANA & ASHVARATNAMUDRA
Garland Squat & Perspective

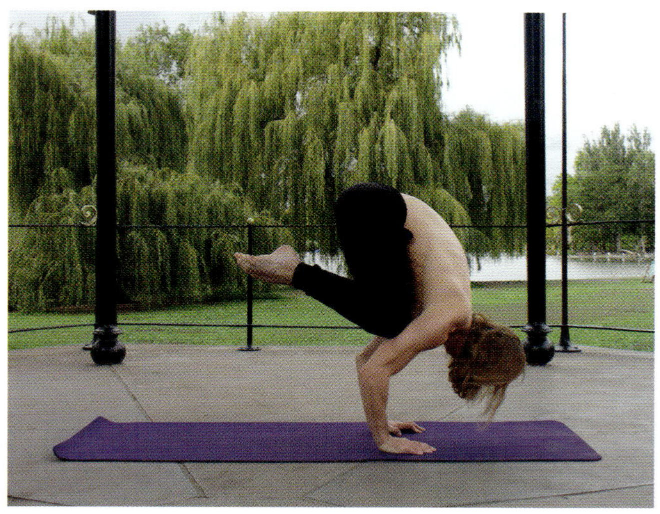

BAKASANA
Crow

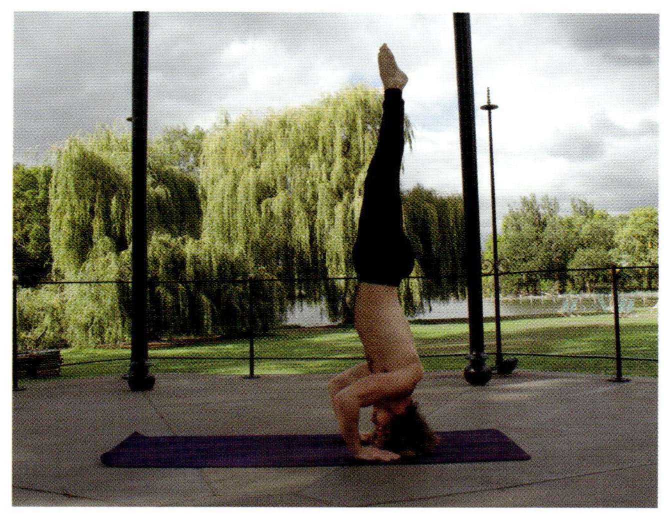

TRIKONASIRSASANA
Three-Pointed Headstand

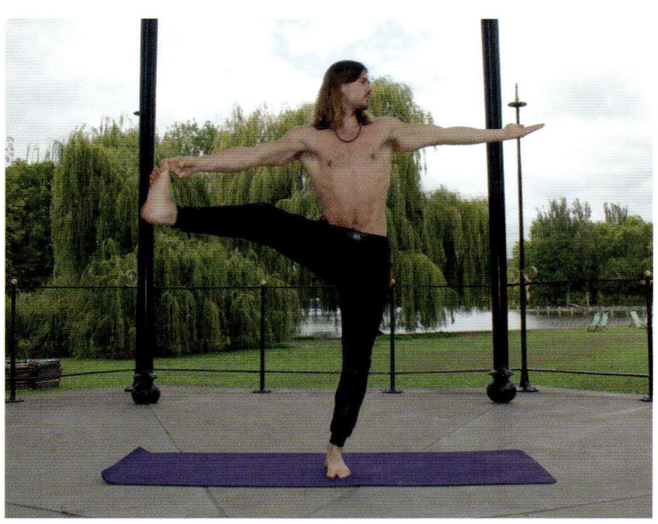

UTTHITA HASTA PADANGUSTHASANA
Extended Hand-to-Toe

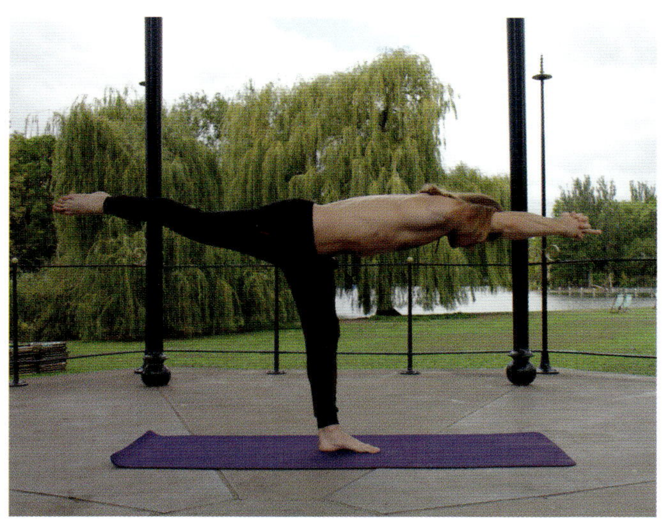

VIRABHADRASANA TRINI & GADAMUDRA
Warrior III & Stability

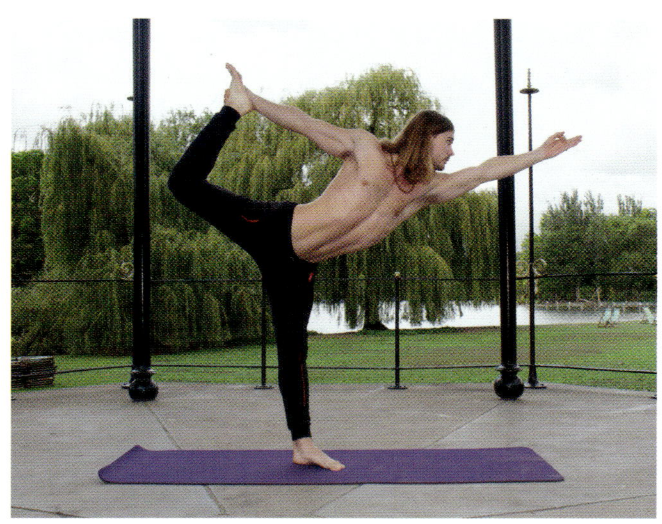

NATARAJASANA
Dancer

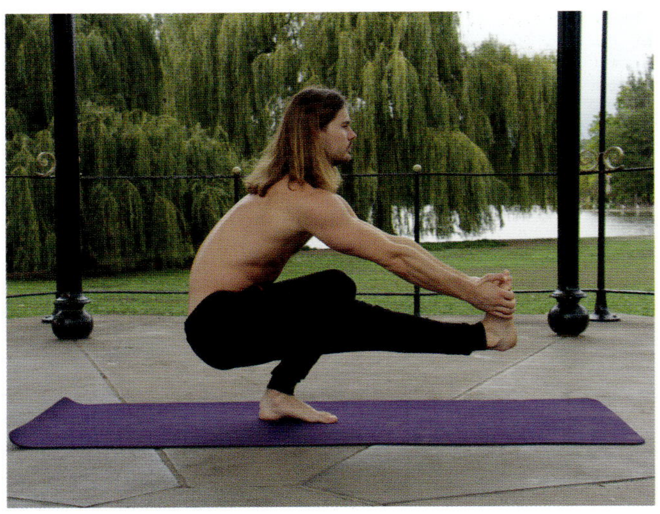

UTTHITA PADA MALASANA
Foot-to-Heel Squat

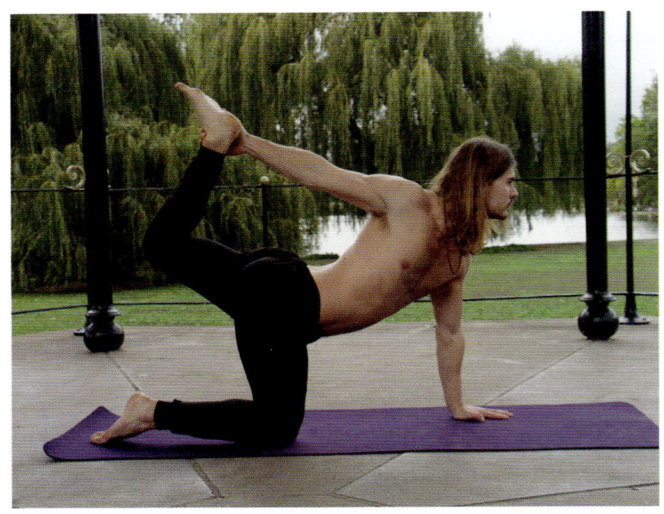

PARIVRTTA BHARMANASANA
Twisted Tabletop

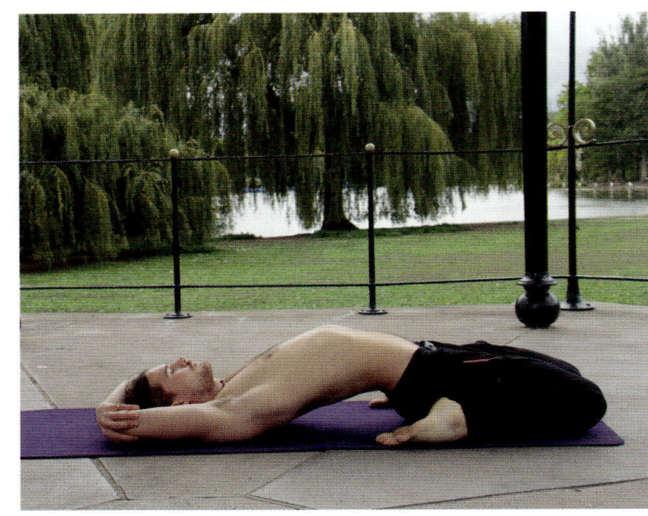

SUPTA VAJRASANA
Reclined Thunderbolt

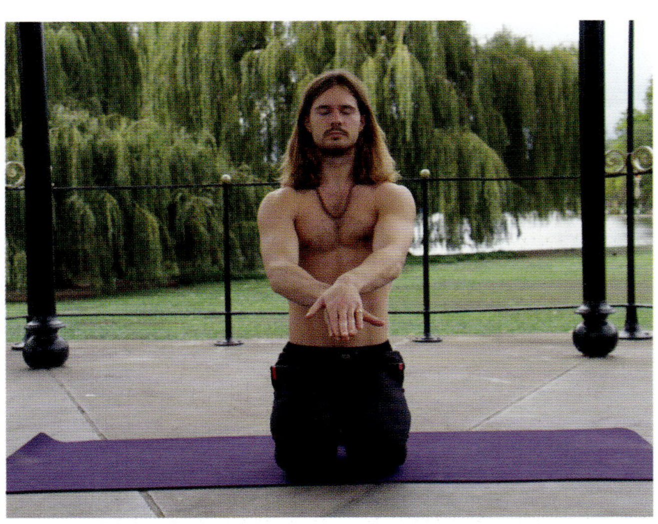

PRAPADASANA & MATSYAMUDRA
Toe Balance & Integration

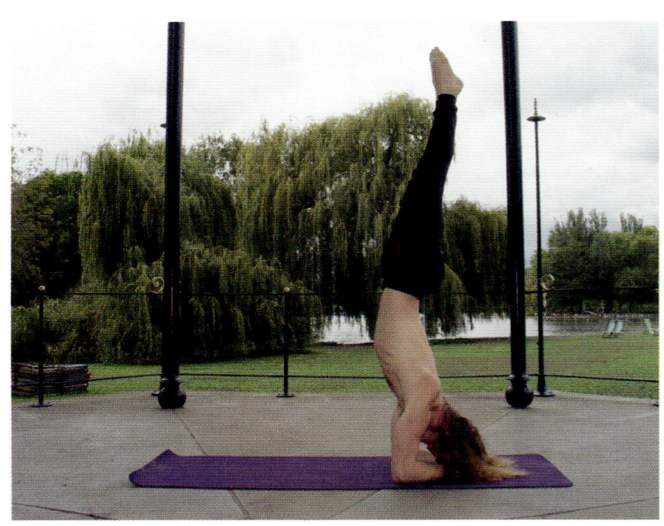

PINCHA MAYURASANA
Feathered Peacock

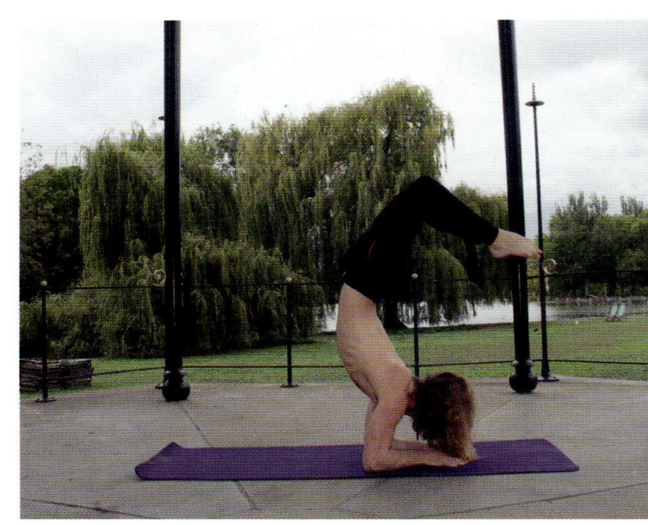

VRISCHIKASANA
Scorpion

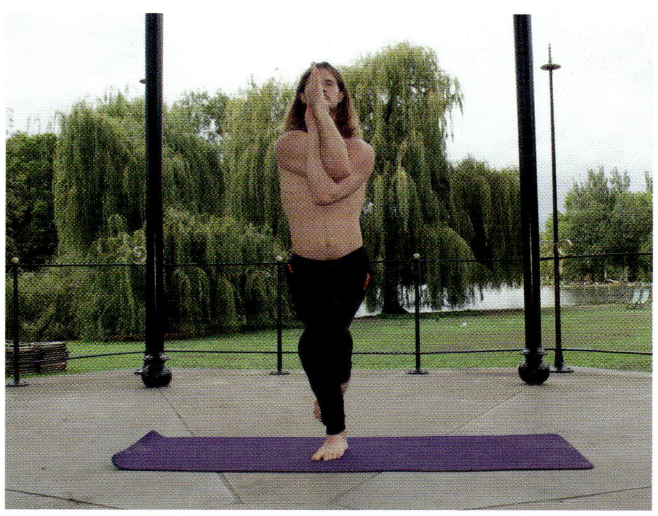

GARUDASANA
Eagle

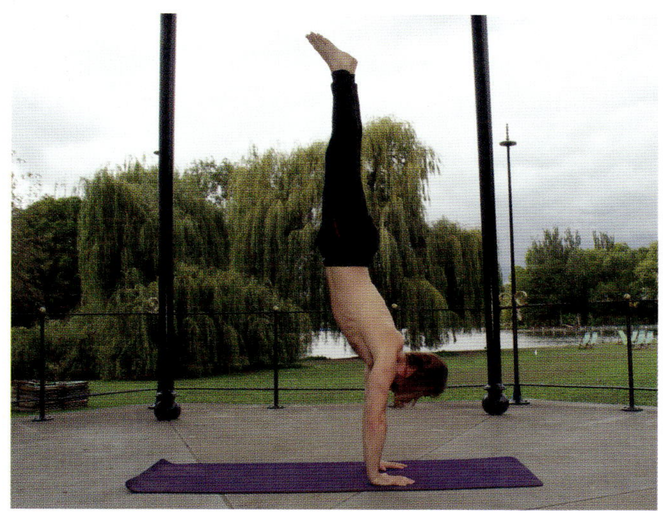

ADHO MUKHA VRKSASANA
Downward-Facing Tree

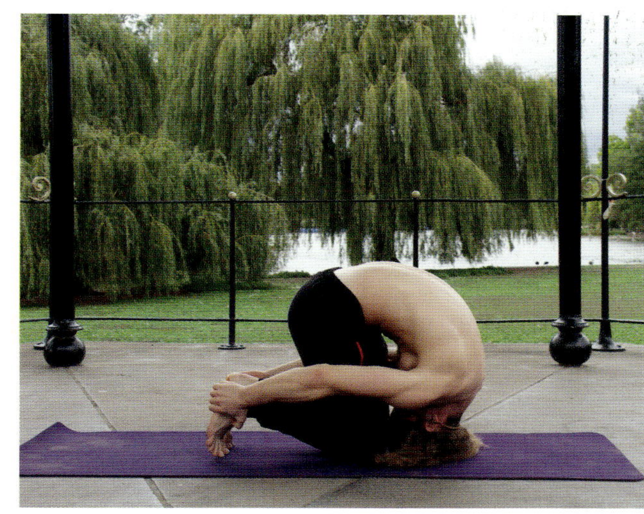

SASANGASANA
Rabbit

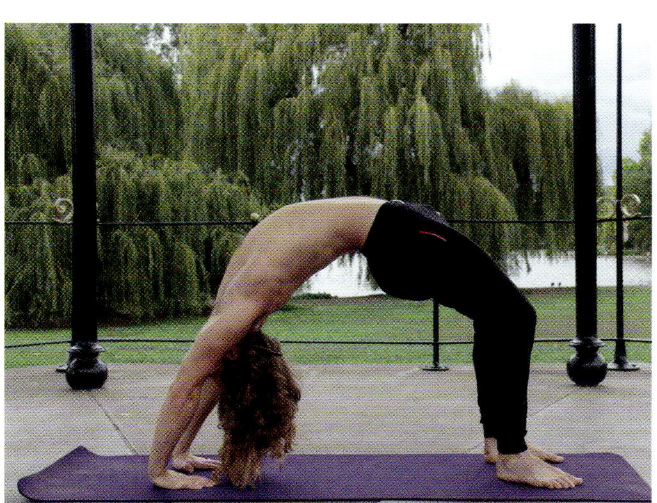

CHAKRASANA
Wheel

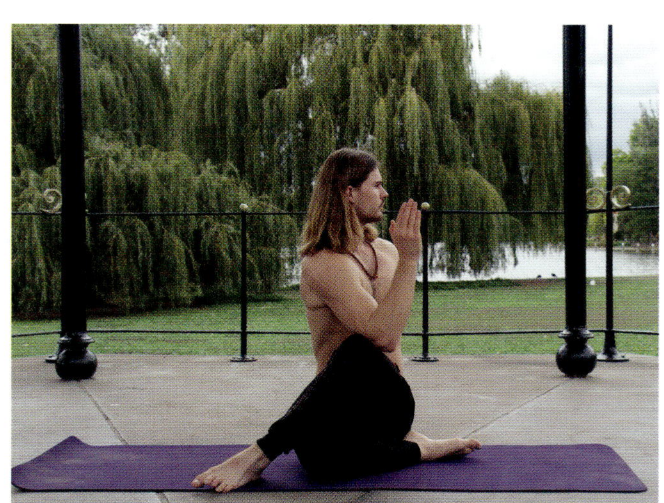

ARDHA MATSYENDRASANA
Half Lord of the Fish

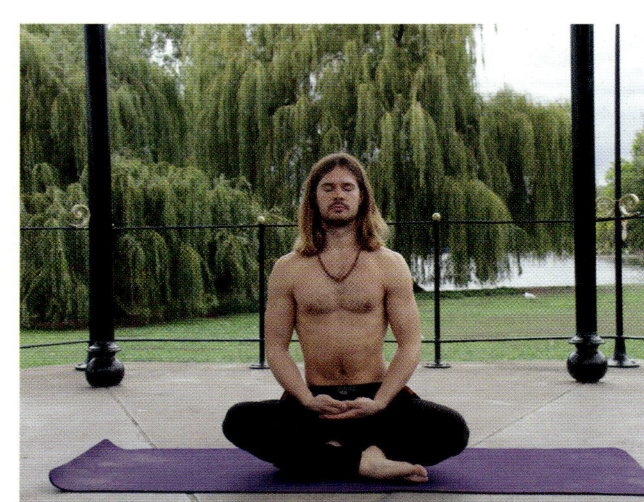

SIDDHASANA & BHAIRAVAMUDRA
Seated Accomplished & Wildness

BRAHMA VRISHABHA · Taurus

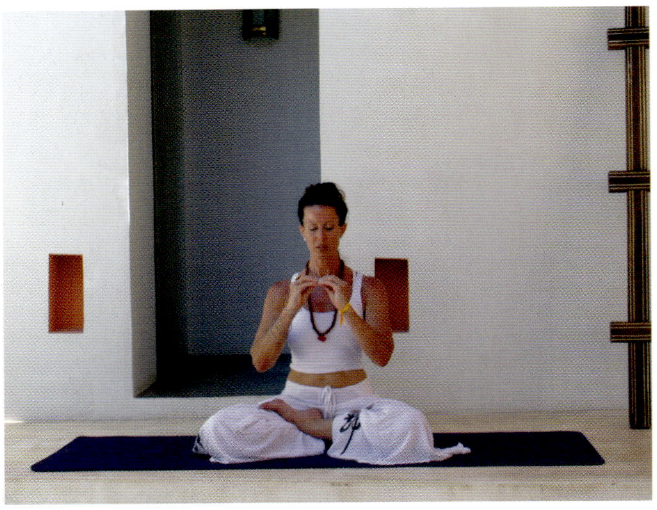

ARDHA PADMASANA & SUMUKHAMUDRA
Half Lotus & Coordination

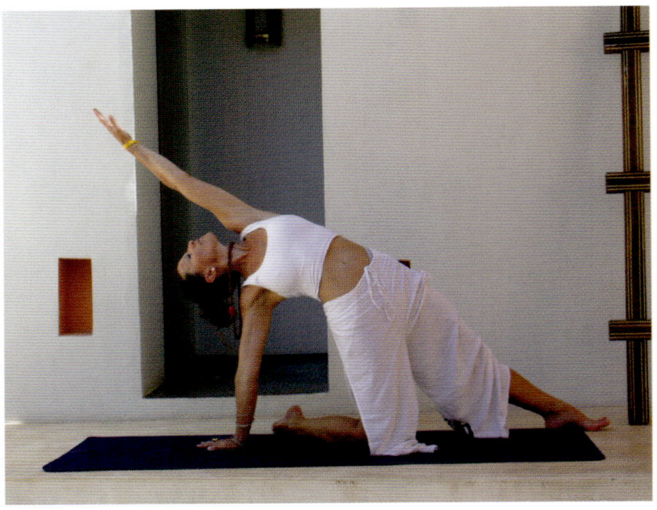

CAMATKARASANA
Enraptured Heart

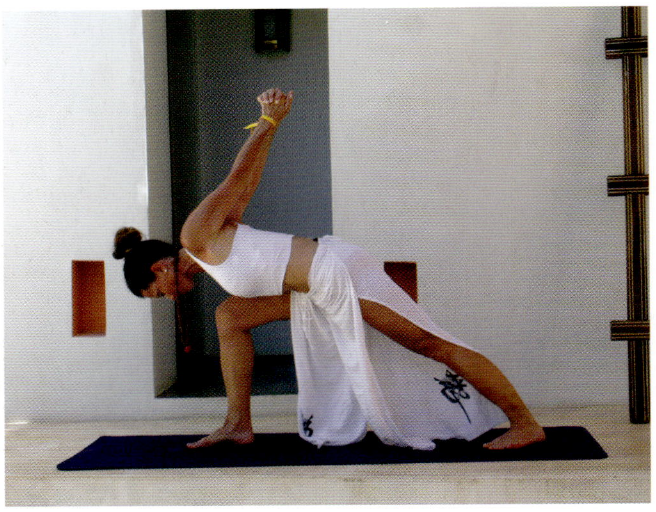

BADDHA VIRABHADRASANA
Humble Warrior

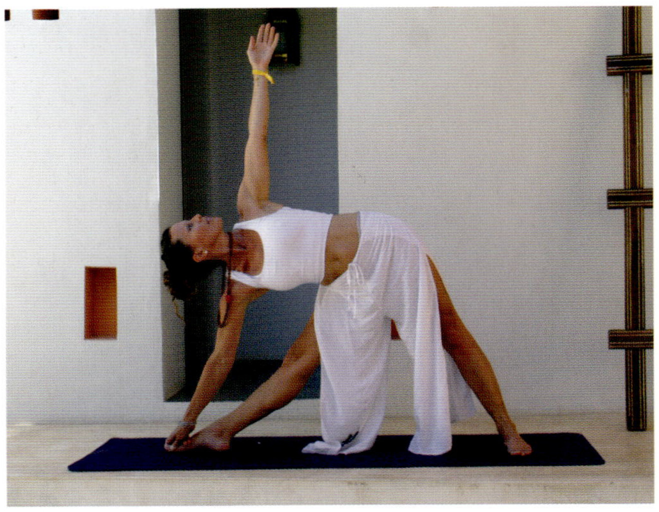

PADA TRIKONASANA
Toehold Triangle

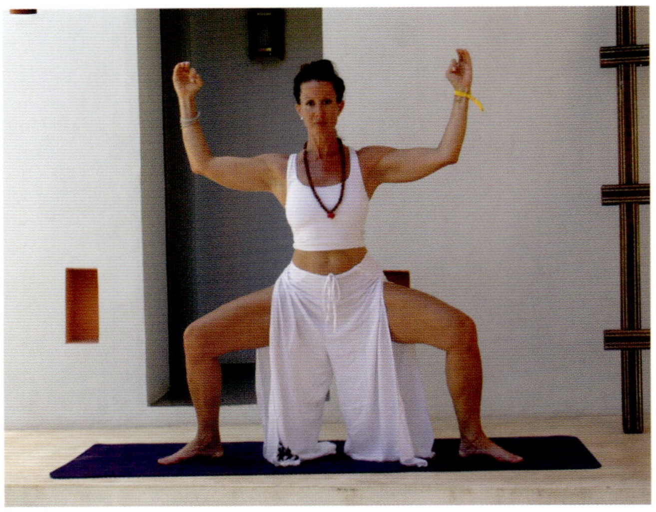

UTKATA KONASANA & KAMAJAYIMUDRA
Goddess & Restraint

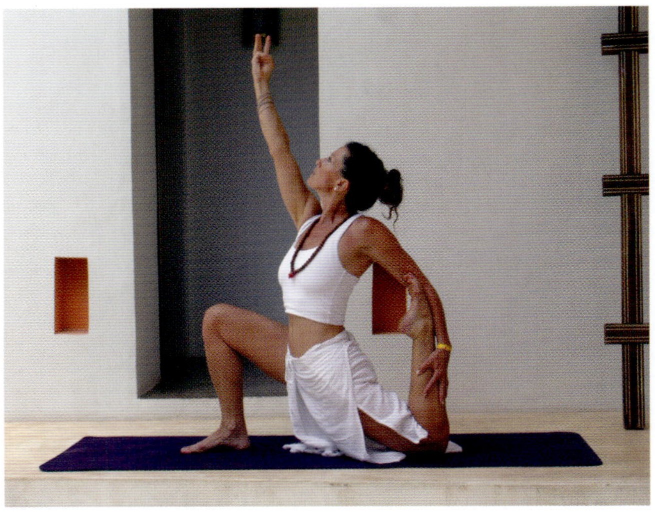

BADDHA ANJANEYASANA & TRISHULAMUDRA
Bound Crescent Low Lunge & Dissolving

In Brahma Vrishabha, we are in the settled season of elemental earth. This constellation of beautiful upright, seated, and standing asanas nurtures a sustainable practice. By finding pleasure through movement as in dance, we are able to sustain our practice into varied shapes mirroring the beauty of the natural world. The mudras bring a sensory approach to the coordination of asymmetrical movement, restraint of past limitations, dissolving disconnecting boundaries, and offering a fresh and soaring sense of freedom. This solidifies loyalty through self-care and consolidation of the present moment by keeping us more in the body and less in the mind.

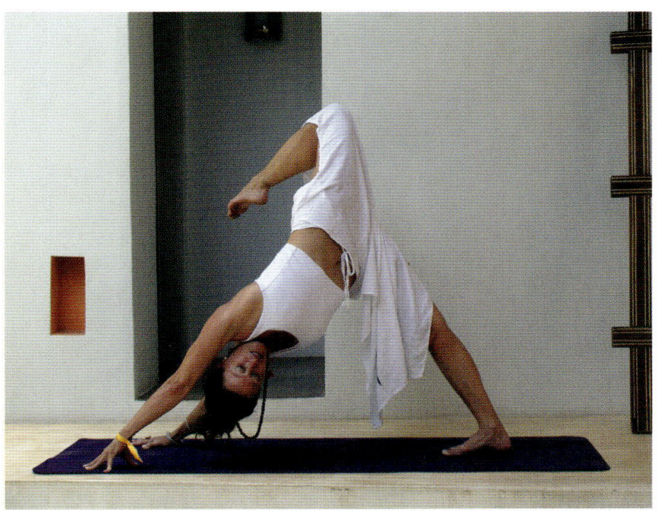

TRI PADA ADHO MUKHA SVANASANA
Three-Legged Downward-Facing Dog

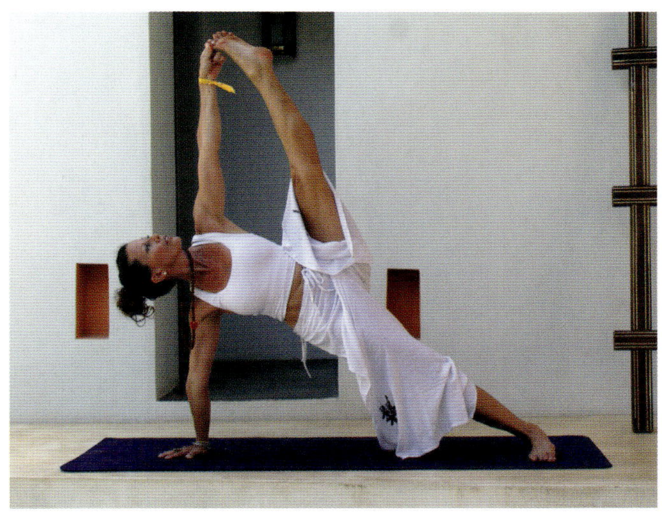

VASISTHASANA PADANGUSTHASANA
Side Plank Toehold

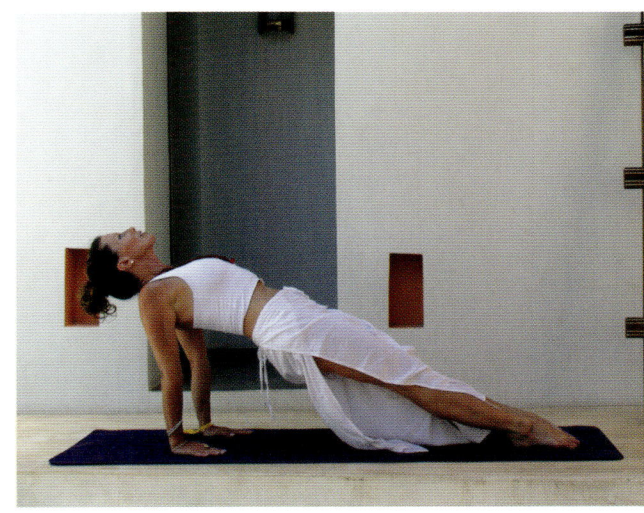

PURVOTTANASANA
Upward Plank

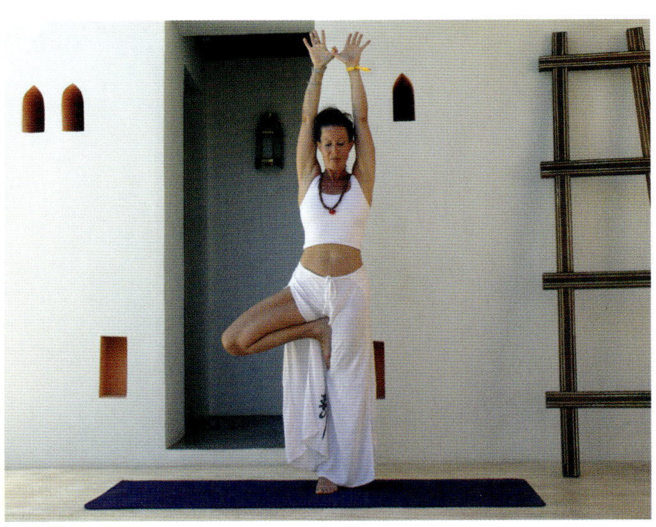

VRKSASANA & GARUDAMUDRA
Tree & Soaring

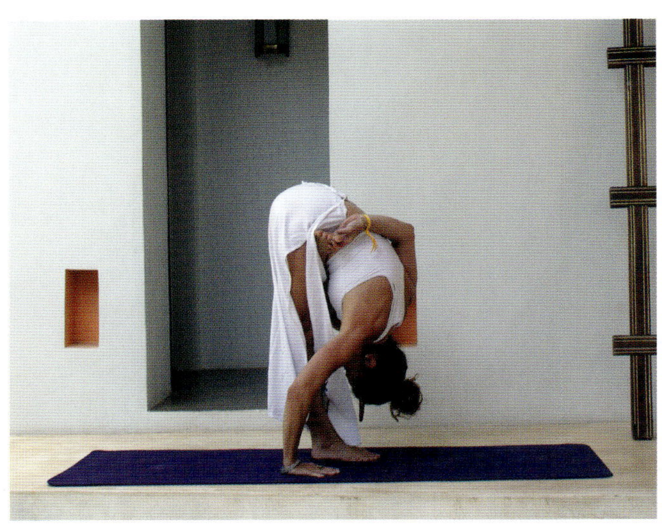

ARDHA BADDHA PADMOTTANASANA
Half Lotus Tree

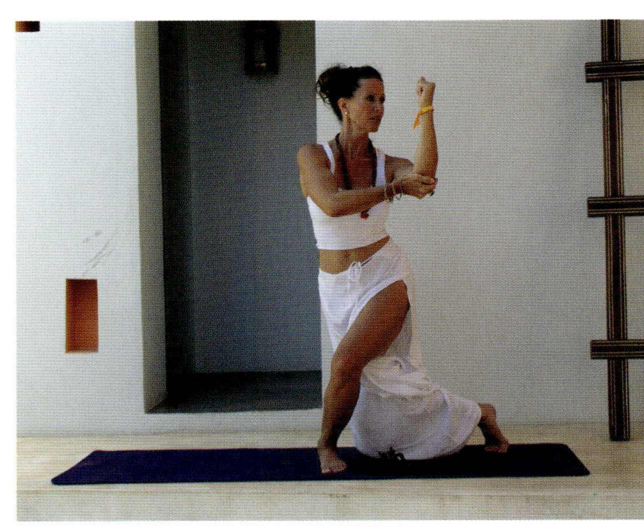

PARSVA BHANGASANA & MUDGARAMUDRA
Palm Tree & Loyalty

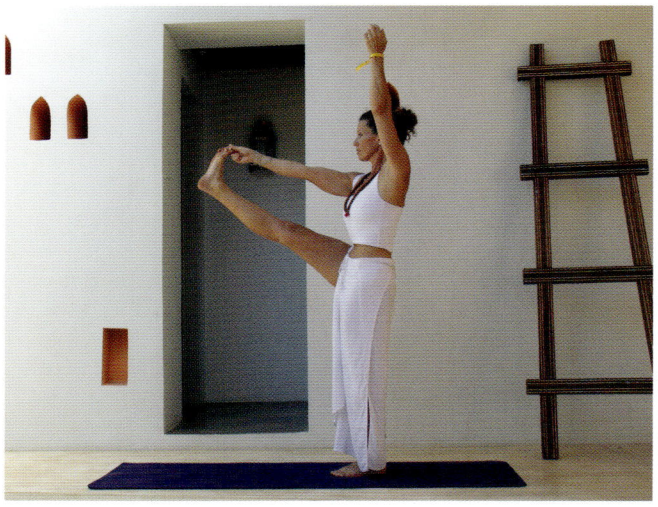

UTTHITA HASTA PADANGUSTHASANA
Extended Hand-to-Toe

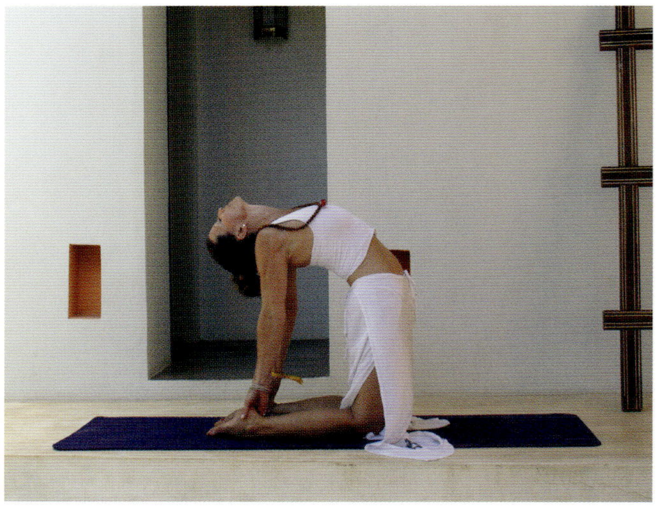

USTRASANA
Camel

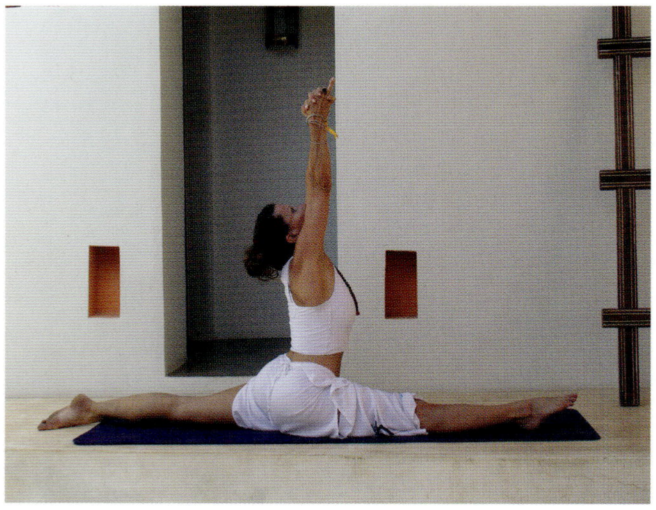

HANUMANASANA & CHAKRAMUDRA
Splits & Consolidation

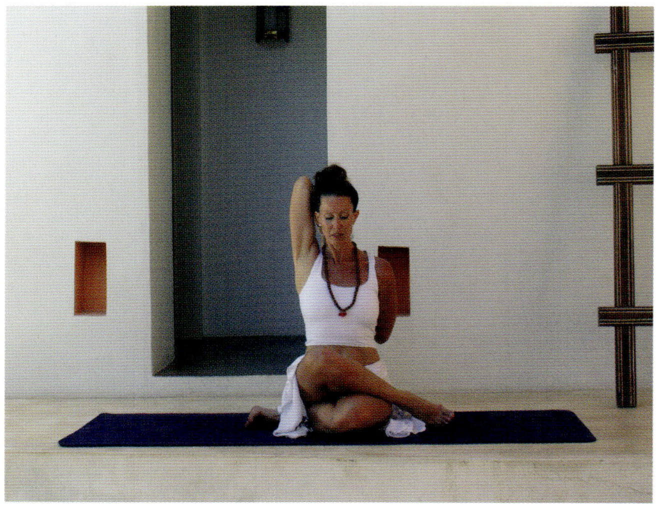

BADDHA GOMUKHASANA
Bound Cow Face

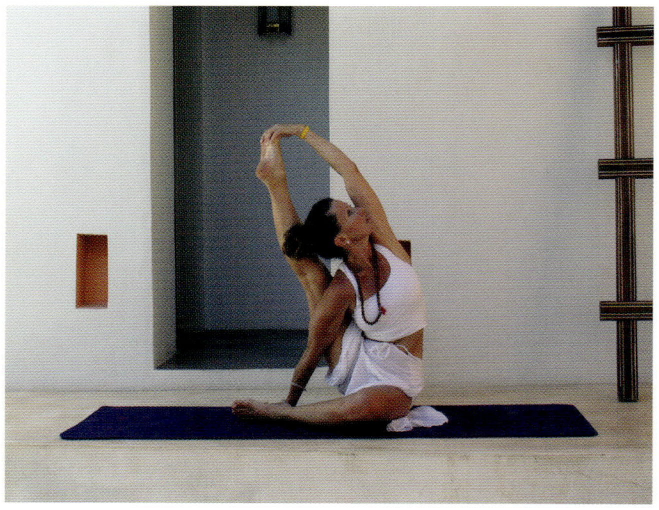

PARIVRTTA SURYA YANTRASANA
Compass

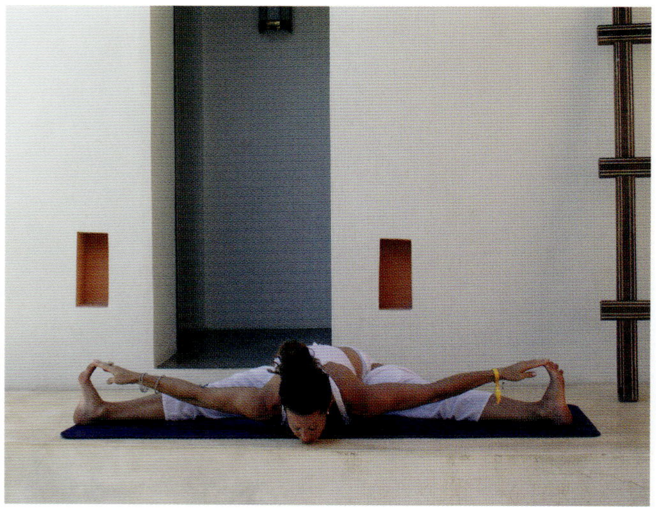

UTTANA SAMAKONASANA
Forward-Folding Straddle Splits

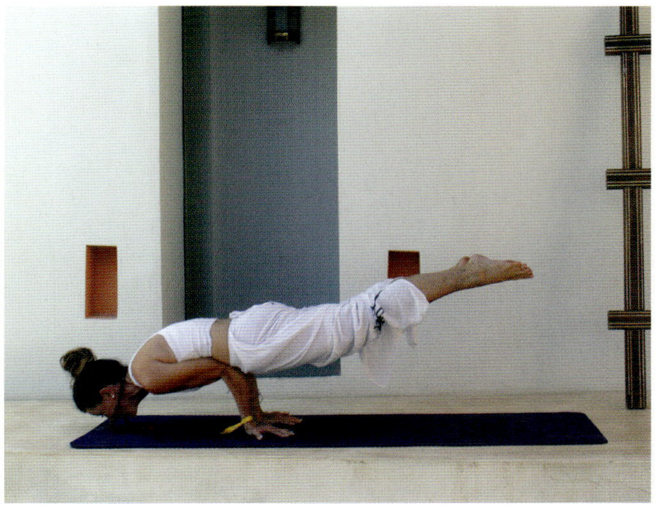

MAYURASANA
Peacock

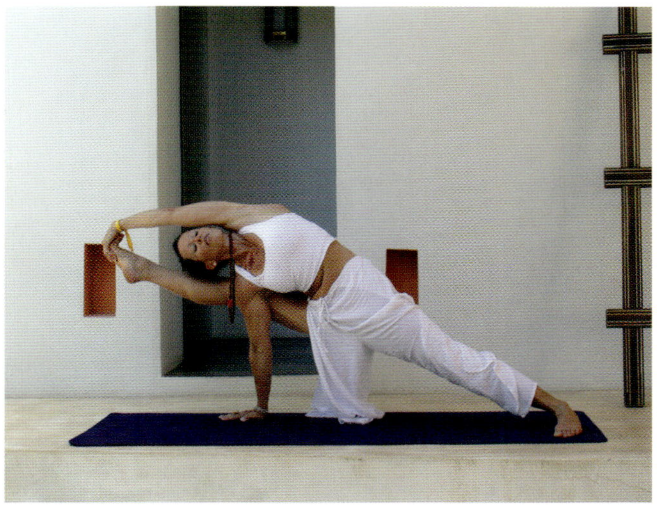

VISVAMITRASANA
Twisted Arm Balance

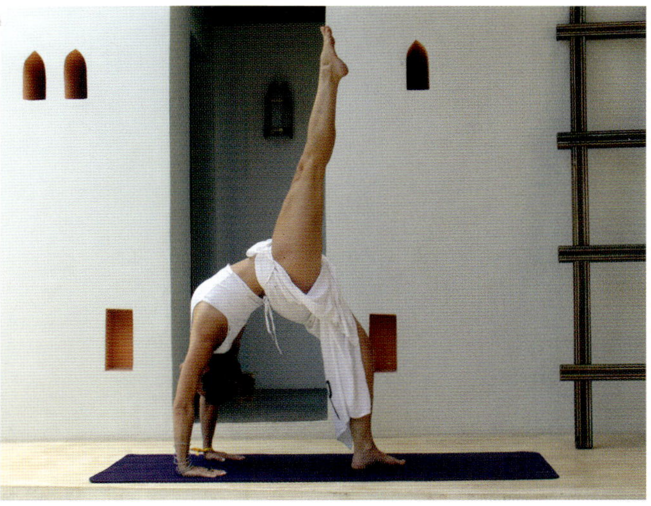

EKA PADA URDHVA DHANURASANA
One-Legged Wheel

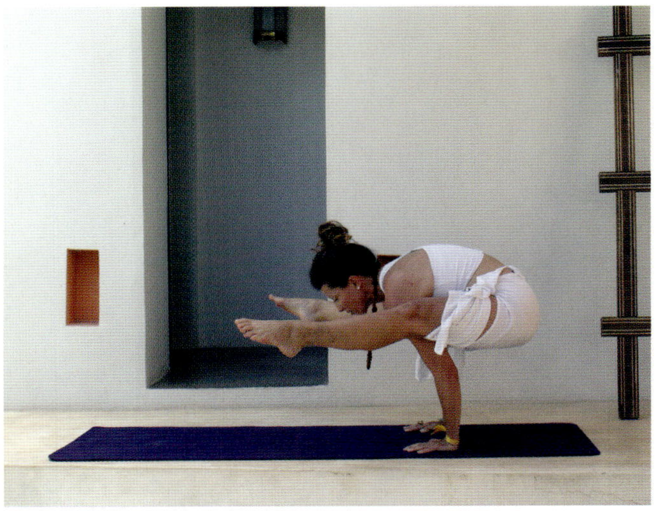

TITIBASANA
Firefly

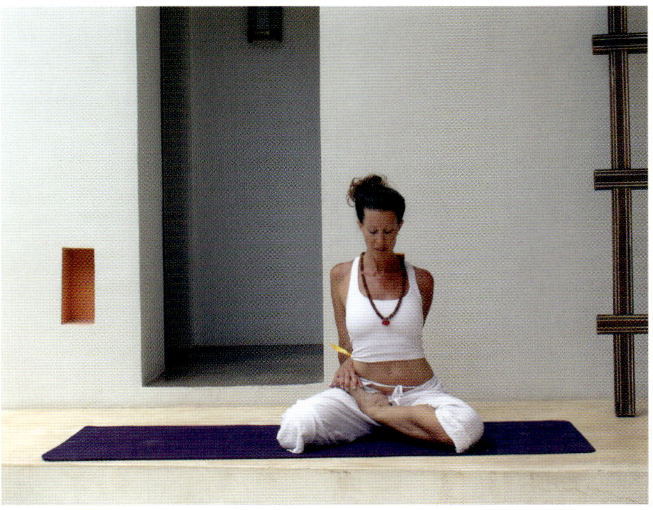

ARDHA BADDHA PADMASANA
Half-Bound Lotus

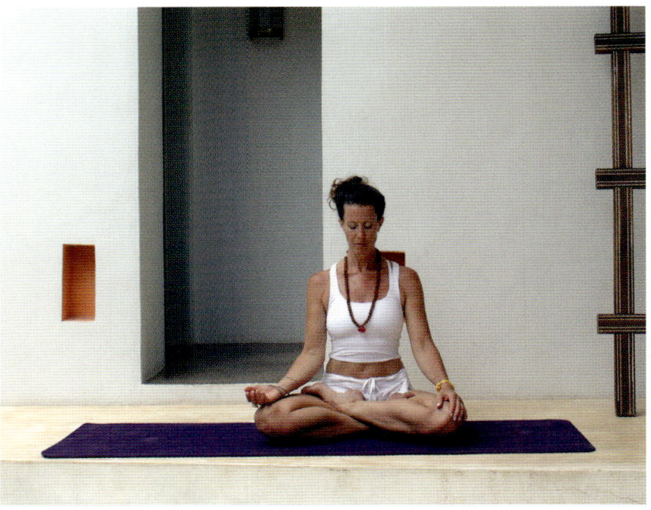

PADMASANA
Lotus

REST & REJUVENATE

In Brahma Mithuna / Gemini, we are in the shifting season of elemental air, so we are focusing on using the mind in a guided way to settle into deeper states of relaxation. In Brahma Karkata / Cancer, we are initiating the season of elemental water, which corresponds with the volume of liquid moving through the labyrinths of our body. As infants, we were around 80 percent water, but as adults that number reduces down to around 60 percent. The Brahma Yoga asanas in this chapter act as an aqueduct in this process to reflectively bring stillness to the body. We aim to be childlike in our practice so we can receive and restore any imbalances from living and live in the purity of our presence.

By taking a restorative approach through Brahma Yoga, we can experience profound relaxation and restoration of both the mind and body. In the various supine poses, we can begin to release physical and mental tension and rest deeply. By holding the asanas, some for several minutes, we can be passive, allowing the body to loosen and sink into deeper relaxation. This reduces stress levels, improves sleep, reduces turbulent moods and anxiety, and boosts the immune system.

In these gentle postures, we create a perfect atmosphere for well-being. We do so by intentionally moving the body languidly and slowing down the breathing rate to calm the mind. Consciously releasing discomfort in the body leads to a sense of relaxation. Furthermore, the combination of asanas and controlled breathing can help reduce stress and anxiety, resulting in a more relaxed state of mind for meditation. It is in this meditation, through gentle somatic movement, that we can receive the benefit of feeling physically and mentally relaxed, rested, and rejuvenated. For example, child's pose helps stretch the hips, thighs, and ankles while calming the mind. The asanas where we lift the legs help improve circulation. Rest poses, such as savasana, let us release physical tension and relinquish incessant thinking, which help bring deep calmness. The seated forward folds help stretch the back, legs, and hips while also calming the body.

There are also plenty of supine yoga poses, which reduce pressure on the spine. When lying on your back, the spine is supported and relieved of any weight while reducing strain in the muscles and tissues. The emphasis is to minimize tension in the neck, back, and hips. This has a calming effect on the nervous system. It gently activates the parasympathetic response, which slows down the heart rate, decreases blood pressure, and aids rest and recovery. The asanas we do in this chapter diffuse the sympathetic response, which activates during times of stress, prepares the body for action, and keeps you unnecessarily alert.

Compared to some of the more movement-based practices offered throughout this book, by being more still here, we can become the great observer, mindfully acting as the guardians of our cells. Our cells rejuvenate through a self-cleansing process called autophagy, where we clear out metabolic waste and damaged components to maintain the cells' overall health. Practicing Brahma Yoga can also help increase self-awareness, inner peace, and acceptance, which improves our moods through observing our processes.

BRAHMA YOGA SUTRAS

BRAHMA MITHUNA • Gemini

- My mind and body are in attunement with Nature, so freedom is available to me in every moment.
- When I experience presence, I live in the space between my thoughts.
- When I have clarity, I can begin again every time.
- Brahma Yoga knows that deep within, I am a conscious being living consciously, and this knowledge brings me absolute assimilation.
- My mind reaches its highest state of serenity when it is withdrawn from all forms of attachment.
- I am a prism through which I see the world. A refracted mind sees a broken world, so I always choose peace.
- When I give away everything I know, I keep receiving from the beyond.
- I observe but do not second-guess others' thoughts.
- When I listen to my intuition, my being can be more spontaneous and natural and effortlessly flow.

BRAHMA KARKATA • Cancer

- I experience rejuvenation when I accept that my home truly resides within me, so every place I visit is an extension of this assurance.
- My crowning thoughts come best when I renounce my limitations, reconcile that everything is impermanent, and find peace within.
- What brings me to you is us, and with that, we can achieve anything together. So in this oneness we have union.
- I am in harmony nestled in Nature. I am protected from anyone or anything trying to control or oppress me, as I can never truly be owned.
- I welcome restoration, as I am more than my history.
- In my tranquility, I know there is no need to take when I can receive.
- Hearts, like atoms, are bonded beyond the restraints of time and space.
- Brahma Yoga prepares me to know that I do not need the validation of others to be complete.
- I am heartfelt, and my emotions are genuine.

The greatest threat is not fear of the
unknown, disapproval, or change.
The greatest threat is indifference.

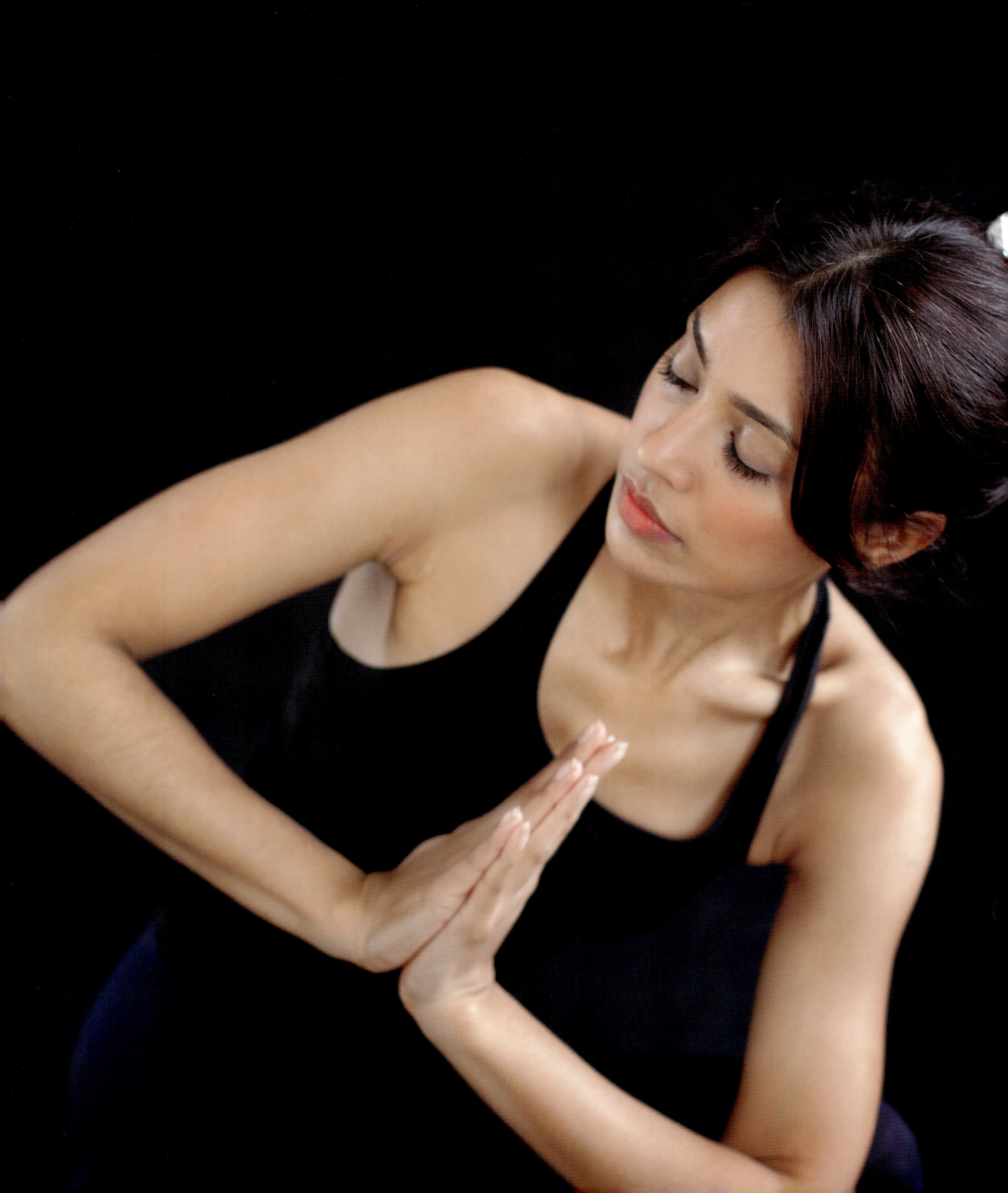

In stillness,

you will find serenity.

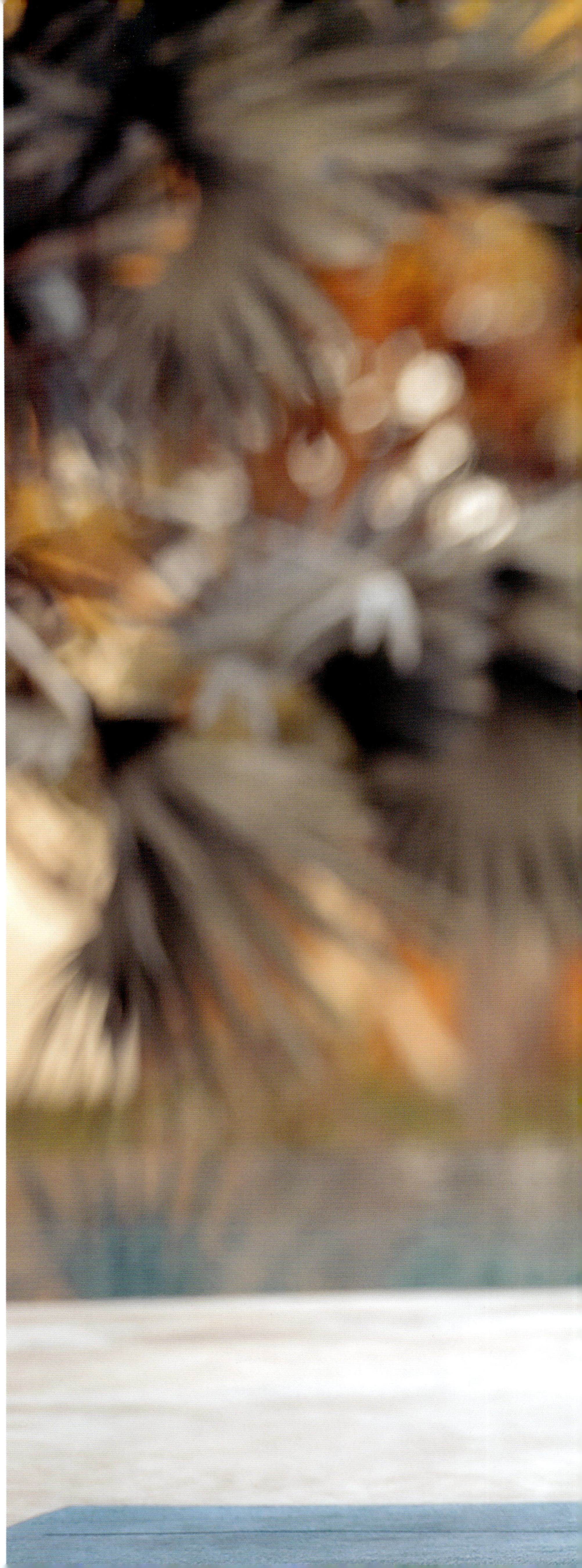

BADDHA ANJANEYASANA · Bound Crescent Low Lunge

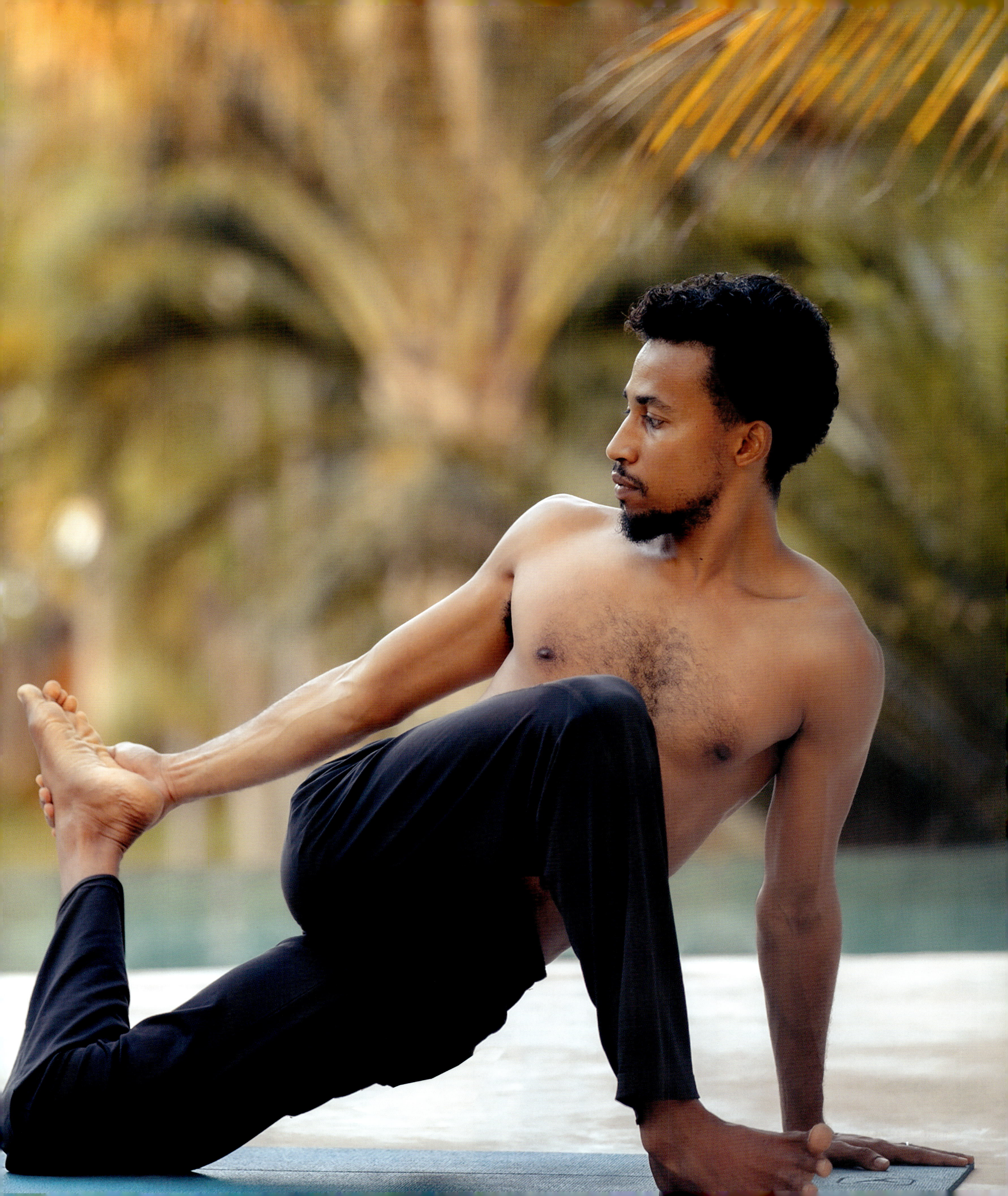

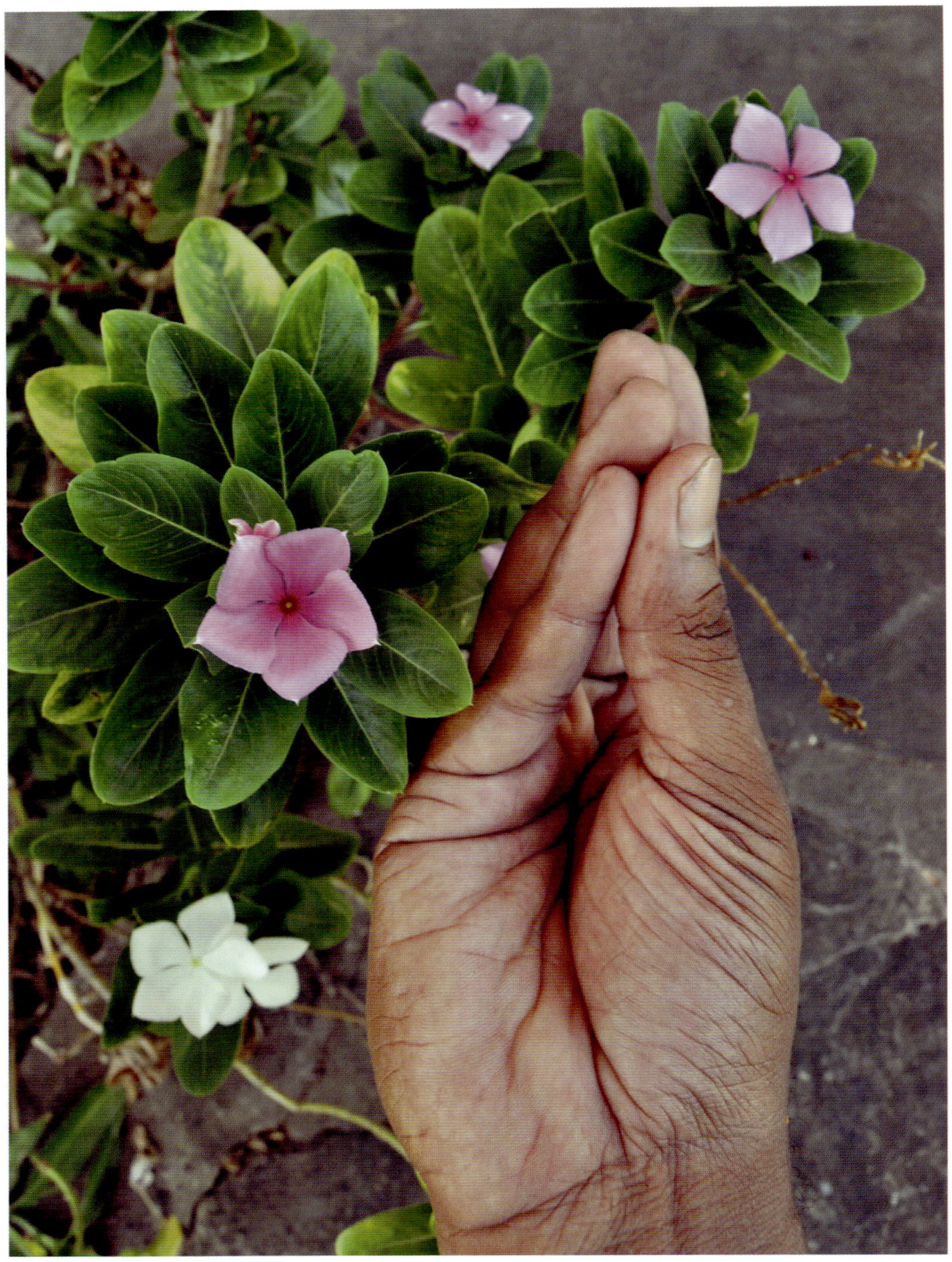

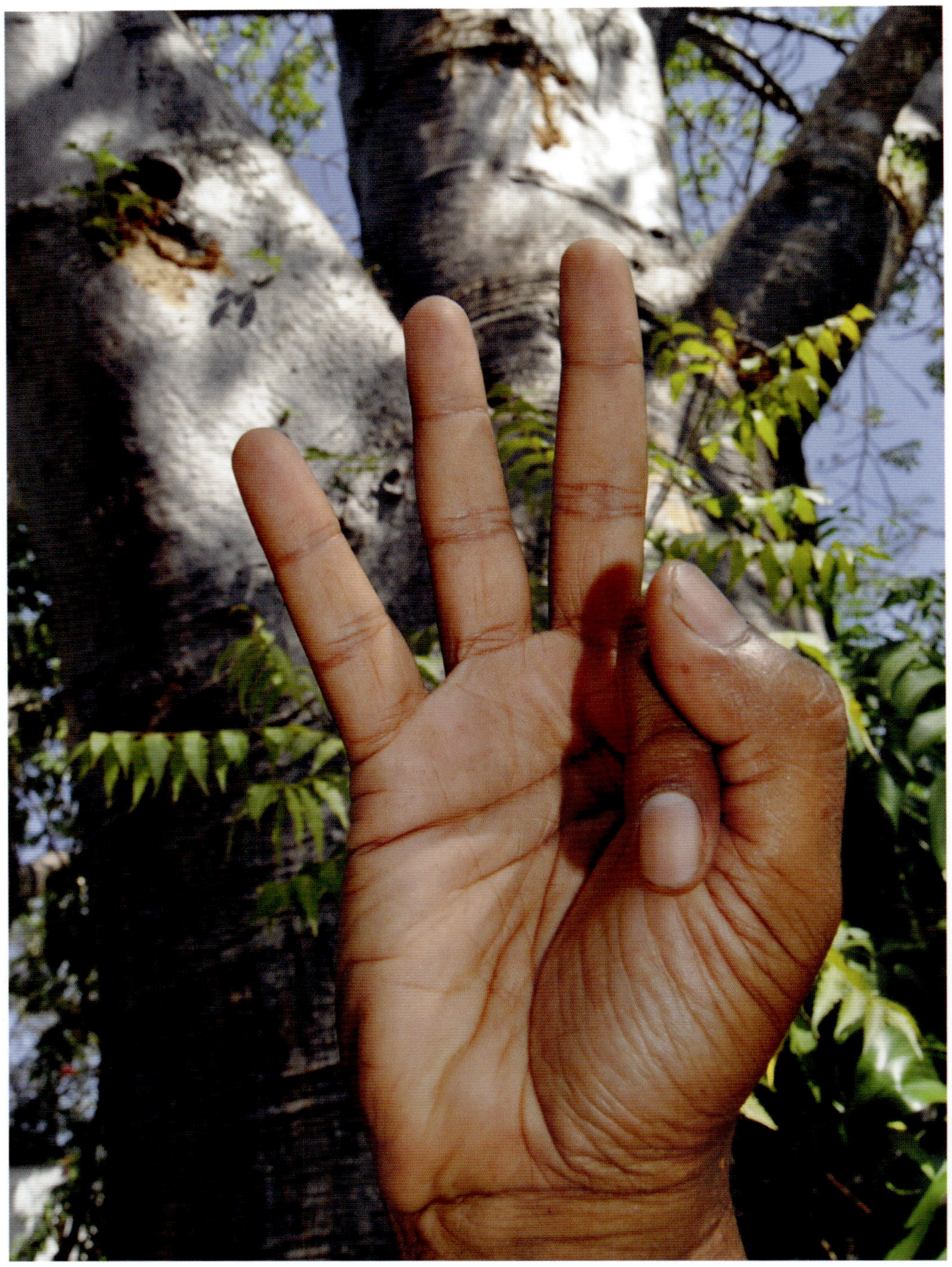

▲ **SHUKRIMUDRA** • Attunement *(left)* **VAYUMUDRA** • Serenity *(right)*

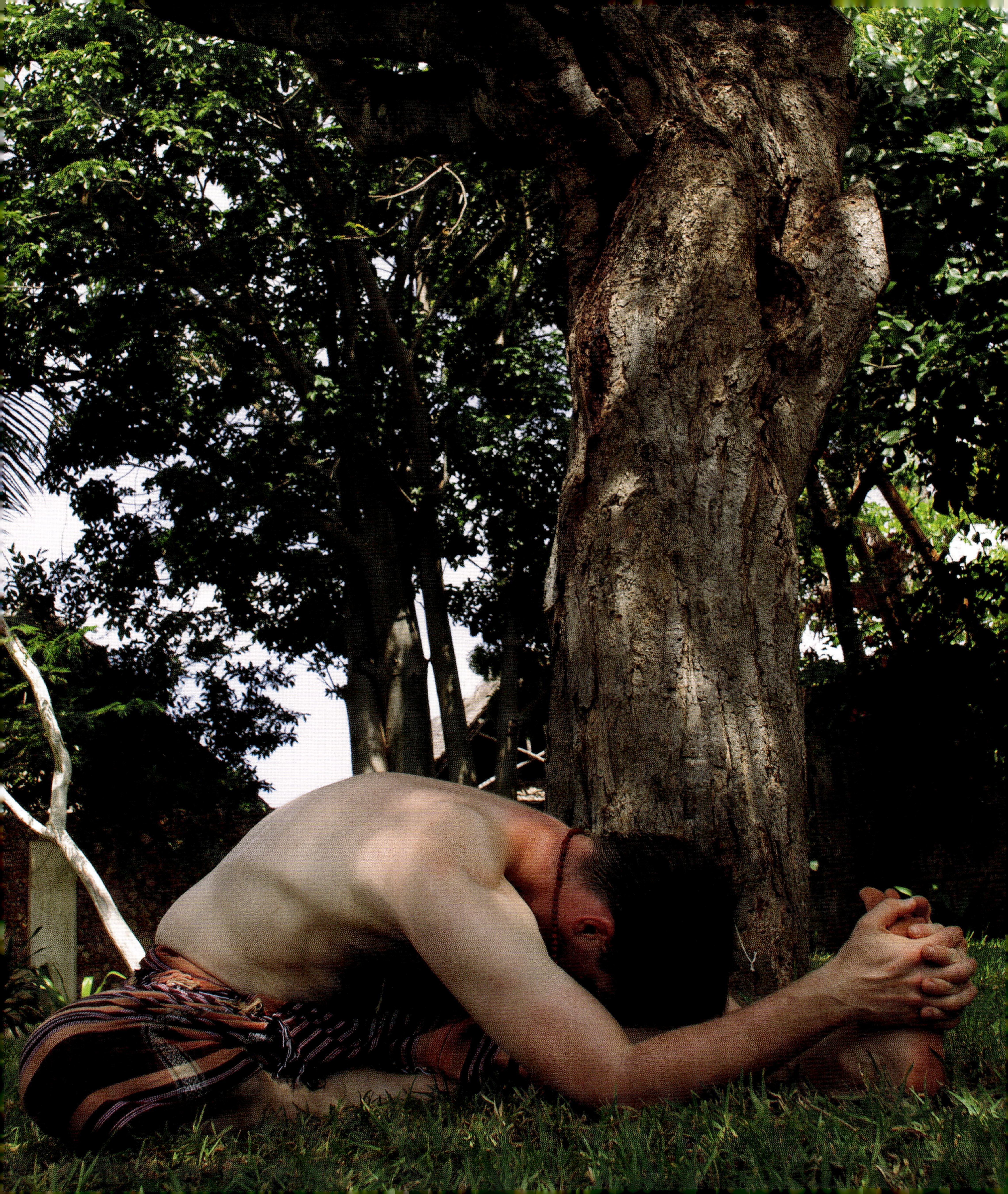

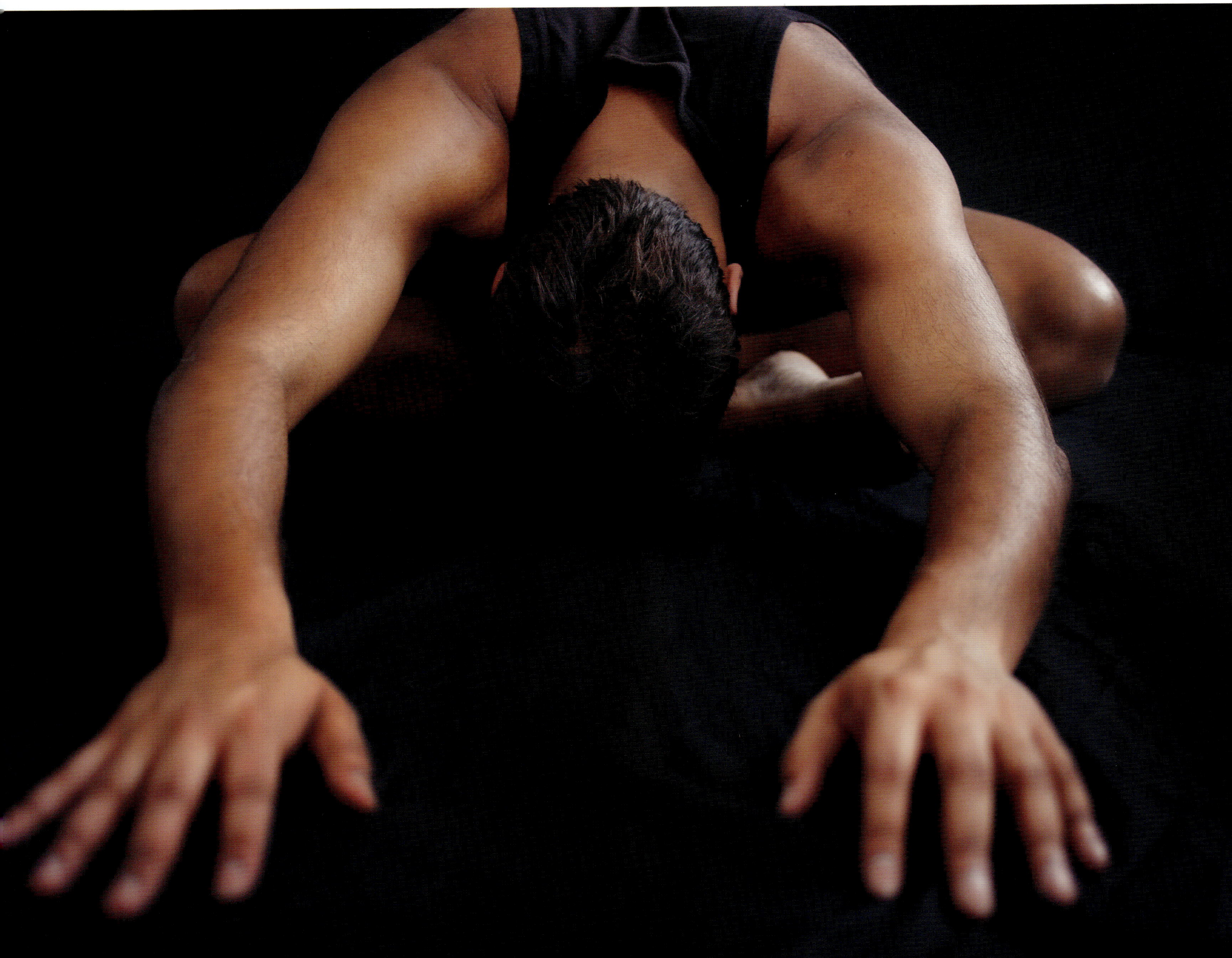

SUKHA UTTANASANA · Easy Seated Forward Fold

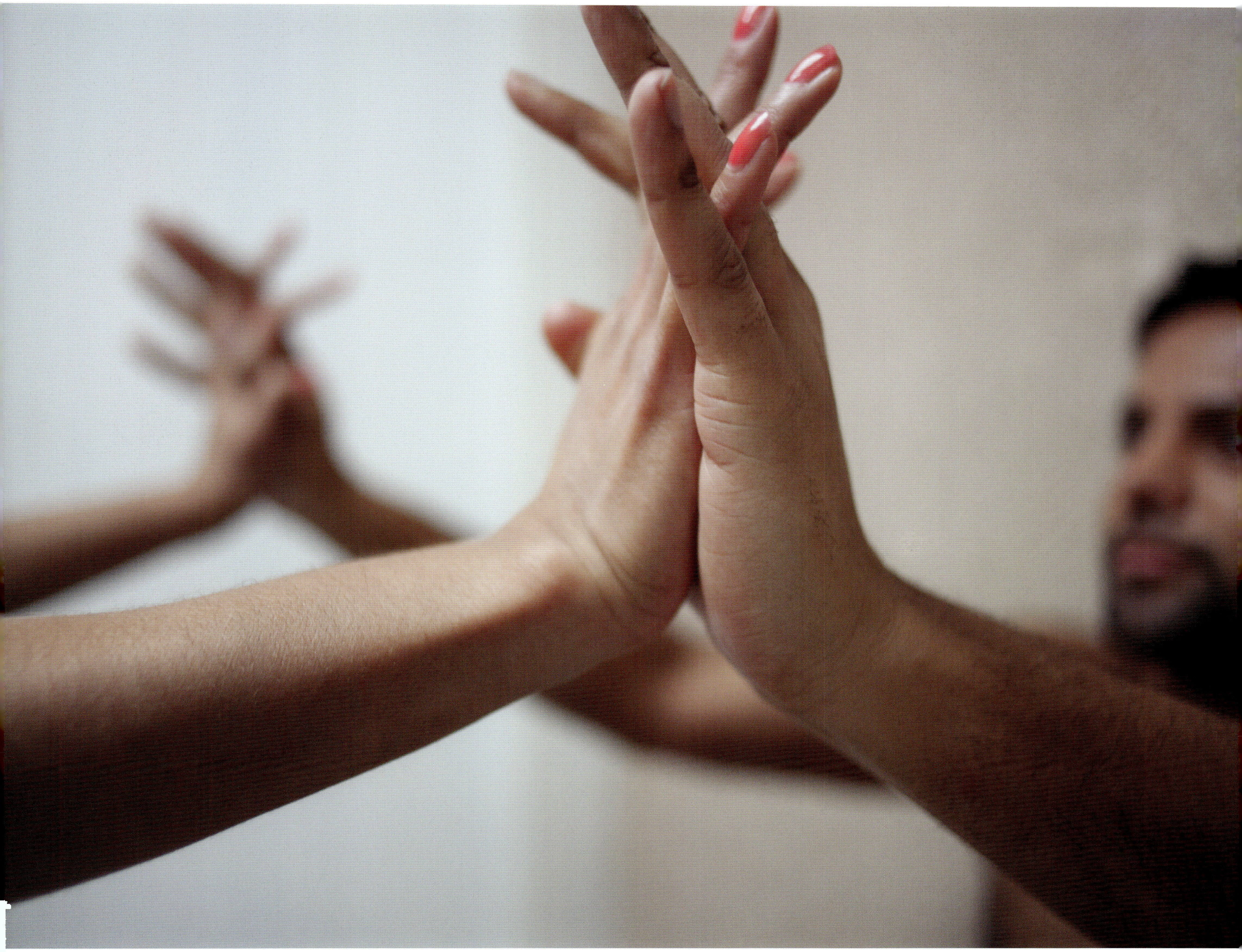

The space I am trying to get to is right inside of me.

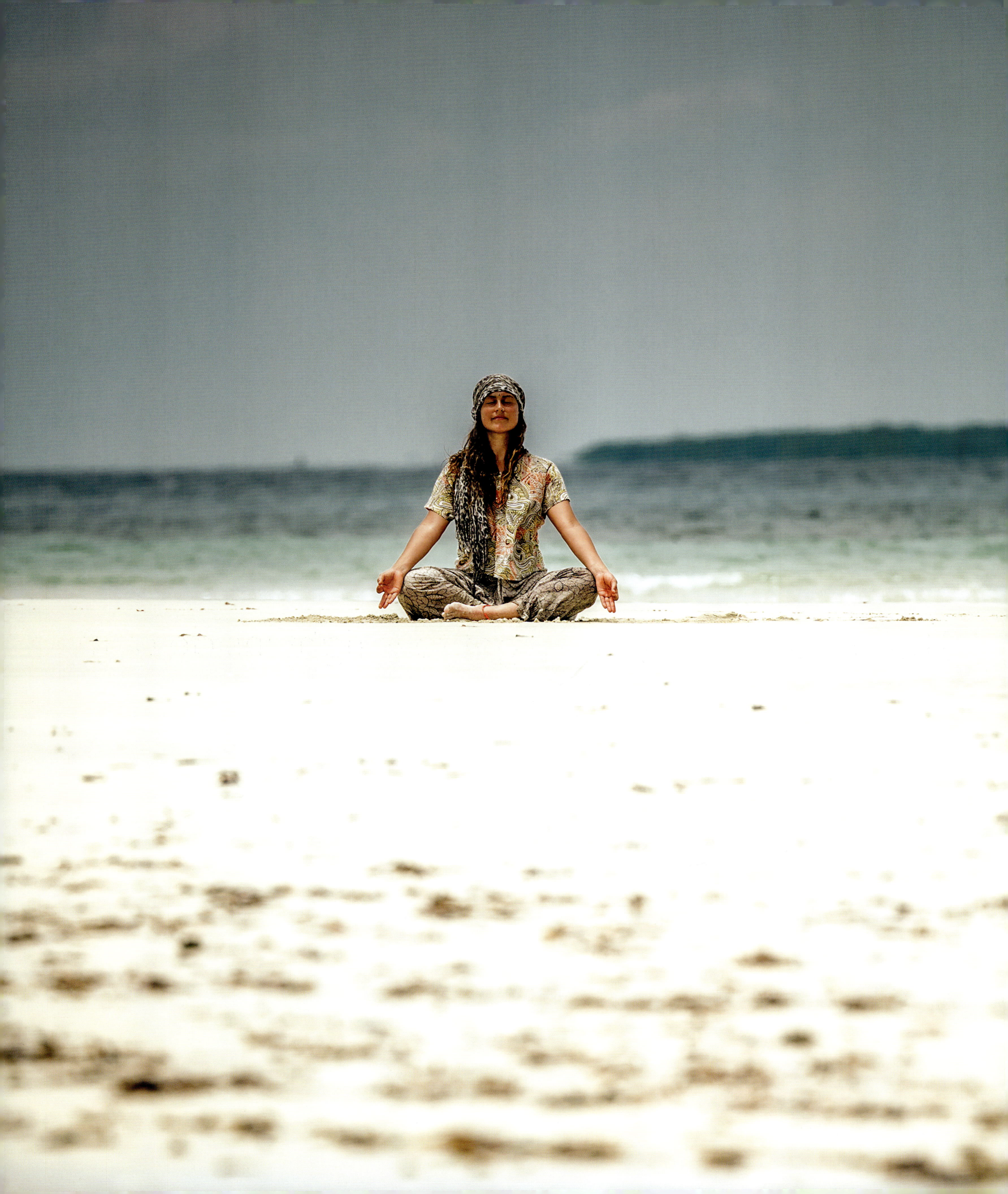

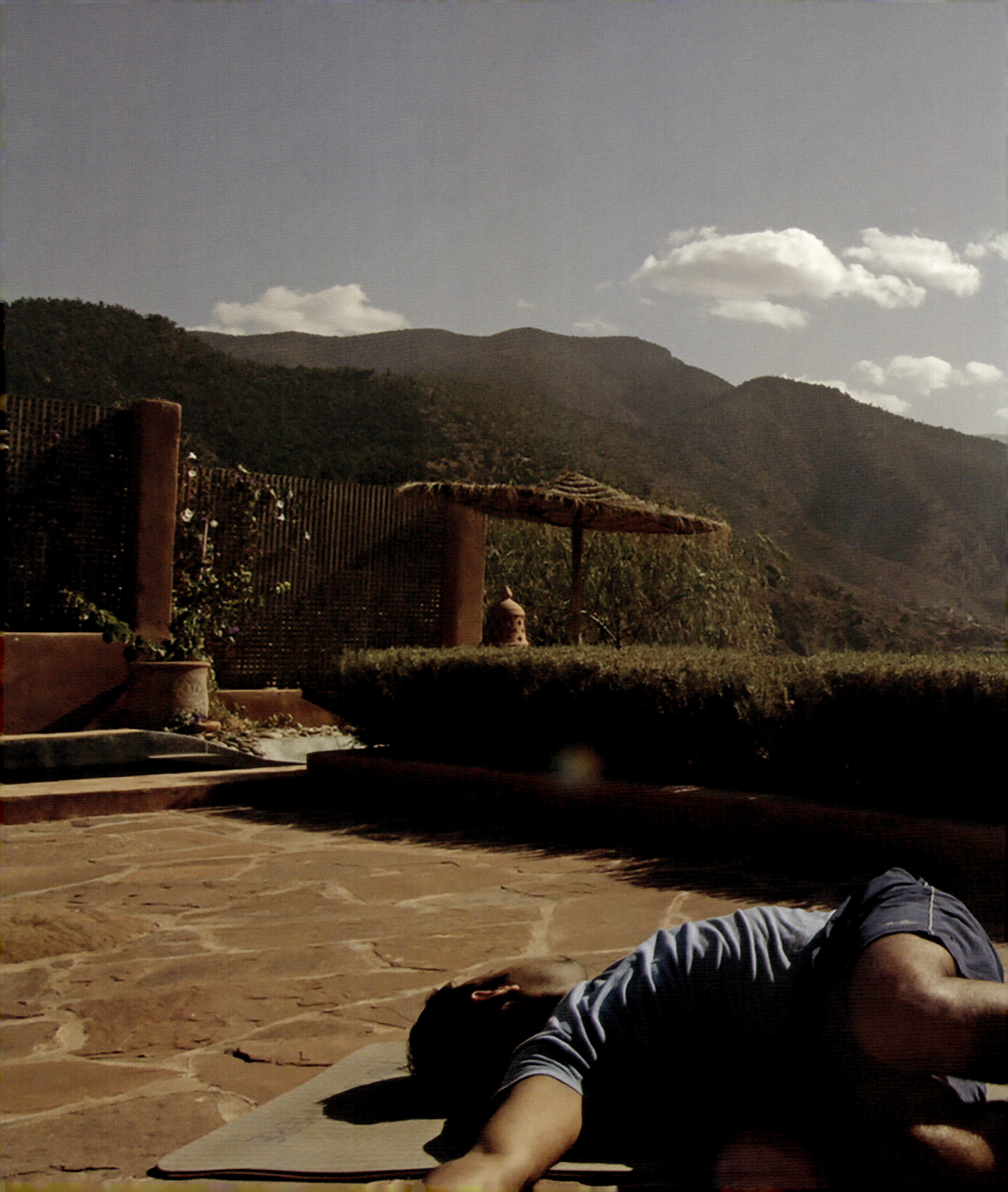

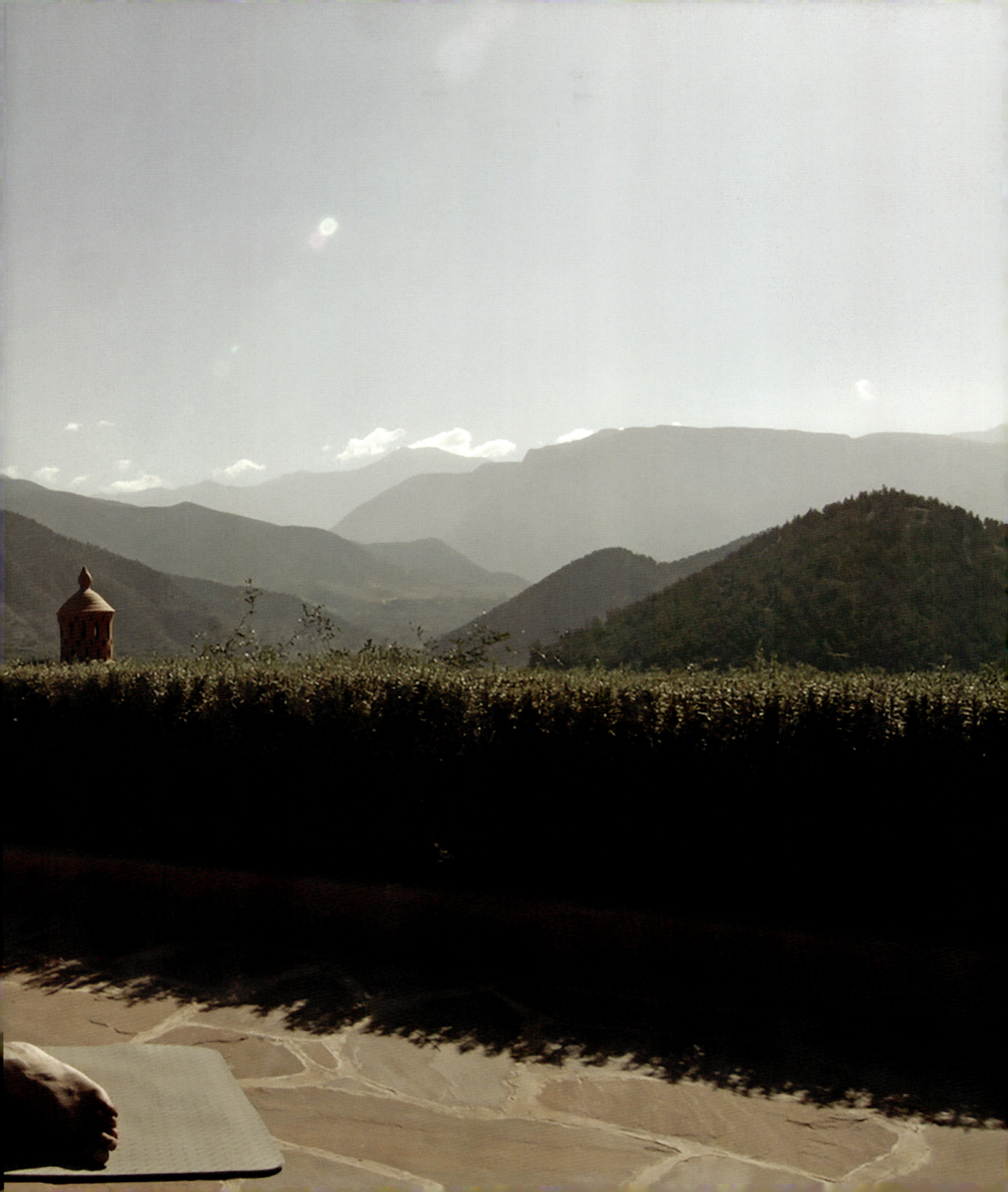

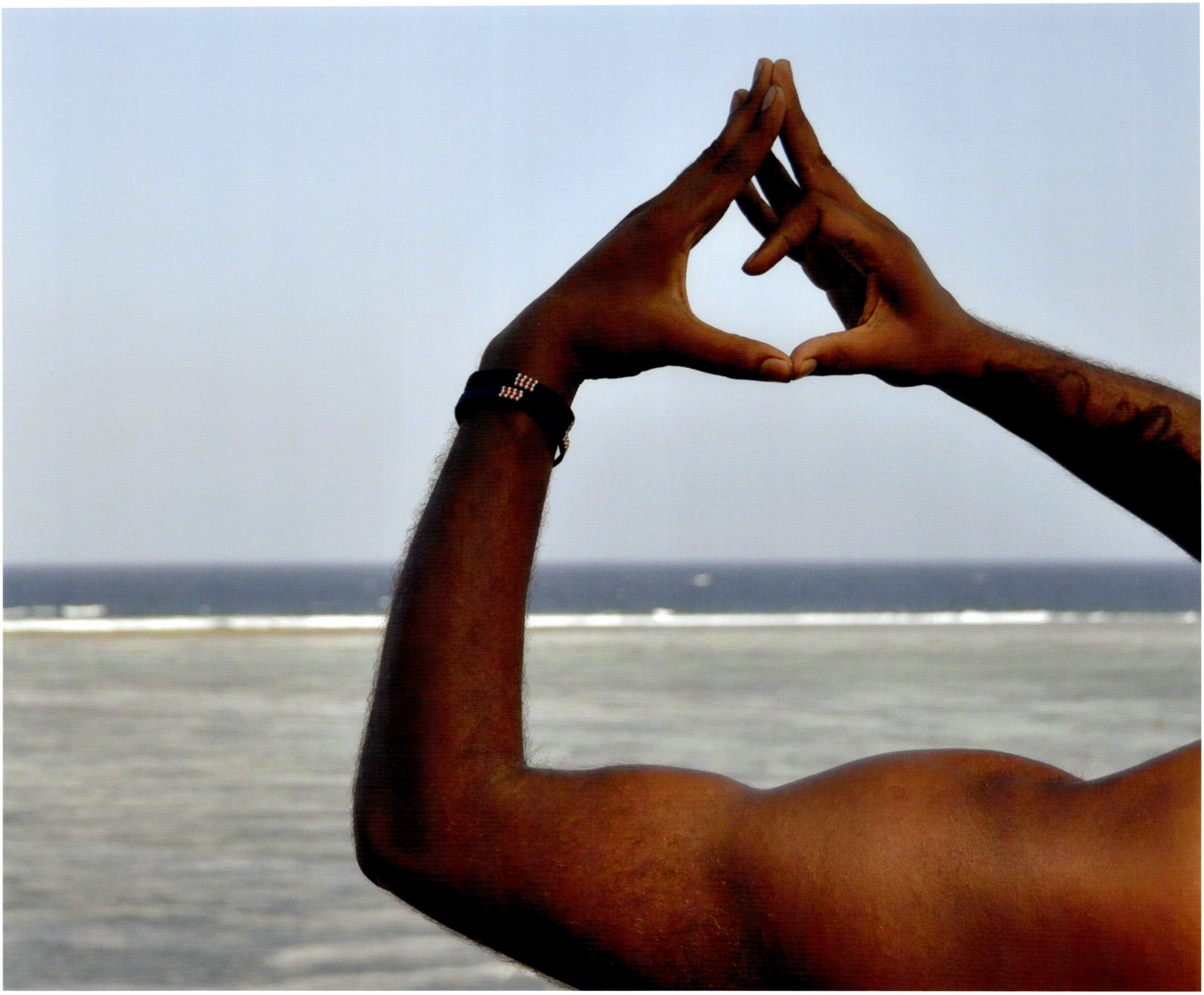

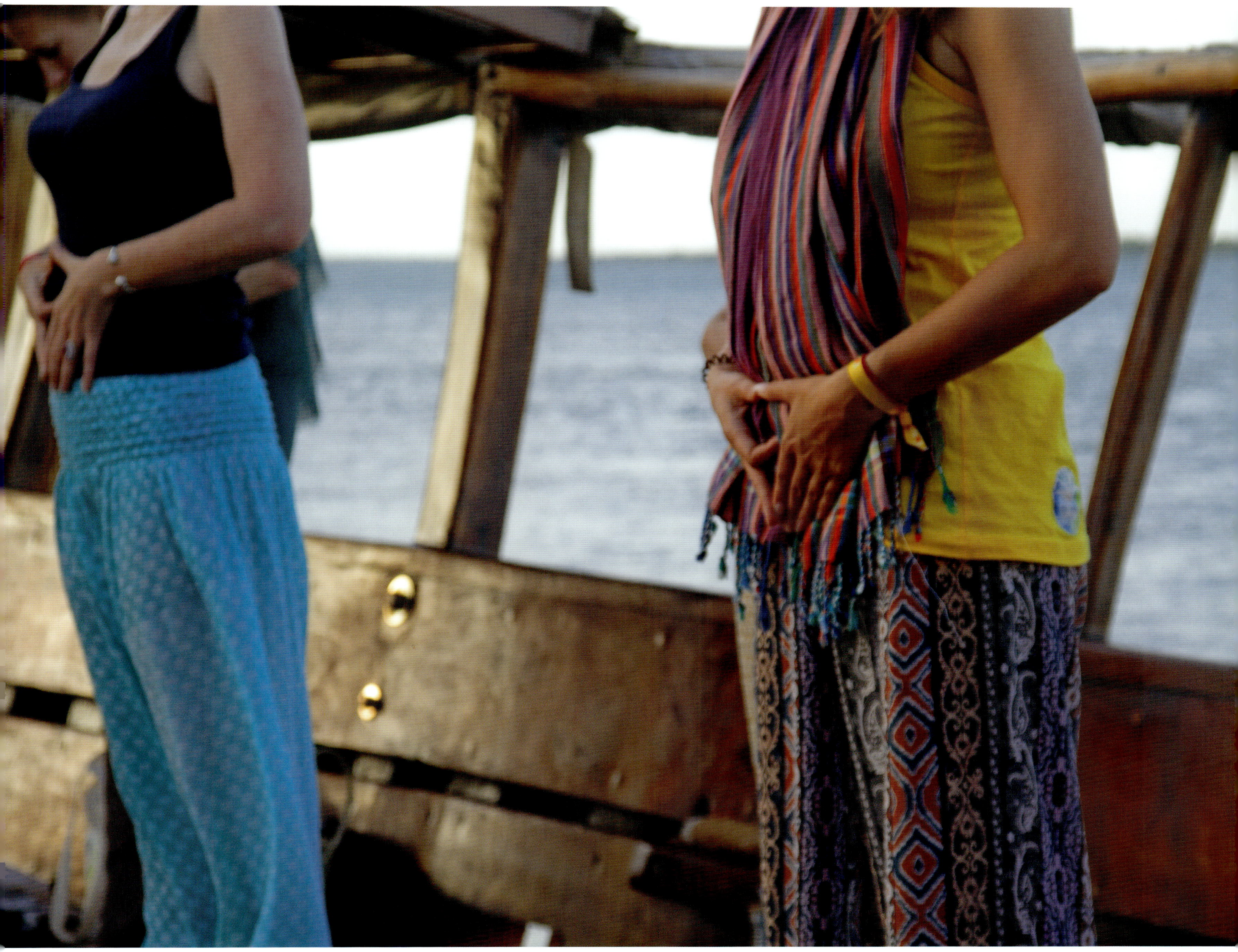

The promise of spring will forgive the harshness of winter every time.

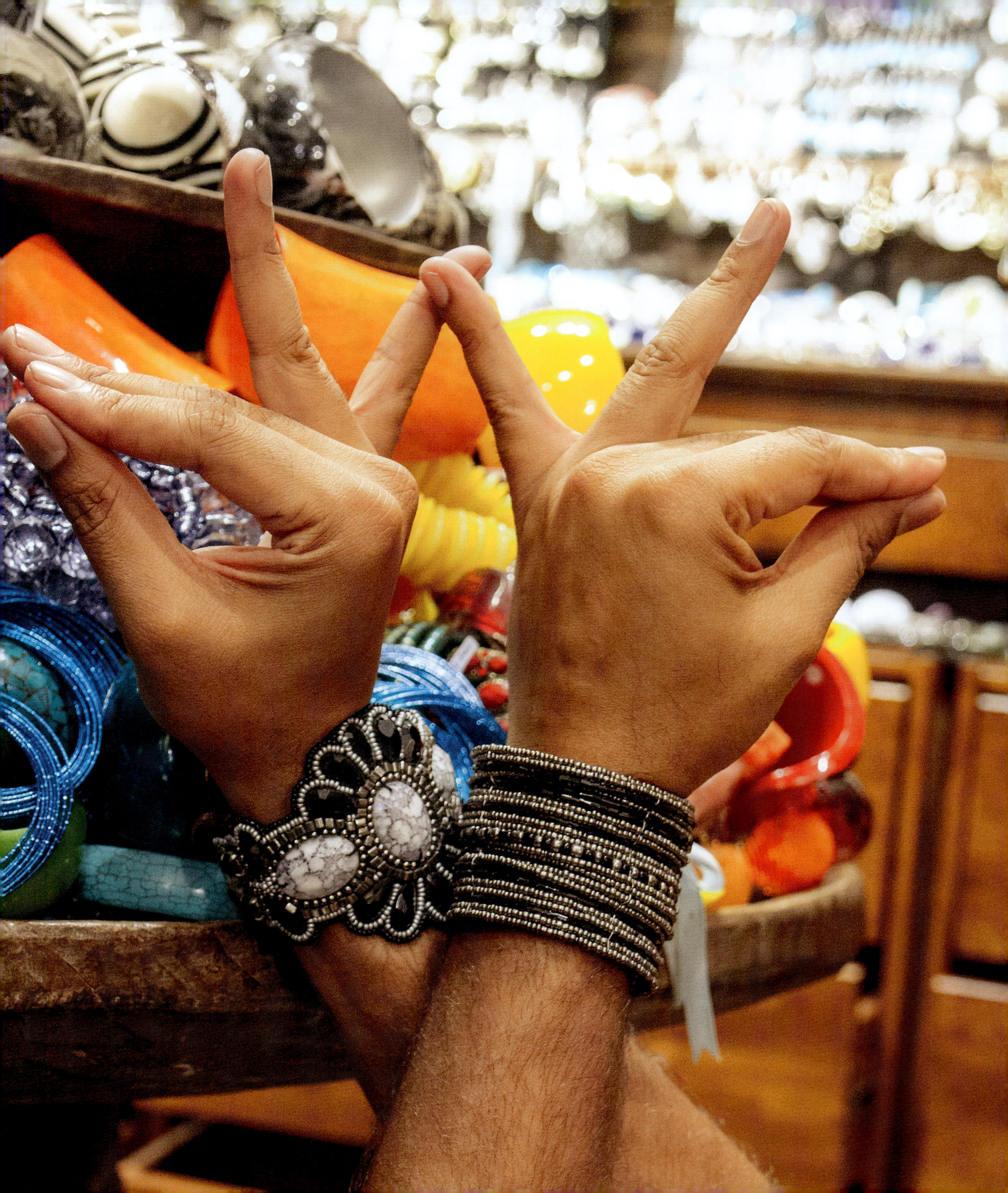

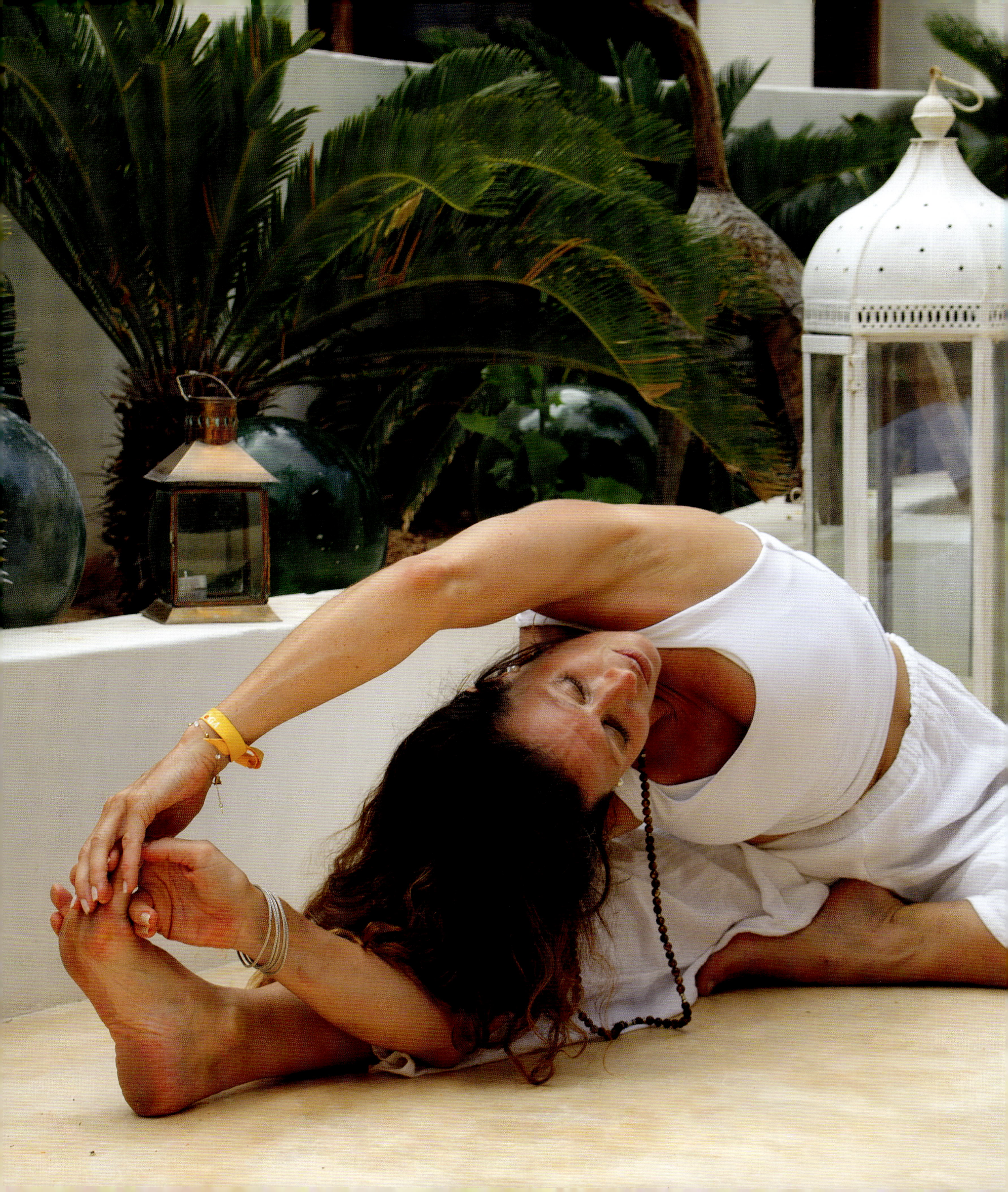

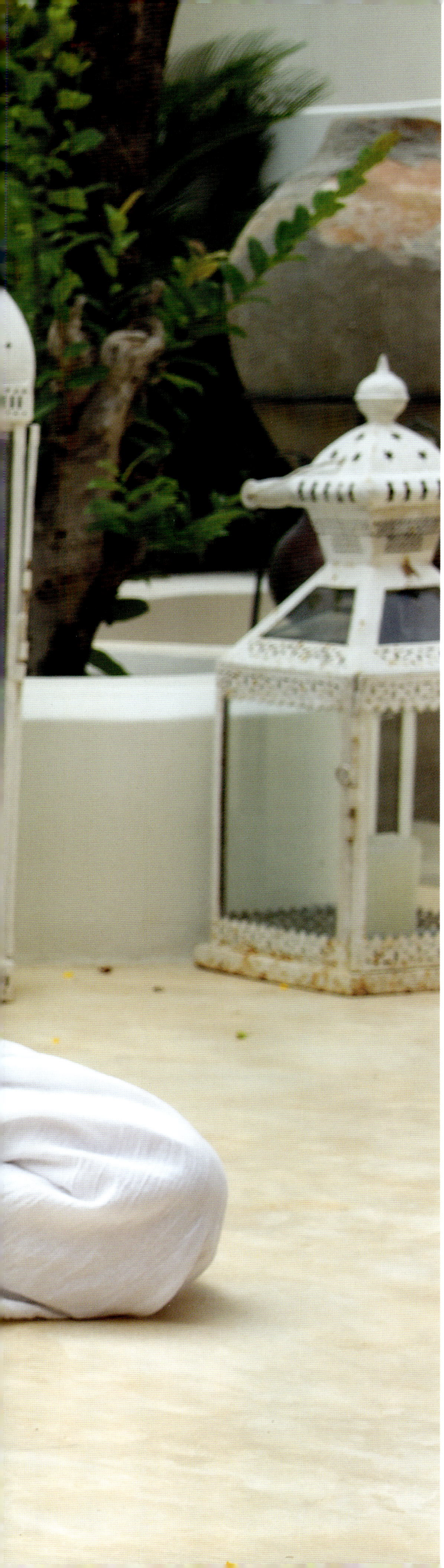

To pause is not the
same as to stop.

PARIVRTTA JANUSIRSASANA · Twisted Head-to-Knee Forward Bend

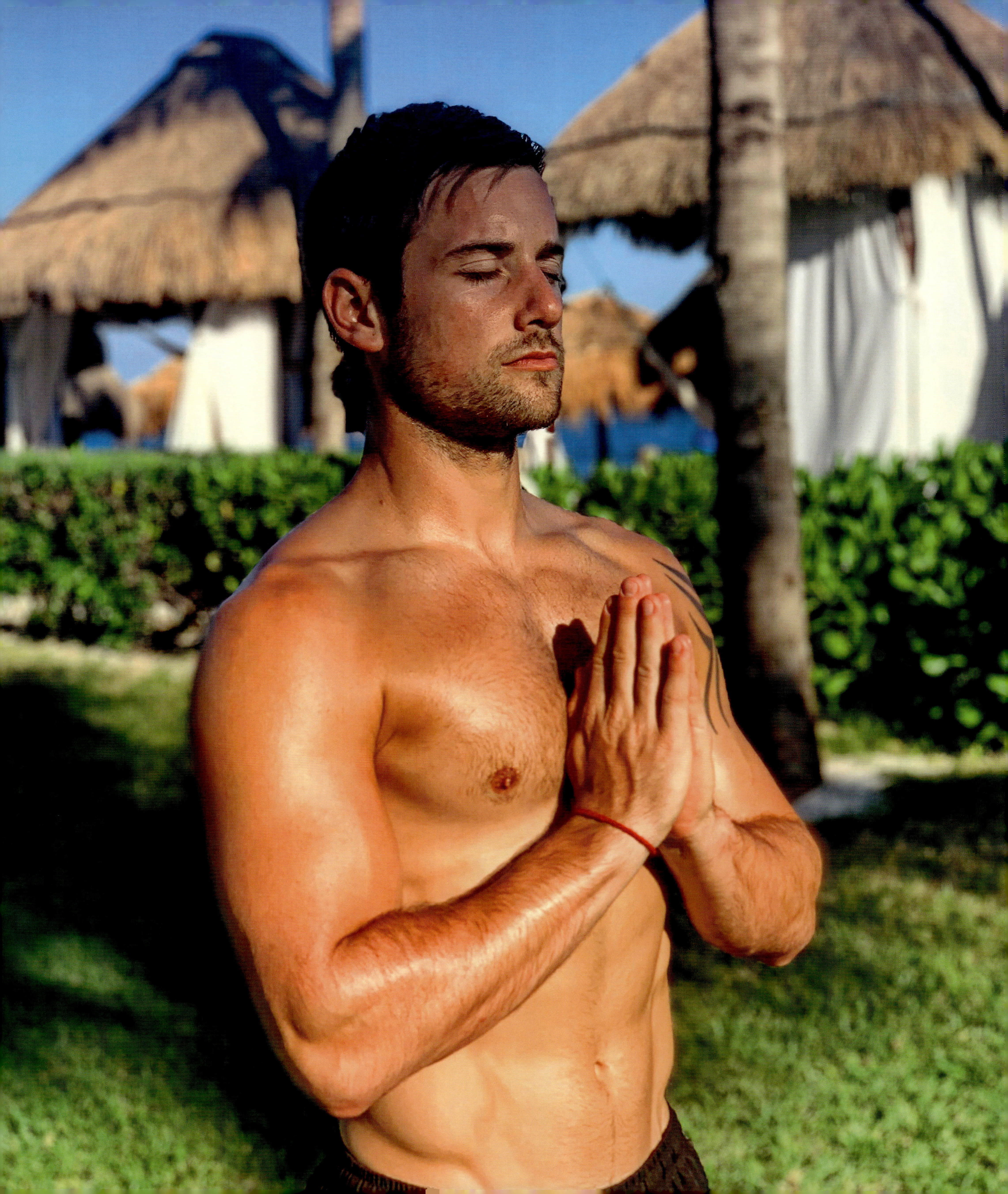

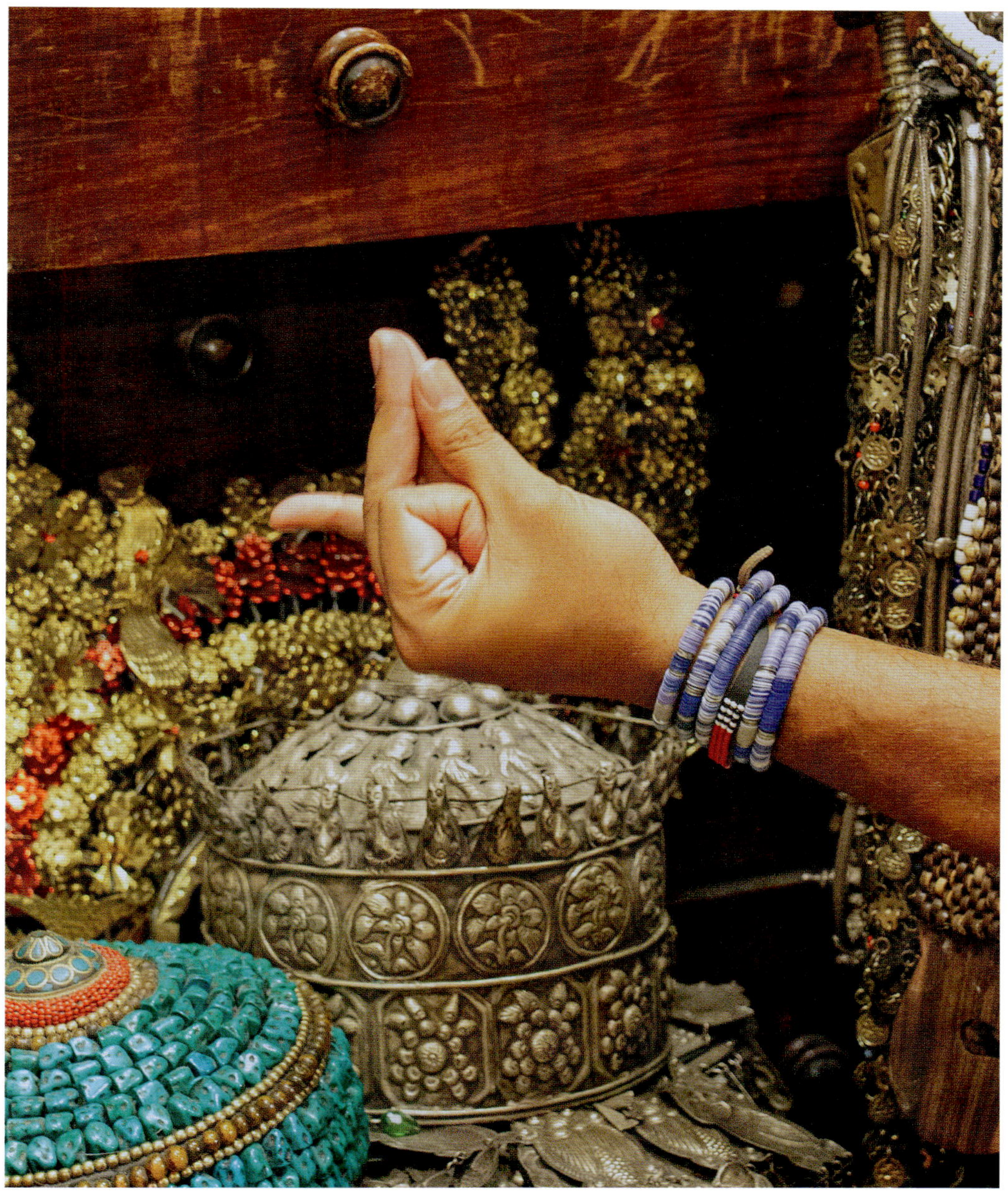

DHYANA ANJALIMUDRA • Love Meditation

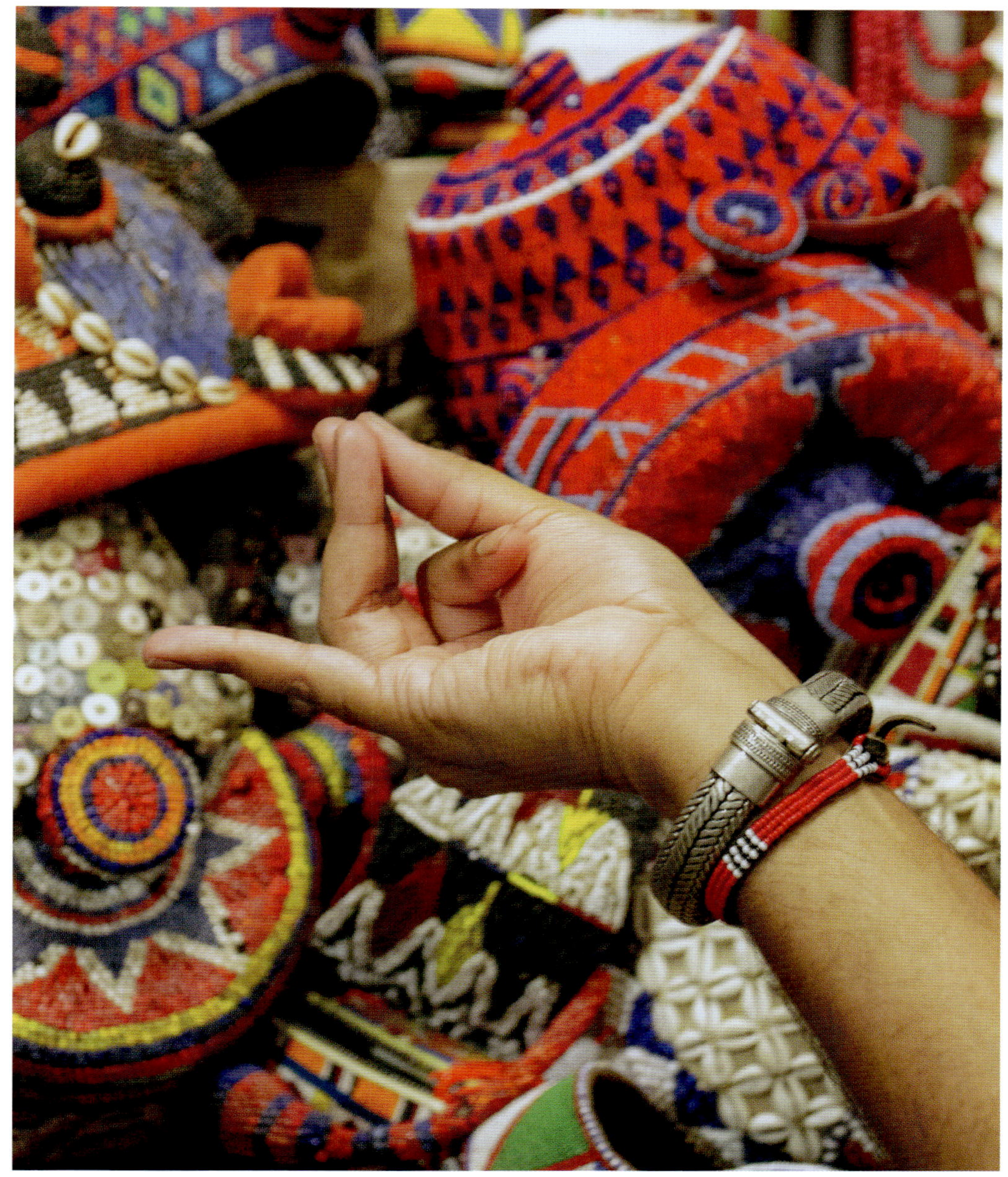

▲ HRIDAYAMUDRA • Tranquility *(left)*   MRITSAMJIVANIMUDRA • Restoration *(right)*

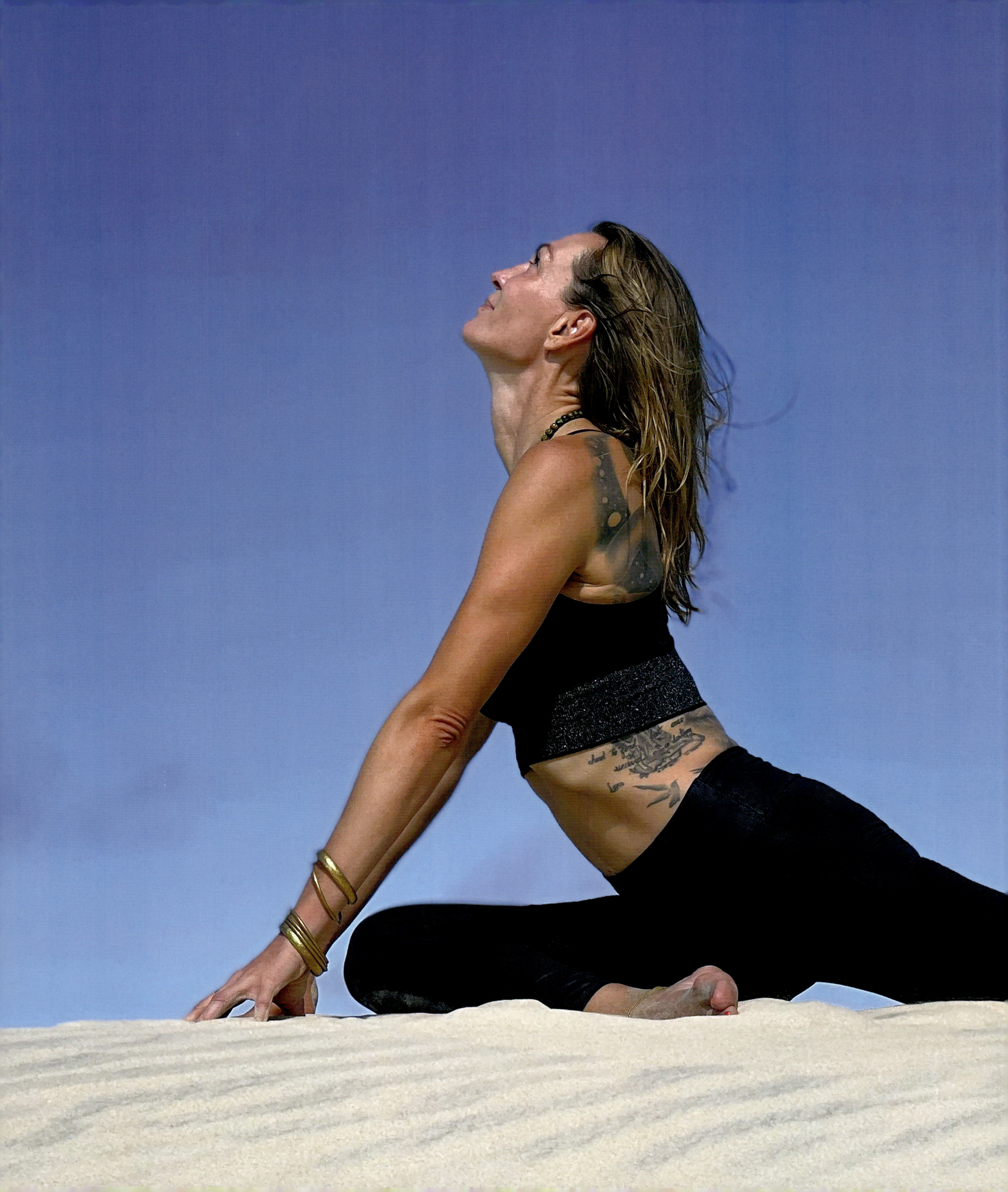

UTHANA SONASVAINASANA · Rising Swan

People often regret their words

but rarely their silence.

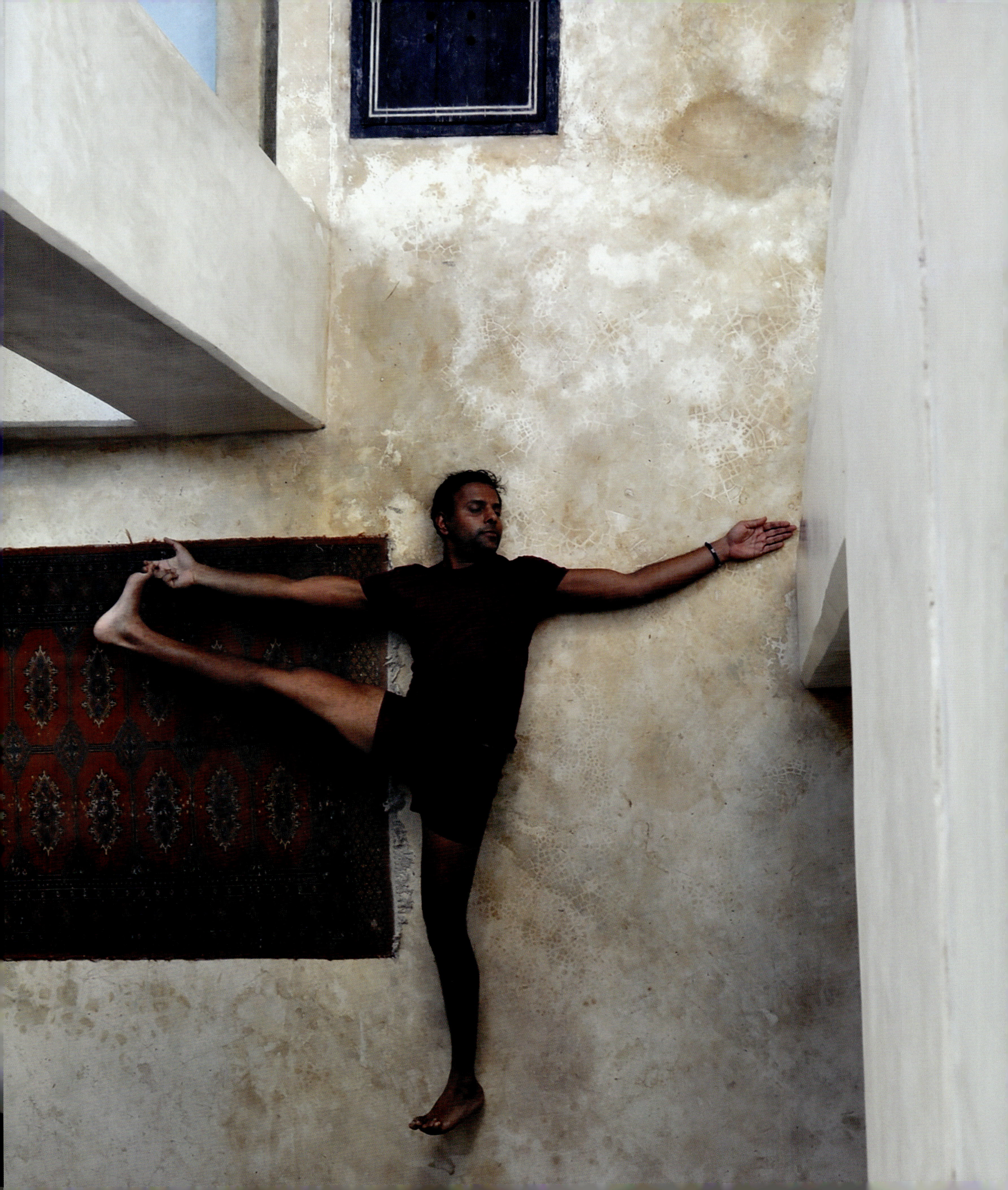

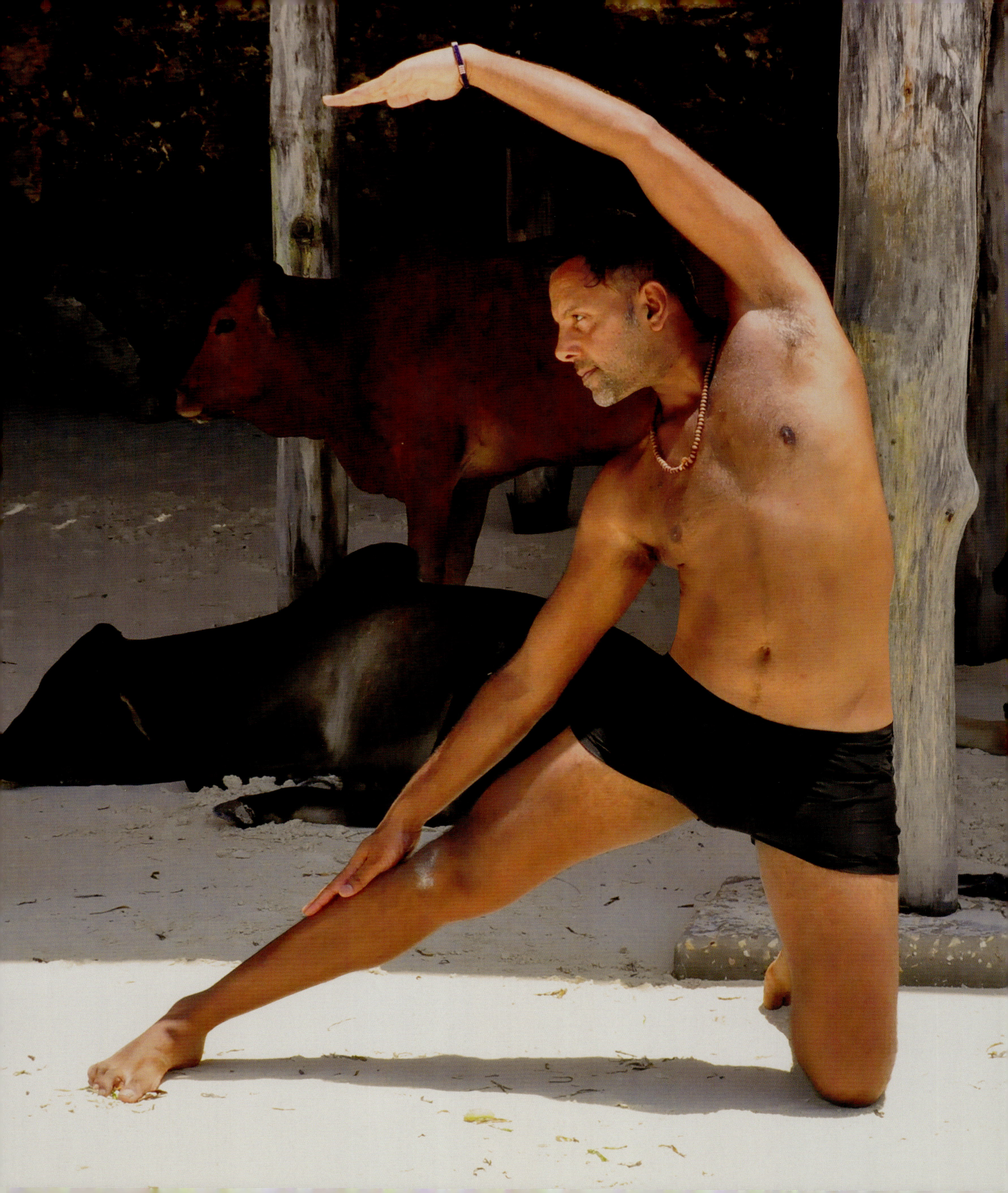

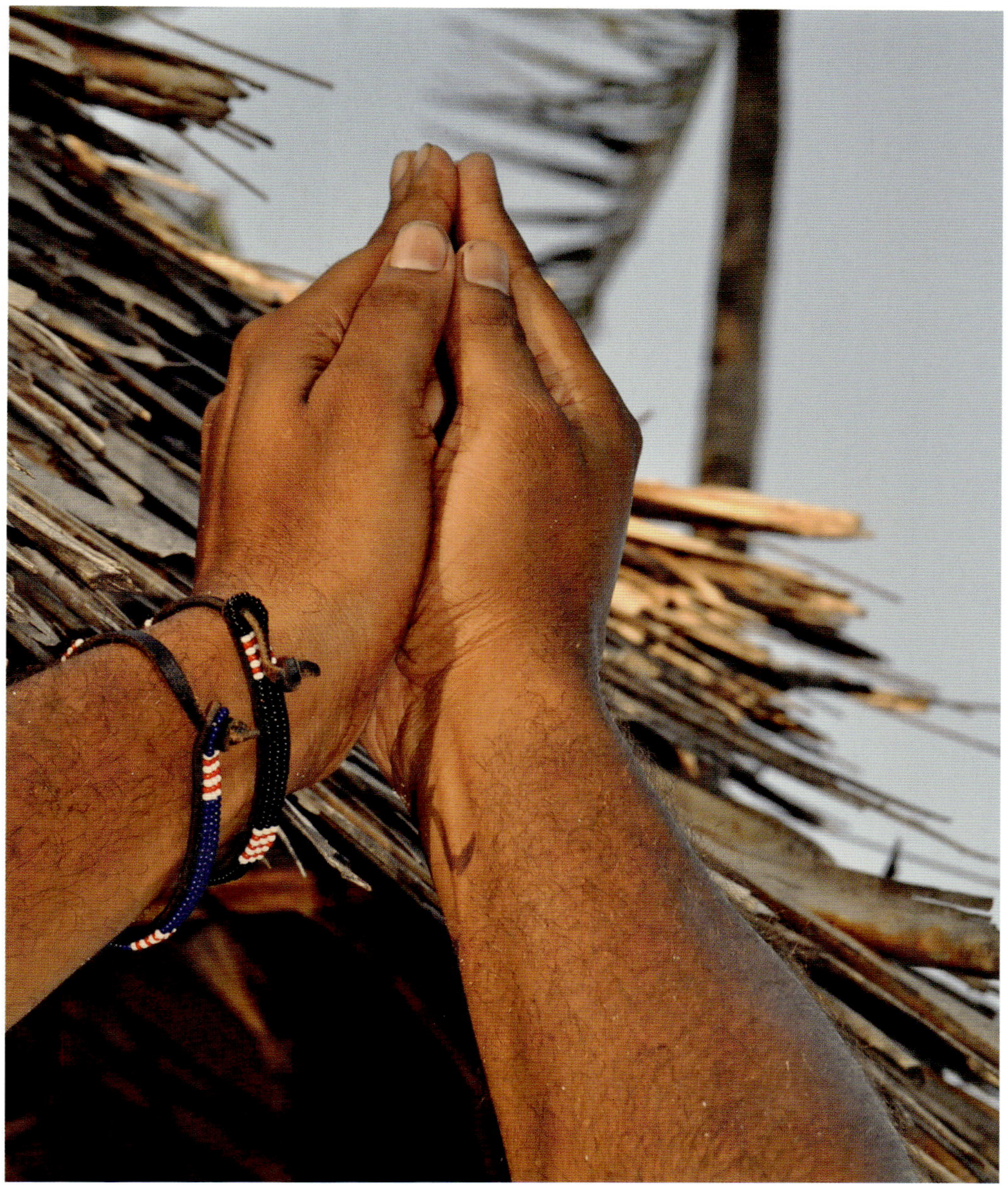

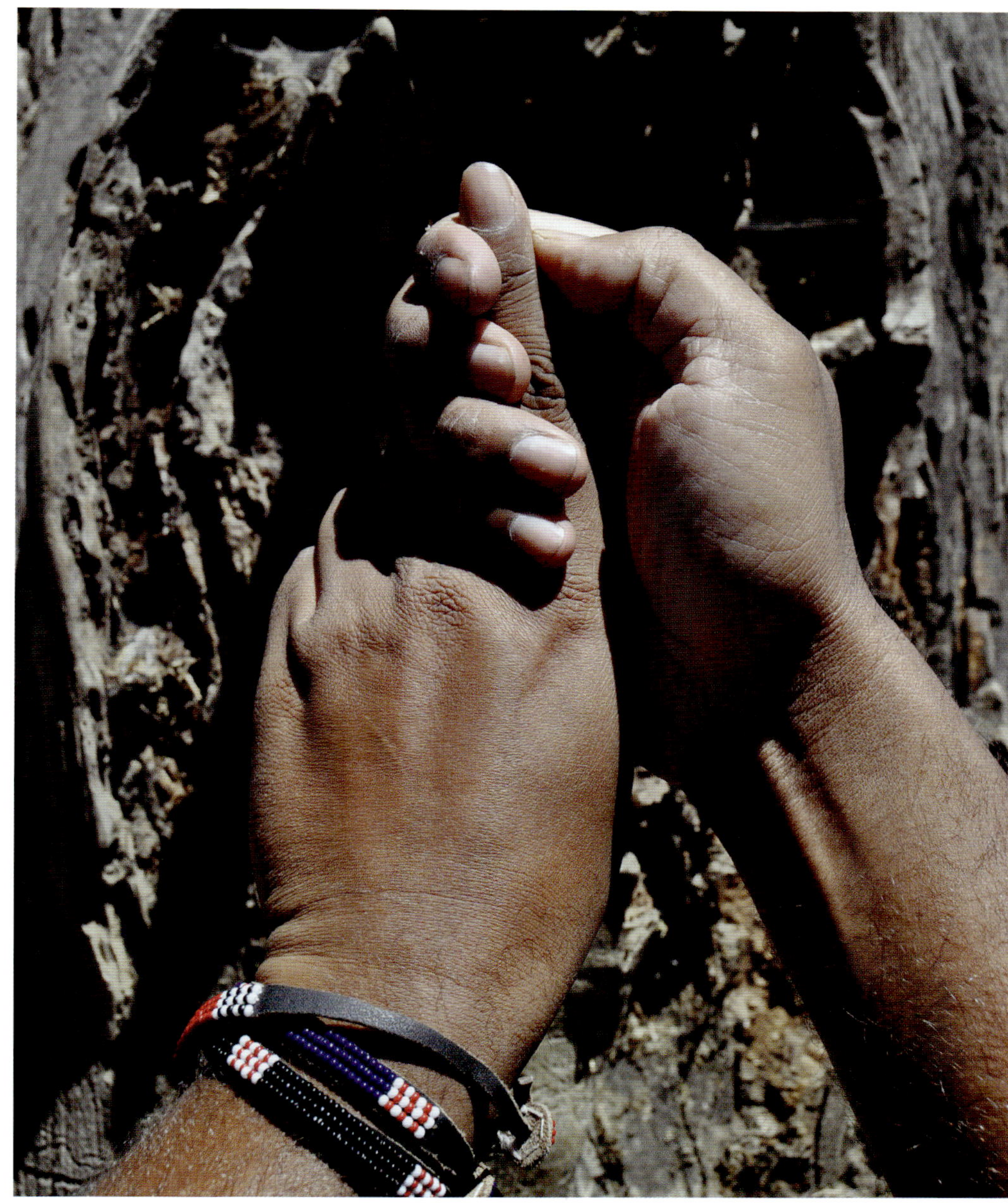

PARIGHASANA · Gate

▲ SAMPUTAMUDRA · Presence *(left)* AJNACHAKRAMUDRA · Clarity *(right)*

Take a journey
to discover your
own inner nature.

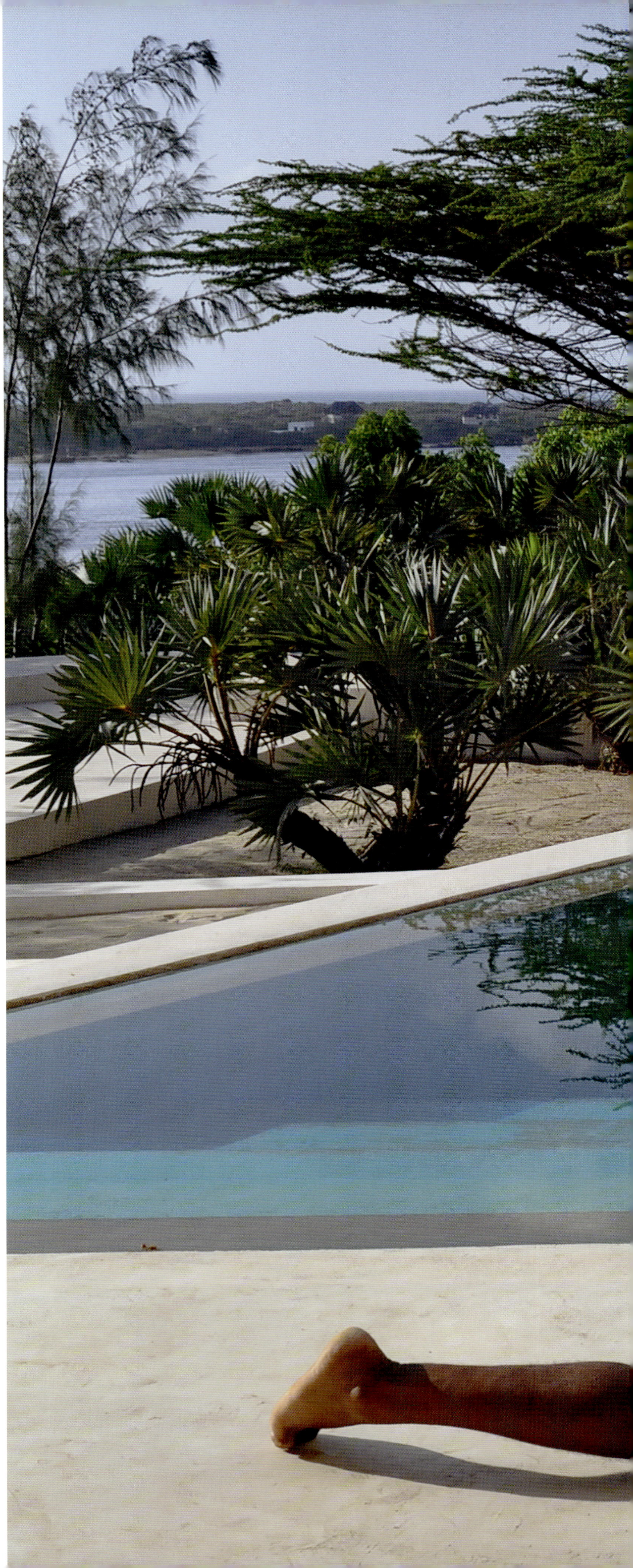

HASTA SONASVAINASANA · Reaching Swan

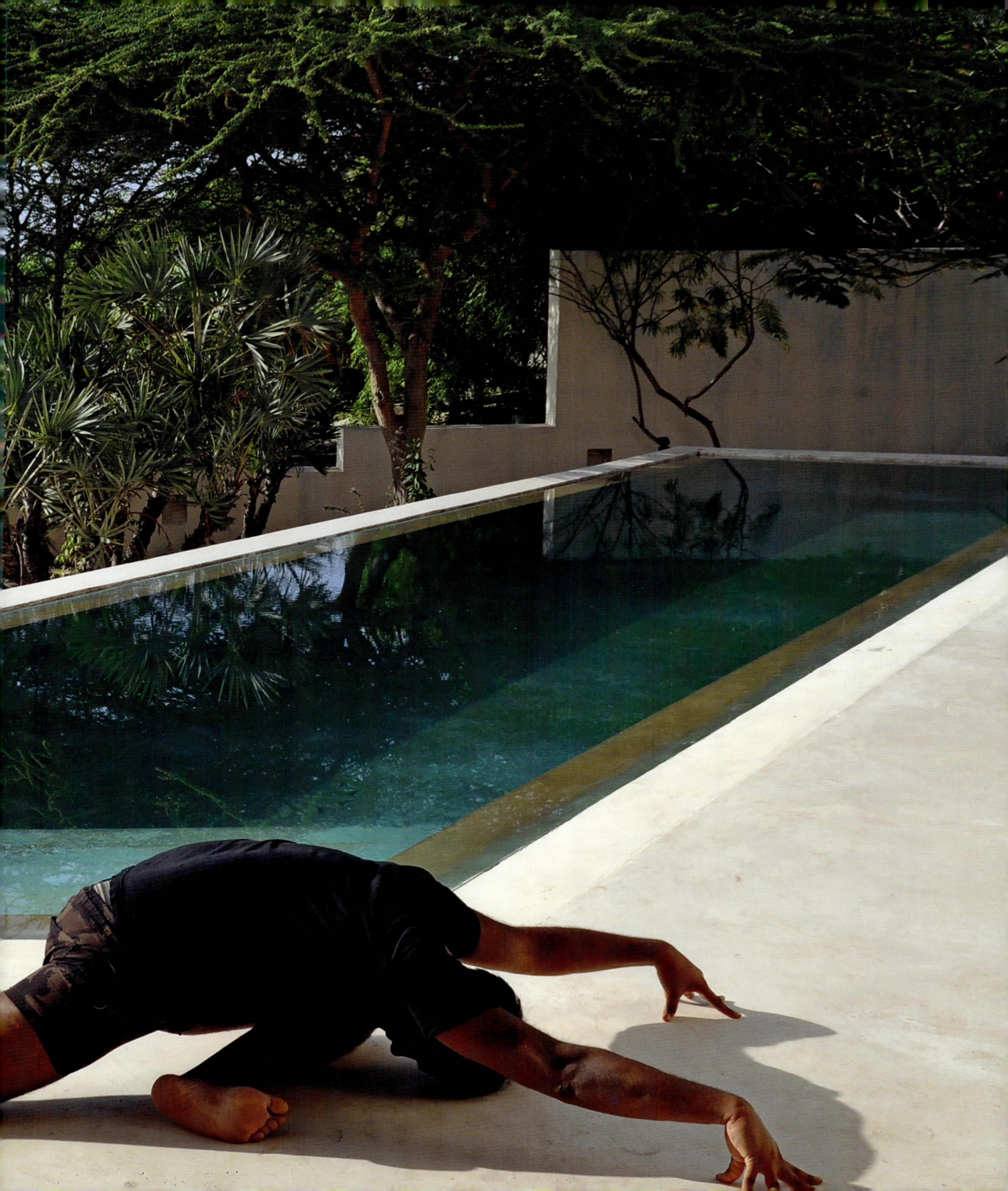

BRAHMA MITHUNA • Gemini

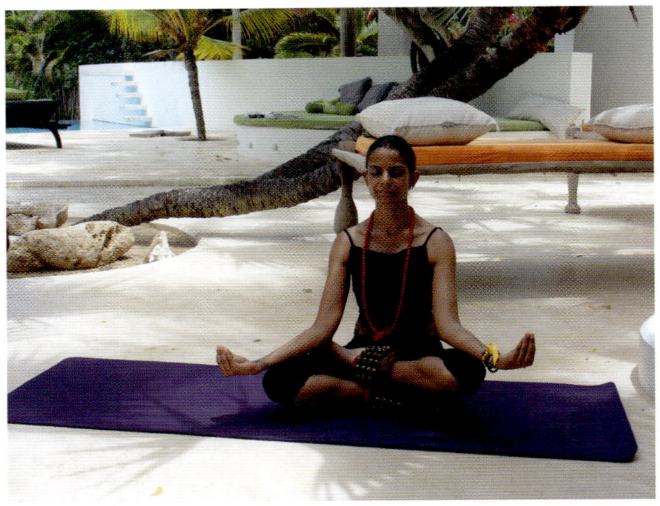

ARDHA PADMASANA & SHUKRIMUDRA
Half Lotus & Attunement

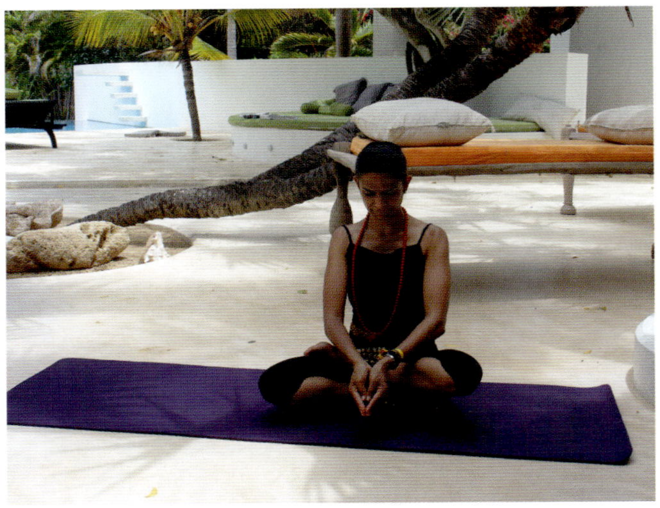

ARDHA PADMASANA & SAMPUTAMUDRA
Half Lotus & Presence

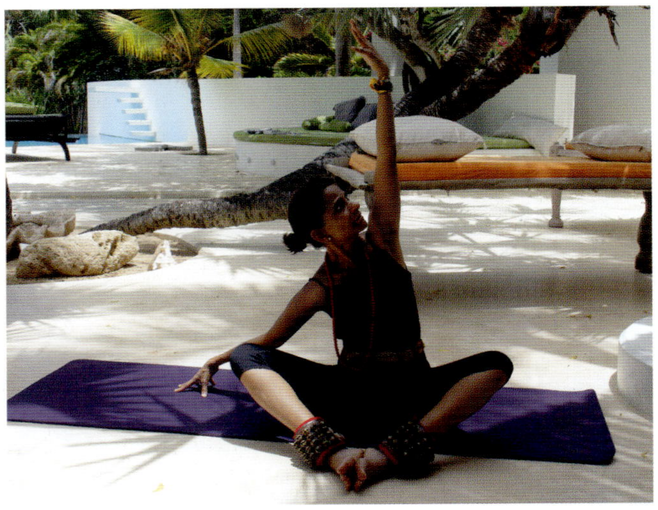

PARSVA SUKHASANA
Seated Side Bend

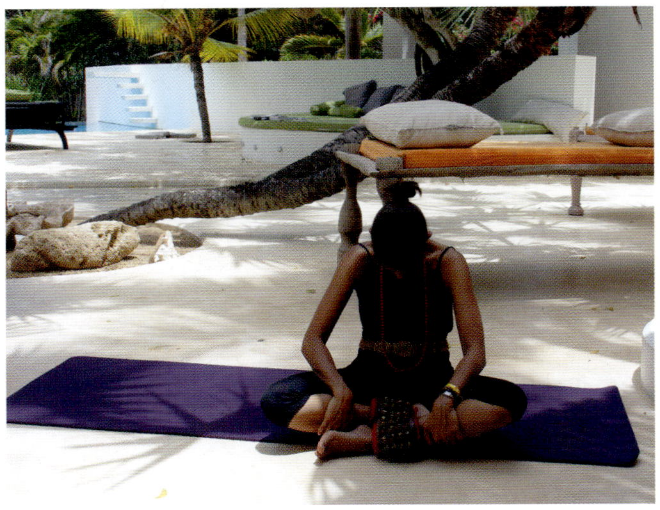

SUKHASANA MARJARYASANA BITILASANA
Seated Cat Cow

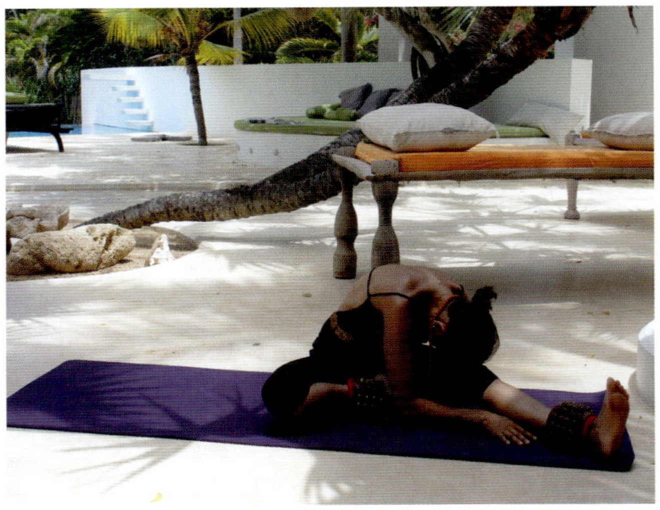

JANUSIRSASANA
Head-to-Knee Forward Bend

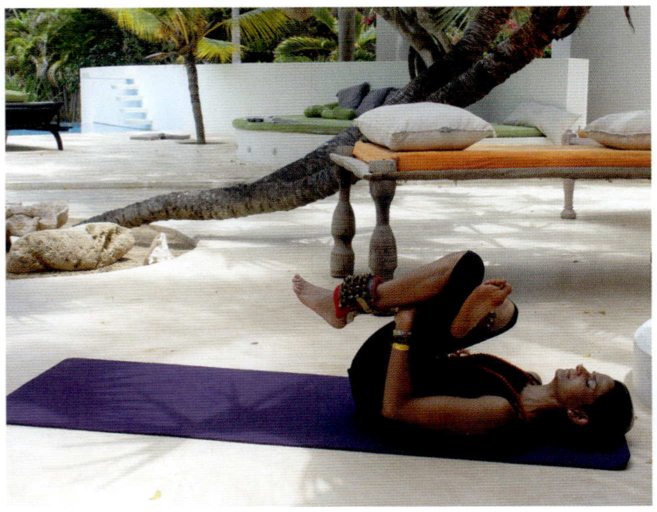

SUPTA KAPOTASANA
Reclining Pigeon

In Brahma Mithuna, we are in the shifting season of elemental air. This constellation of asanas guides you through the unfolding of gentle restful supine stances. Giving the body and mind space to rest and rejuvenate allows the central channel of energy in the spine to adapt and flow with less effort. This shifts the intellectual mind into retreating from the demands of thinking. The mudras help us in the attunement of the spaces between thoughts, which brings presence. In this waking restfulness, clarity results in assimilation of all states of mind, inviting you to submit to serenity and awaken intuition.

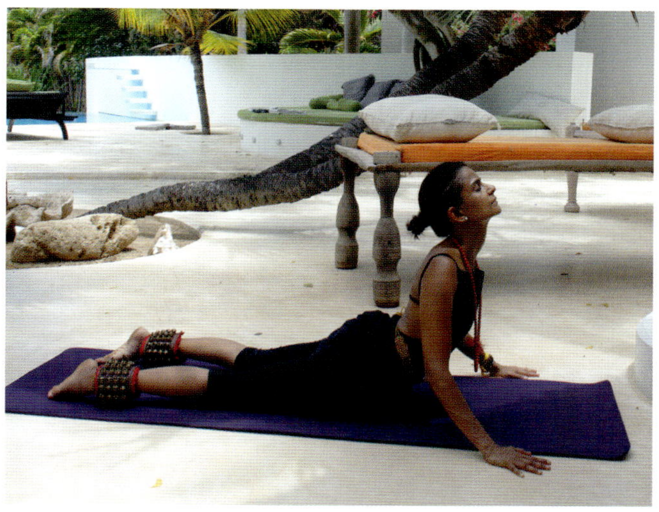

UTTHITA NIRAVALASANA
Seal

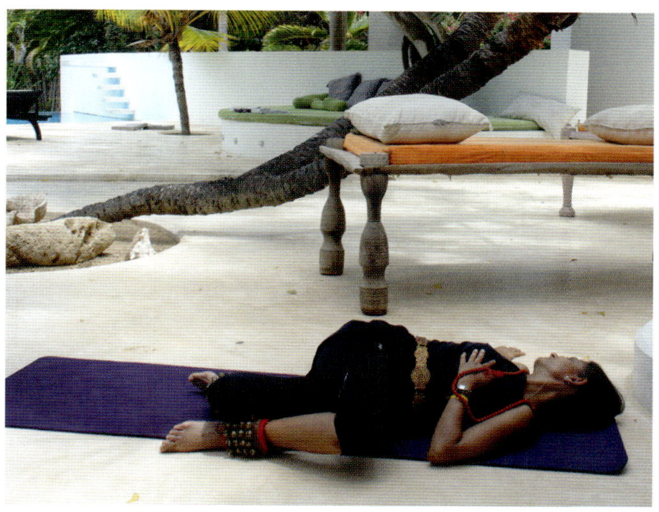

PARIVRTTA SUPTA KAPOTASANA
Reclining Twisted Pigeon

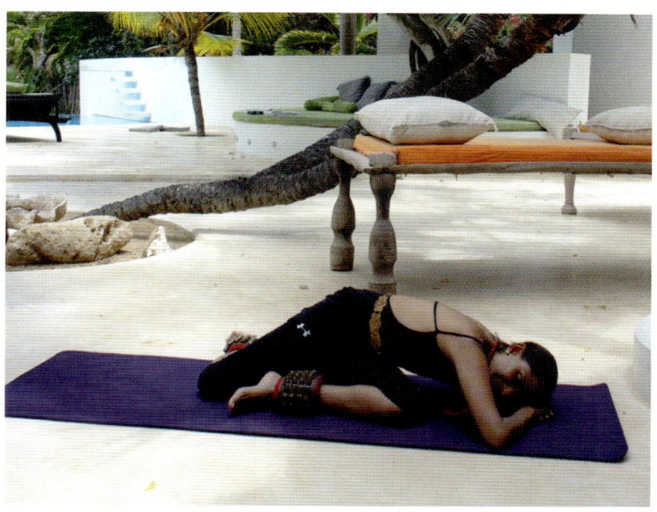

SWASTIKASANA
Resting Auspicious

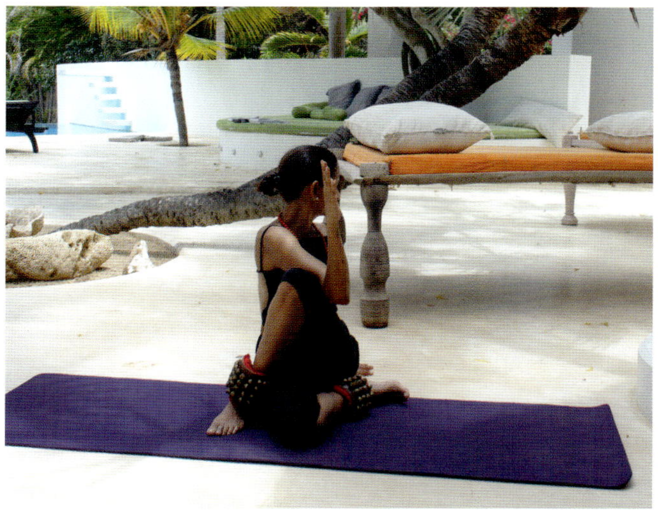

ARDHA MATSYENDRASANA
Half Lord of the Fish

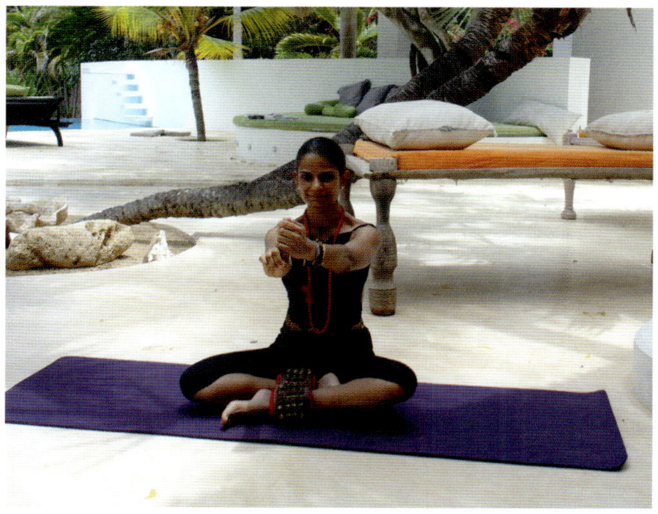

SIDDHASANA & AJNACHAKRAMUDRA
Seated Accomplished & Clarity

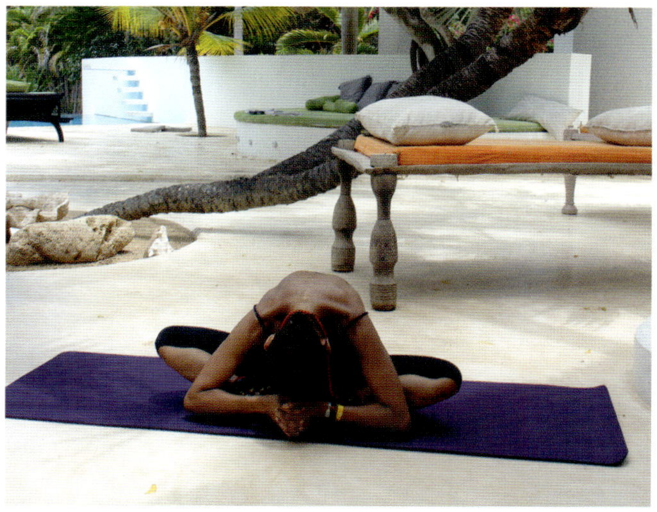

BADDHA KONASANA
Cobbler

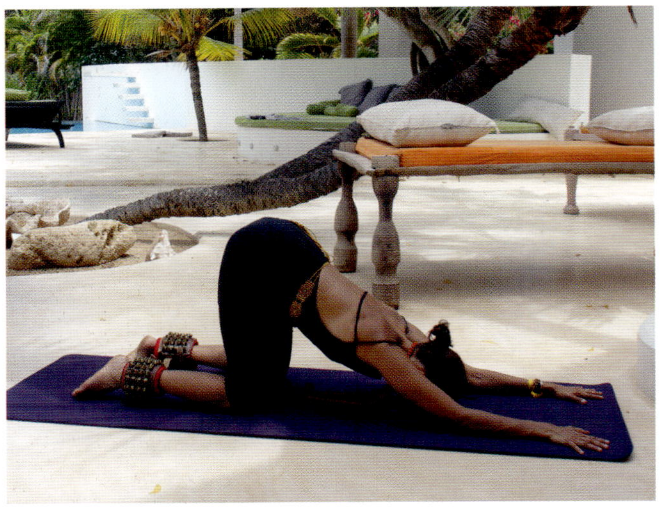

UTTANA SHISHOSANA
Puppy Dog

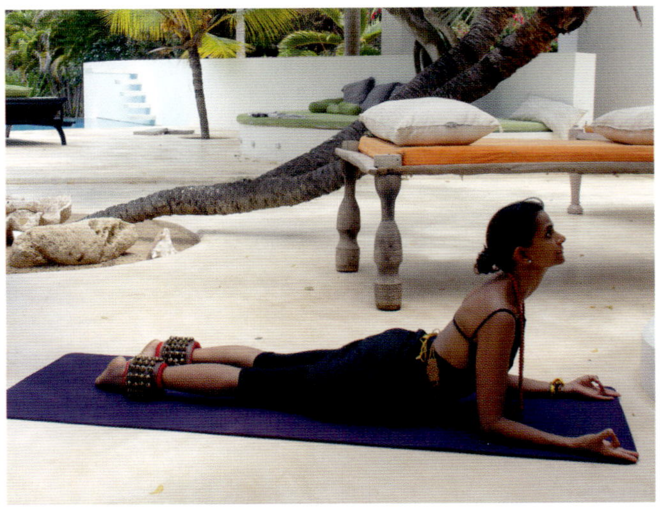

NIRAVALASANA & PRITHVIMUDRA
Sphinx & Assimilation

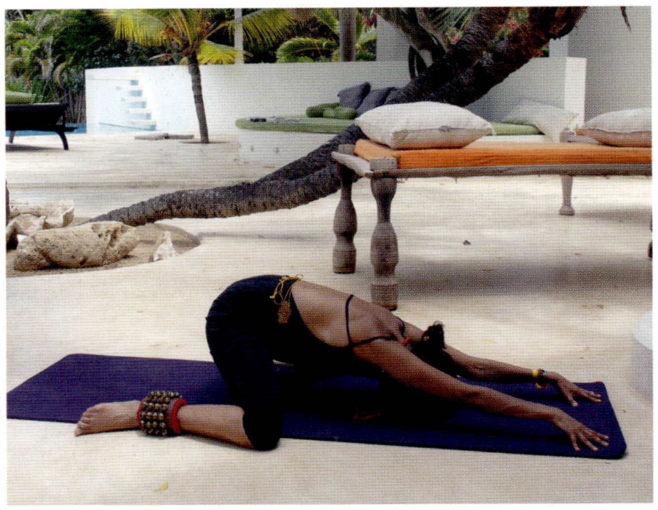

SHISHU BHEKASANA
Baby Frog

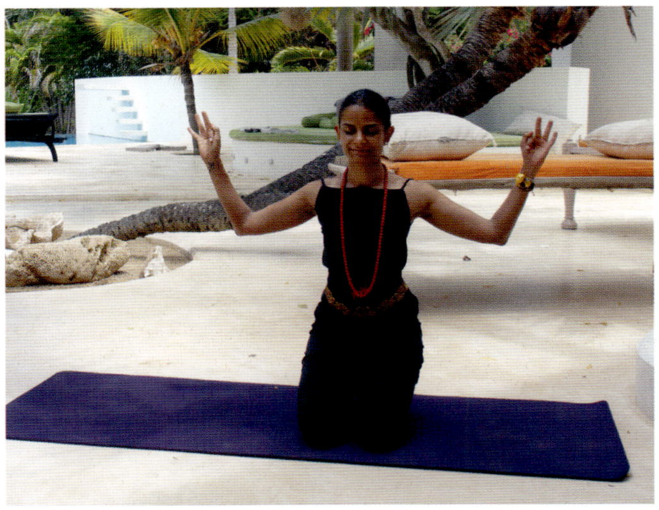

VAJRASANA & VAYUMUDRA
Thunderbolt & Serenity

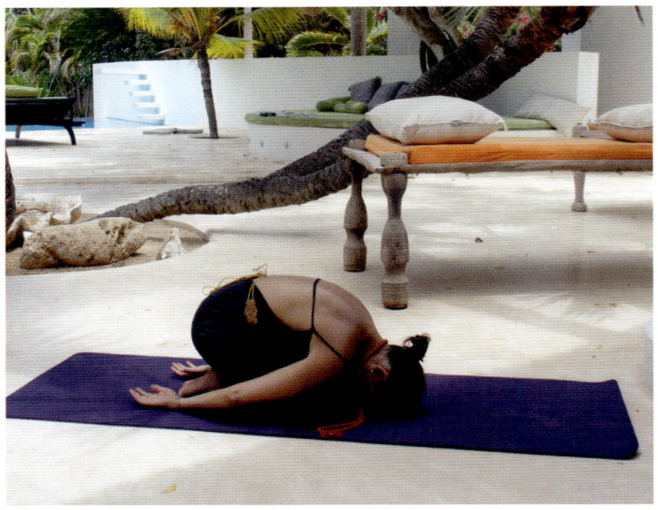

BALASANA
Child's

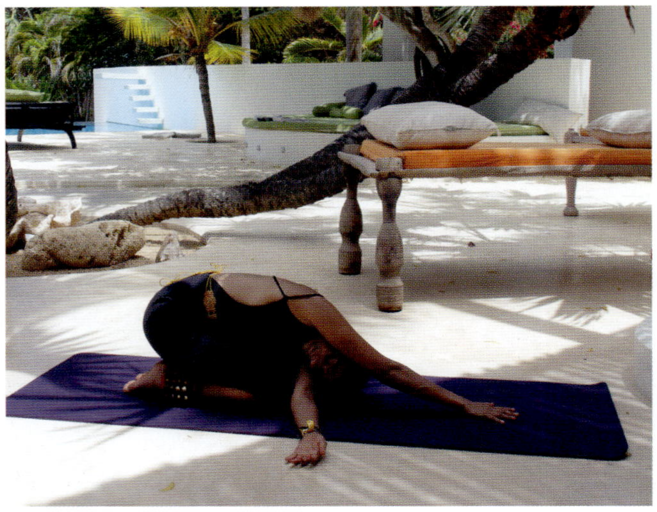

URDHVA MUKHA PASASANA
Thread the Needle

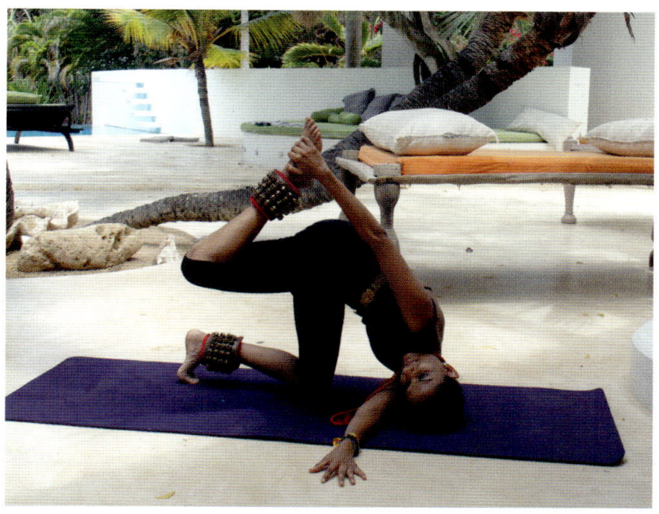

EKA PADA URDHVA MUKHA PASASANA
Silk Loom

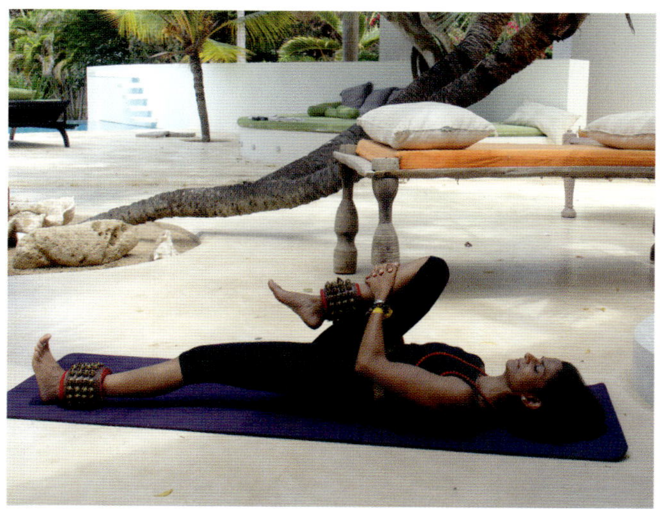

APANASANA
Wind Removing

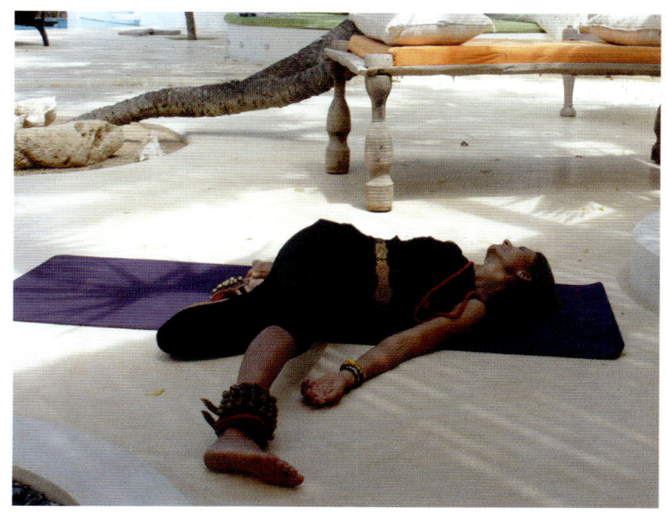

GHODASANA
Centaur

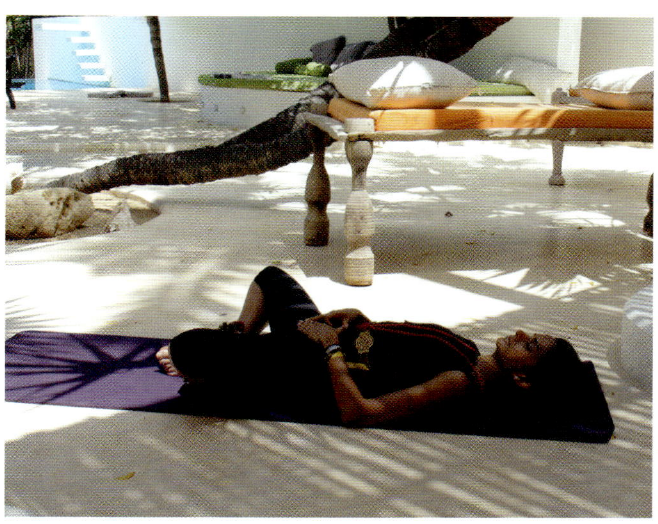

SUPTA BADDHA KONASANA & SHANKHAVARTAMUDRA
Supine Cobbler & Intuition

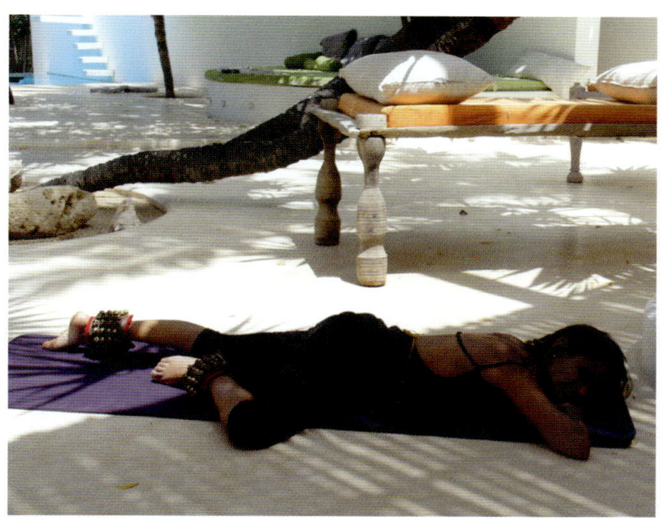

YANG SAVASANA
Resting Recovery

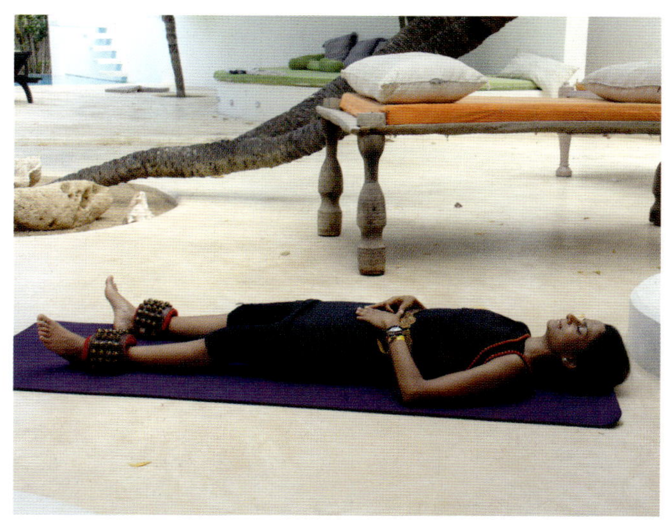

SAVASANA
Resting

BRAHMA KARKATA • Cancer

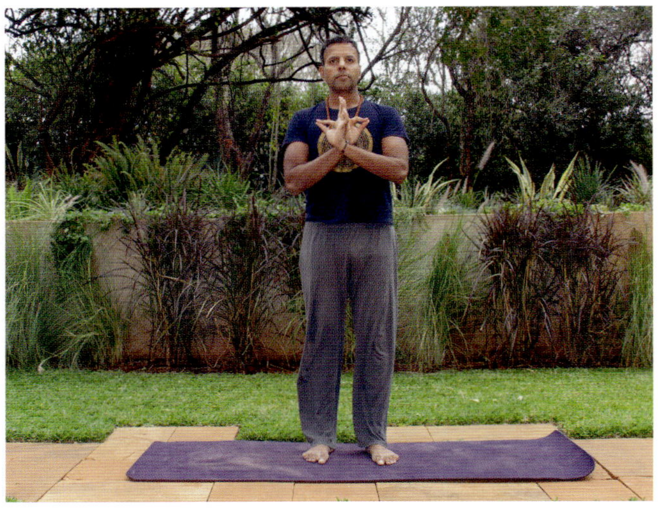

SAMASTHITI & ABHAYAHRIDAYAMUDRA
Equal Standing & Rejuvenation

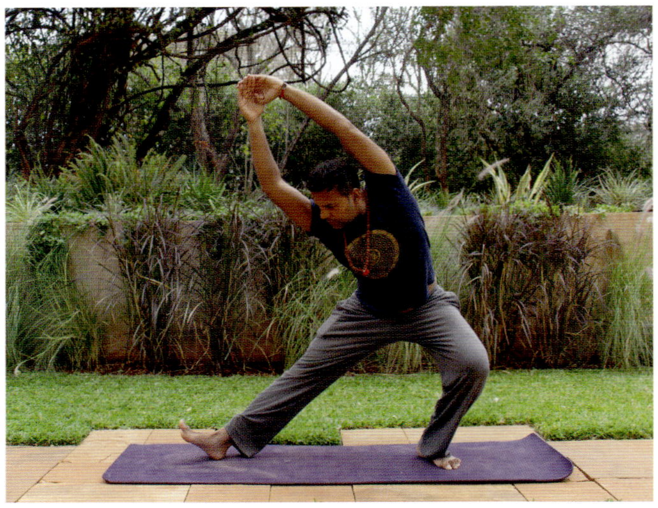

PARSVA URDHVA HASTASANA & KIRITAMUDRA
Standing Half Moon & Crowning

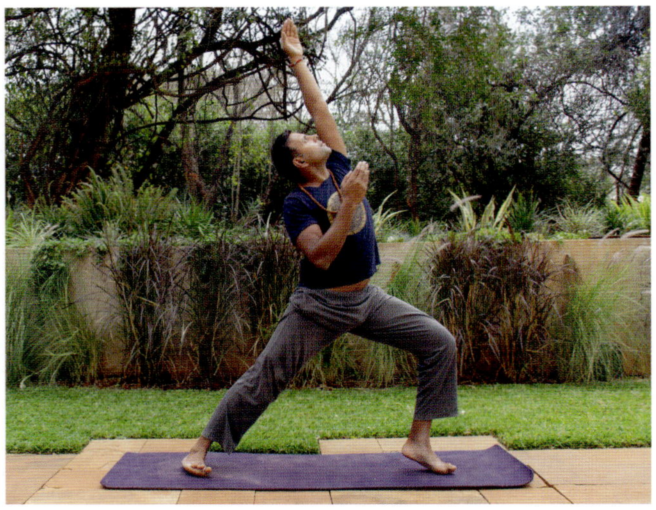

ARDHA UTKATA KONASANA
Half Goddess

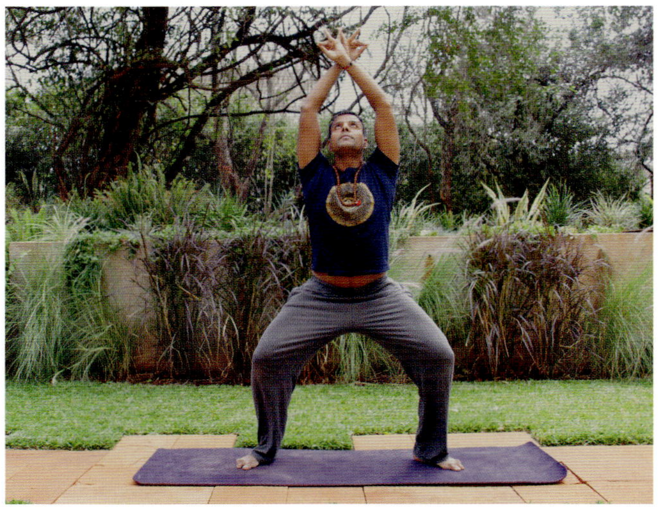

UTKATA KONASANA & KILAKAMUDRA
Goddess & Union

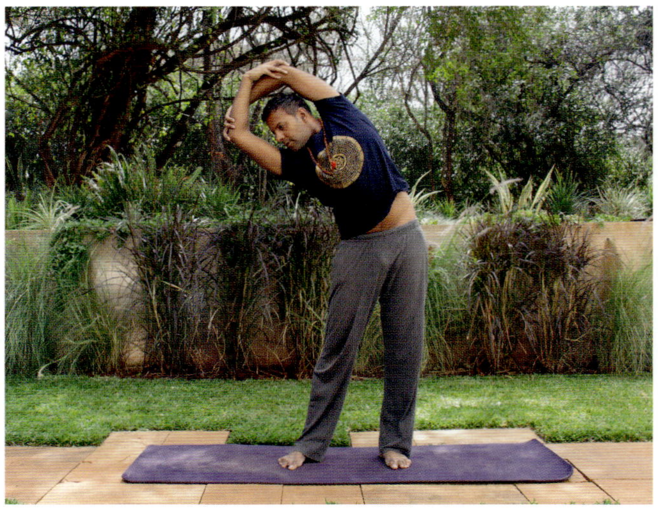

PARSVA URDHVA KOHANEESANA
Standing Half-Moon Elbow

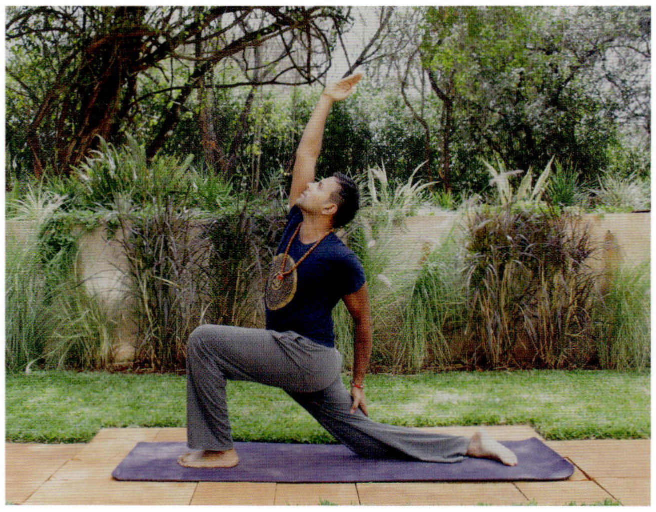

ANJANEYASANA
Low Lunge

In Brahma Karkata, we are initiating the season of elemental water. This constellation of asanas encourages fluid movement, treating the body as an irrigation system, gently guiding the fascia and connective tissues and supporting the structural alignment of our bones. Through somatic movement, we deepen the mind-body connection to listen for signals of any imbalance. Guided breath work oxygenates nutritious blood to vital organs and consequently all systems of the body. The mudras bring rejuvenation and a crowning sense of union to all aspects of the self. This creates a nurturing safe space of harmony, restoration, and tranquility.

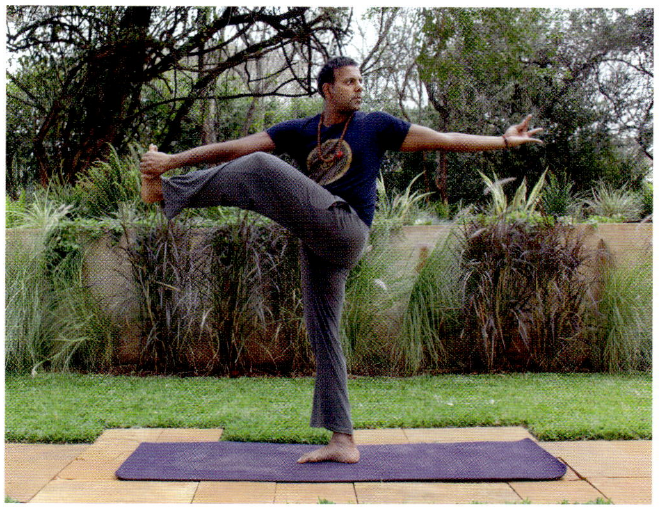

PAUDHASANA & BHRAMARAMUDRA
Plant & Harmony

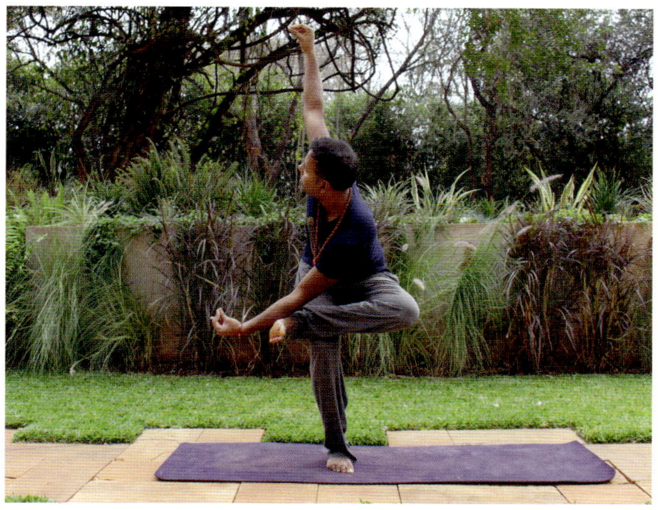

JIRAAFASANA & MRITSAMJIVANIMUDRA
Giraffe & Restoration

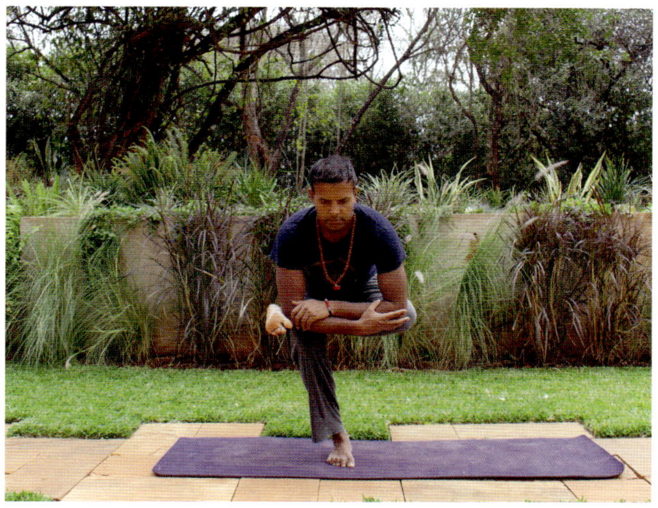

TADA KAPOTASANA
Standing Pigeon

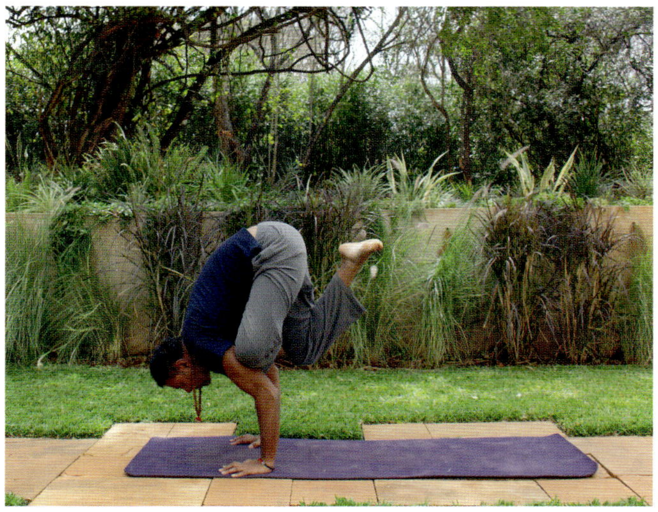

EKA PADA GALAVASANA
Flying Pigeon

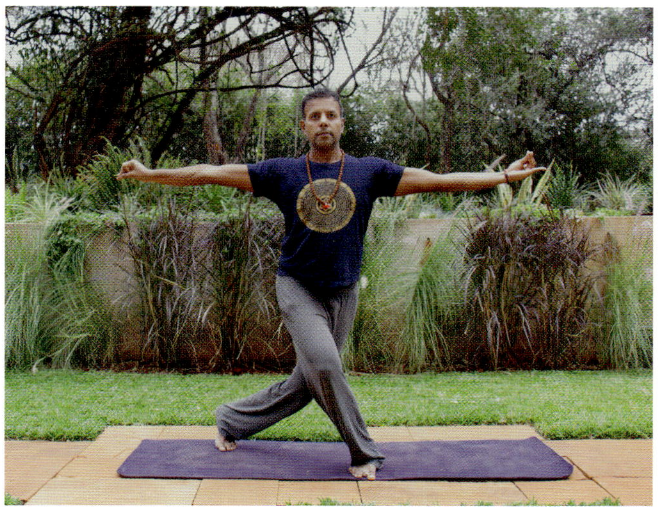

VIMANASANA & HRIDAYAMUDRA
Flight & Tranquility

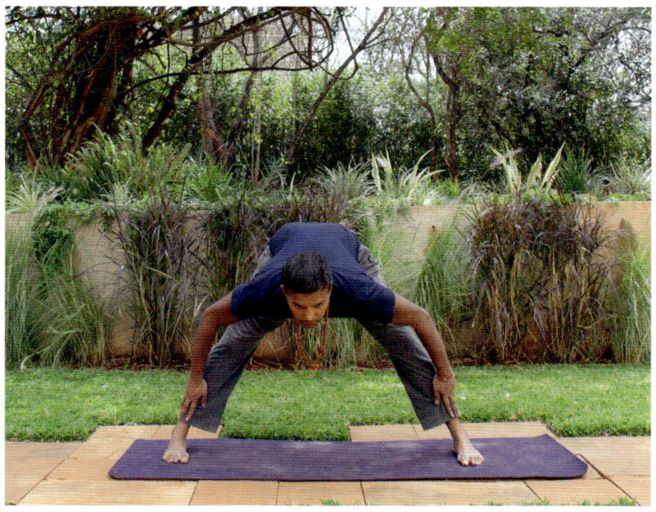

PRASARITA PADOTTANASANA EKAM
Wide-Legged Standing Forward Bend I

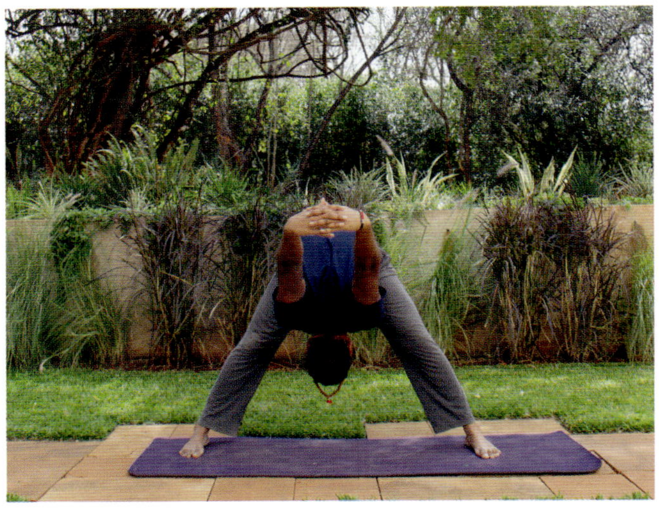

PRASARITA PADOTTANASANA TRINI
Wide-Legged Standing Forward Bend III

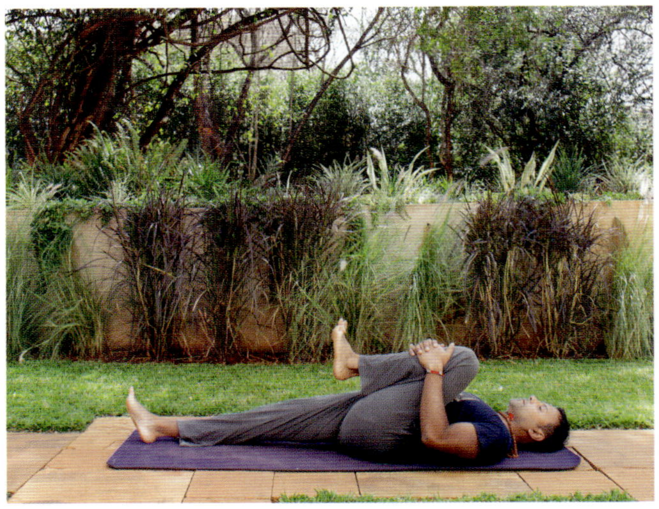

APANASANA
Wind Removing

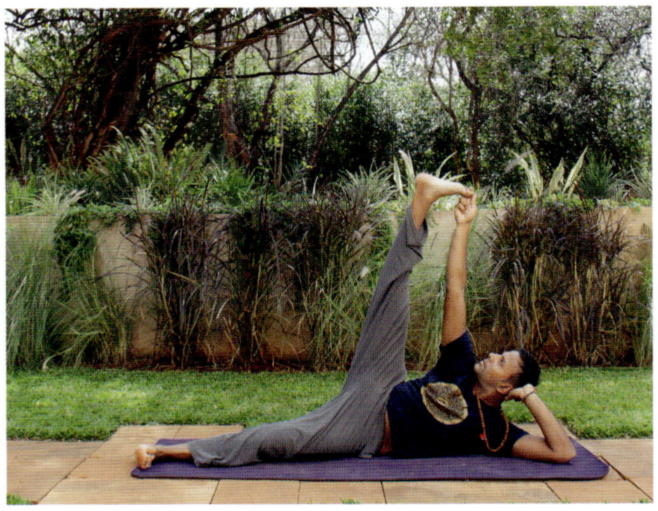

ANANTASANA
Sleeping Vishnu

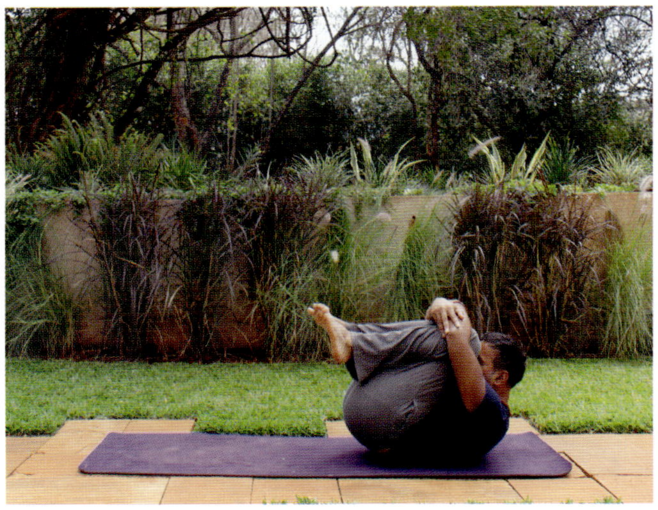

PAVANAMUKTASANA
Wind Relieving

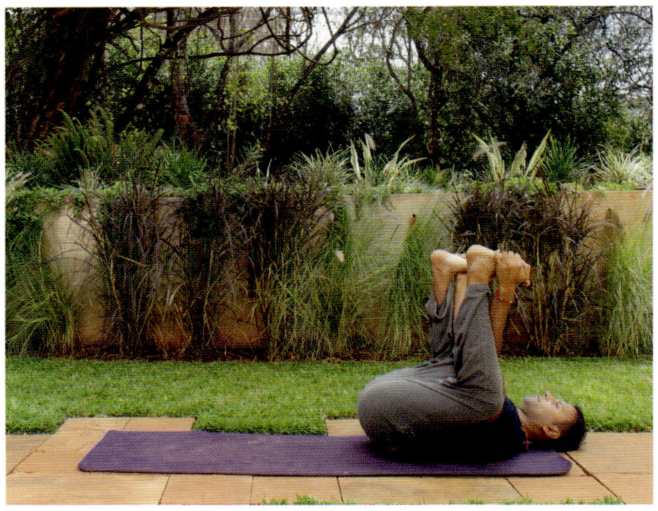

ANANDA BALASANA
Happy Baby

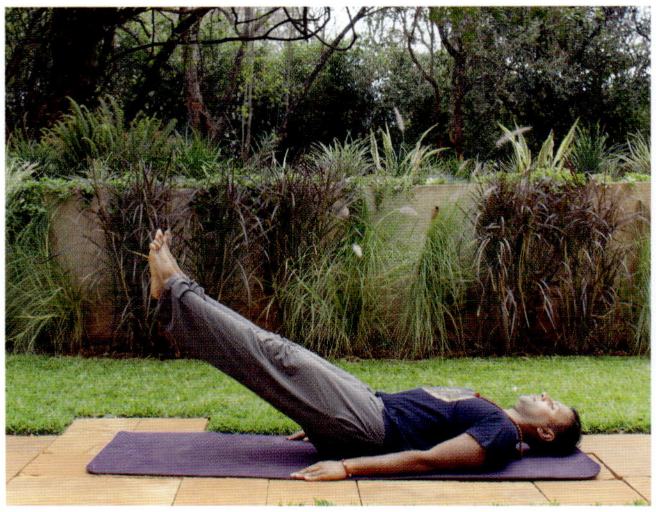

UTTANA PADASANA
Raised Legs

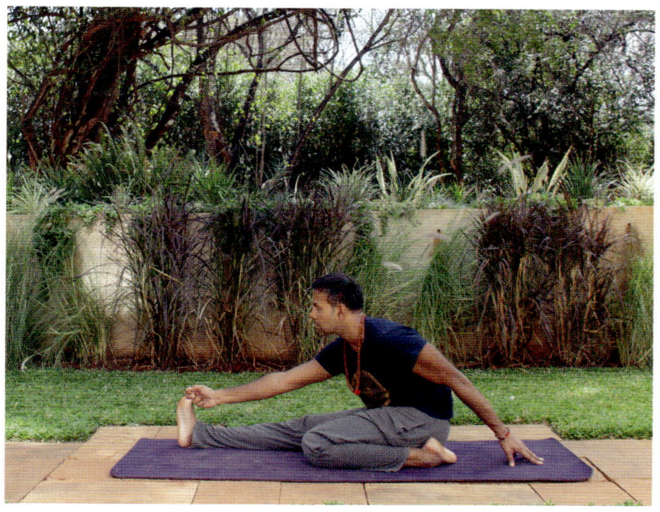

TRIANGA MUKHAIKAPADA PASCHIMOTTANASANA
One-Legged Folded Forward Bend

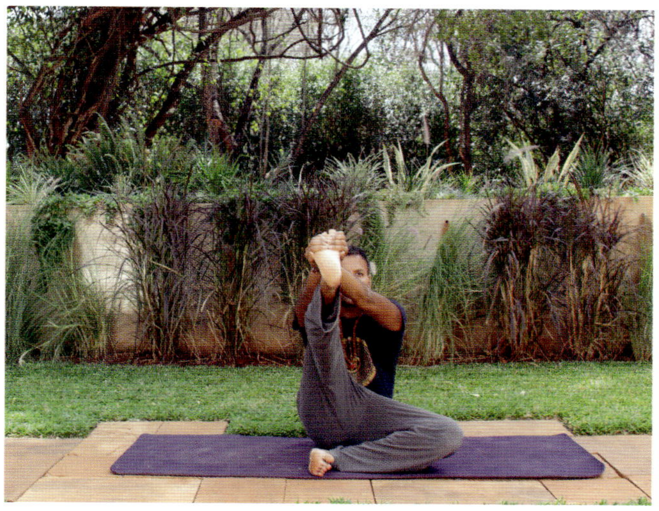

KROUNCHASANA
Heron

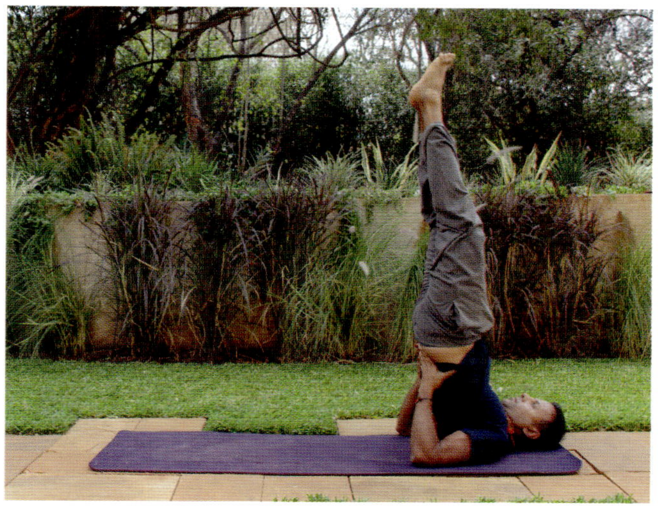

SARVANGASANA
Shoulder Stand

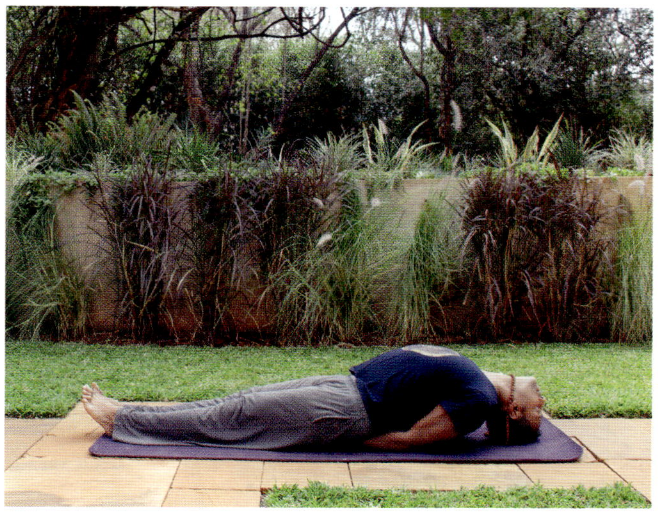

MATSYASANA
Fish

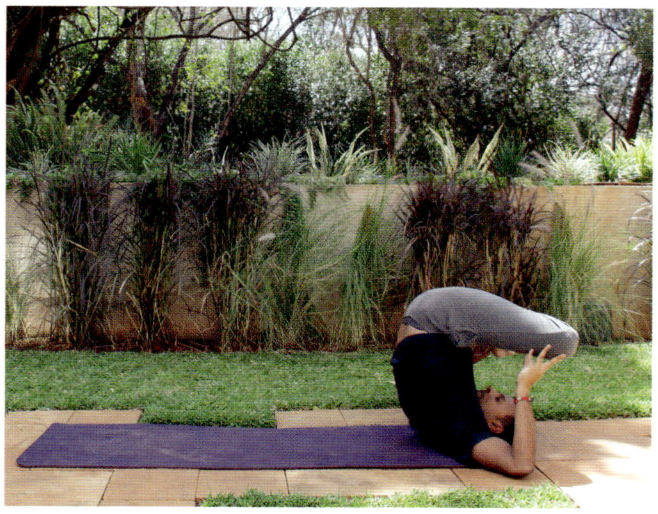

URDHVA PADMASANA
Upward Lotus

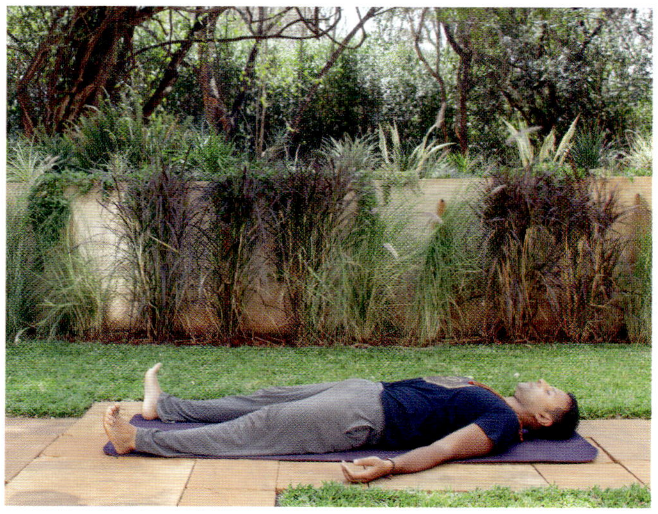

SAVASANA
Resting

BOOST VITALITY

In Brahma Simha / Leo, we are in the settled season of fire. Our ancestors' discovery of fire changed the pathway of humanity. We were able to isolate the fire element to bring warmth, illuminate the night, and protect ourselves against danger. In Brahma Kanya / Virgo, we are in the shifting season of earth, which is our ability to build and change the way we work the land. In modern times, we have turned into a sad, sedentary species. The constellation of sequences in this chapter gets us moving and continues our human journey along a more elevated path. You reap what you sow in the body, and this can inspire you to live a healthier, more wholesome life.

In a world where everything seems available immediately, we live in impoverished minds and treat our bodies without the care they really need. Your body is always talking to you, and when you are ill, it is shouting louder so you can hear. Perhaps we should start by listening to the body more and the fractious mind less. By moving away from the survival mode that life puts us in through stress, we can cultivate a better way of living, with yoga bringing physical agility and mental clarity. This creates a sense of liveliness, robustness, and an overall positive mood.

Brahma Yoga offers asanas such as twists and intricate binds that help improve our health and well-being. The asanas offered in this chapter bring vitality in helping improve circulation by increasing blood flow and stimulating the lymphatic system. By cleansing our system regularly, we stimulate and improve the digestive system and eliminate waste and toxins from the body. Practicing yoga asanas that focus on the torso, then move outward to the limbs, helps move the flow of blood through the digestive organs, which can help support the liver to naturally detoxify.

Also, it is estimated that around 70 percent of waste is eliminated through our lungs just by the process of breathing, so we can directly and instantly boost vitality by increasing the oxygen levels in our blood through conscious breath. Over time, and with regular practice, you will improve respiratory function, increase your lung capacity, and strengthen the supportive respiratory muscles. Poses such as camel and advanced variations can also help open up the chest.

According to Brahma Yoga, the elixir of youth that vitality brings has nothing to do with your actual age. What is important is how you choose to live your life each day, hour, minute, and moment. The asanas in this chapter will help you improve cardiovascular health. This lowers blood pressure, improves heart rate variability, and increases cardiovascular endurance, which can help reduce the risk of heart disease and stroke as we age. This will inoculate you from some of the usual ailments and chronic health conditions that can impact longevity. The asanas improve our practice in a precise way, and the inversion balances boost our confidence and concentration levels.

Practicing Brahma Yoga enriches our lives by enabling us to create our own personalized rituals. By living better, we can increase our life span, improve our quality of life, maintain our cognitive function, and drastically reduce the risk of depression, anxiety, and loneliness.

BRAHMA YOGA SUTRAS

BRAHMA SIMHA • Leo

- All time exists now, and I am present and ready for life with all its vitality.
- I seek interconnectedness with all of life, and my truth resonates well with the right people.
- When I understand the inception of my desires, I can experience bliss and pleasure without craving, fixation, shame, or dependency.
- I nurture preservation while time listens patiently to the drones and demands of destiny's desire.
- Having greater awareness can bring me inner peace. I can and must take love right inside to activate positive changes in my life.
- I know that the best journeys meet at the intersection of doing things differently, taking chances, and ultimately trusting.
- I cannot be broken, and I am stronger than anything that can happen to me.
- By living my innateness, I am abundant, full of radiance, and can unlock the great secrets of life.
- Brahma Yoga helps me recognize the inherited privilege of being human, so I have benevolence for animals, plants, all sentient beings, and minerals. I care for their dignity and use on our shared planet.

BRAHMA KANYA • Virgo

- Through the purification of my thoughts, I process my emotions without unreasonably leaning on others.
- I believe in blossoming, and I inspire others and myself to be the best we can be.
- My virility is not only biological or existential. It is both sacred and sensual, so I am purposefully a lover of all of life.
- I am directly connected to my source and origin.
- The universe is filled with fertility and is cyclical, and all elements are in a state of constant change and evolution. My dreams are by my side; they form beneath the unseen.
- Brahma Yoga enables me to incorporate habits into my own personalized ritual, and through reflection, empowers me to enrich my life.
- In simplicity, I can find my purity.
- When I give love to myself fully, I can receive love and abundance from others without expectation.
- Although I may seek order, reality is abstract and subjective. If I dig deep, I will see that I live in a world of ideas and the structure of elements are simply reified into different forms.

I will not allow myself to be threatened

by any darkness that seeks to

realize itself through my process.

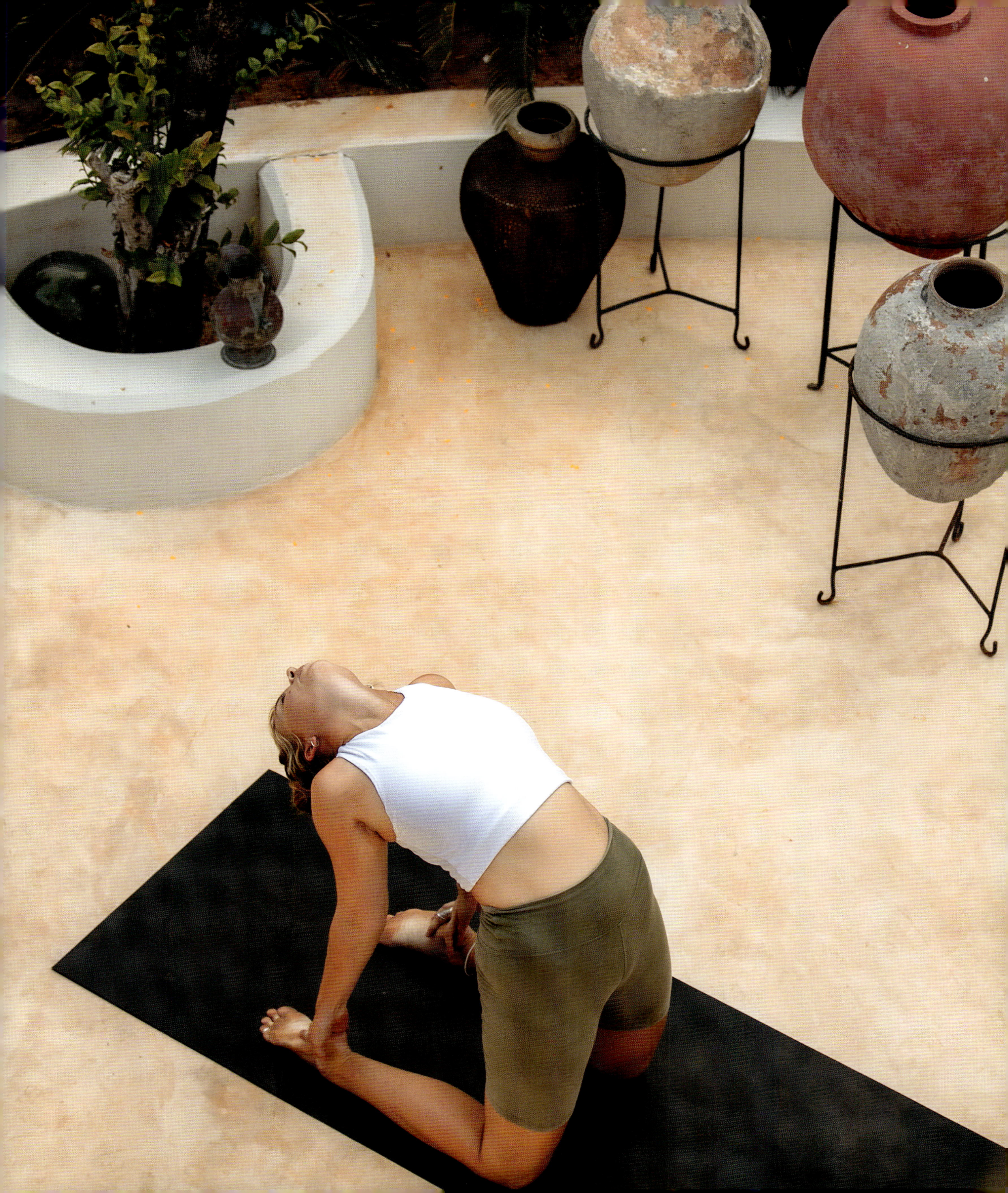

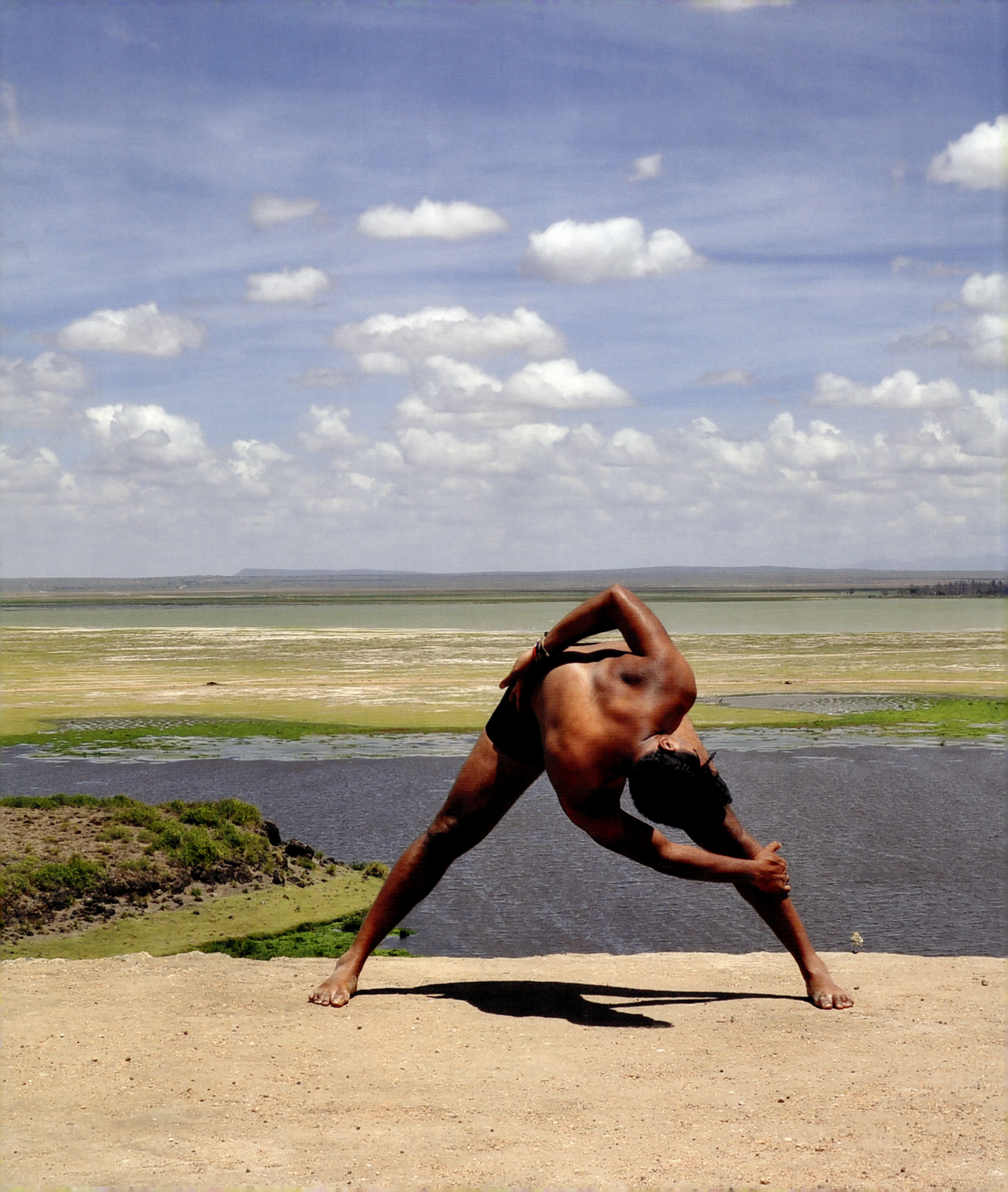

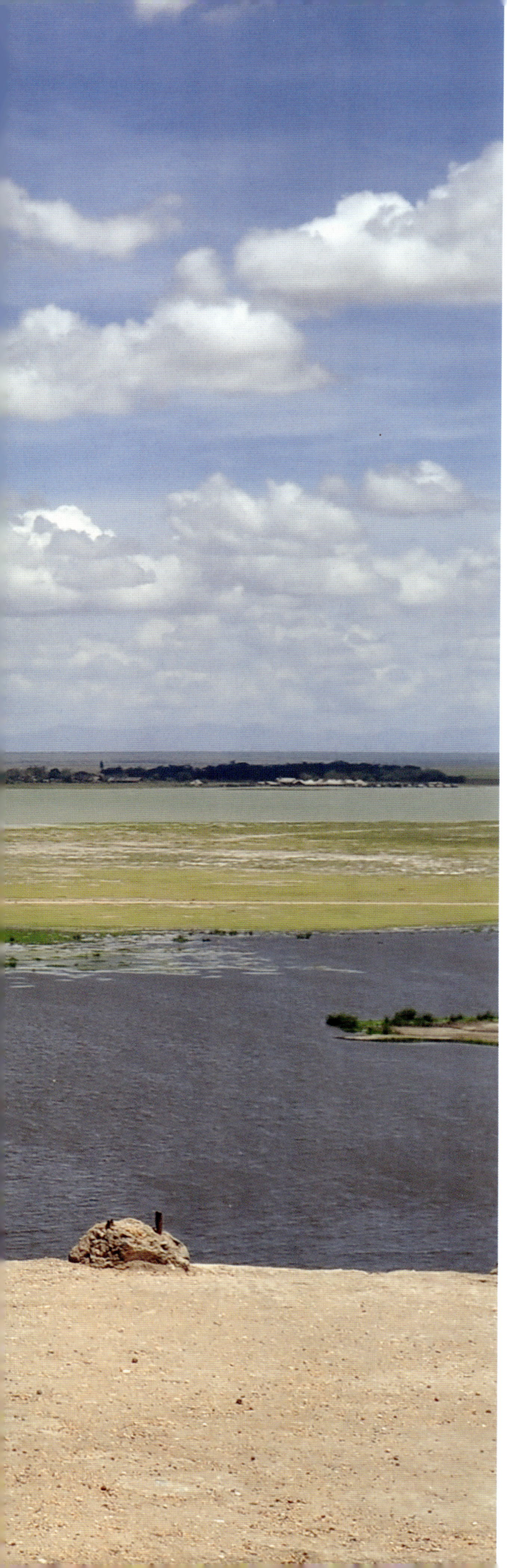

BADDHA PARIVRTTA PRASARITA PADOTTANASANA • Bound Twisted Wide-Legged Standing Forward Bend

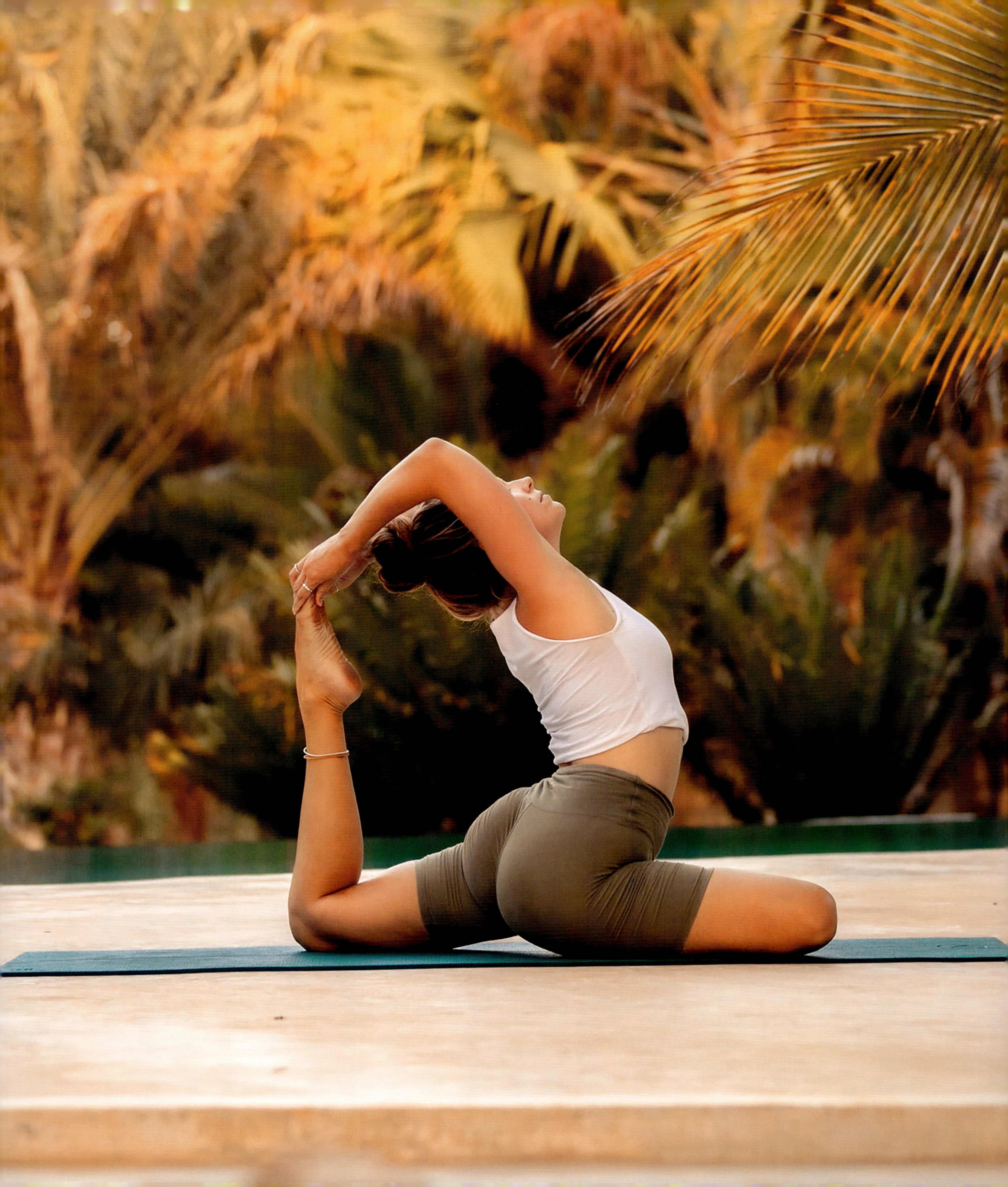

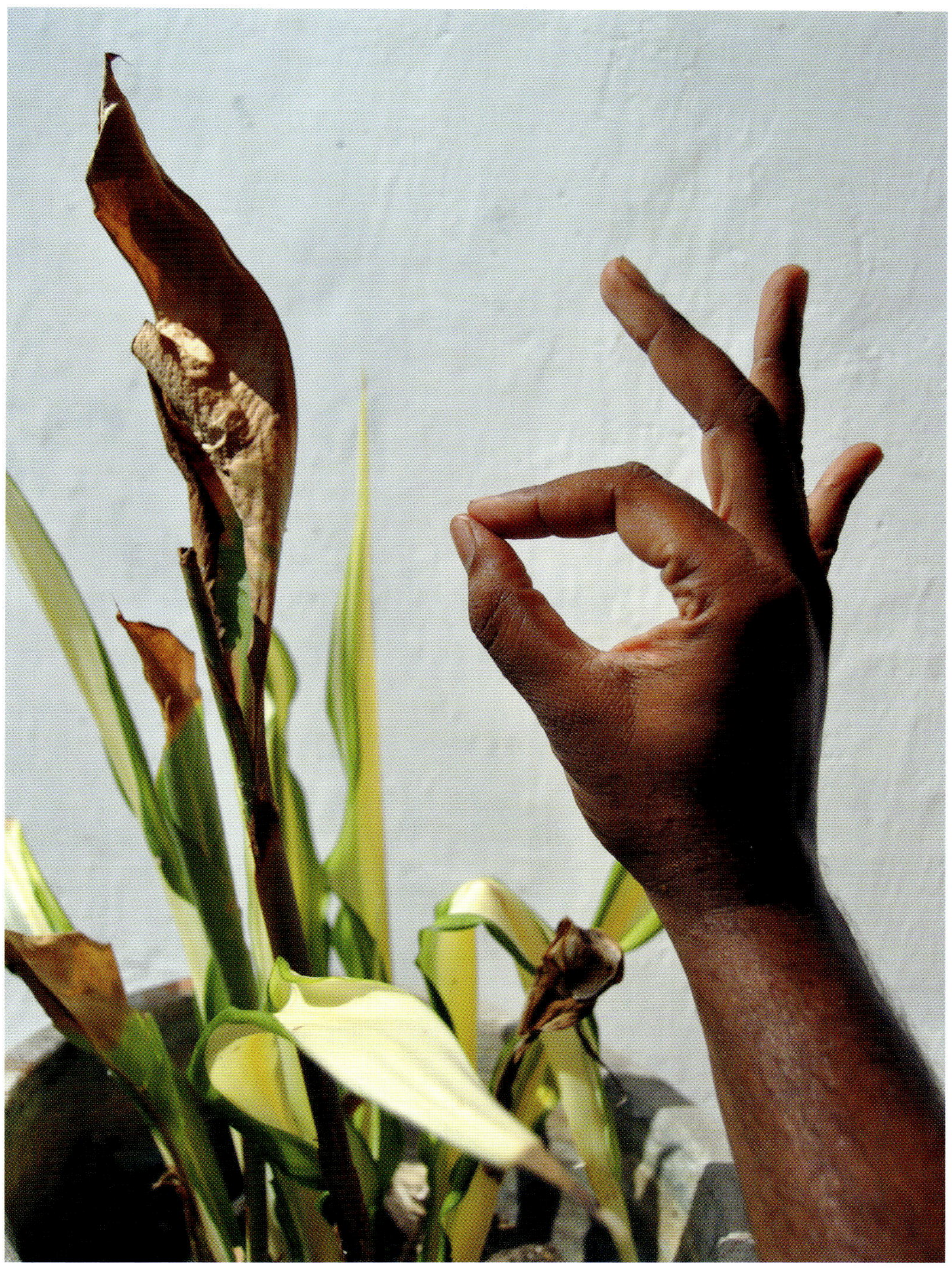

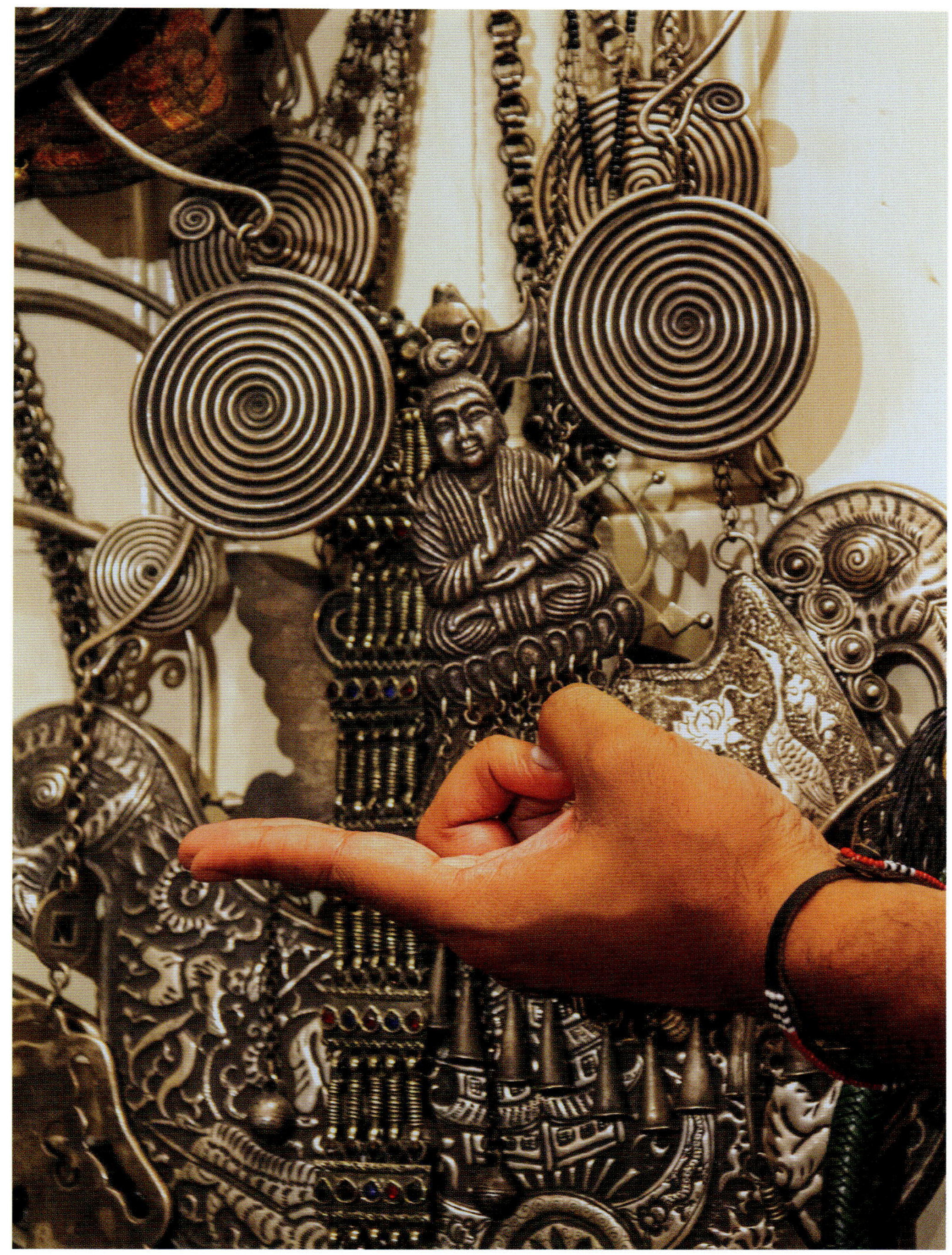

EKA PADA RAJAKAPOTASANA • King Pigeon

▲ **CHINMUDRA** • Awareness *(left)* **PRANAMUDRA** • Vitality *(right)*

I celebrate as my cells are

being rebuilt, replenished, and reformed

through a perpetual cosmic dance.

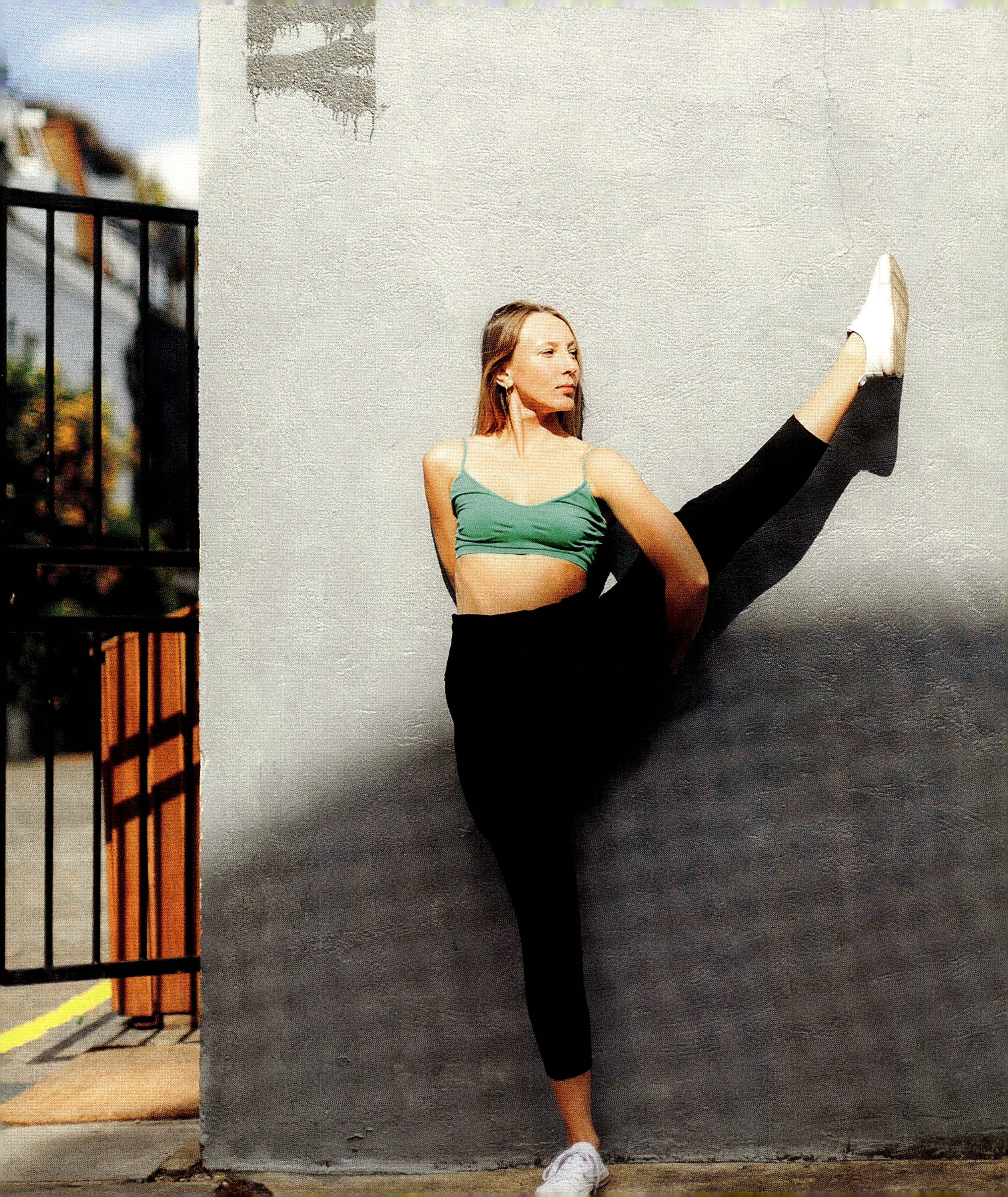

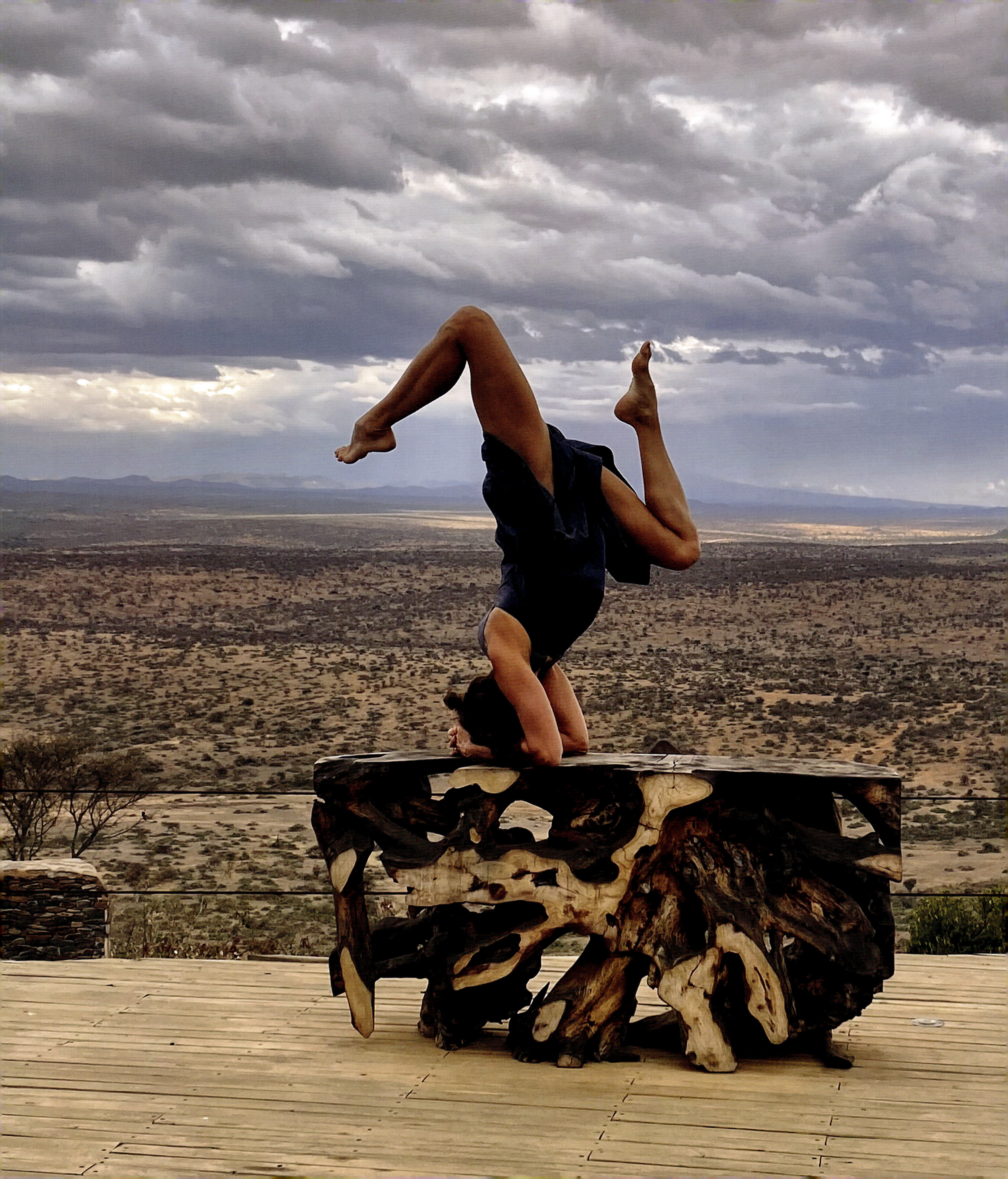

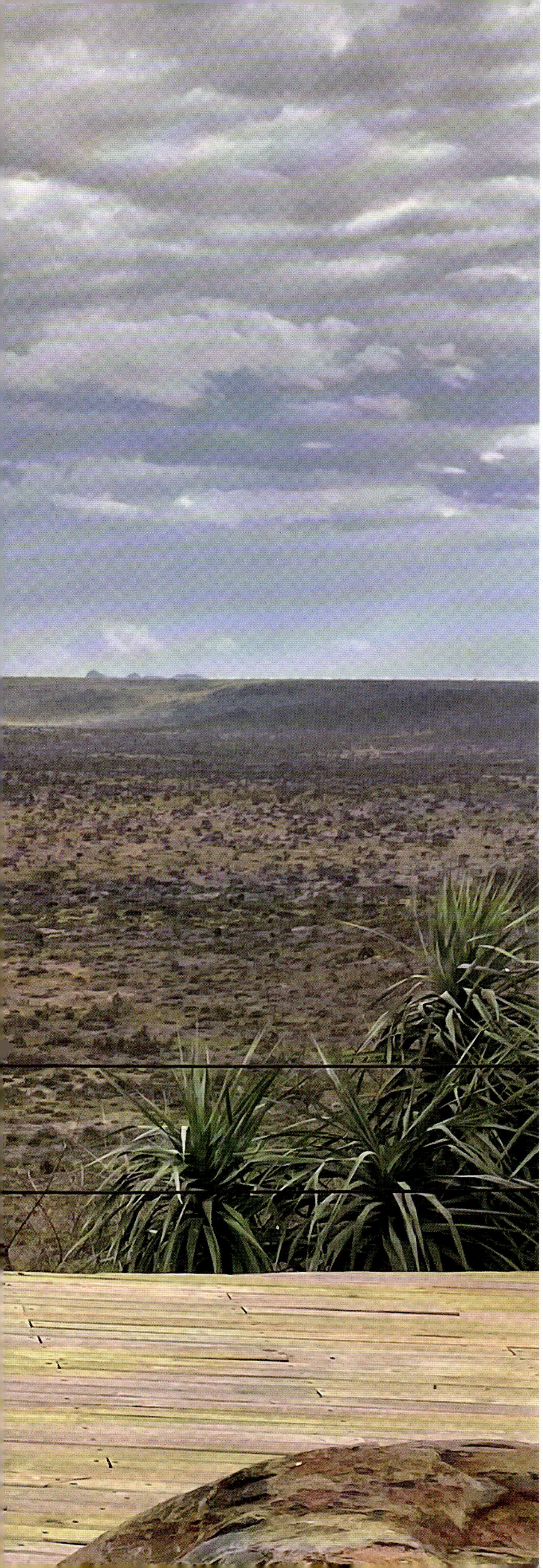

NIRALAMBA SIRSASANA · Extended Headstand

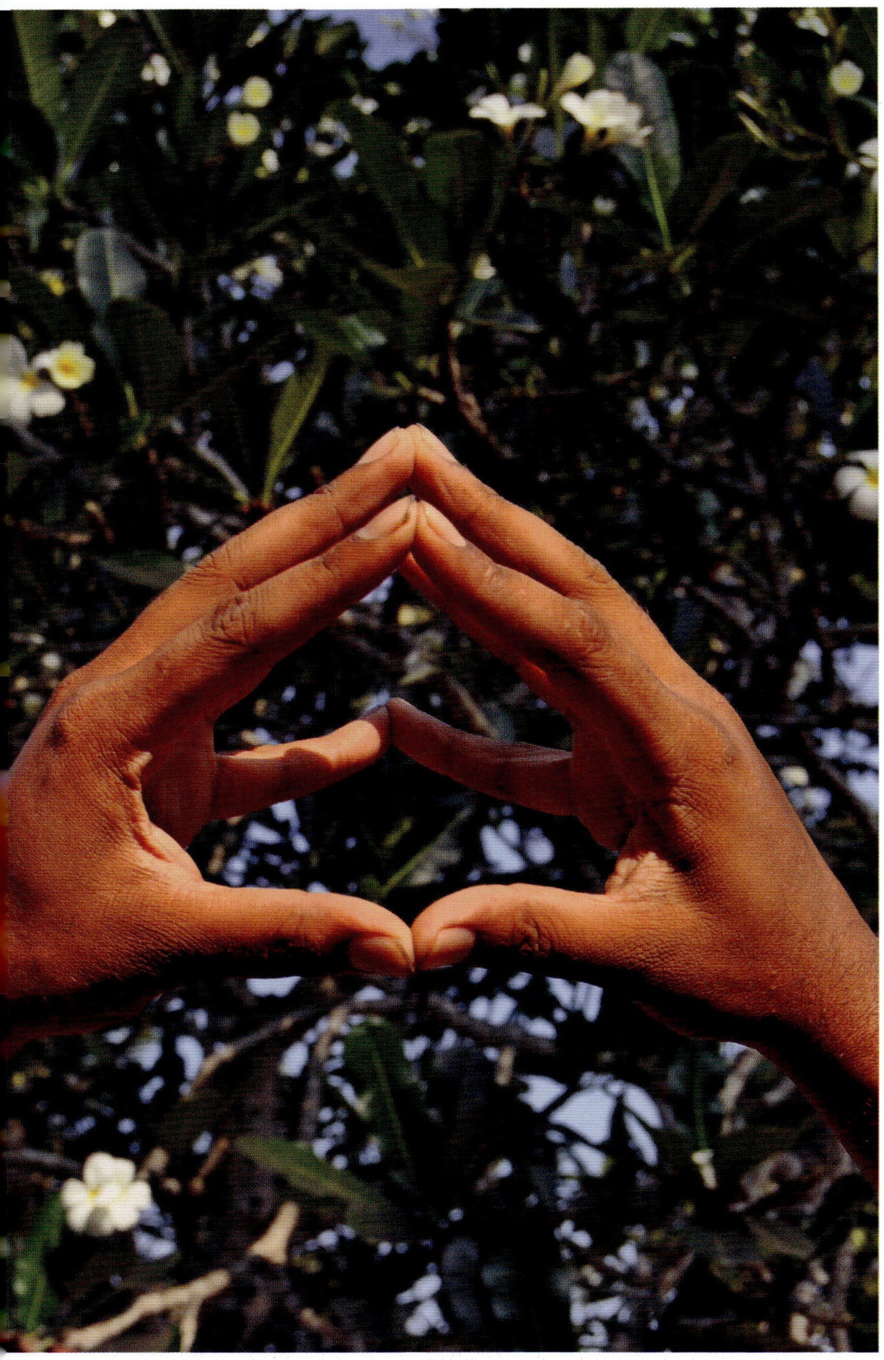

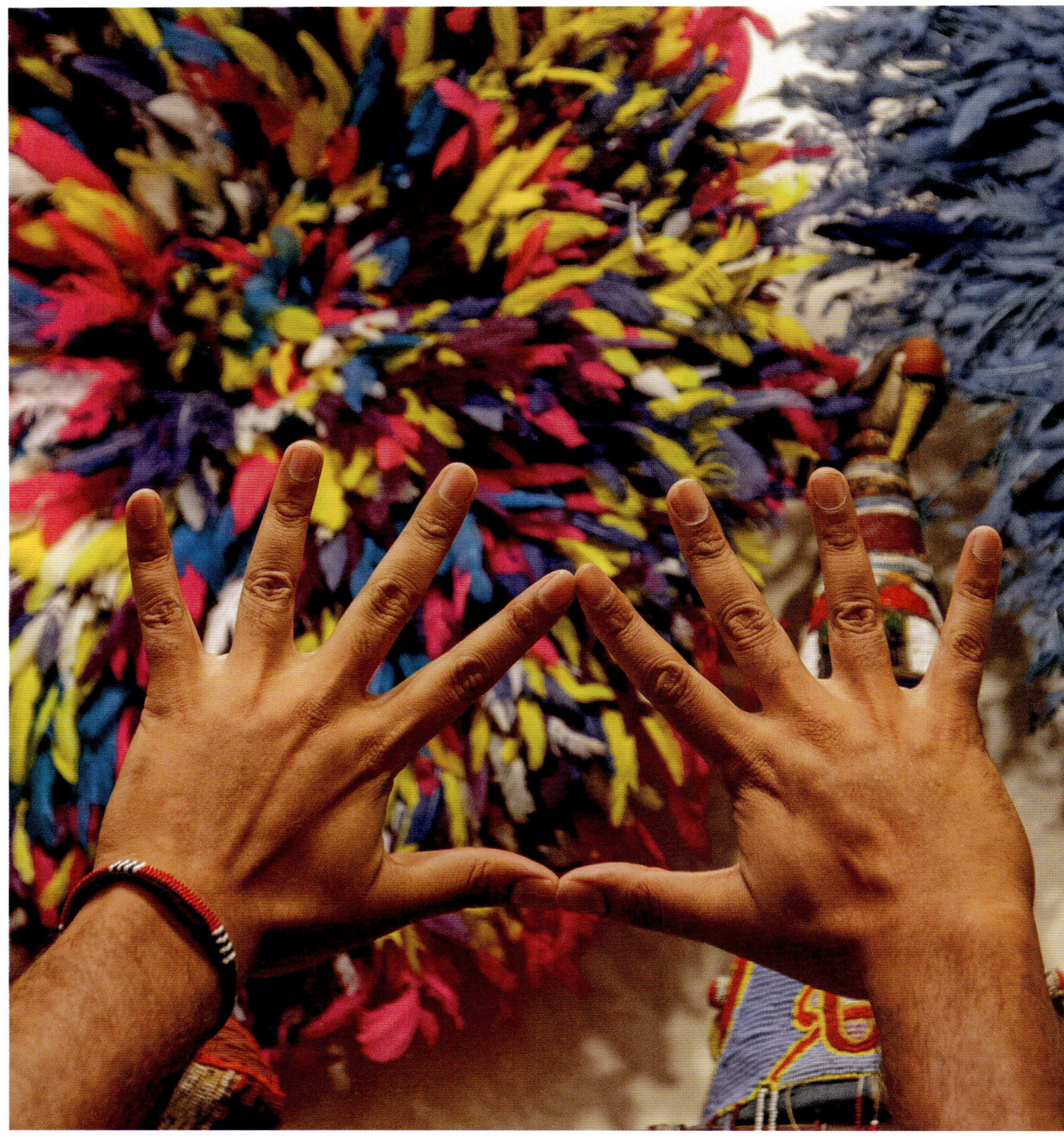

▲ **PANCHAMUKHAMUDRA** • Innateness *(left)* **SAHASARAMUDRA** • Interconnectedness *(right)*

PARIVRTTA BHARMANASANA • Twisted Tabletop

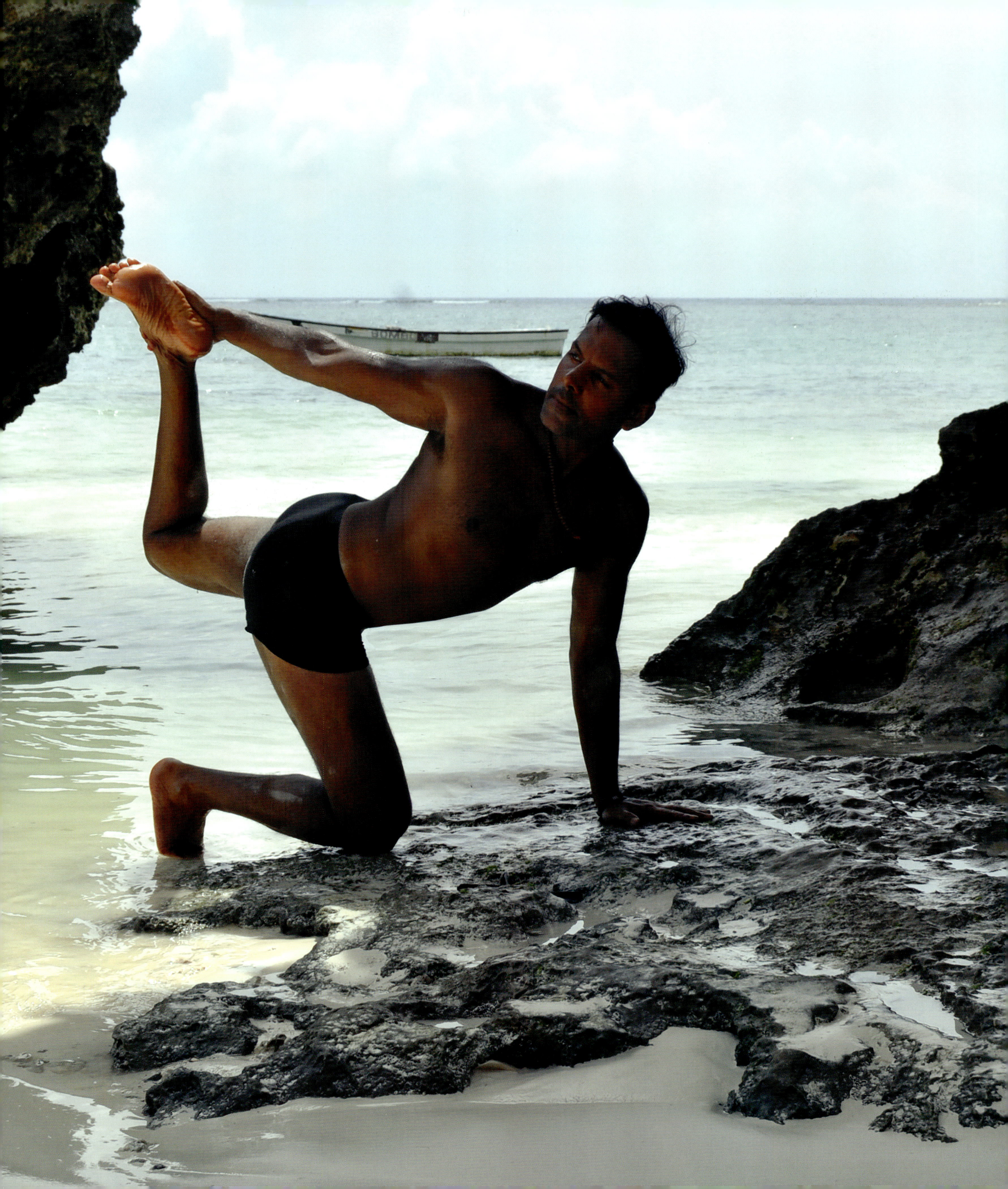

A seed is not yet a tree,

but it has everything it needs to be.

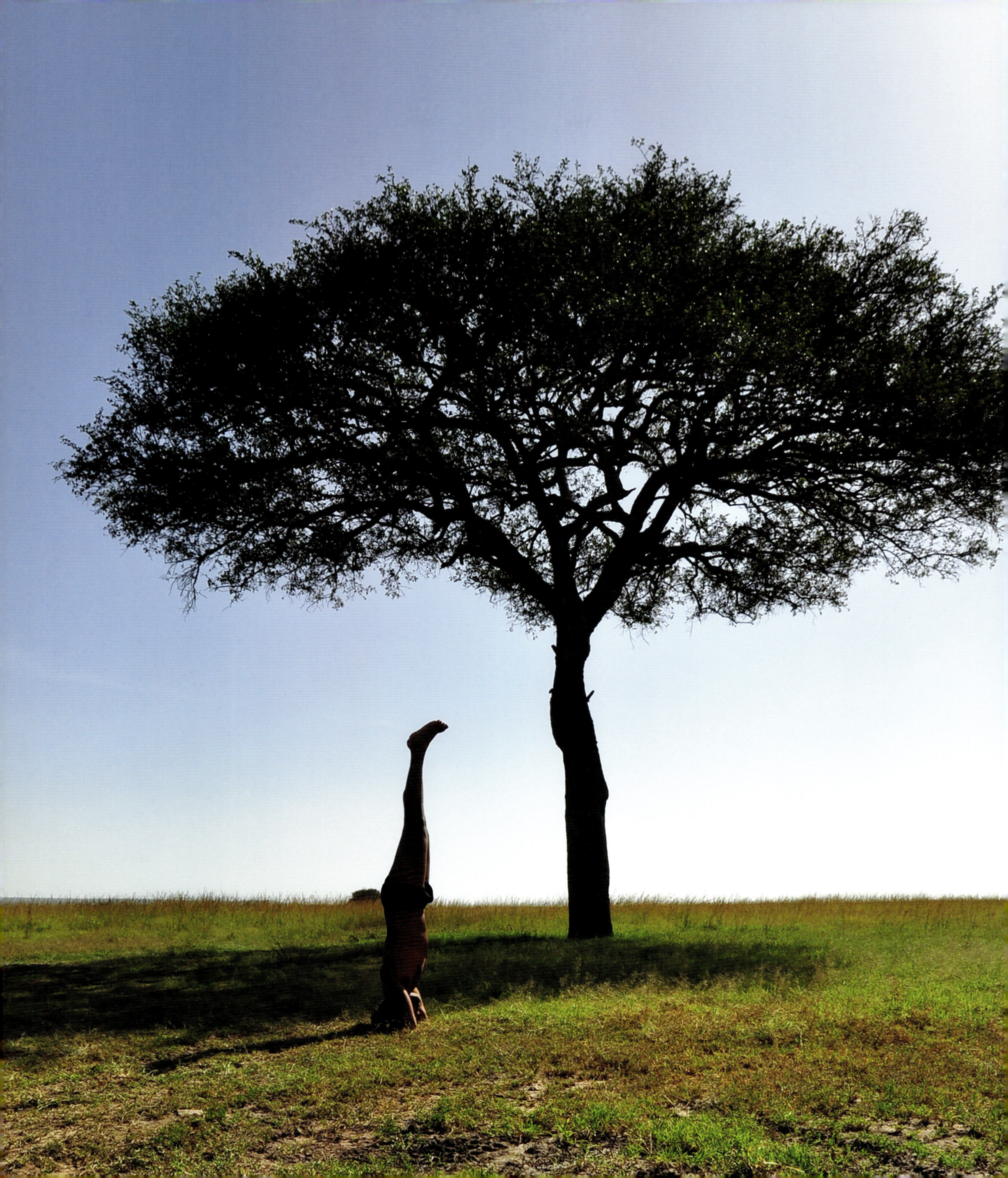

MATSYAANGANASANA · Mermaid

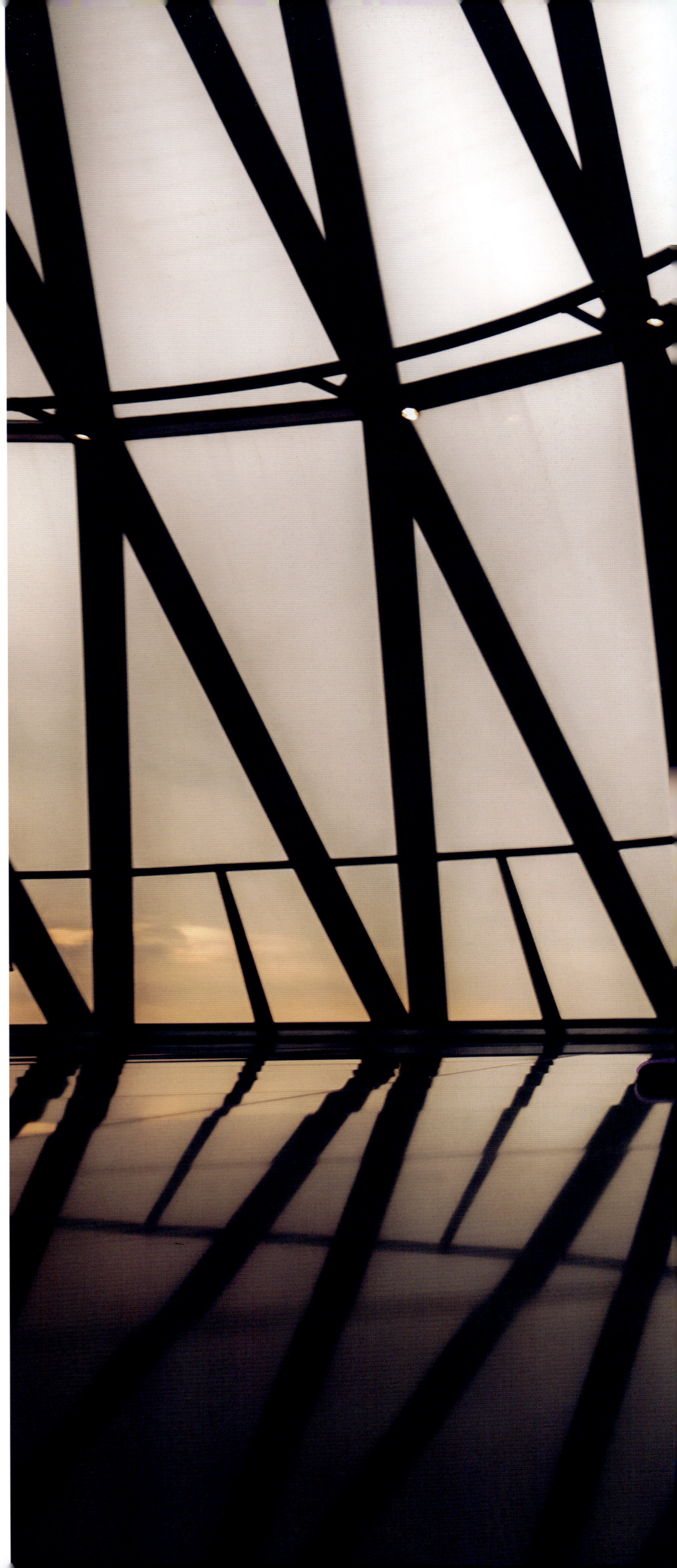

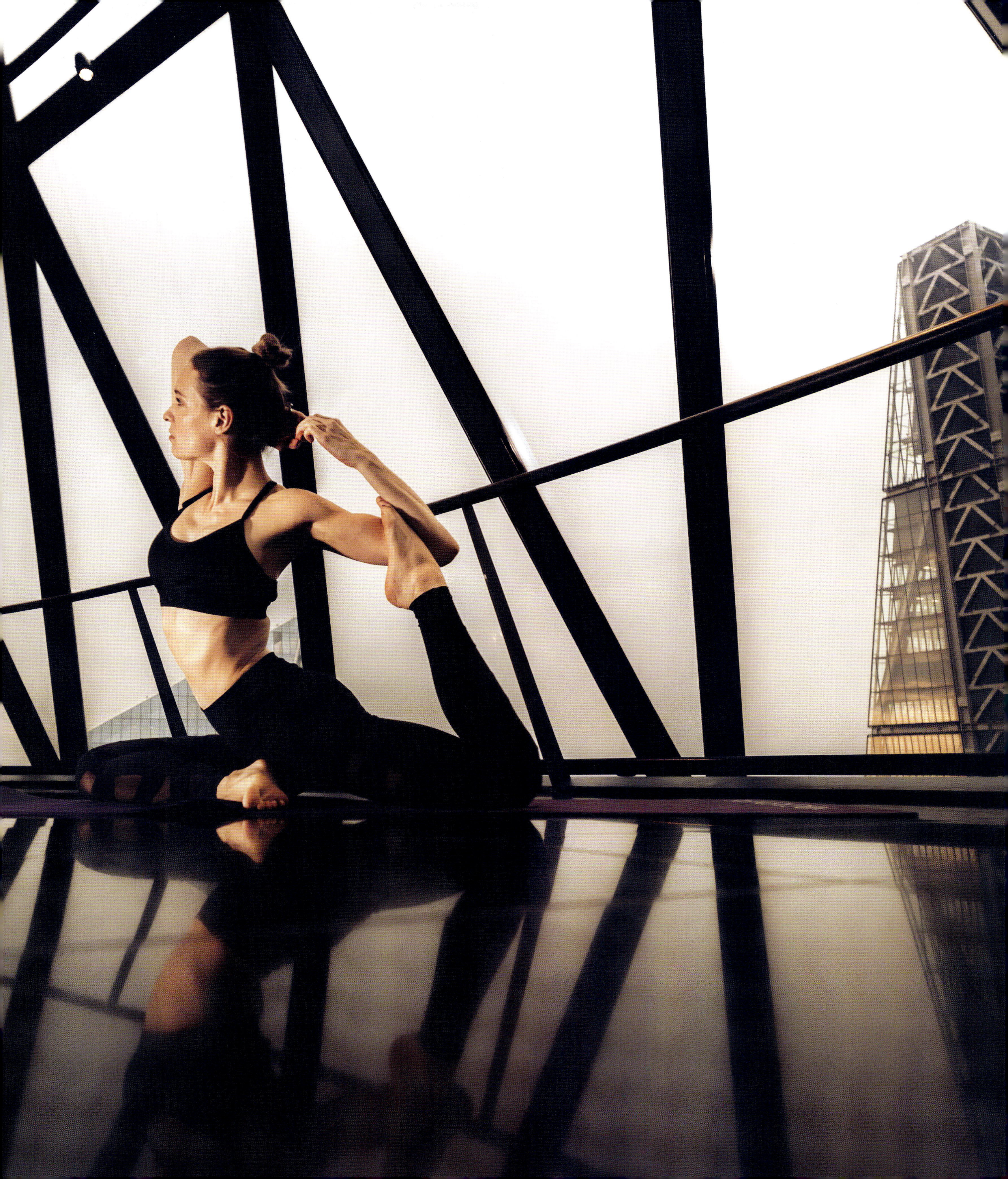

May all that is good in you

meet all that is good in this world.

Everything else can take care of itself.

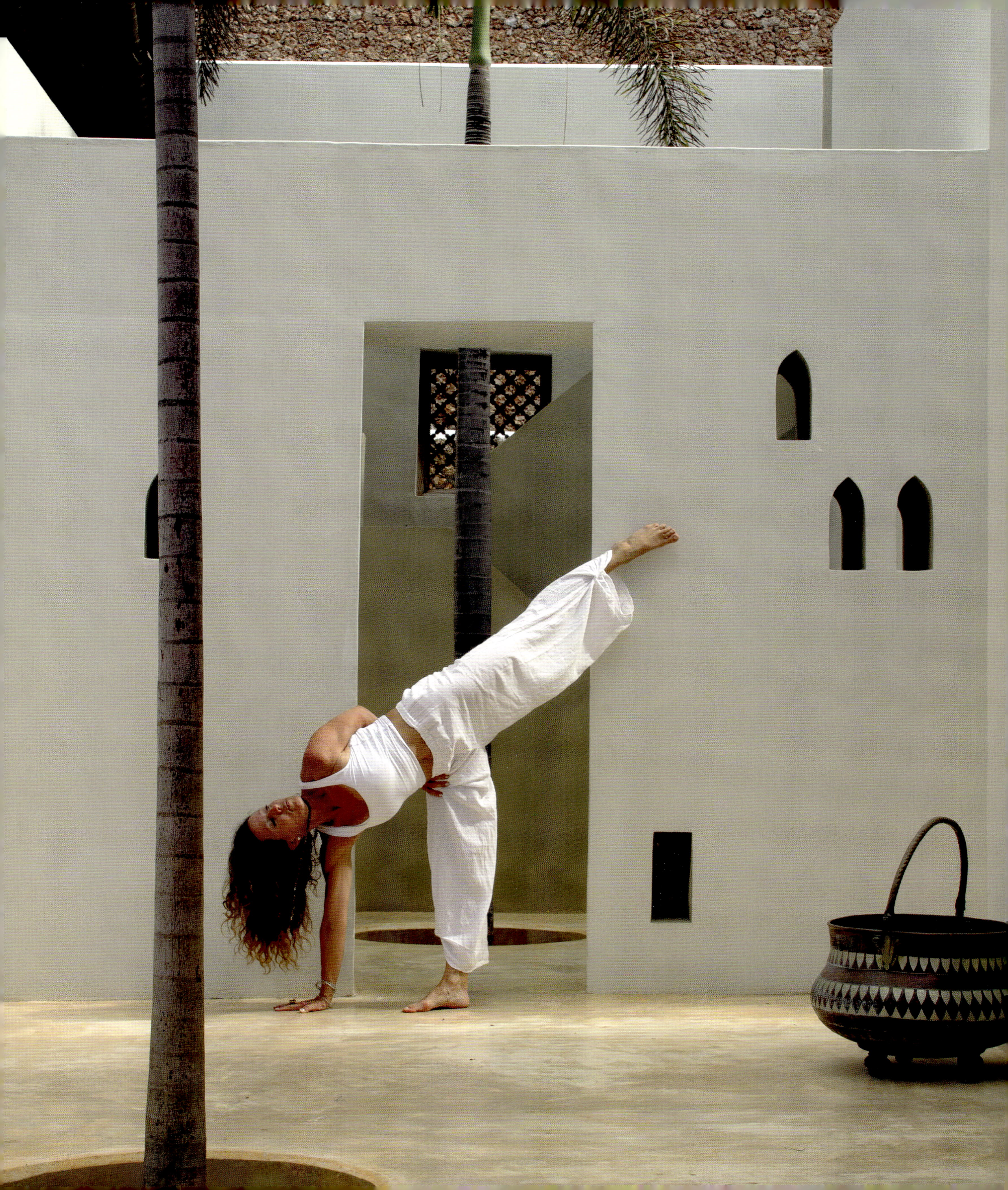

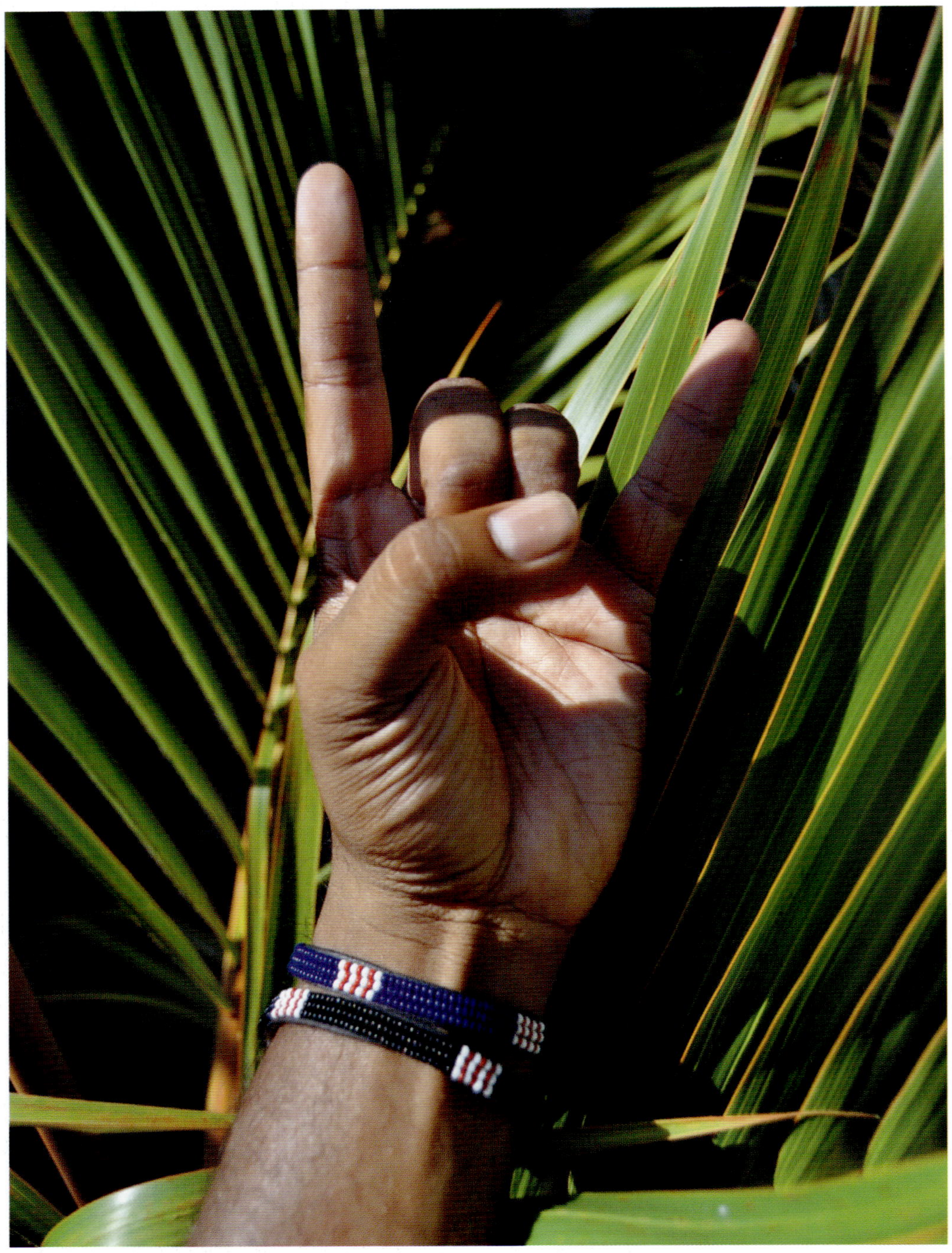

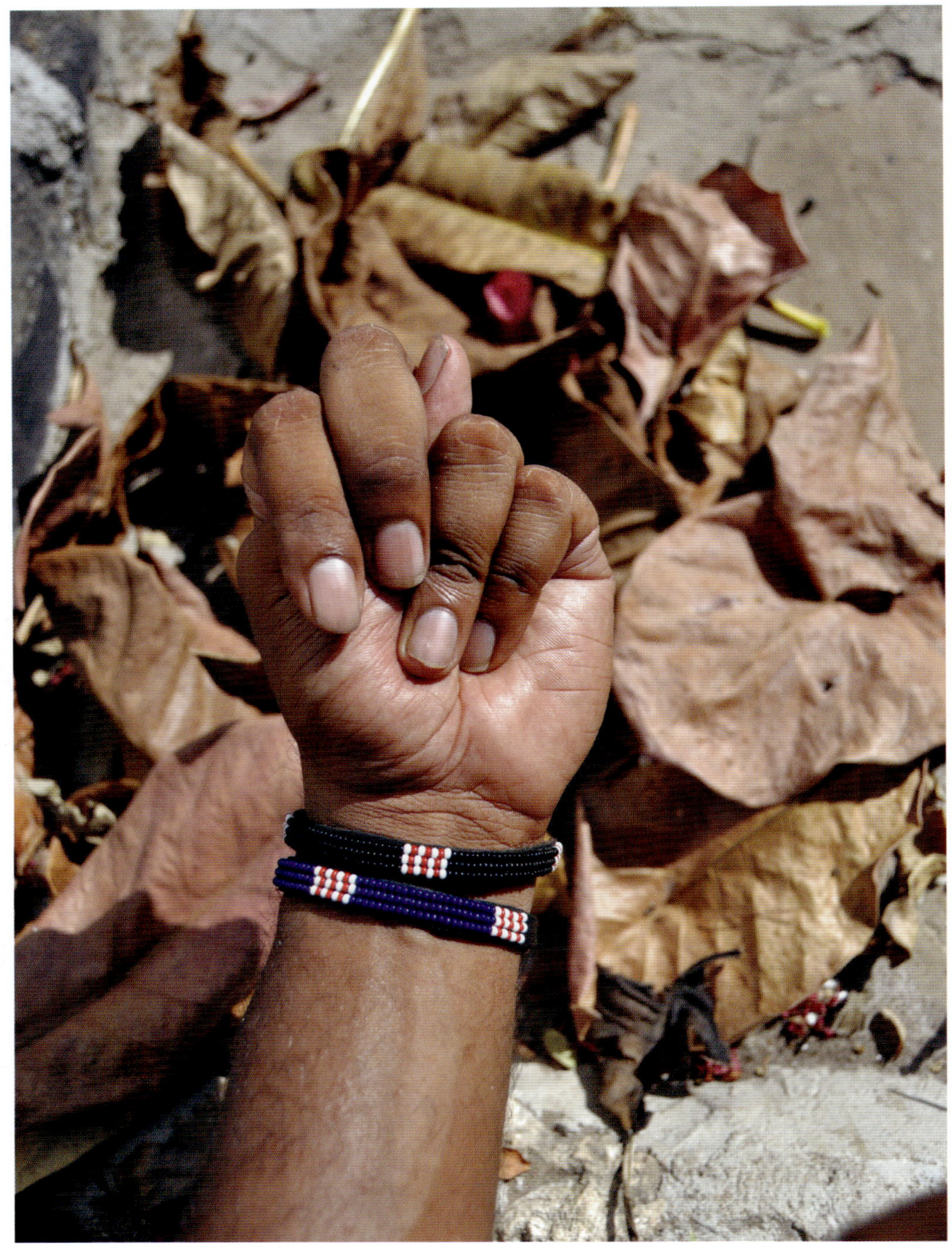

▲ **KARANAMUDRA** · Purification *(left)* **KASHYAPAMUDRA** · Preservation *(right)*

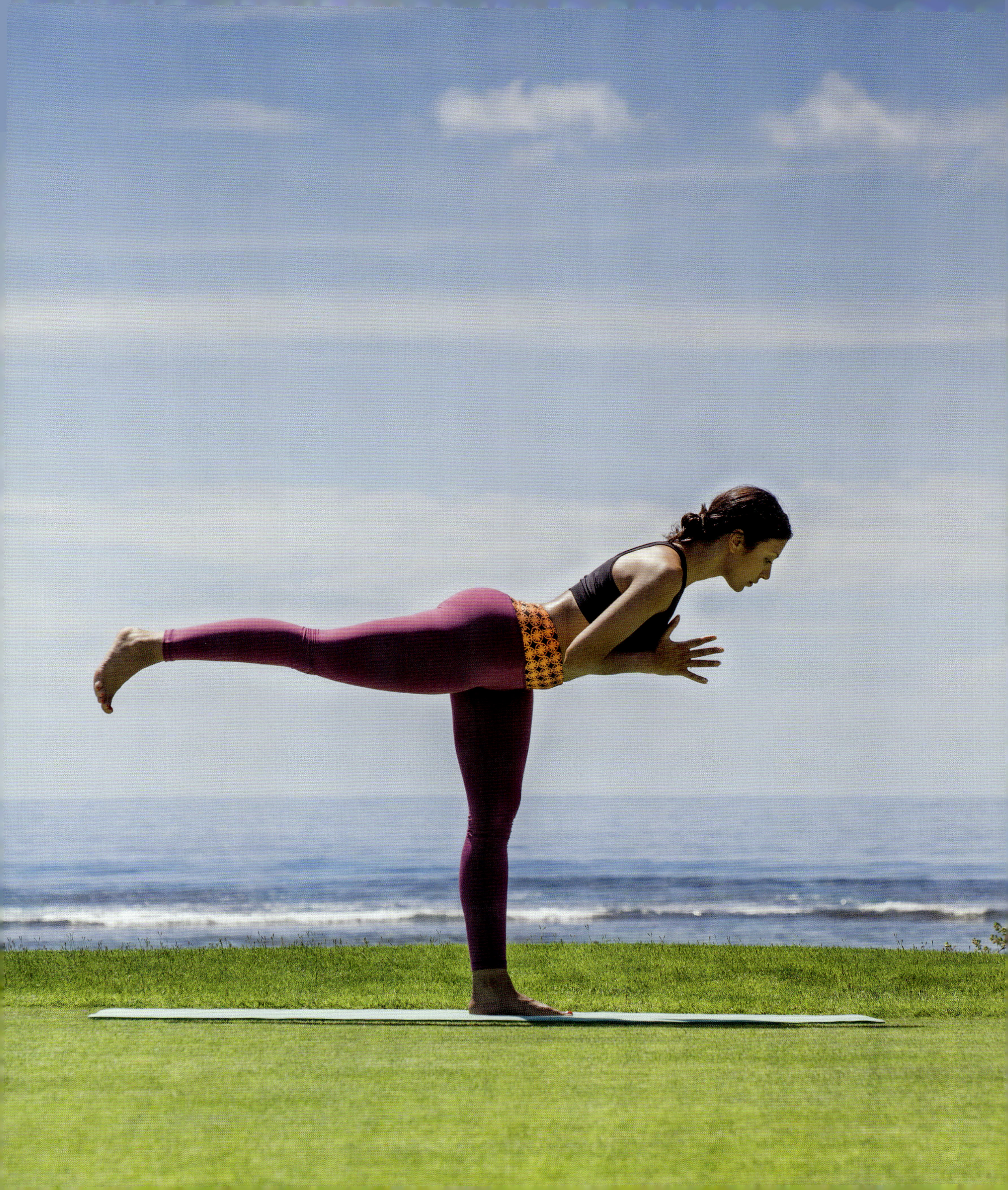

PARIVRTTA BANARASANA · Twisted Lunge

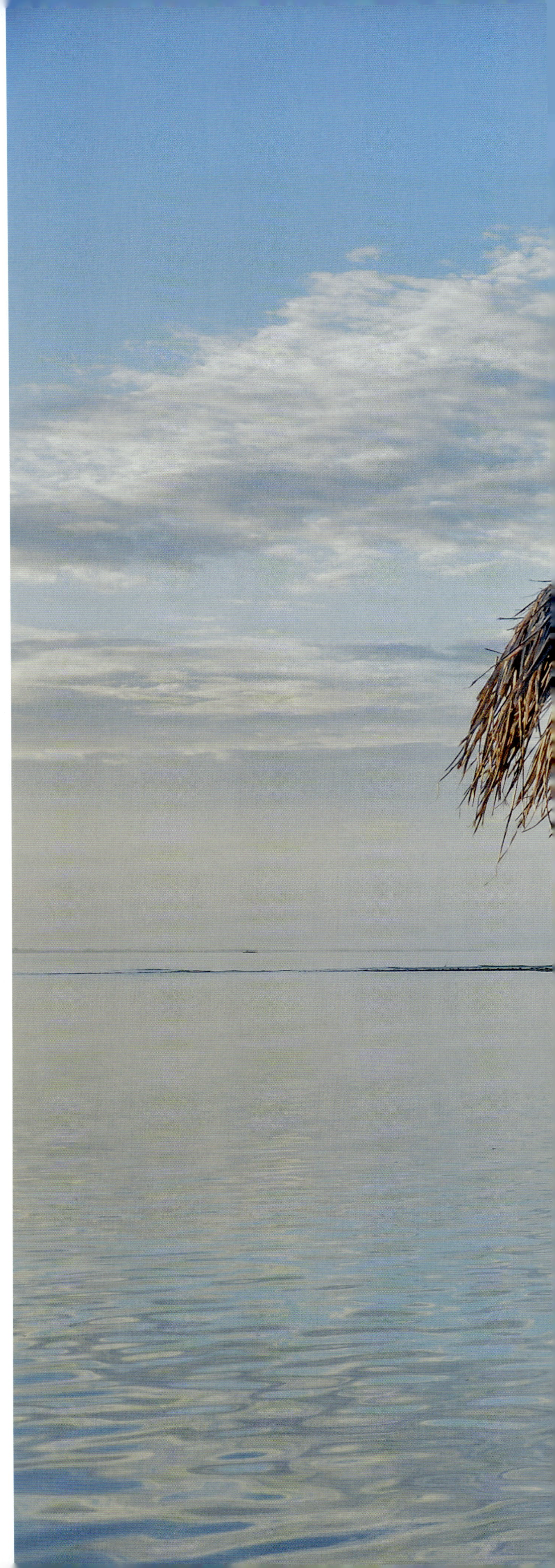

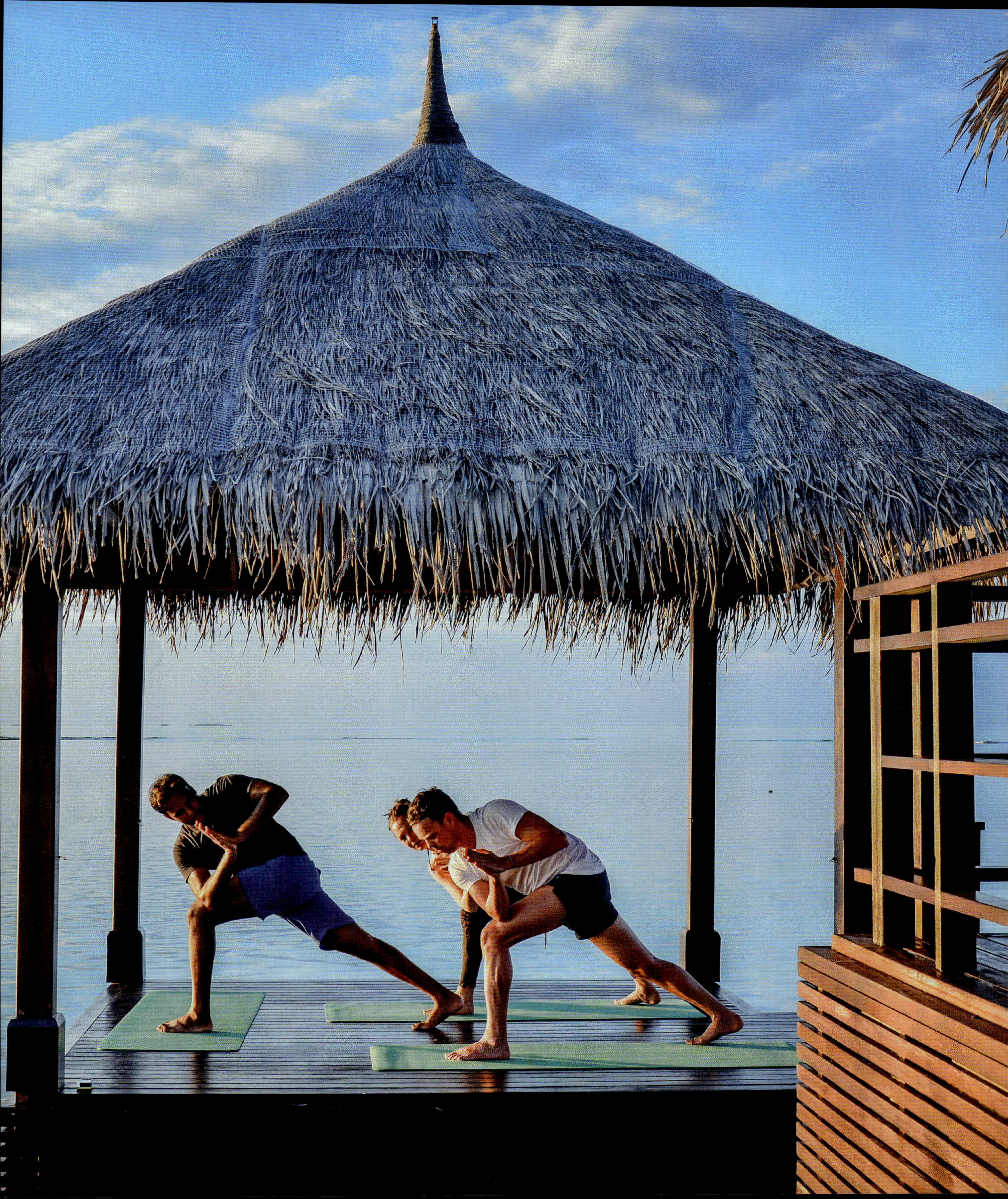

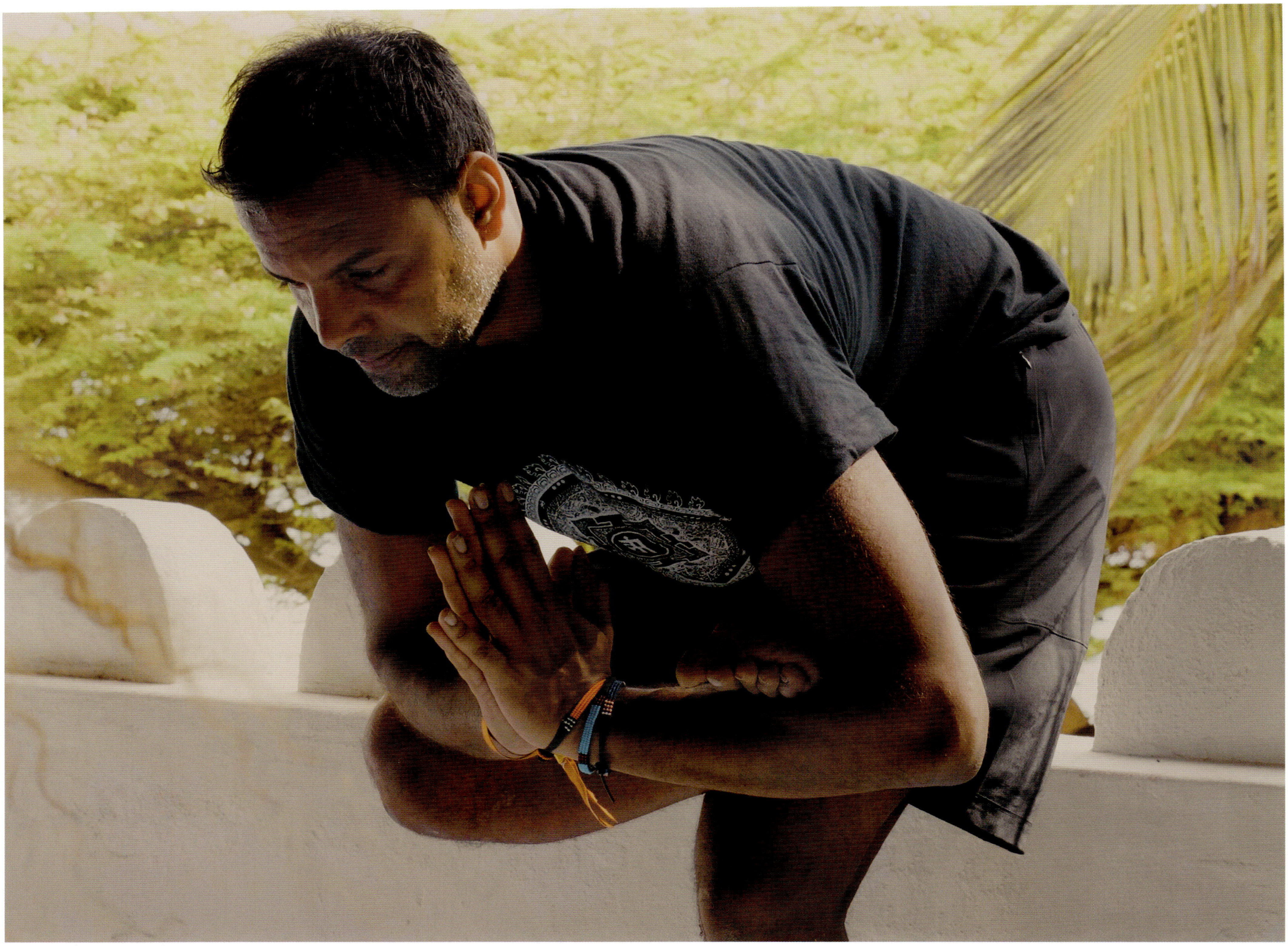

▲ **TADA KAPOTASANA** • Standing Pigeon

JIRAAFASANA • Giraffe

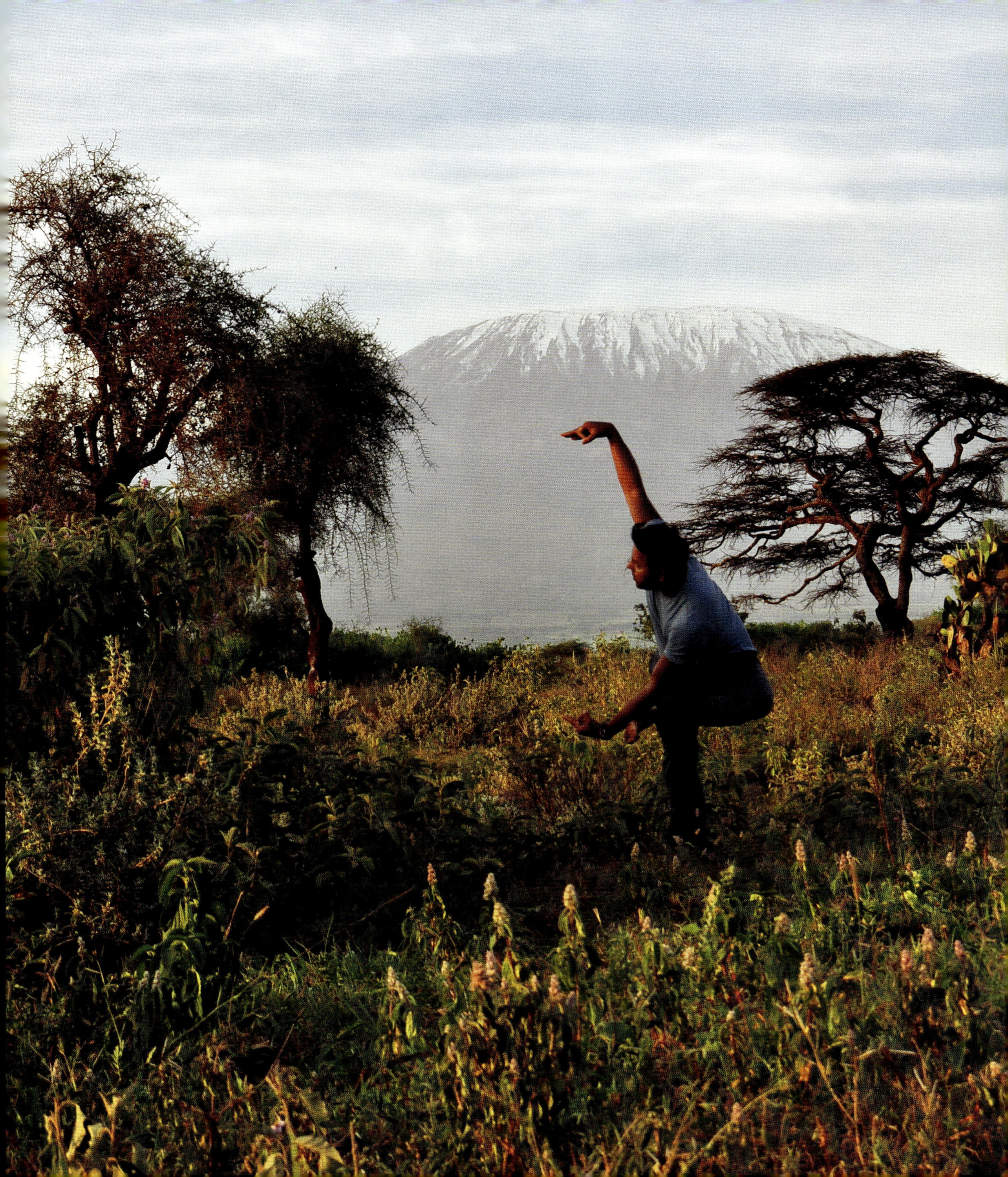

Make sure the food you love loves you back.

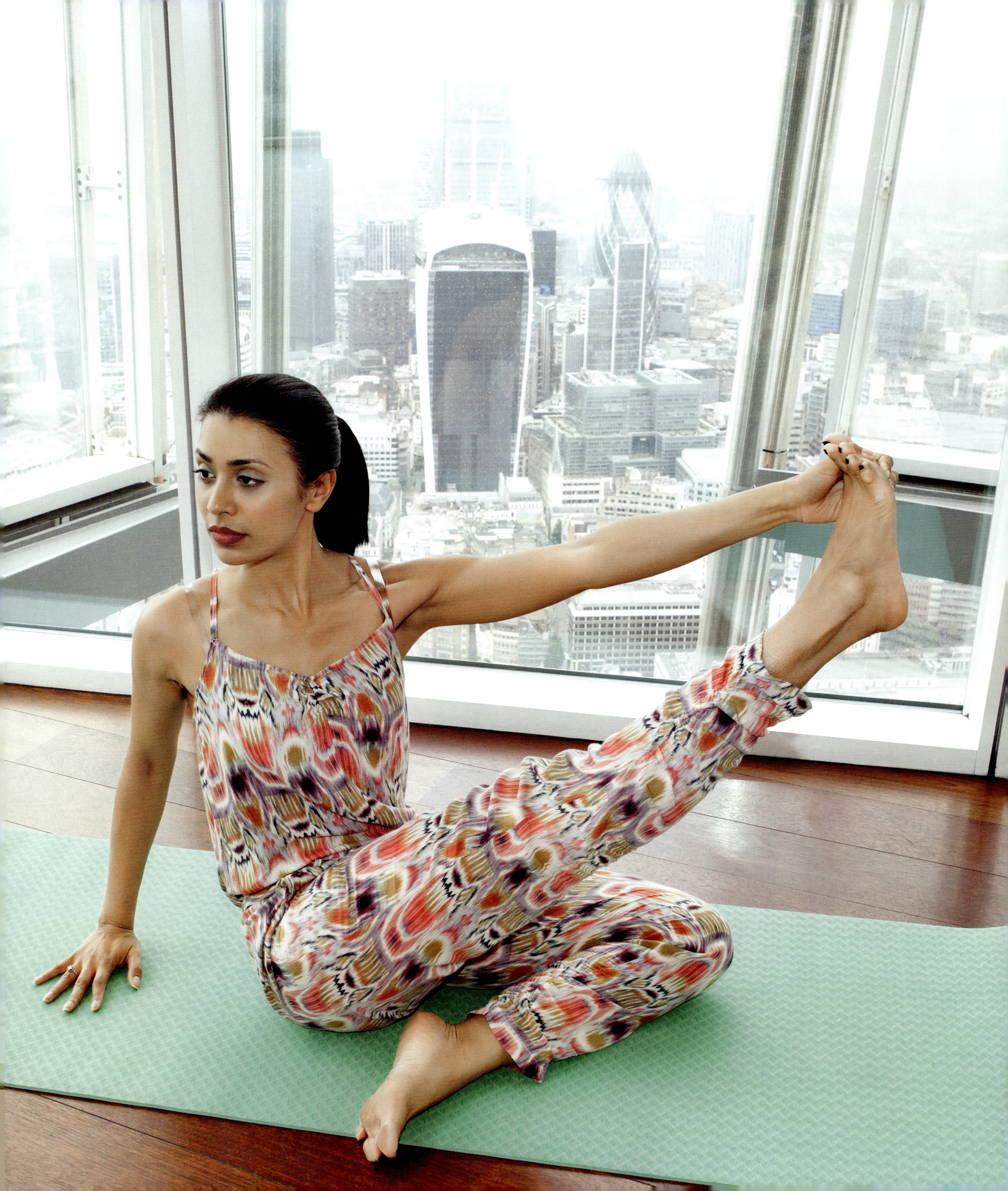

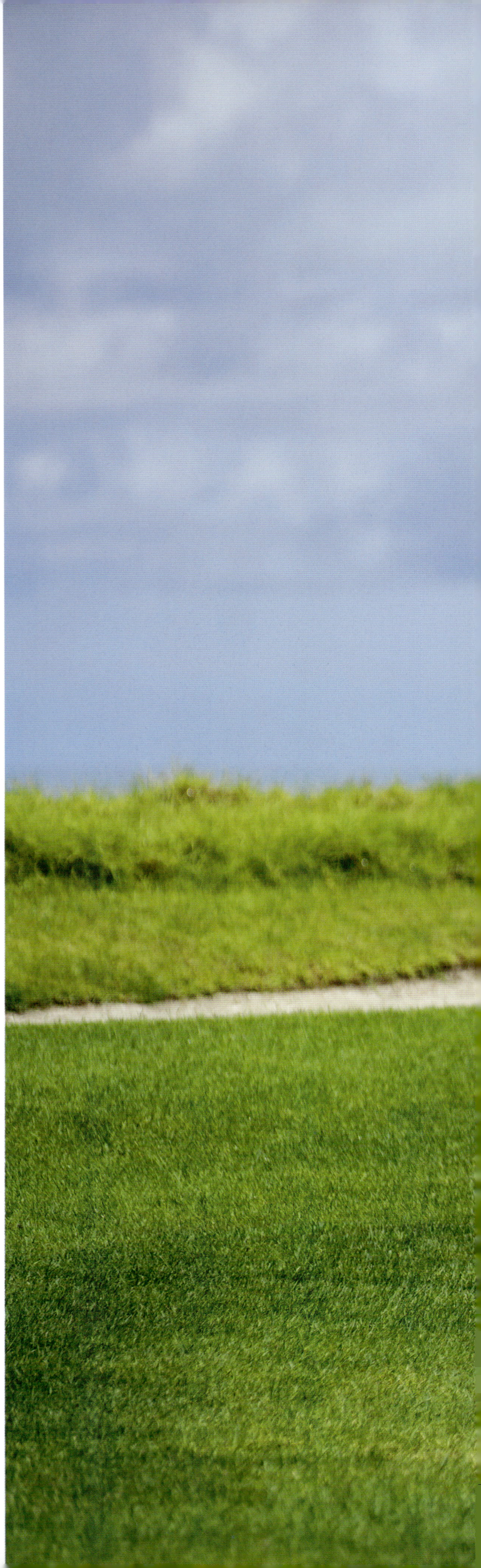

ARDHA USTRASANA · Half Camel

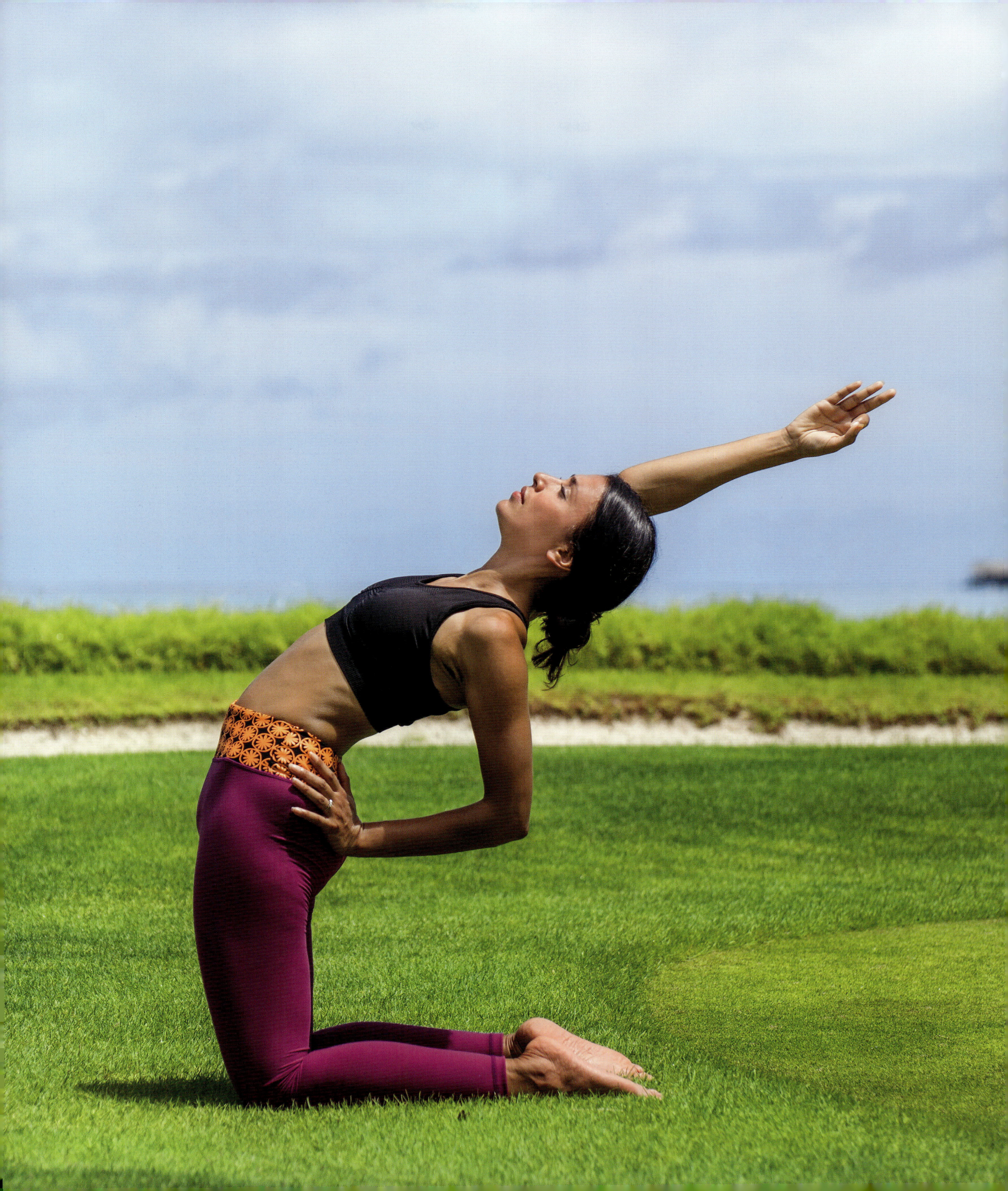

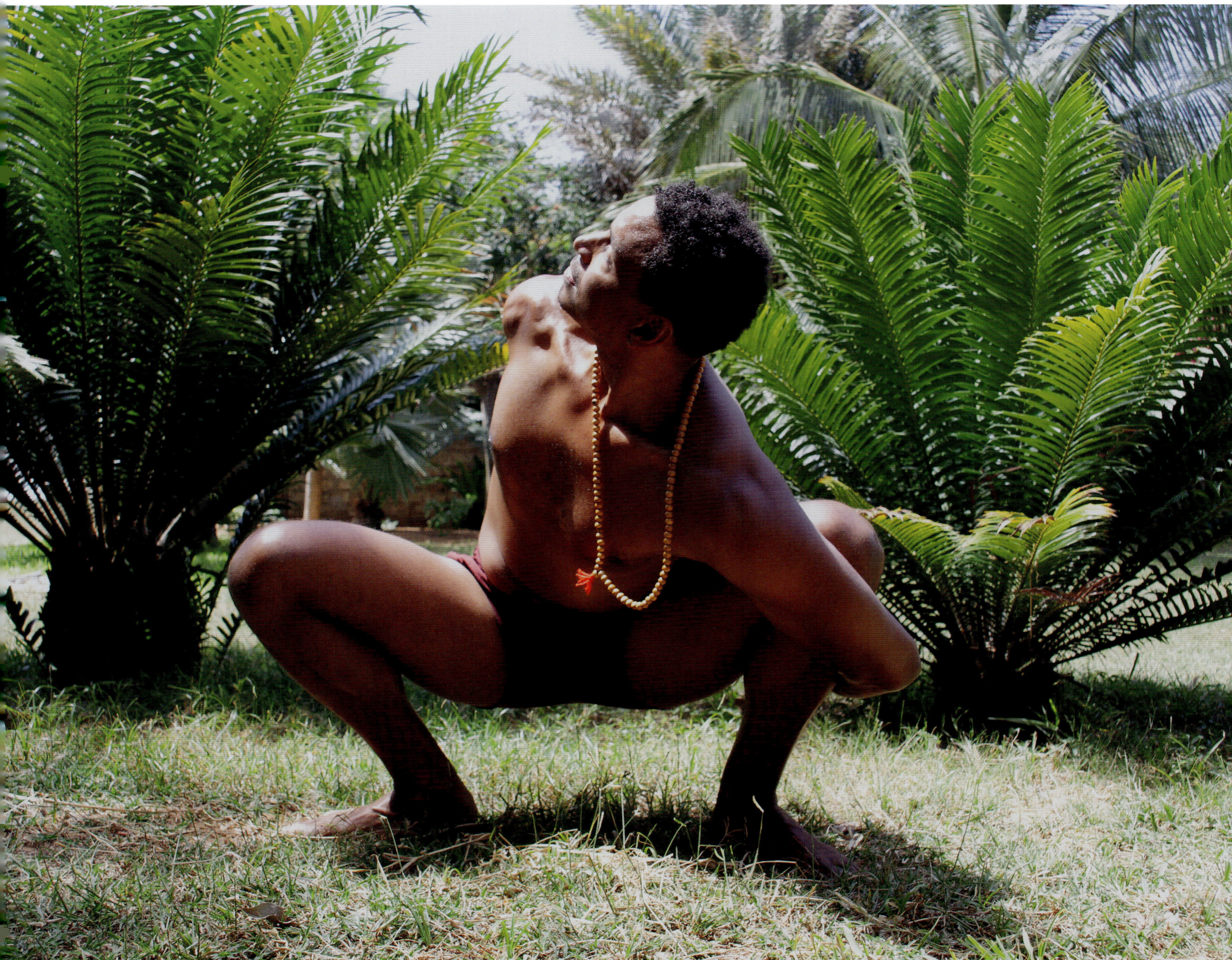

▲ **BADDHA MALASANA** • Bound Garland

PRASARITA PADOTTANASANA EKAM • Wide-Legged Standing Forward Bend I

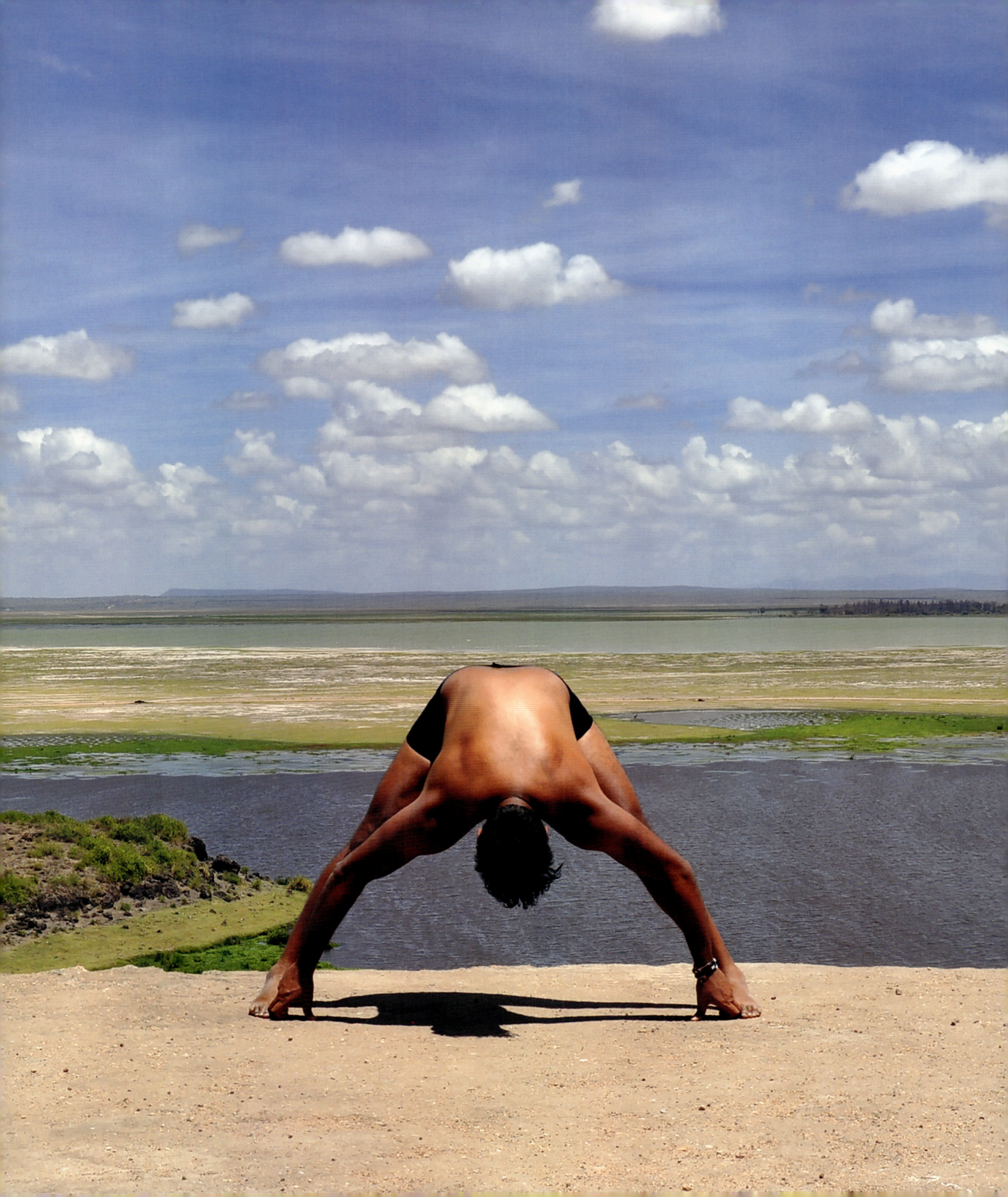

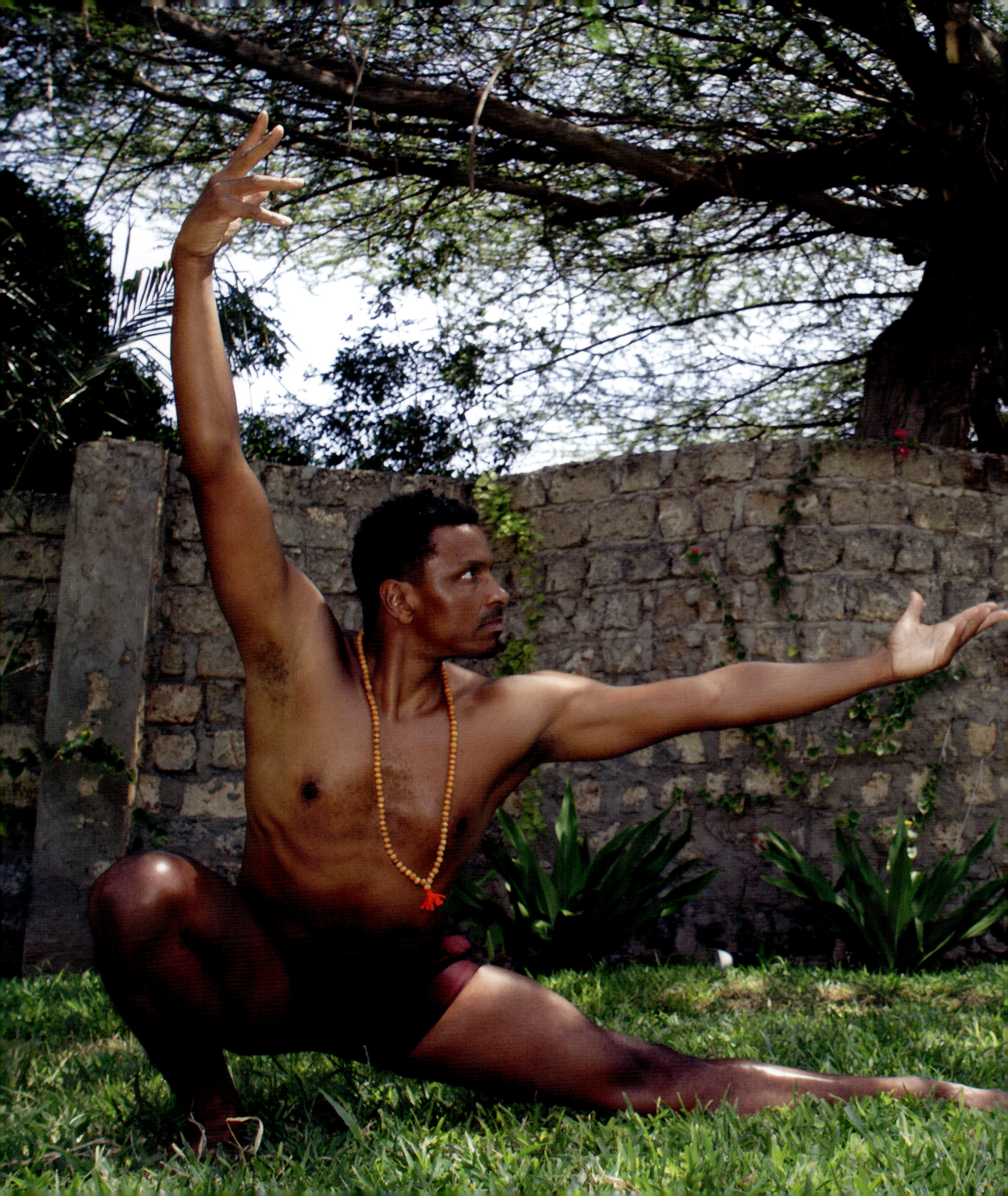

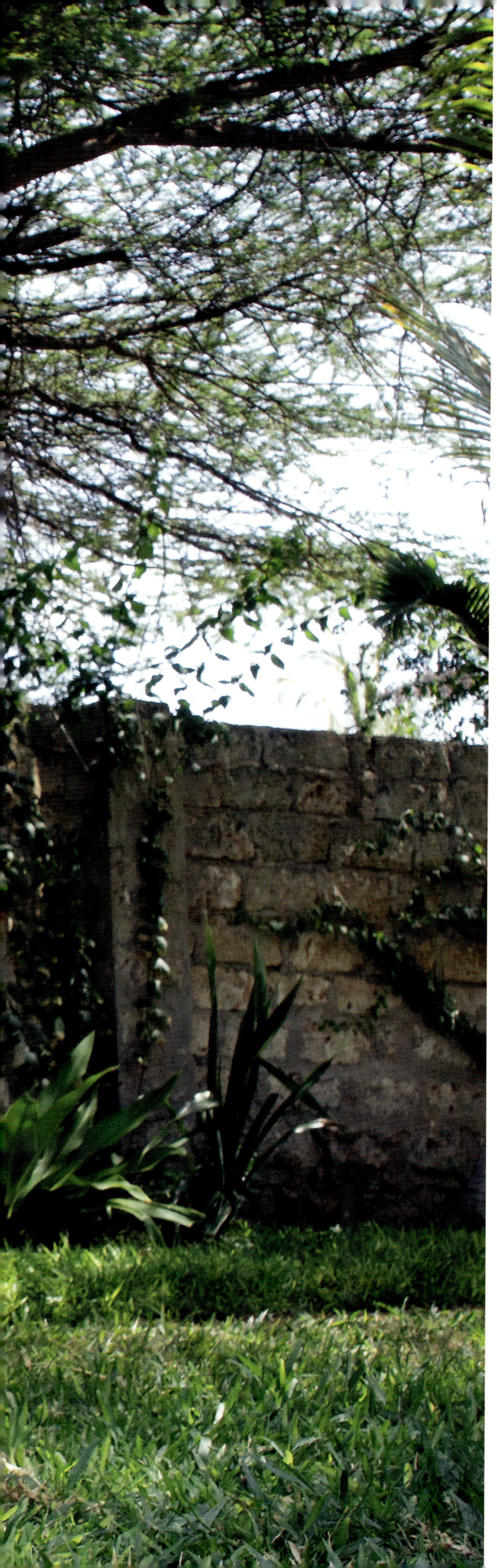

EKA PADA MALASANA · Extended Garland

If your mind was as efficient
as your lungs in taking what it needs
and discarding what it doesn’t,
you would be invincible.

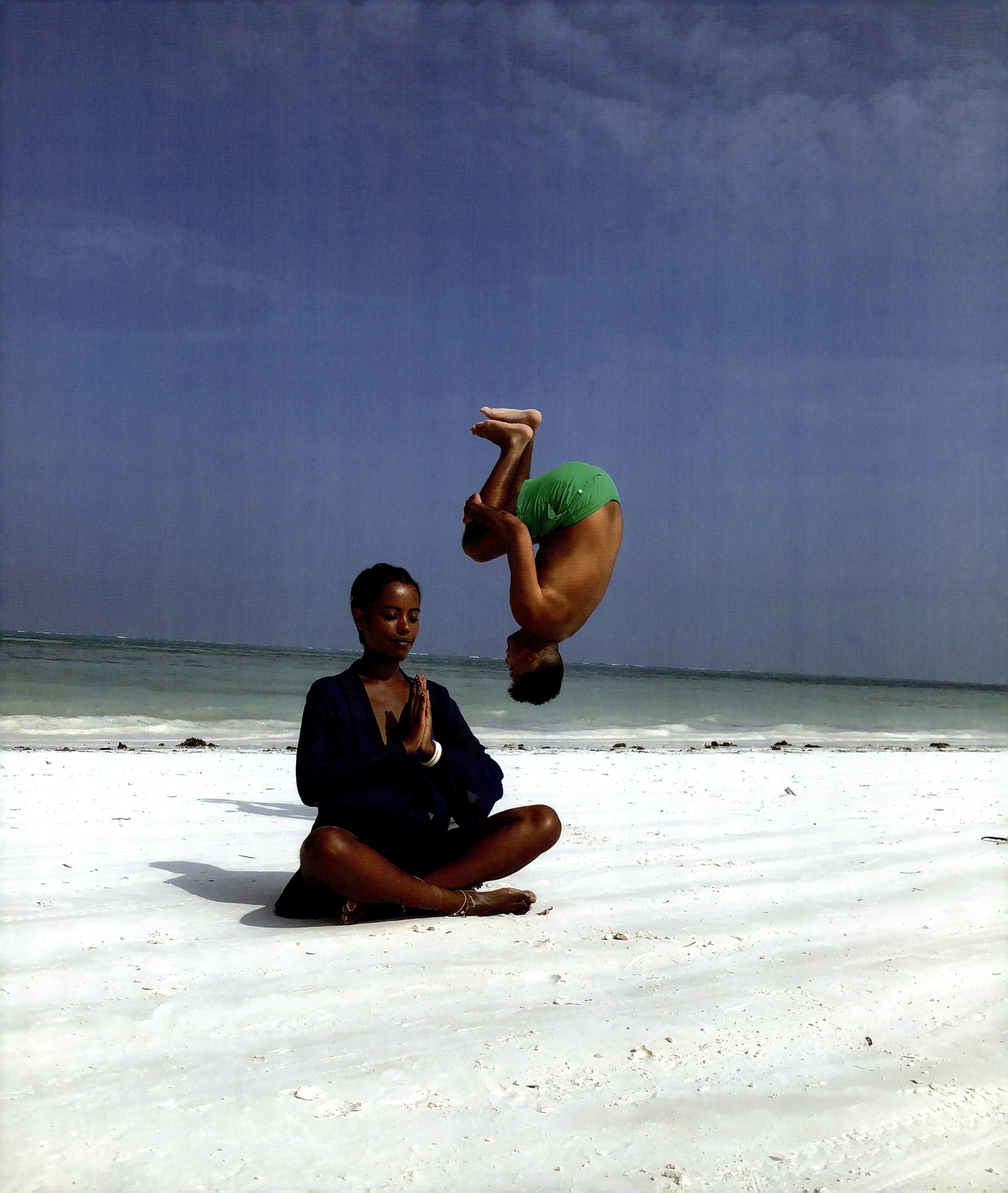

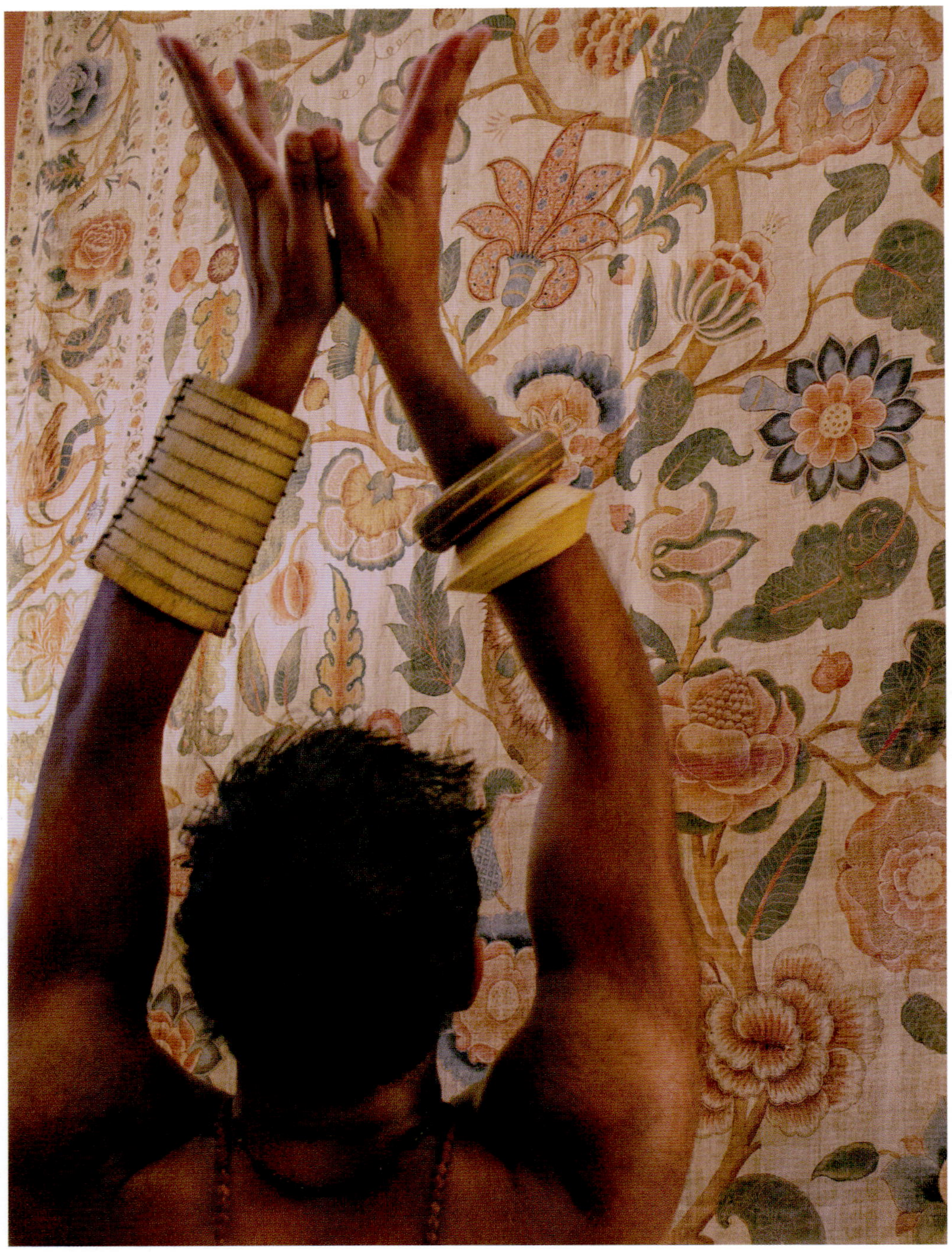

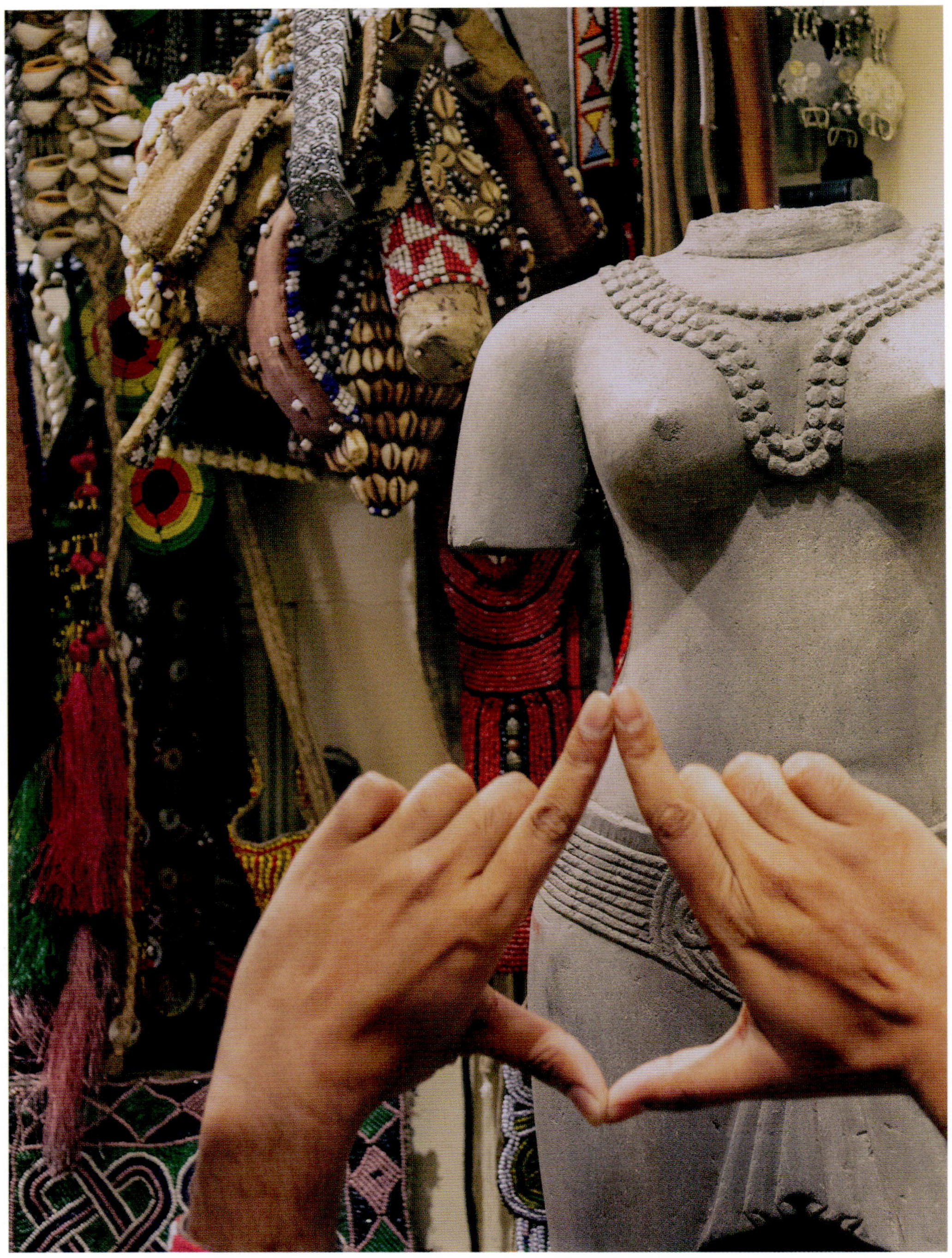

▲ **PADMAMUDRA** • Blossoming *(left)* **YONIMUDRA** • Origin *(right)*

UTTHITA PARIVRTTA UTKATASANA • Revolving Chair

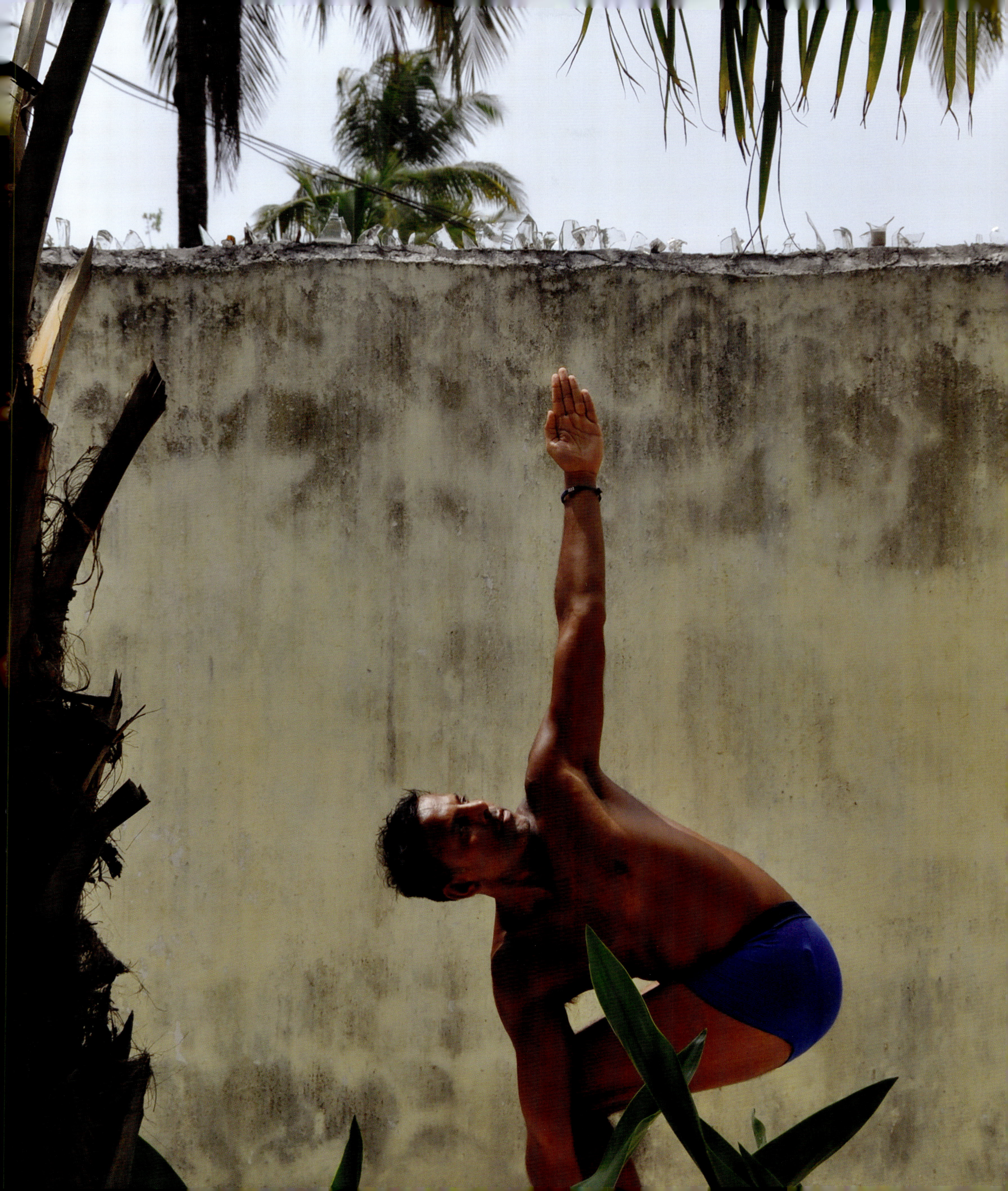

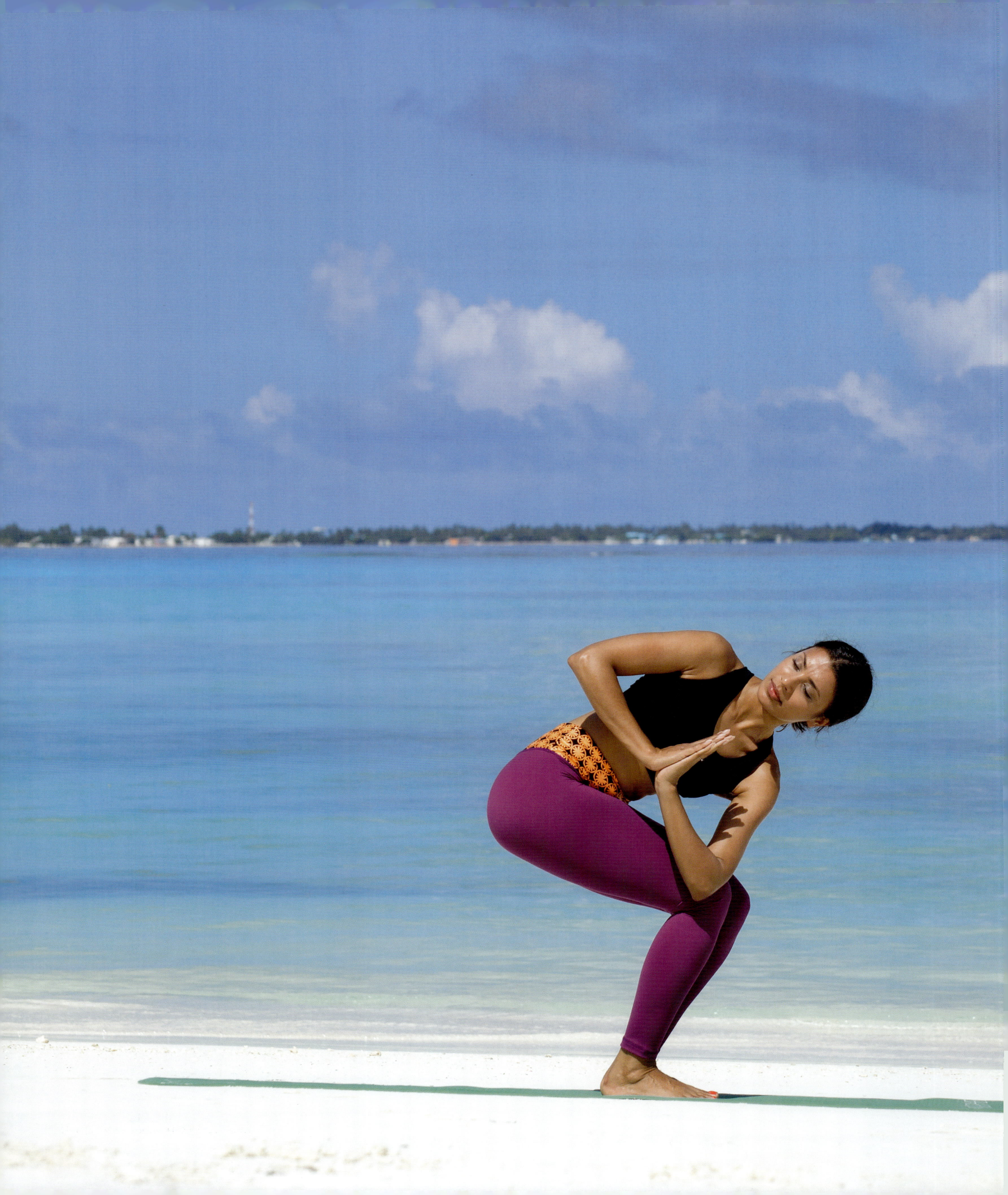

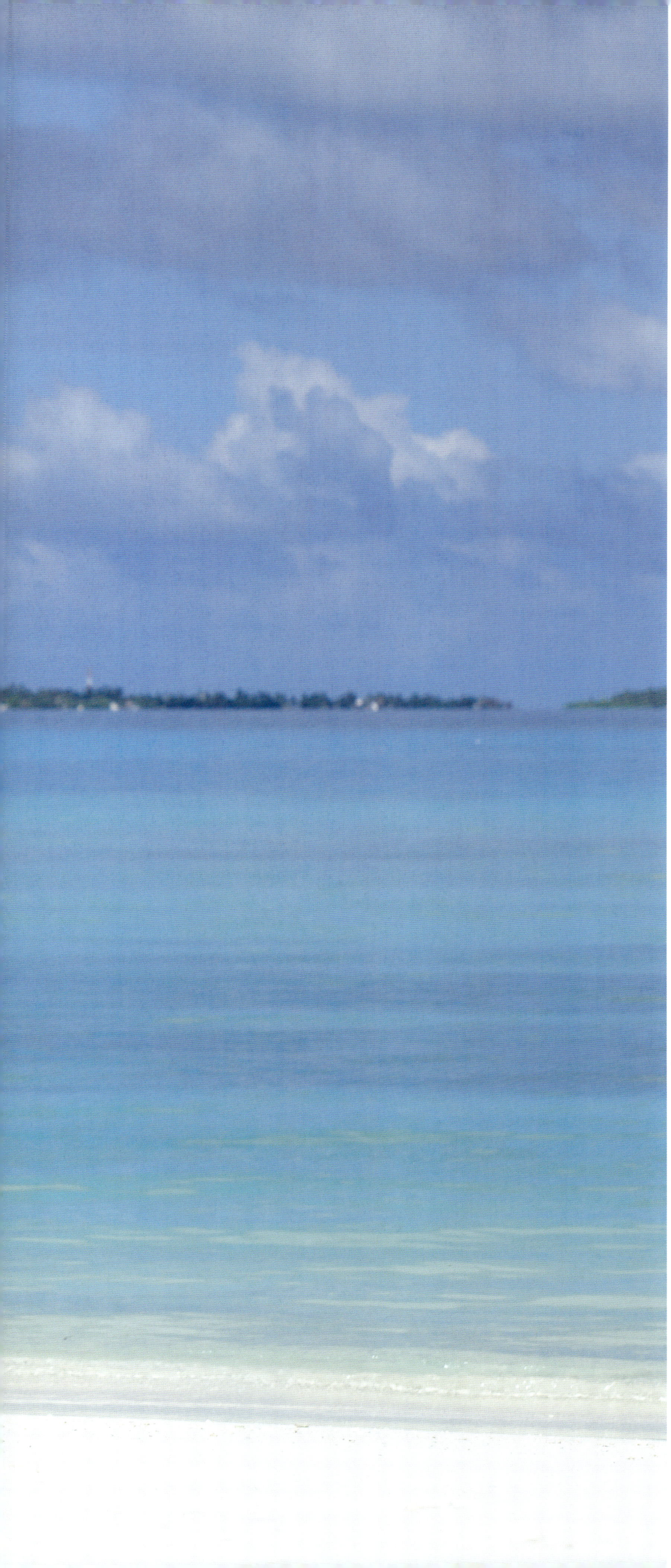

Keep reaching, bonding,

and merging with Nature.

It holds all of Earth's innermost secrets

and ultimately knows your truth.

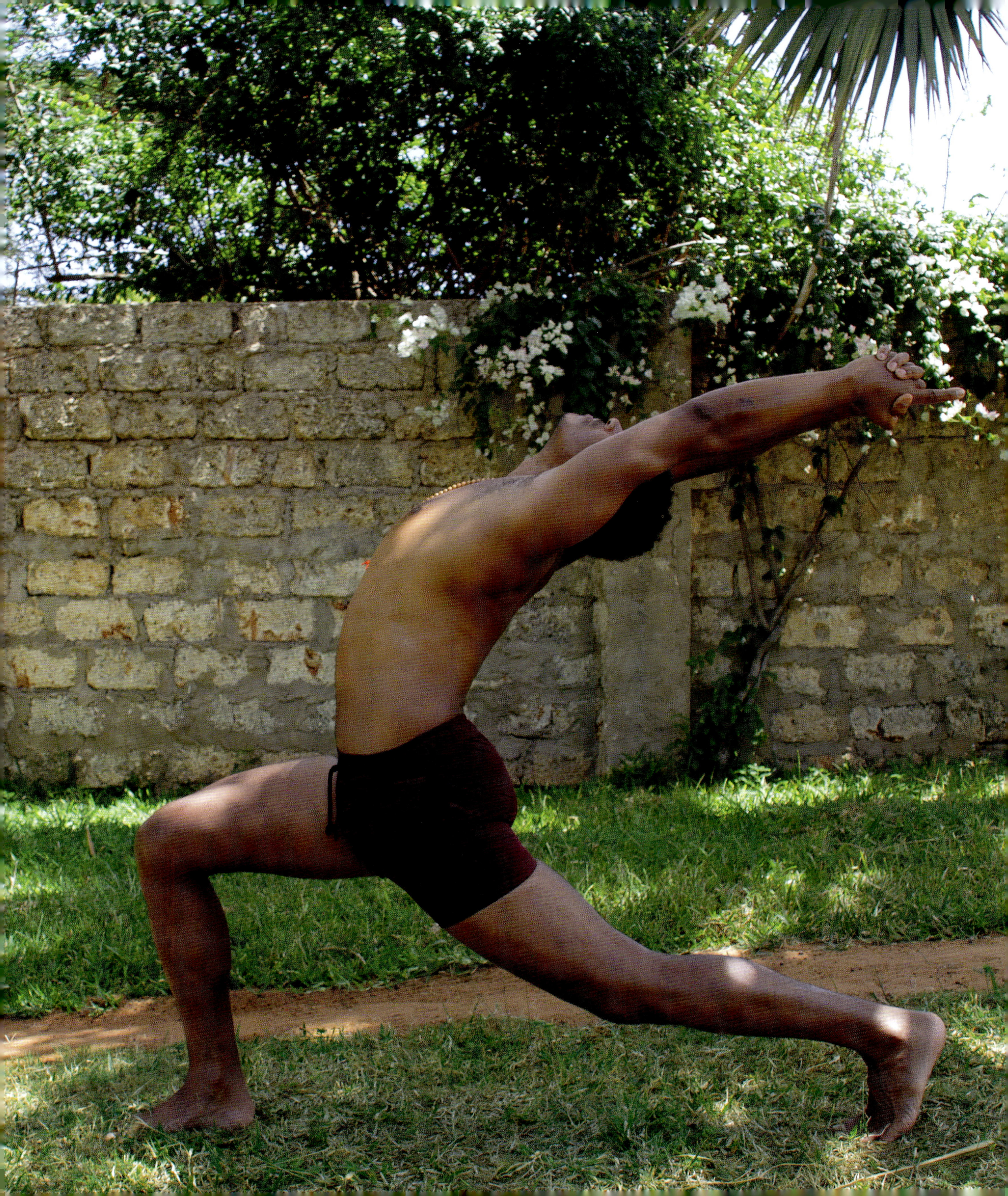

BRAHMA SIMHA • Leo

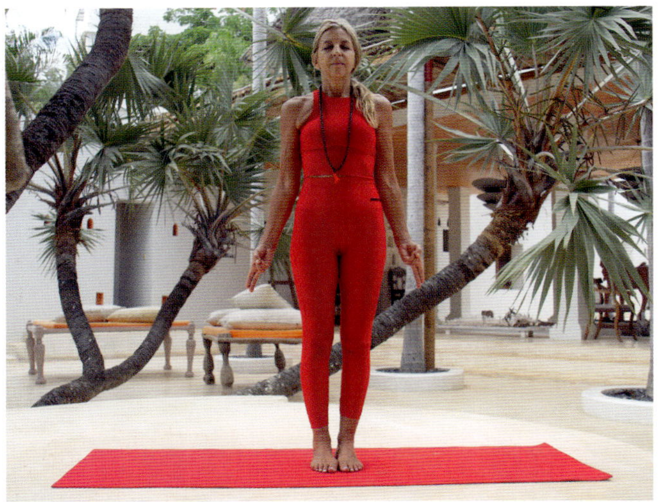

TADASANA & PRANAMUDRA
Mountain & Vitality

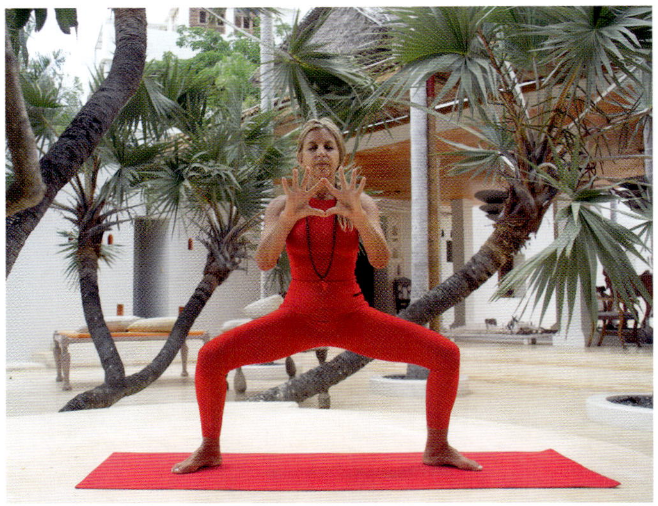

UTKATA KONASANA & SAHASARAMUDRA
Goddess & Interconnectedness

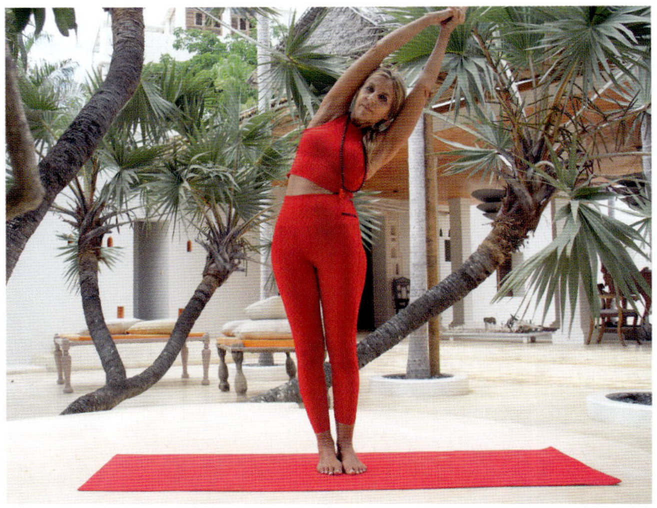

PARSVA URDHVA HASTASANA
Standing Half Moon

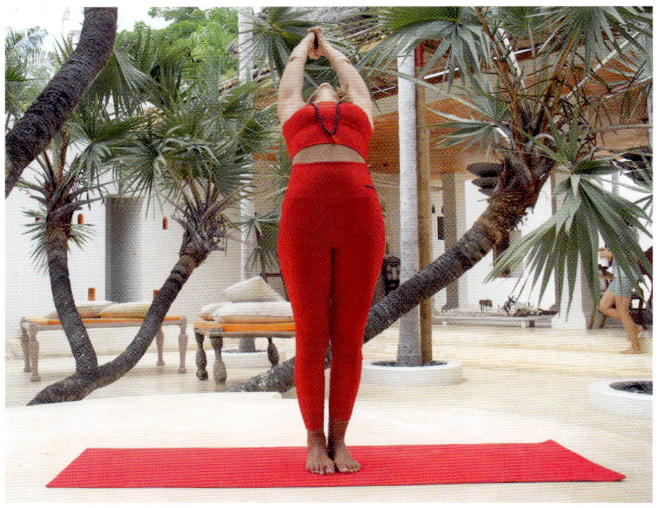

ANUVITTASANA
Standing Backbend

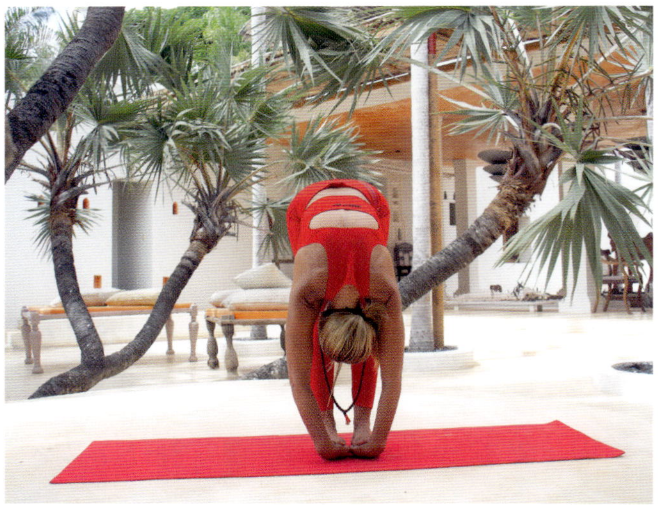

PADAHASTASANA
Hand under Foot

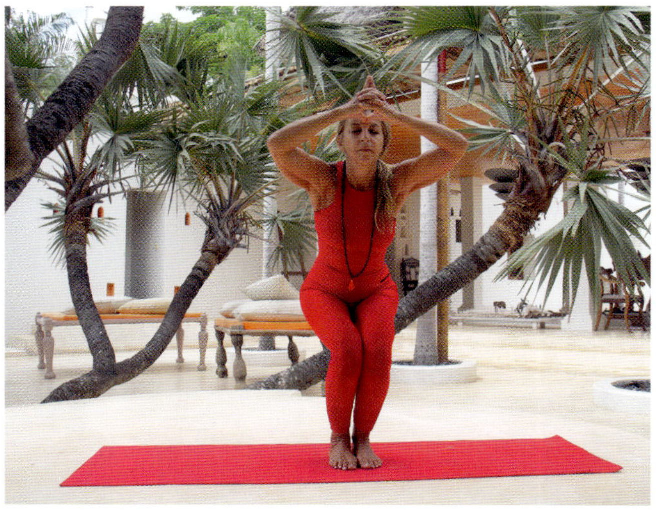

UTKATASANA & UTTARABODHIMUDRA
Chair & Inception

In Brahma Simha, we are in the settled season of elemental fire. This constellation of asanas—such as detoxifying twists, lateral stretches, and adventurous balance poses—culminates in a variety of creative headstand inversions. This creates an emboldened and ambitious practice that feels exciting and rewarding. The mudras bring vitality to the body and interconnectedness of personal power both in body and mind. By following the inception of ideas into movement, we bring about the preservation of well-being. With greater awareness, there is a warmhearted sense of innateness that leaves you feeling radiant and exuberant.

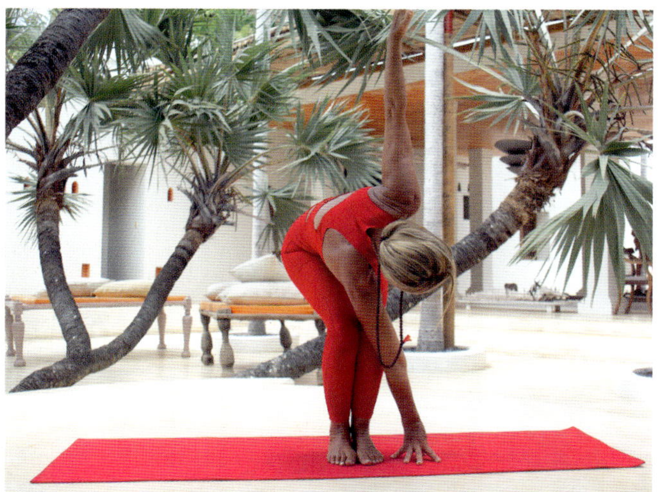

UTTHITA PARIVRTTA UTKATASANA
Revolving Chair

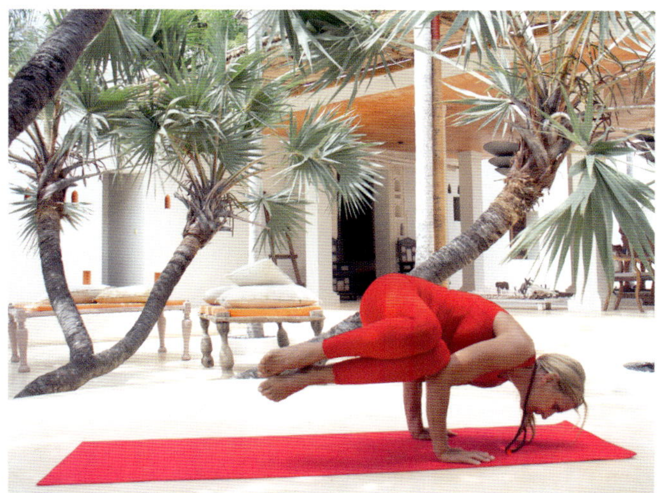

PARSVA BAKASANA
Side Crow

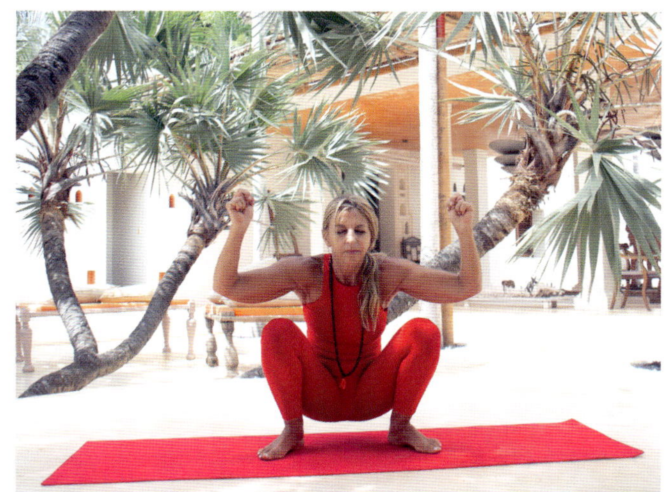

MALASANA & KASHYAPAMUDRA
Garland Squat & Preservation

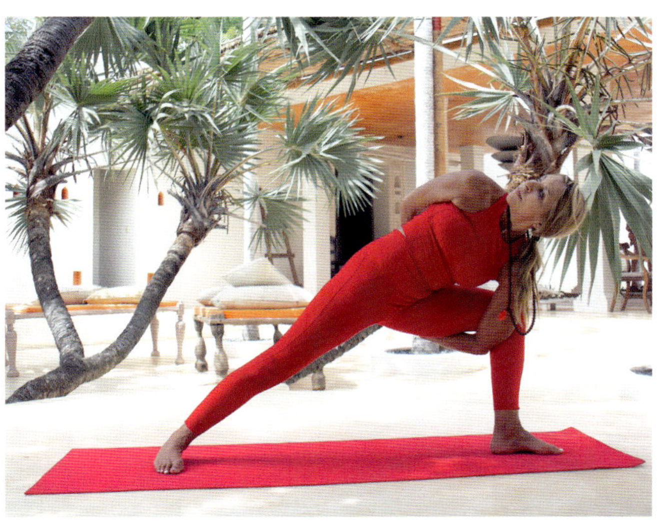

BADDHA UTTHITA PARSVAKONASANA
Bound Side Angle

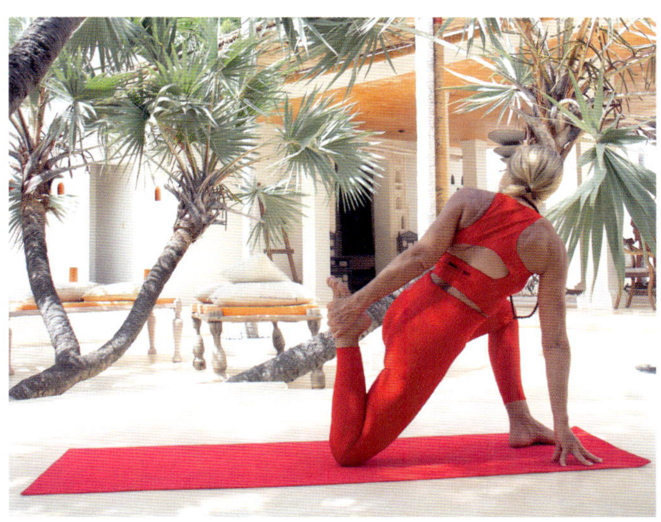

PARIVRTTA ANJANEYASANA
Twisted Crescent Lunge

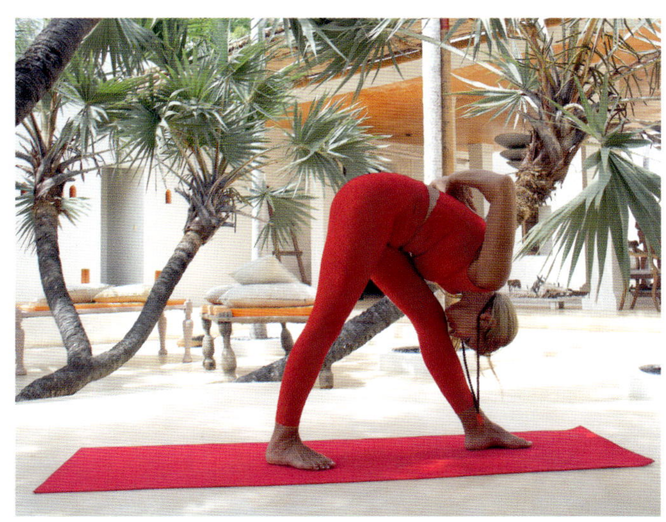

AUNDHA PARSVOTTANASANA
Reverse Pyramid

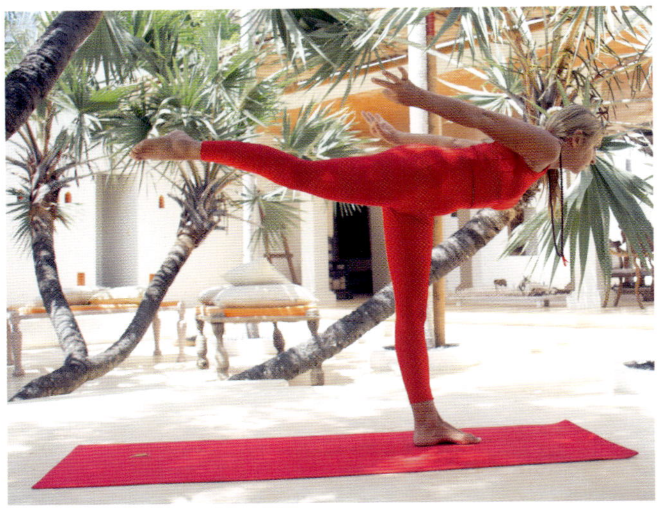

VIRABHADRASANA TRINI & CHINMUDRA
Warrior III & Awareness

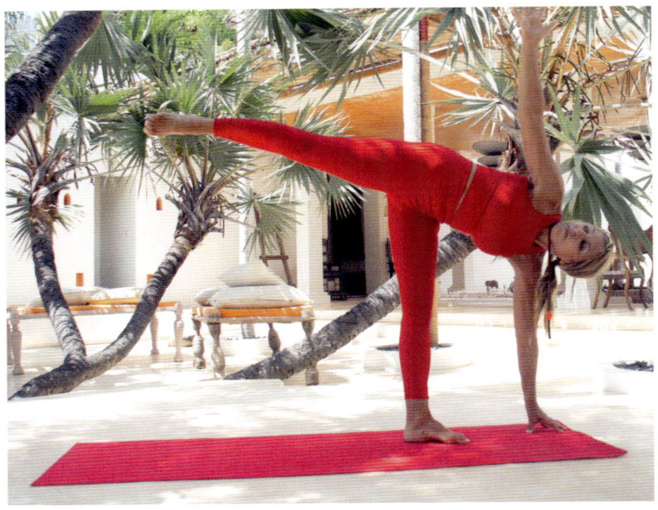

ARDHA CHANDRASANA
Half Moon

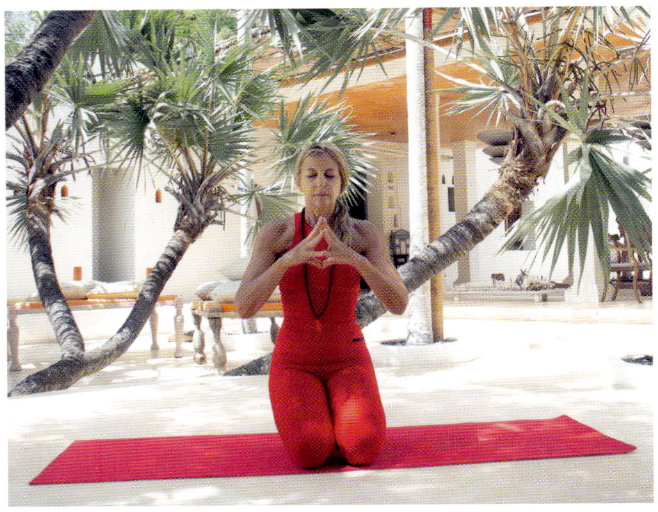

VAJRASANA & PANCHAMUKHAMUDRA
Thunderbolt & Innateness

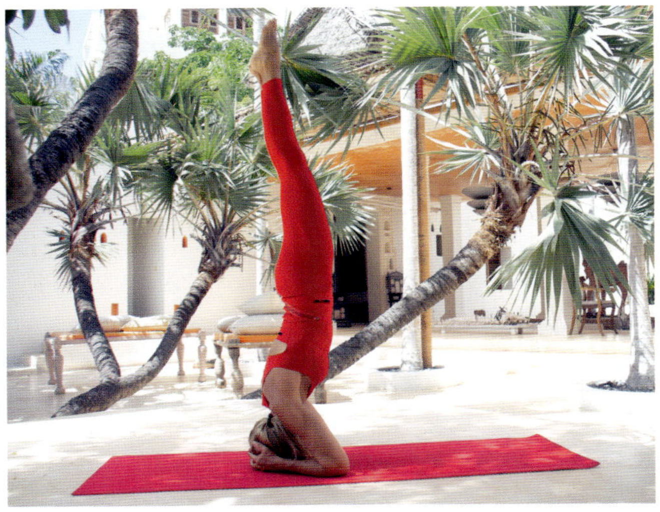

SIRSASANA
Headstand

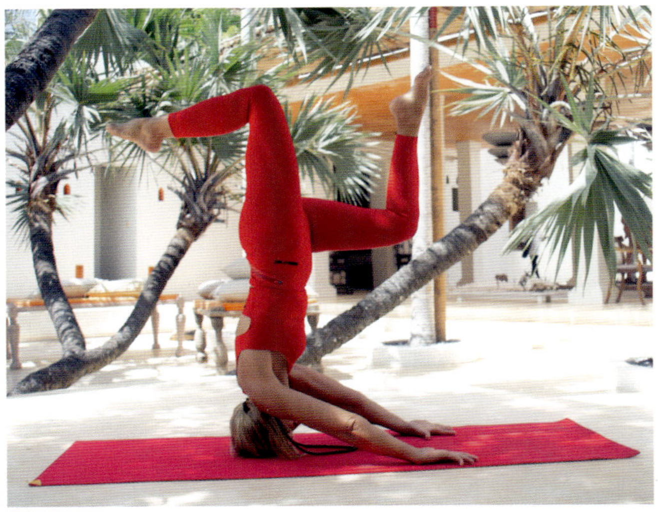

NIRALAMBA SIRSASANA
Extended Headstand

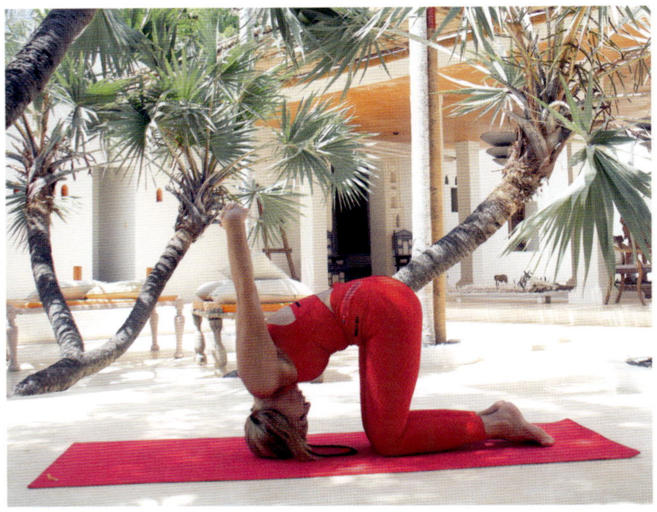

UTTHITA SASANGASANA
Leaping Rabbit

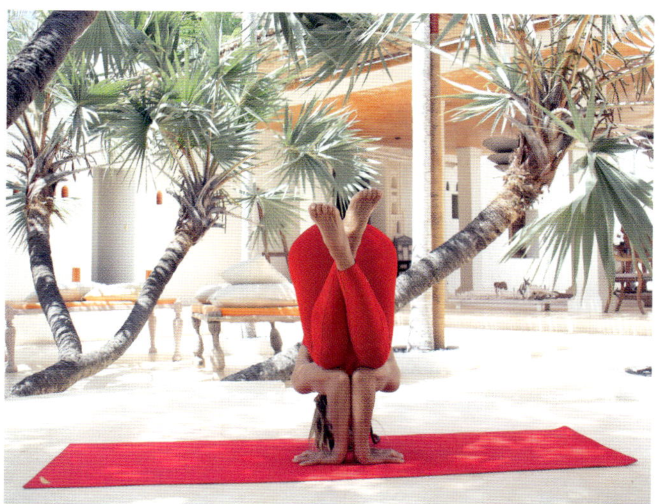

GARUDA SIRSASANA
Eagle Headstand

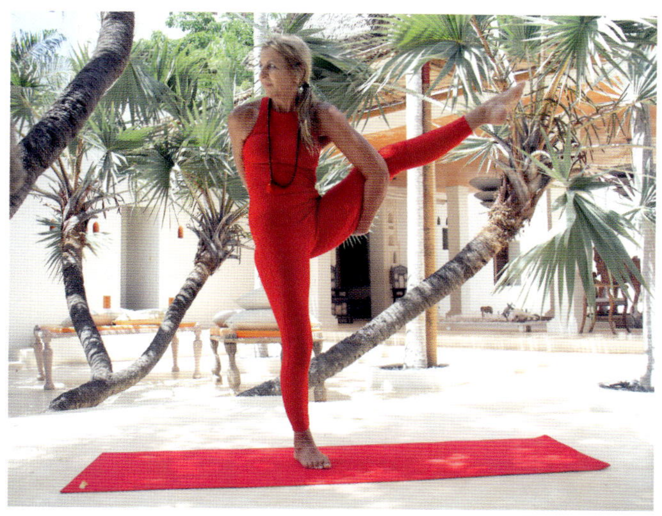

SVARGA DVIJASANA
Bird of Paradise

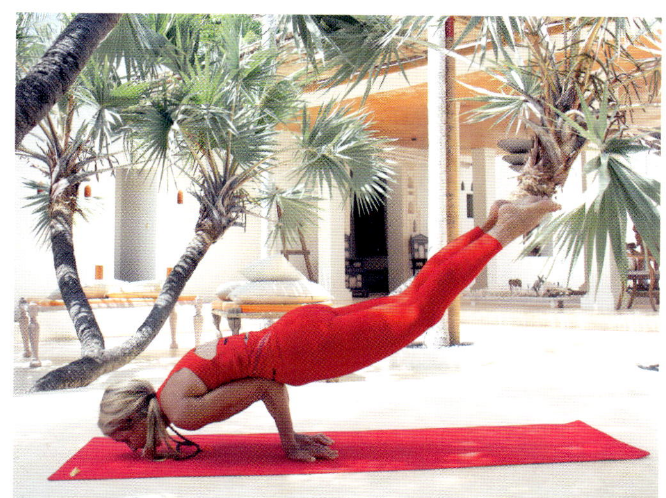

MAYURASANA
Peacock

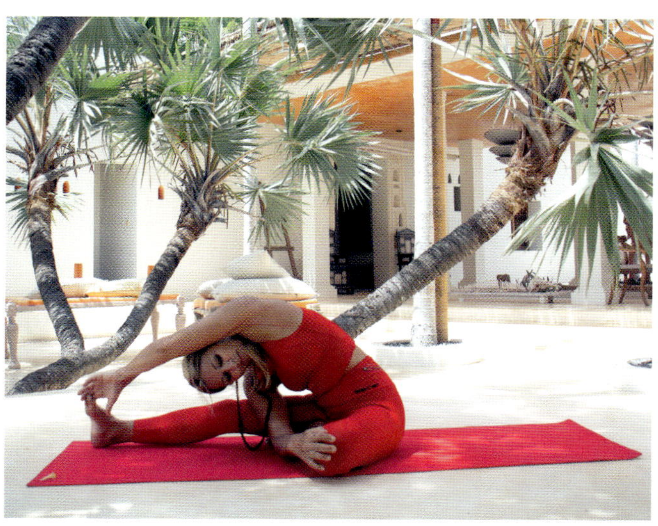

PARIVRTTA JANUSIRSASANA
Twisted Head-to-Knee Forward Bend

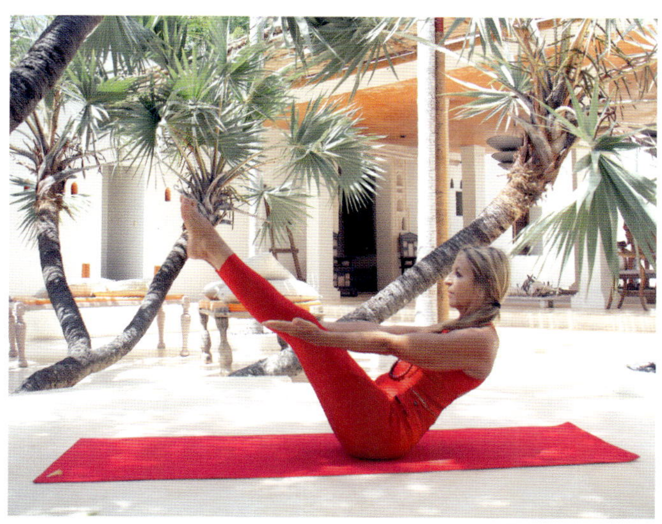

NAVASANA
Boat

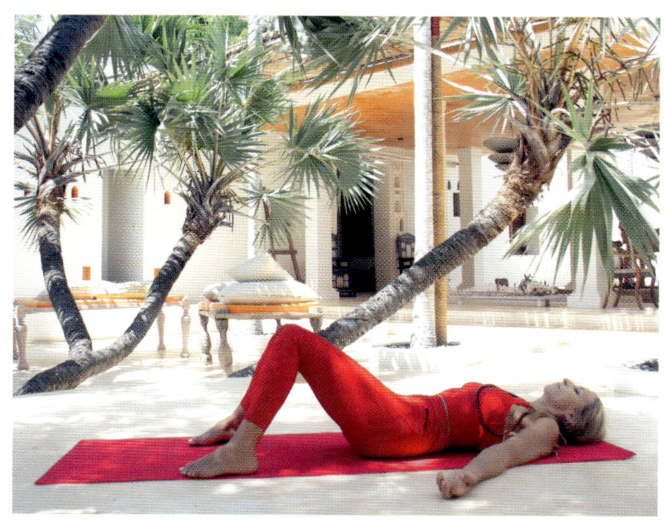

SANTULAN SAVASANA
Balancing Resting

BRAHMA KANYA · Virgo

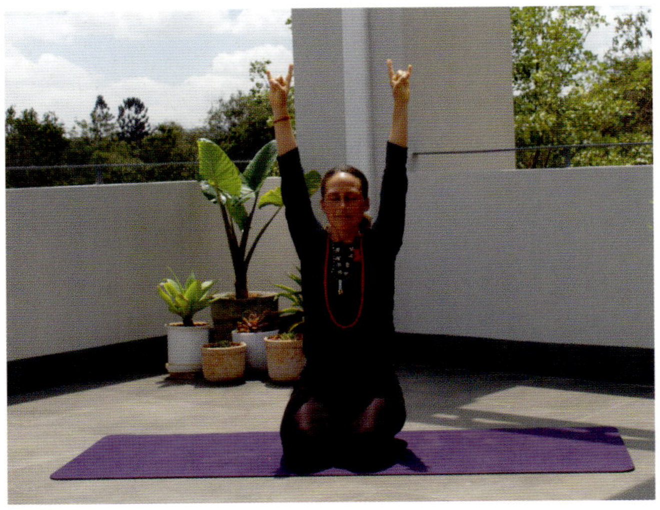

VAJRASANA BHRAMARI & KARANAMUDRA
Thunderbolt Bee Breath & Purification

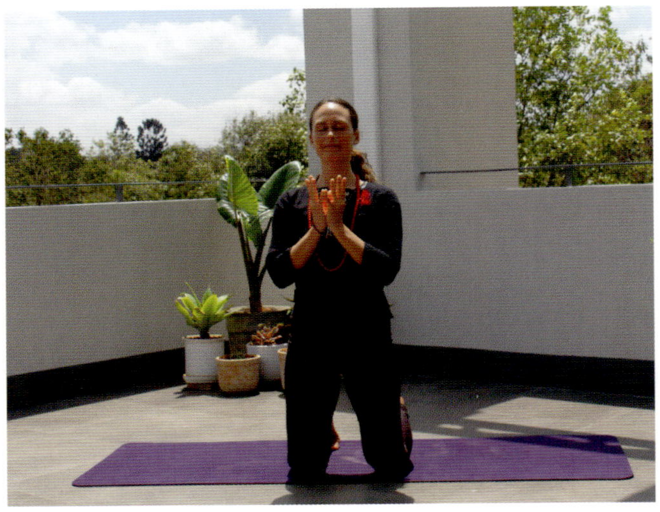

UDAYA VAJRASANA & PADMAMUDRA
Rising Thunderbolt & Blossoming

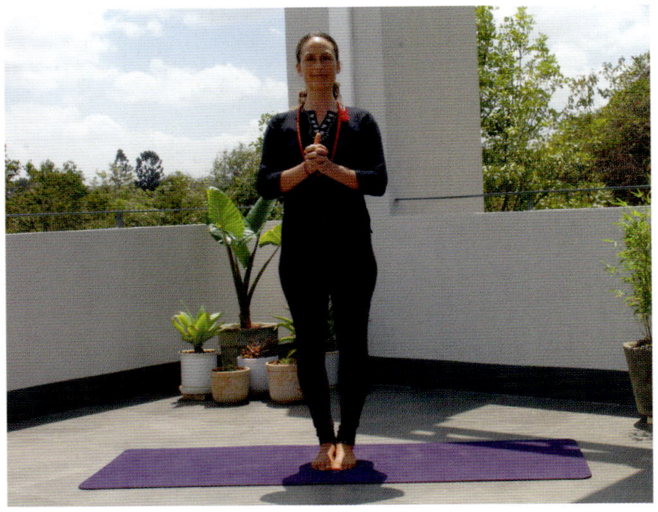

SAMASTHITI & LINGAMUDRA
Equal Standing & Virility

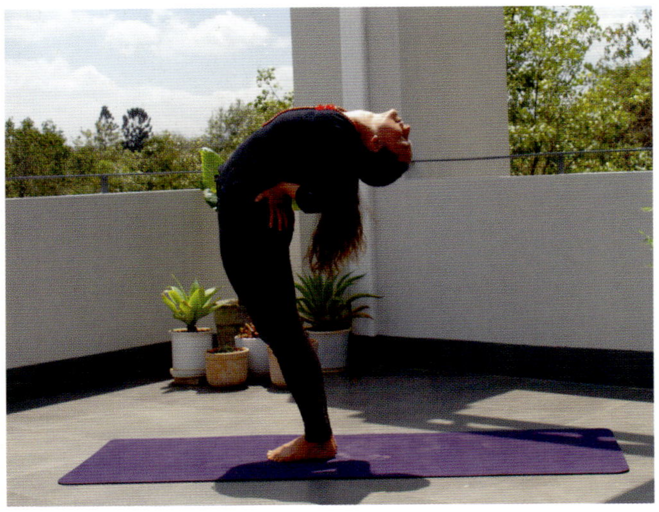

ARDHA CHAKRASANA
Half Spinning Wheel

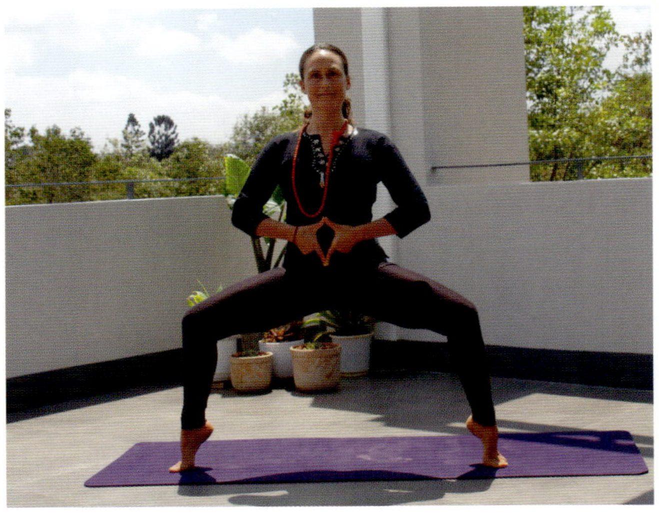

PADA UTKATA KONASANA & YONIMUDRA
Floating Goddess & Origin

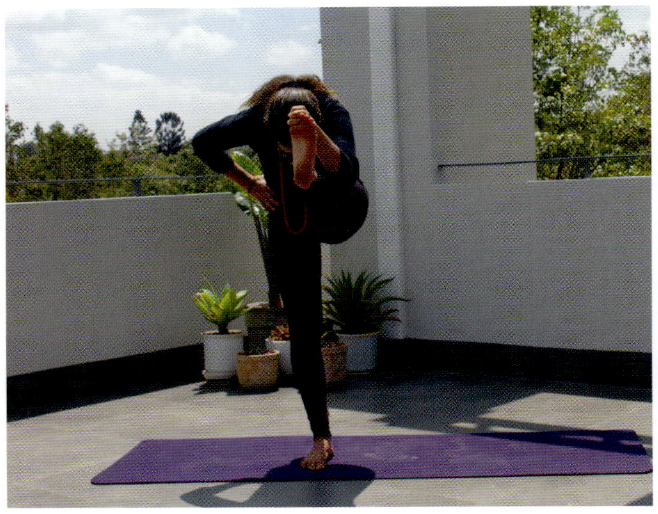

DANDAYAMANA JANUSIRSASANA
Standing Head-to-Knee

In Brahma Kanya, we are in the shifting season of elemental earth. This constellation of asanas explores the intricacies of challenging poses. From the horizon, we start to yield increasingly closer to the earth. The postures are meticulously organized to cultivate a pragmatic approach with intelligent and effective use of breath to support movement. The mudras help the process of purification to aid our becoming and blossoming. We celebrate the virility of nature and its origin and the fertility of the earth. This unlocks the perfect rhythm of abundance with cycles of ecology.

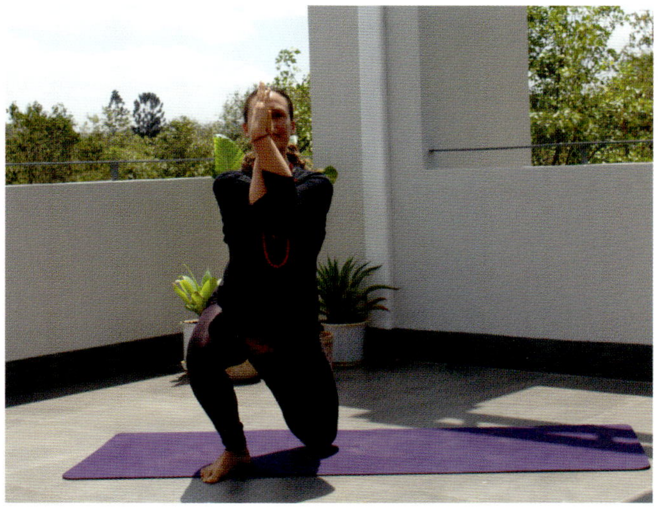

GARUDA VATAYANASANA
Unicorn

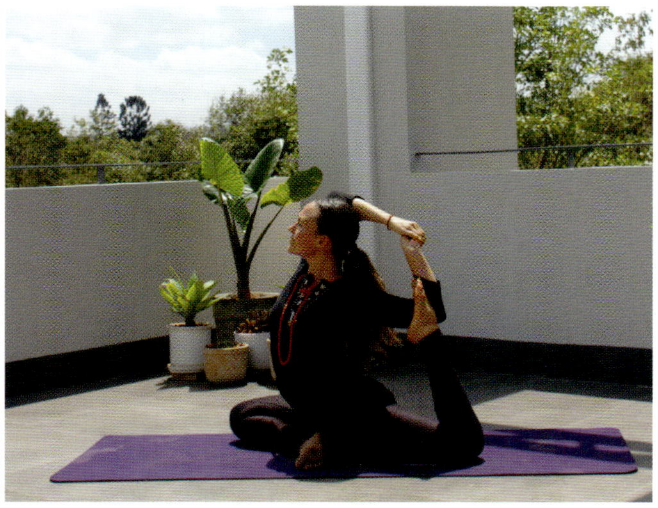

MATSYAANGANASANA & MAKARAMUDRA
Mermaid & Fertility

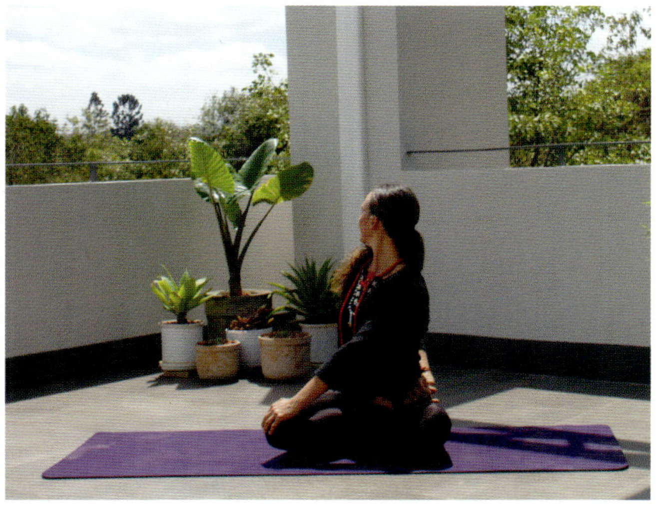

BHARADVAJASANA
Twisting Sage

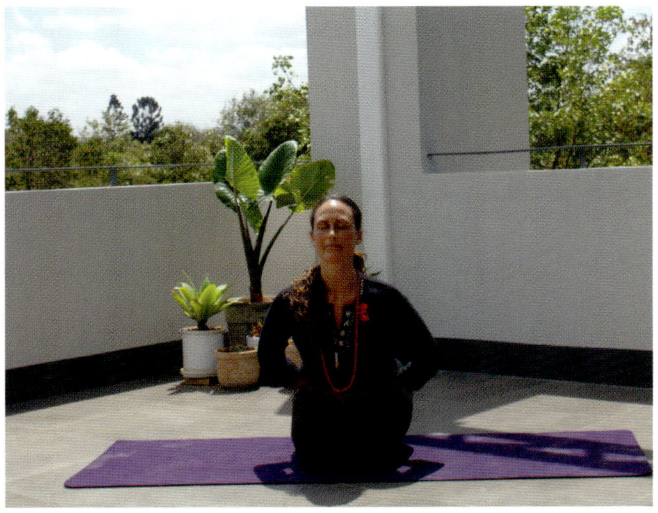

MANDUKASANA
Tadpole

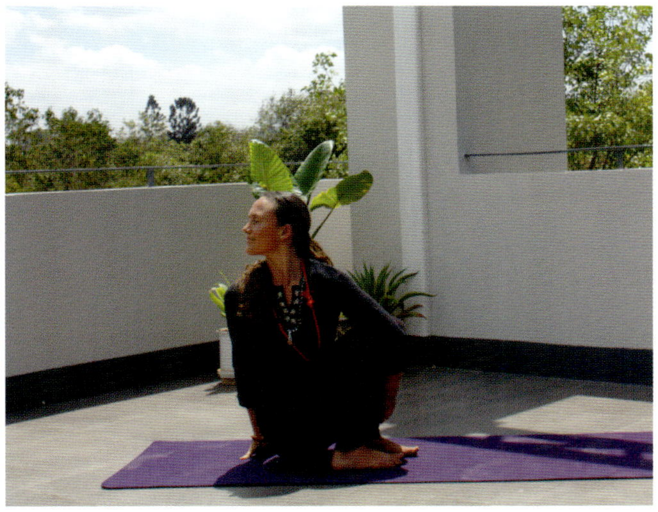

PASASANA
Rope Twist

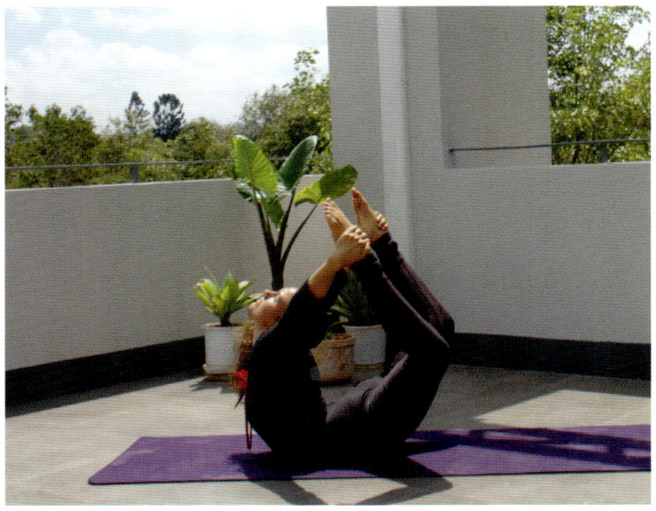

DHANURASANA
Bow

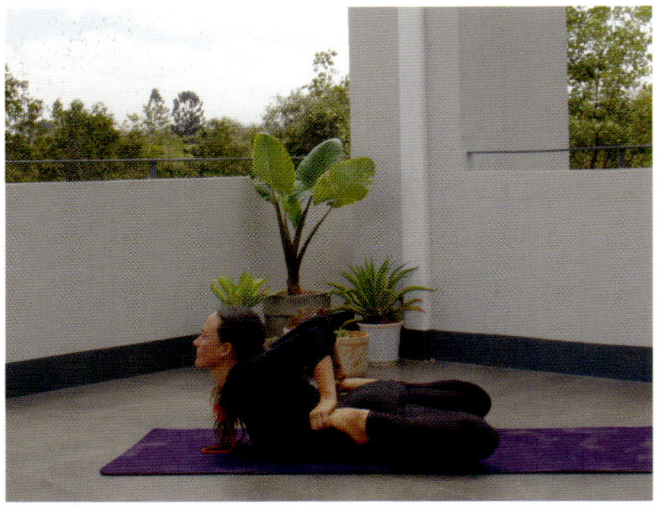

BHEKASANA
Frog

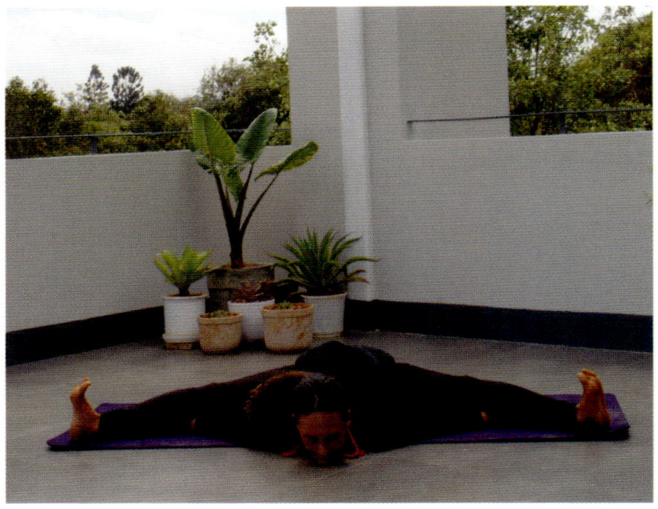

KURMASANA
Turtle

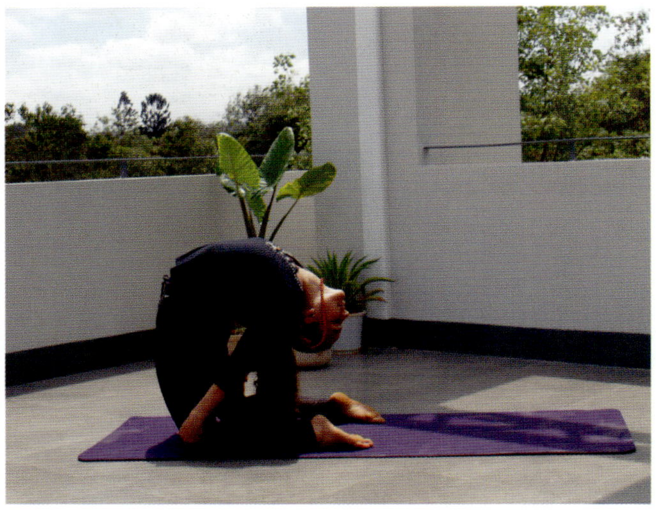

LAGHU VAJRASANA
Small Thunderbolt

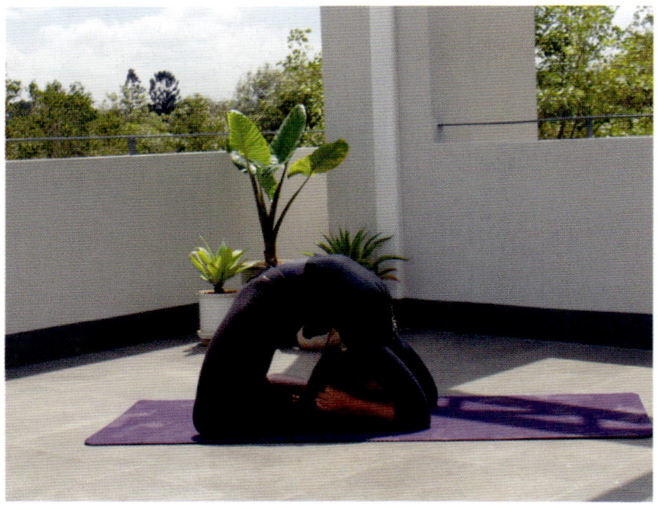

KAPOTASANA
Royal Pigeon

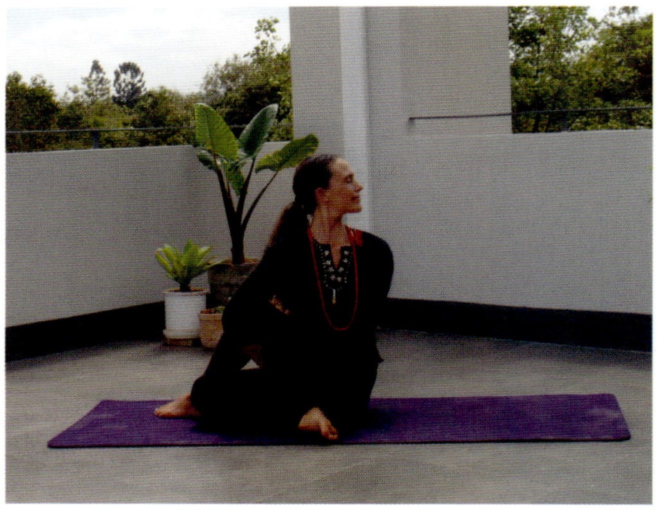

BADDHA ARDHA MATSYENDRASANA
Seated Bound Twist

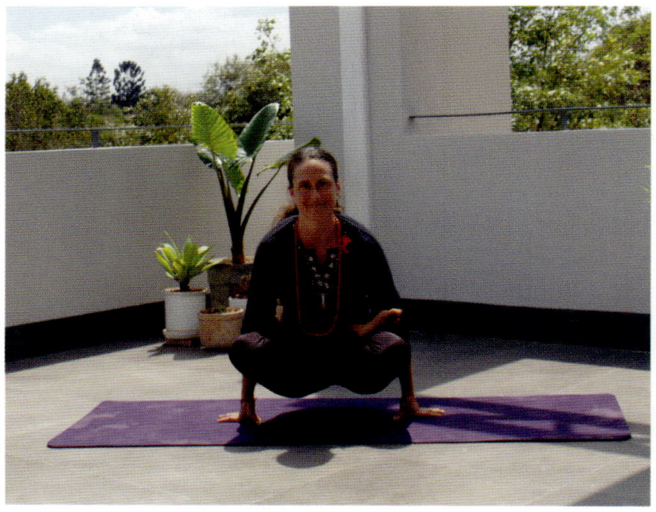

TOLASANA
Floating Lotus

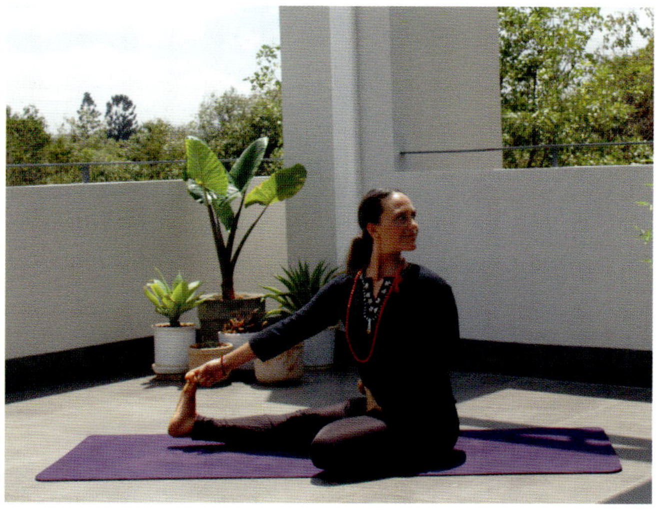

UPAVISTHA VRKSASANA
Rooted Tree

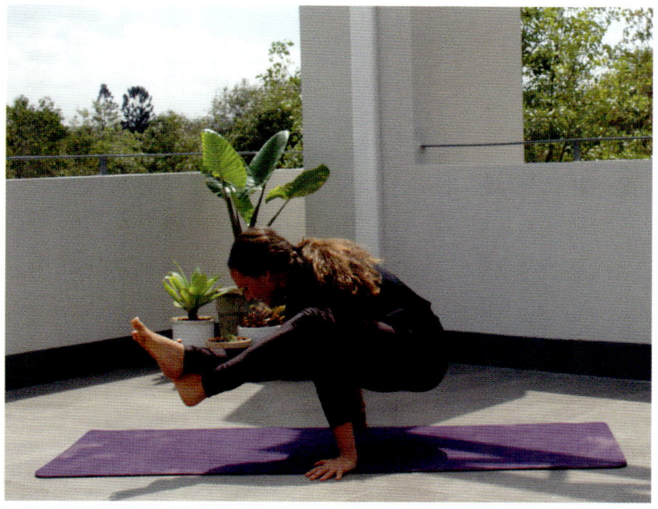

EKA HASTA BHUJASANA
Dancing Elephant

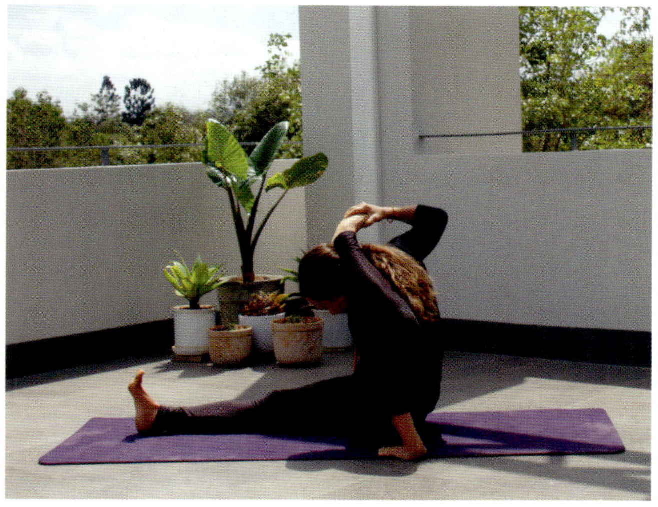

EKA PADA SIRSASANA
Legs behind Head

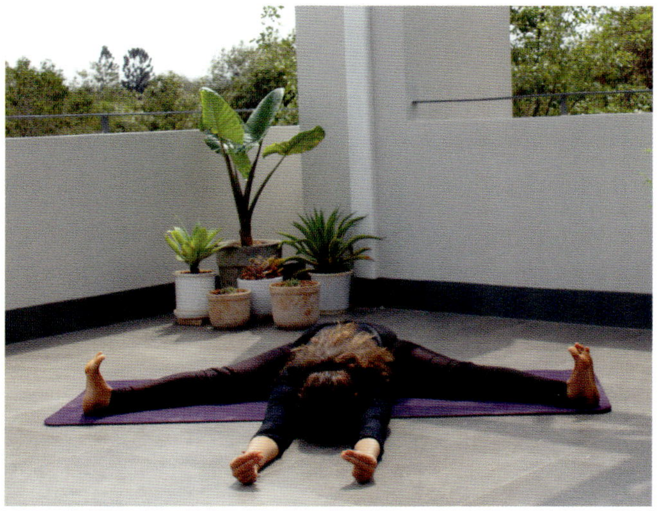

UPAVISTHA KONASANA & KUBERAMUDRA
Wide-Angle Seated Forward Bend & Abundance

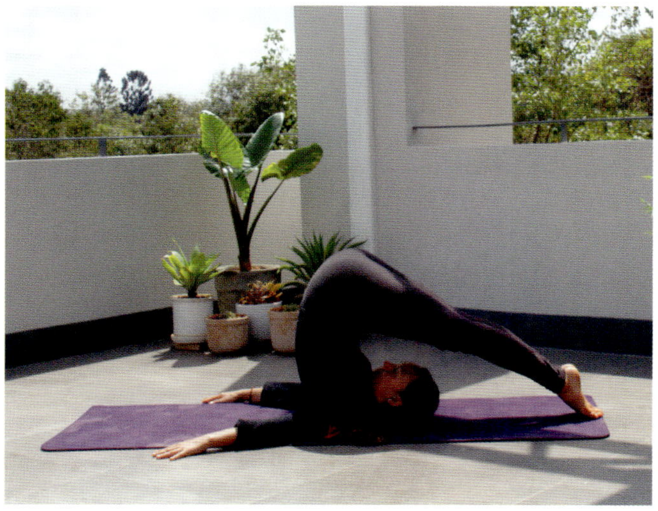

HALASANA
Plow

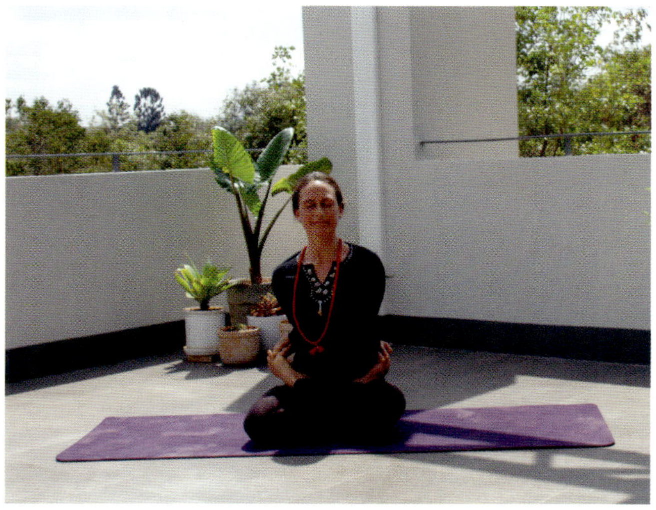

BADDHA PADMASANA
Bound Lotus

INCREASE ENERGY

In Brahma Tula / Libra, we are initiating air, which represents the beginning of a new cycle and is a catalyst for change and a desire for balance, beauty, and harmony. In Brahma Vrishchika / Scorpio, we are in the settled season of water, like a mysterious reflective lake. It represents the middle phase of a cycle, where the initial inspiration and potential have, through productivity, led to prosperity. And we can hold on to what has been created. The combination of these two signs is ideal for this chapter on increasing energy.

In Brahma Yoga, energy means the life force or prana that flows not only through your body but also through the entire cosmos. Traditional yoga believes that the flow of energy in the body, which is a channel, can become blocked or stagnant through living. In Brahma Yoga, we believe that the body is not merely a channel but also a conduit. Furthermore, I truly believe that with a dedicated yoga practice, you will be not only a conduit but also a portal—a gateway to higher consciousness capable of enormous vision and beauty that can transform your life and bring wonder to all those who surround you.

Through the asanas in this chapter—and the pranayama breathing techniques such as lion's breath, fire breath, and cleansing breath—we can regulate, harmonize, and balance the flow of energy in the body. We move the spine in all available directions in order to rouse and awaken the energy called kundalini that resides within the central channel called the sushumna nadi. The closest parallel to this that we are familiar with is the spinal cord, in which varied nerve networks travel between the brain and body. Along with the sushumna is the ida nadi, which is a cooling, passive energy channel linked with the moon and the feminine principle. Its breath dominance is the left nostril, and it is associated with the inward, calming, and reflective aspect of our consciousness. The pingala nadi is considered to be the warming, active energy channel associated with the sun and the masculine principle. Its breath dominance is the right nostril, and it is the outward, active aspect of our consciousness. The nasal cycle alternates the flow of air between the two nostrils approximately every 90 minutes. Brahma Yoga will help you breathe fully with awareness and develop a more bihemispheric mind.

Through the dynamic and energetic movement of the sequences in this chapter, we activate and harmonize the energy centers in the body, described as chakras, which means "spinning wheel." In Ayurveda, there are 72,000 nadis that carry the prana life force throughout the human body. This is the reason there are 72 mudras integrated within the asanas of the Brahma Yoga sequences in this book. Each mudra is dedicated to a thousand nadis each.

Through the asanas in this chapter, you will activate and balance your chakras. This will initially cause you to loosen fatigue, lethargy, and tiredness, and eventually, with practice, you will start to see the benefits of increased luminosity in your thinking and a more effortless and vibrant body. The result will be that your willpower expands. You will spontaneously start to experience more creativity, and opportunities will present themselves to you, leading to great transformation.

BRAHMA YOGA SUTRAS

BRAHMA TULA • Libra

- I have great willpower, as I know the sky is my mirror and my spirit is its reflection.
- I am kind, sincere, and compassionate and give others the opportunity to express themselves.
- The universe is in expansion. It is invested in me, and I am its beneficiary.
- I can differentiate between the eternal and the transient with precision.
- I encourage fluidity, as in my essence, I am a lover made to love.
- Brahma Yoga, regardless of what I may have learned from some humans, shows me that love is love without exceptions or conditions.
- Through beauty and truth, there is great transformation to a higher level of consciousness.
- I am a force for good, and I can empathize with others without losing my position and well-being.
- I give others the freedom to be truly who they are.

BRAHMA VRISHCHIKA • Scorpio

- I know the sun made me see it and the moon made me do it, so I calibrate the connection between the masculine and feminine.
- When I am mindful of the pace and capacity of my breathing and how it affects my emotional state and focus, my productivity grows exponentially and compounds.
- Prosperity and powerful energy come to me when my resolve meets my ambition.
- I live with potential and instinct using discernment.
- Inspiration seeks to emerge through me like the colors of a spectrum. Rainbows represent hope and come after rain, which is a source of life.
- Brahma Yoga nurtures me so I no longer hurt myself with negative thoughts.
- There is no need to give all of me to others.
- I am free from any holding patterns or unresourceful cycles that keep me in any comfort zone for longer than required.
- With creativity, I can manifest anything I wish, so there is no need to force anything when I can consider it.

Live with equanimity between the delight
of an idea and the awareness of opportunity.

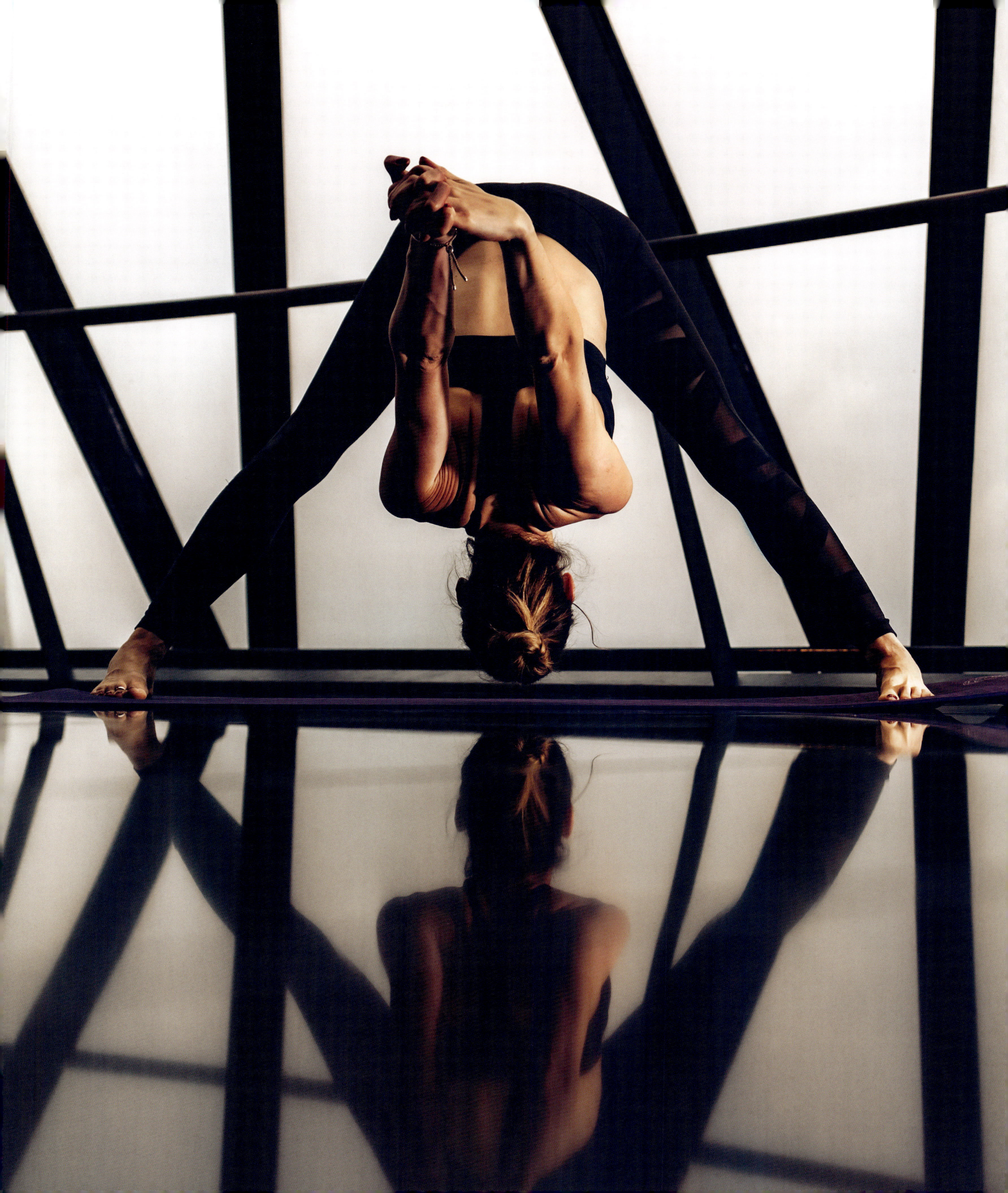

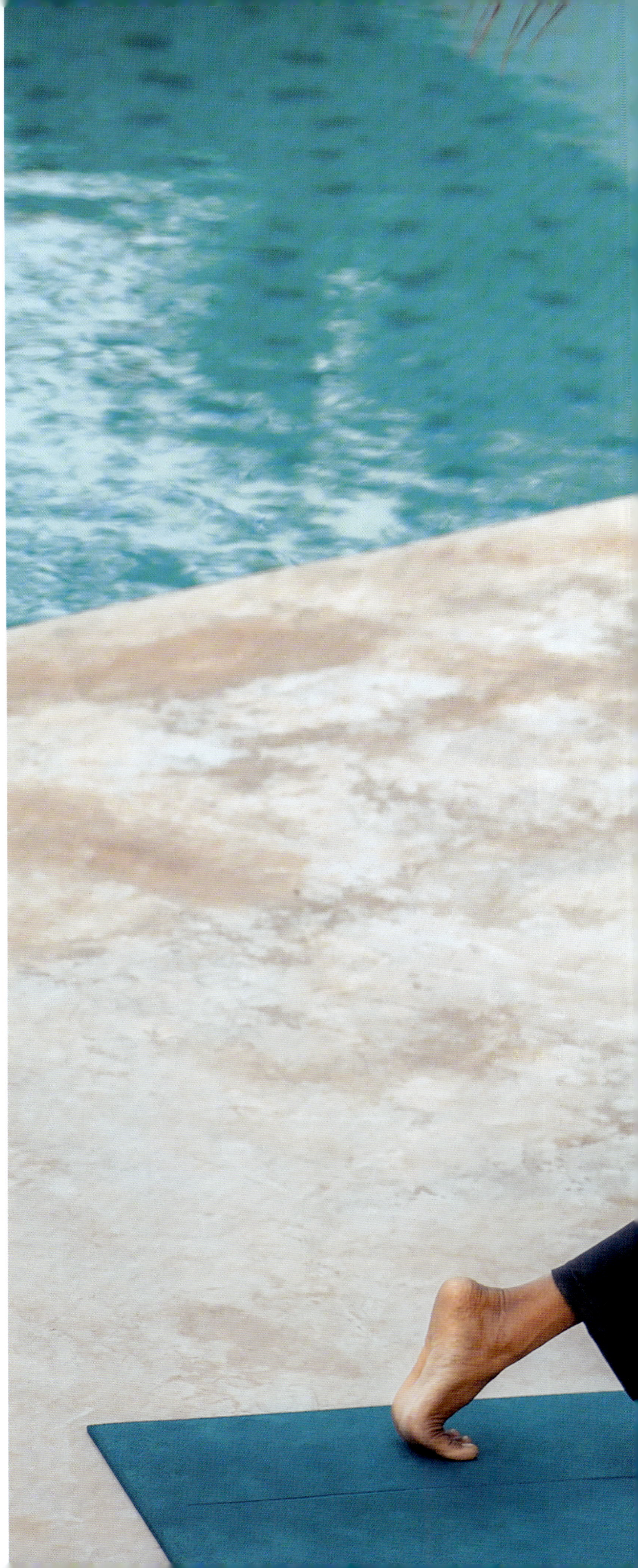

PARIVRTTA BANARASANA · Twisted Lunge

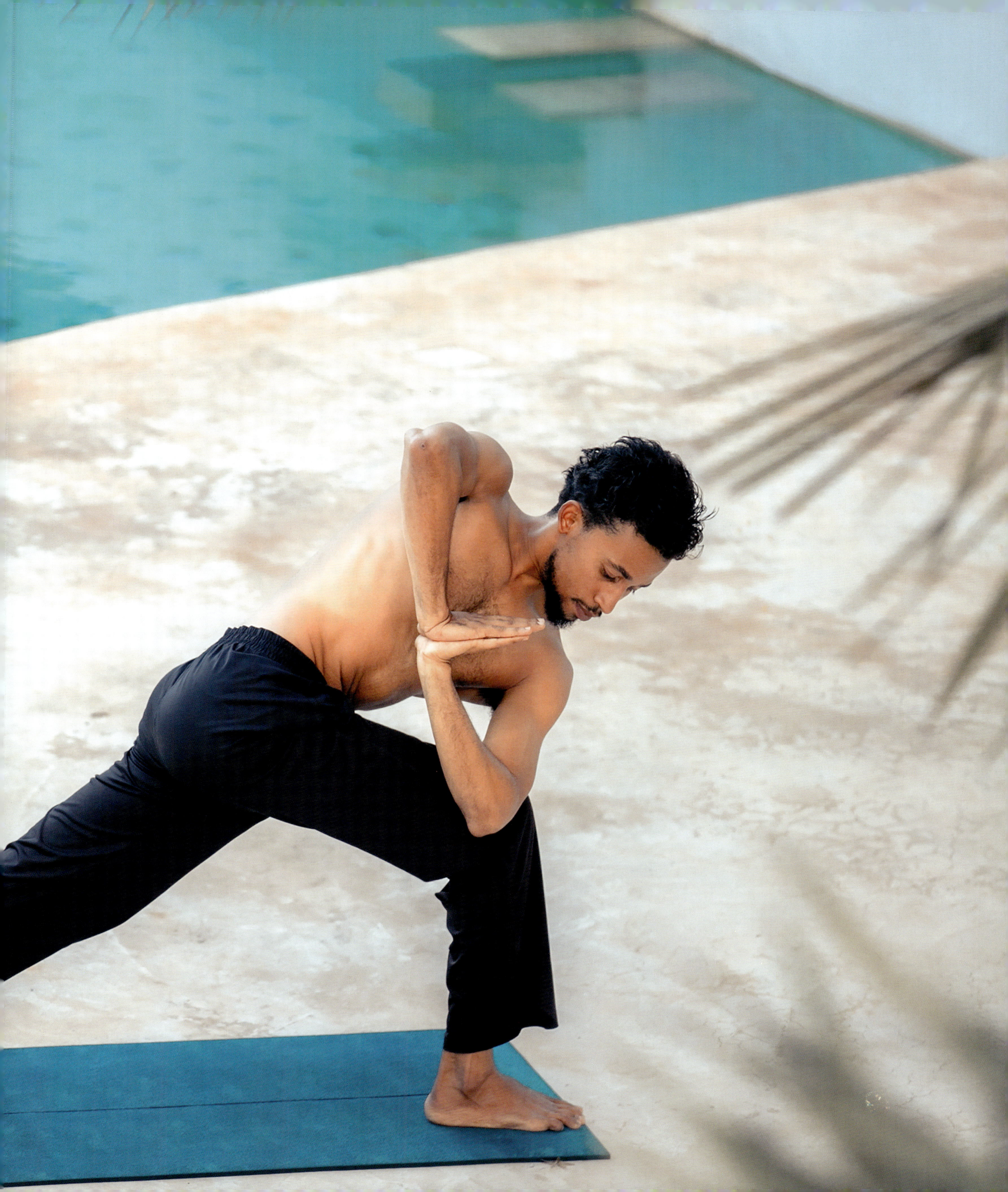

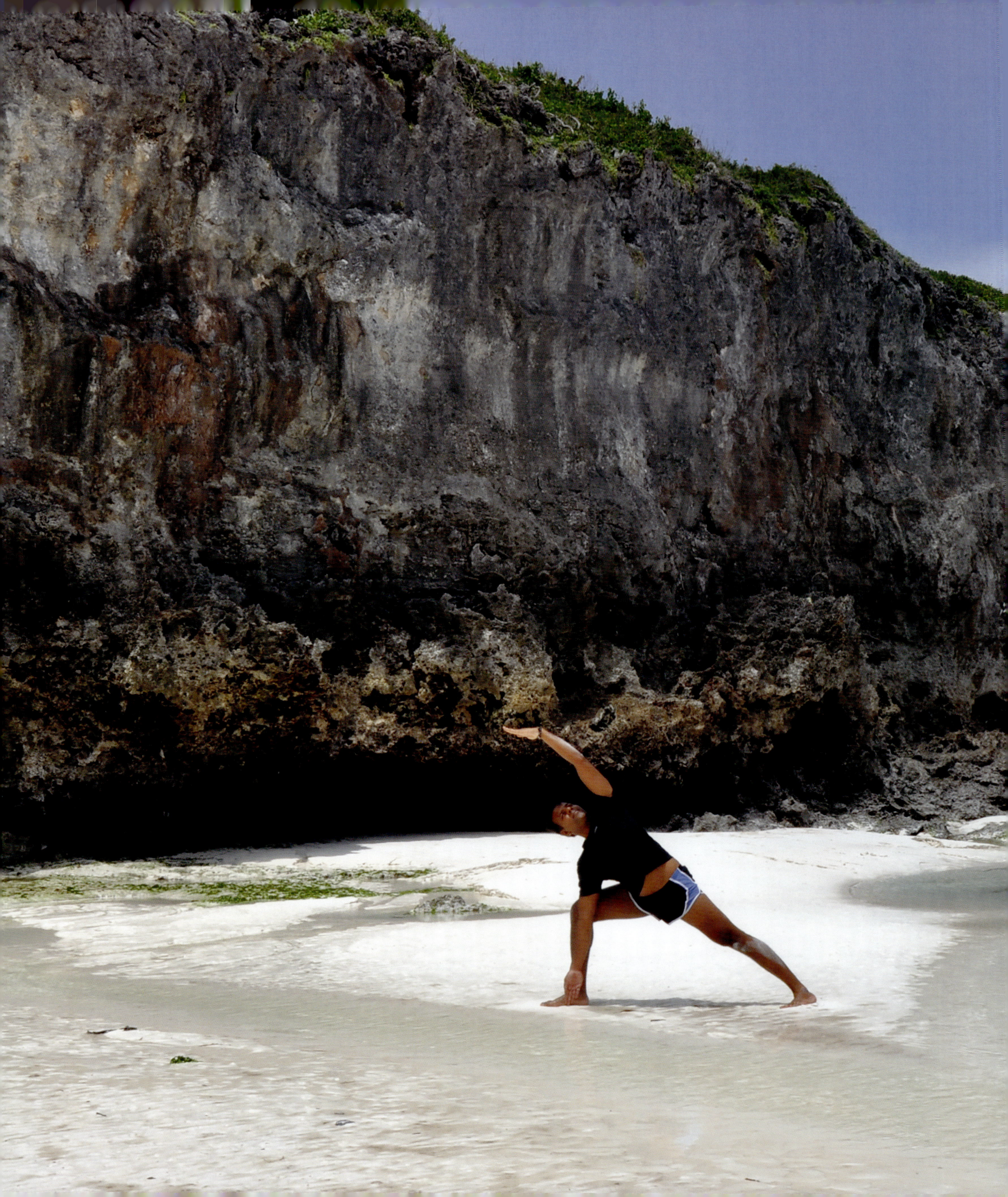

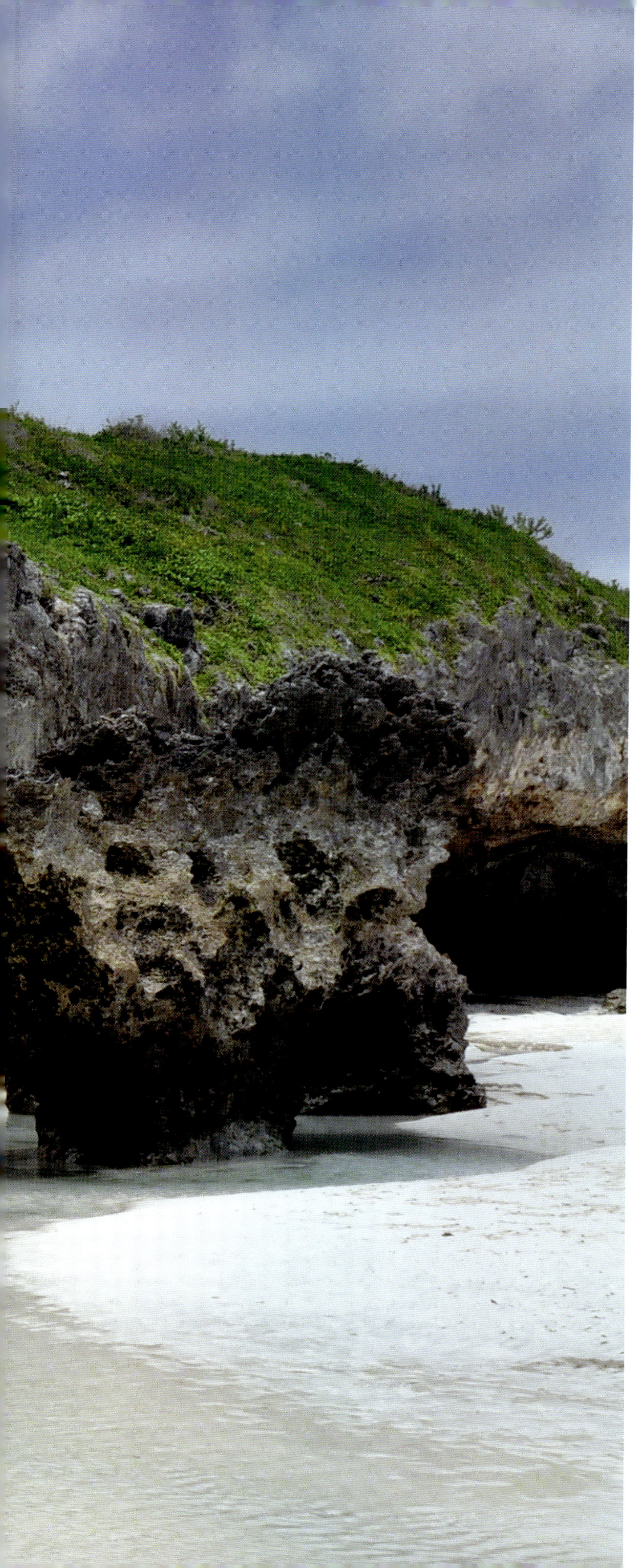

The first language is feeling, not words.

Love transcends words and even language.

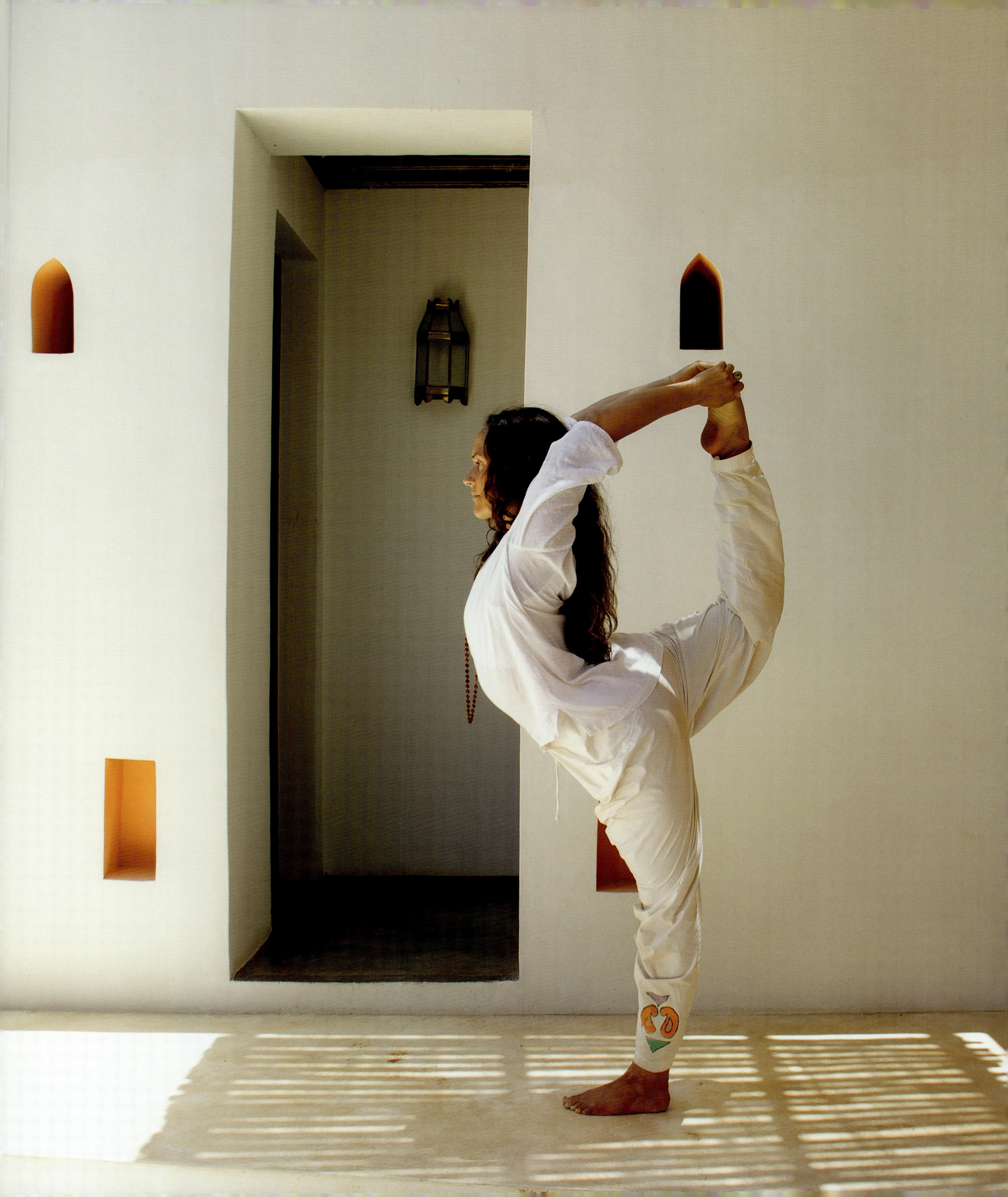

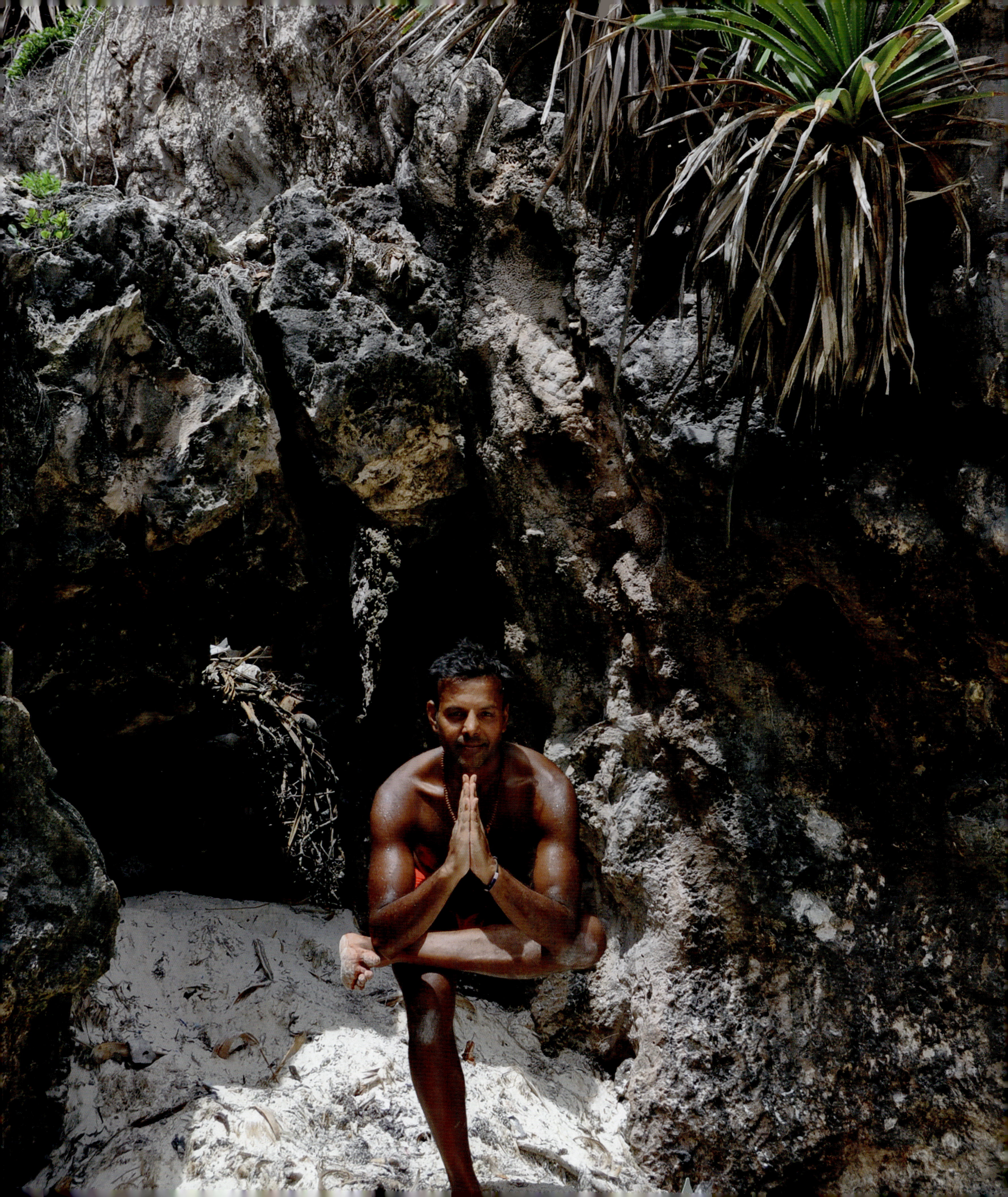

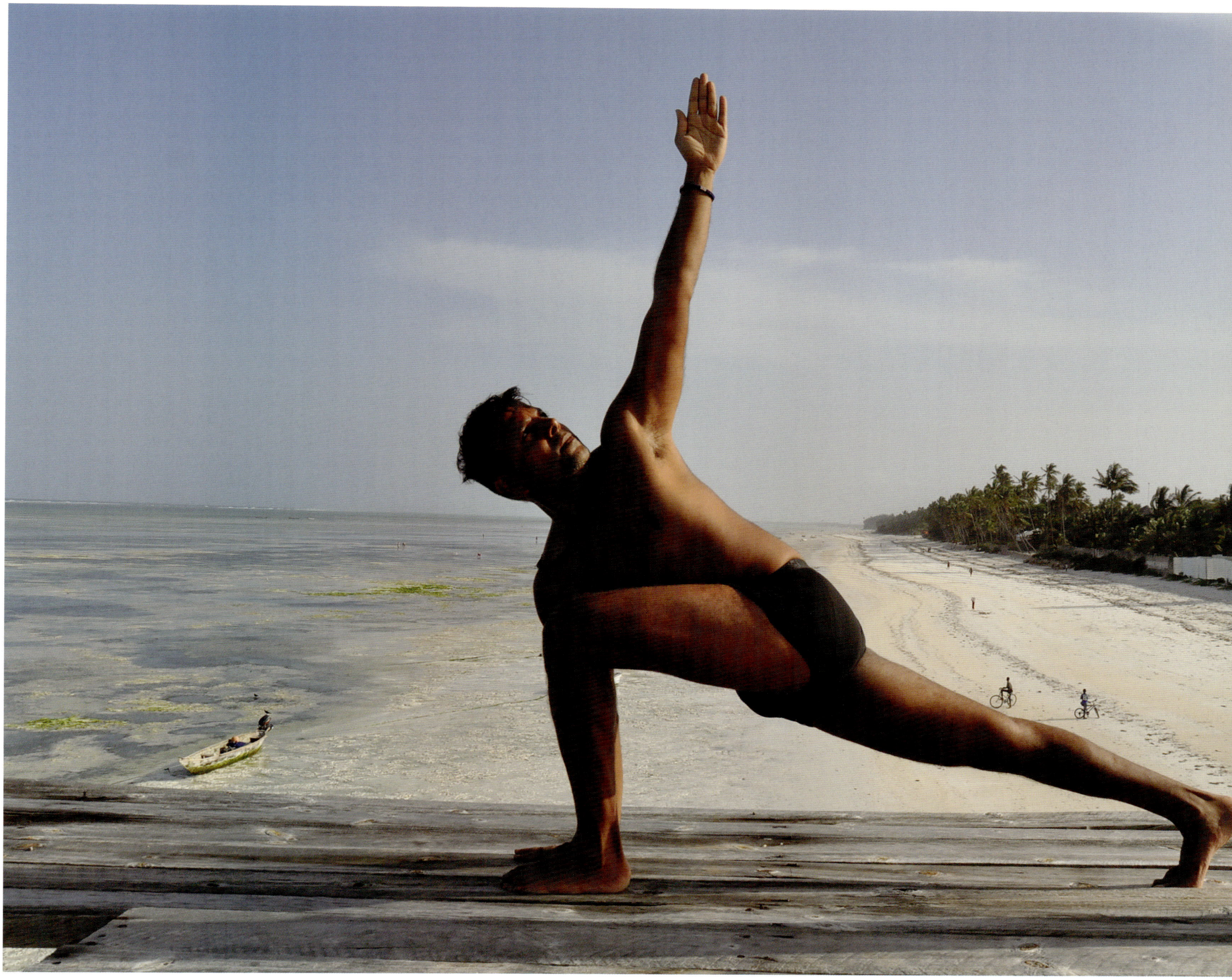

TADA KAPOTASANA • Standing Pigeon

▲ PARIVRTTA HASTA BANARASANA • Raised-Arm Twisted Lunge

Celebrate new beginnings.

NRTYPEDASANA • Dancing Tree

▼ BADDHA UTTHITA PARSVAKONASANA • Bound Side Angle

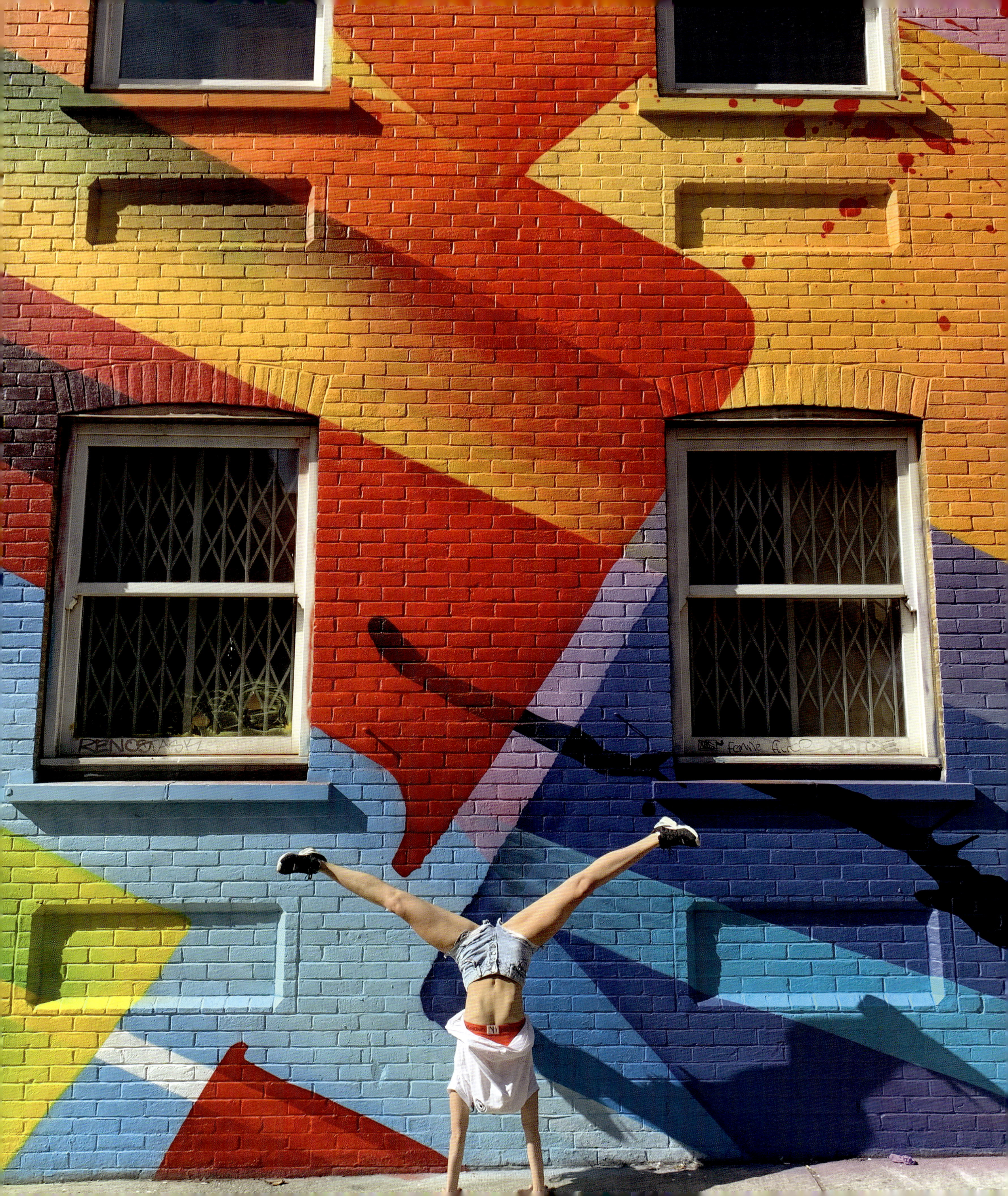

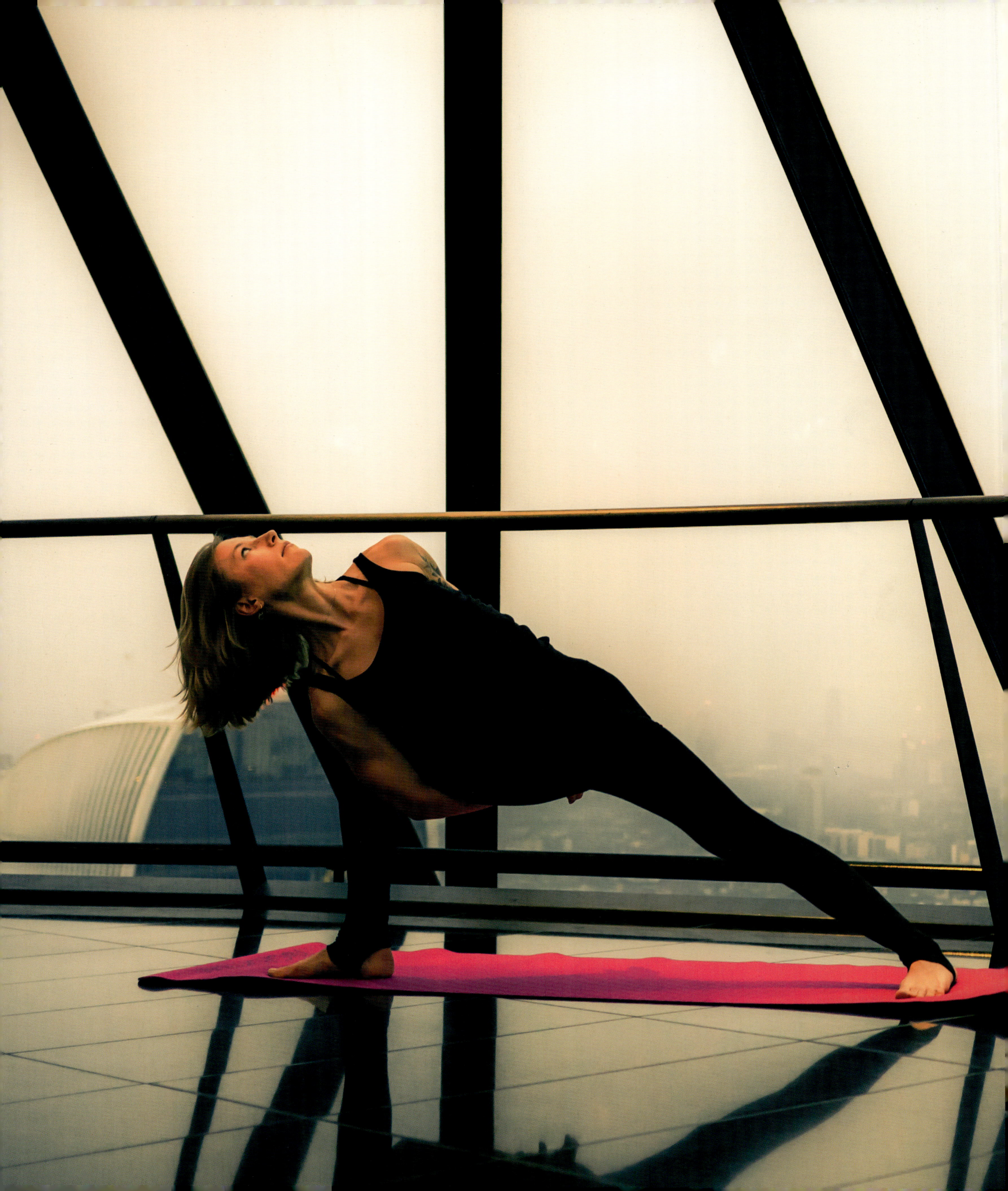

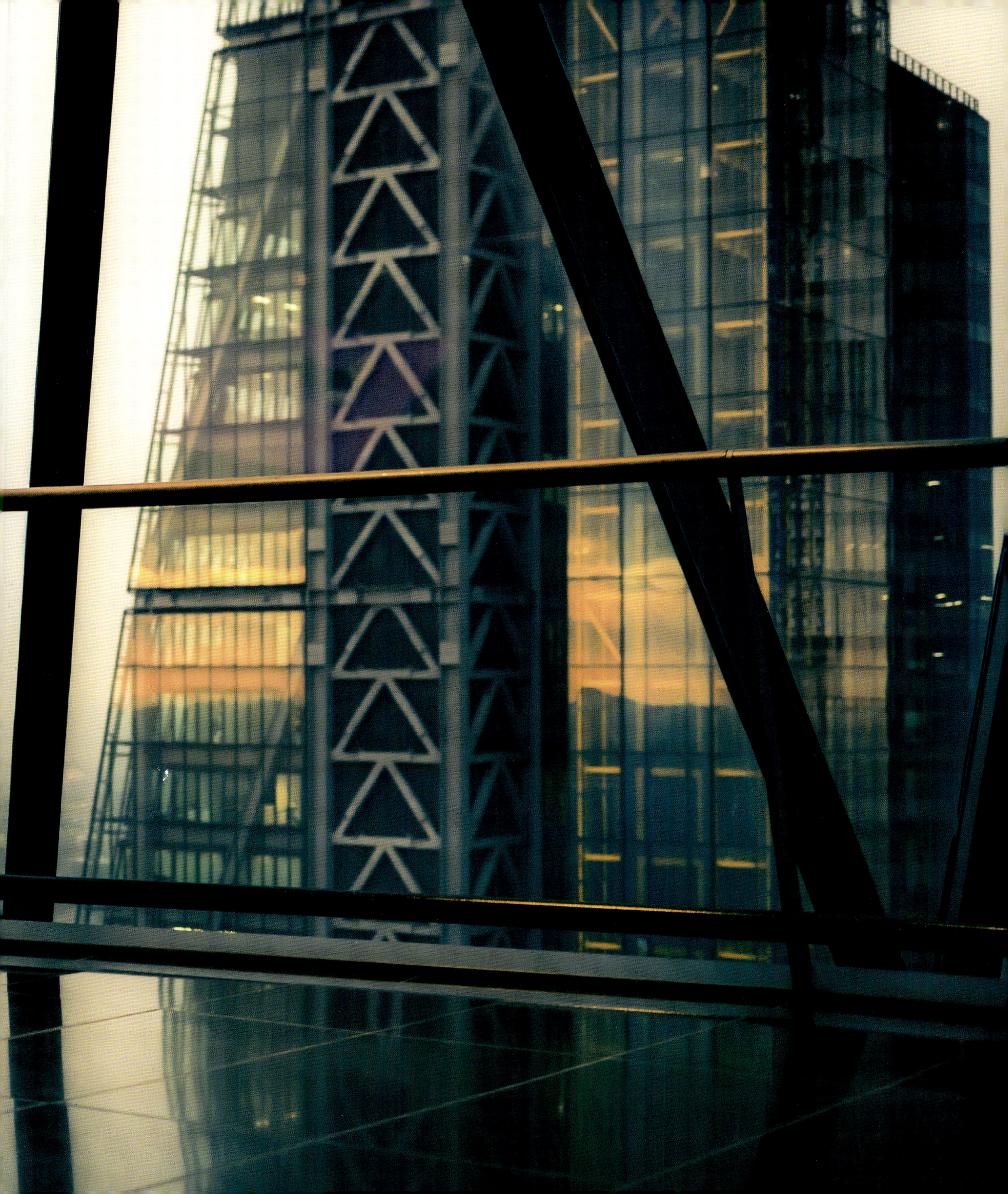

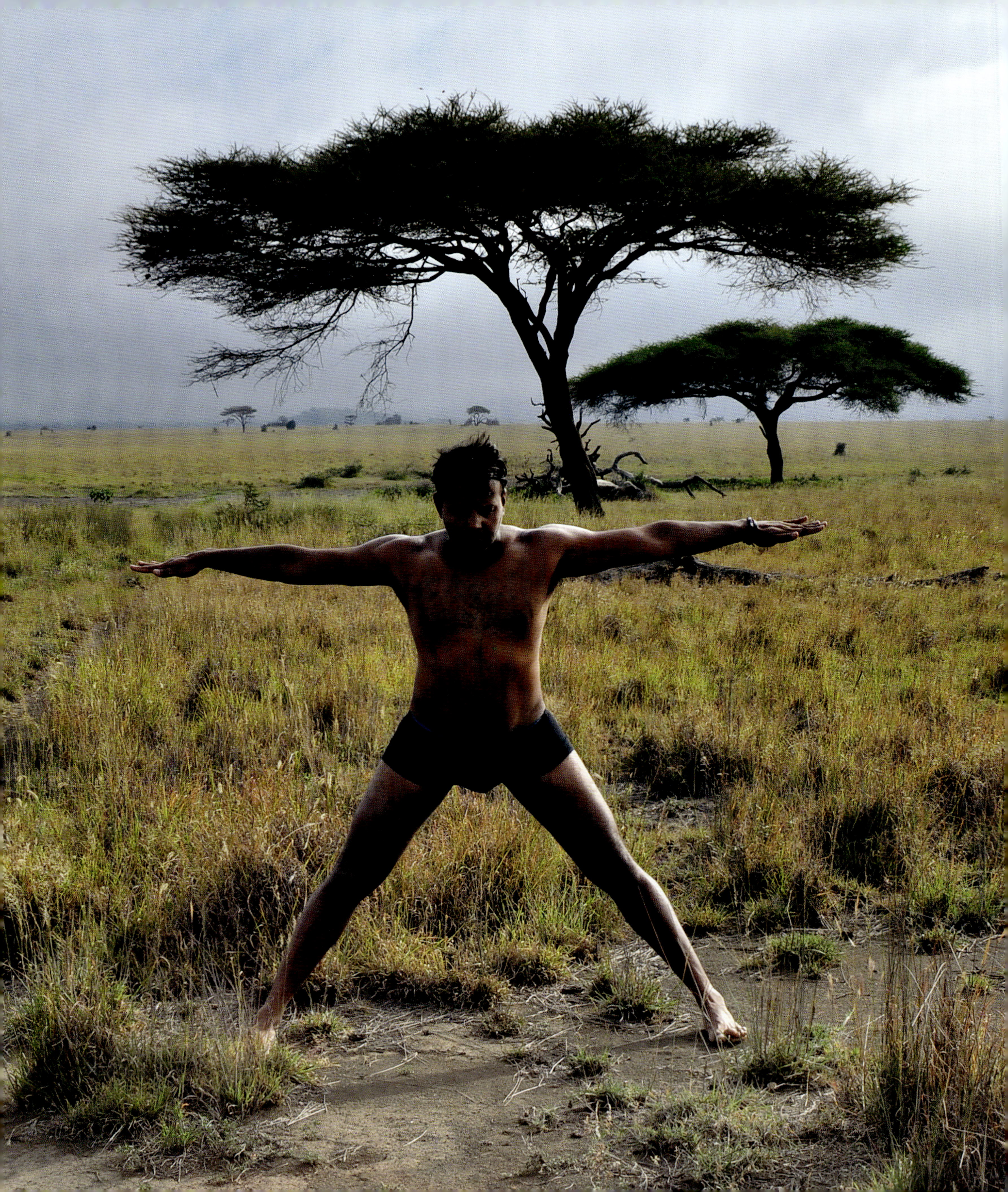

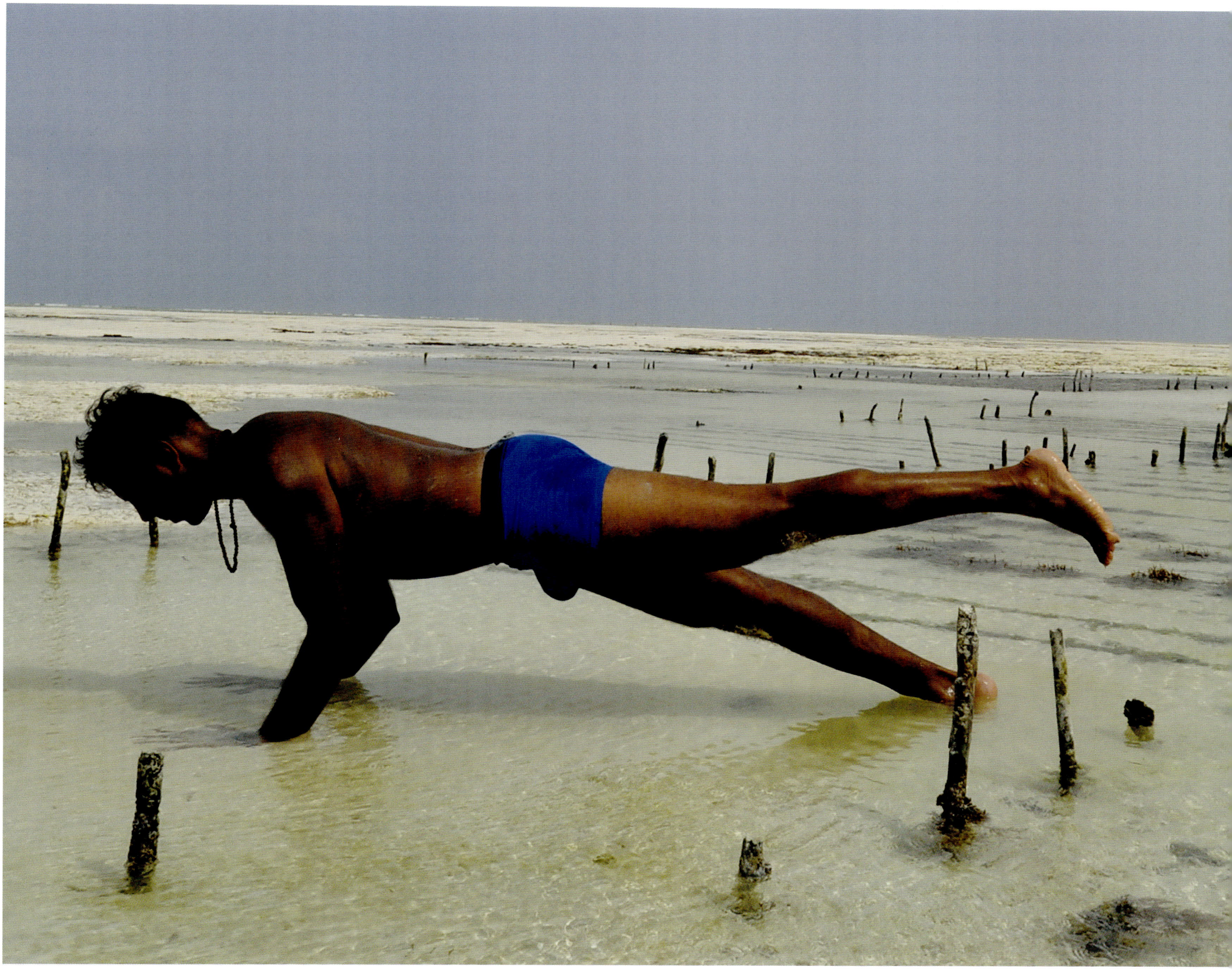

CHANDRA DEVASANA · Moon Angel

▲ **EKA PADA KUMBHAKASANA** · Leg-Lifted Plank

Even happiness is transient, as it needs a reason.

The ultimate state is bliss.

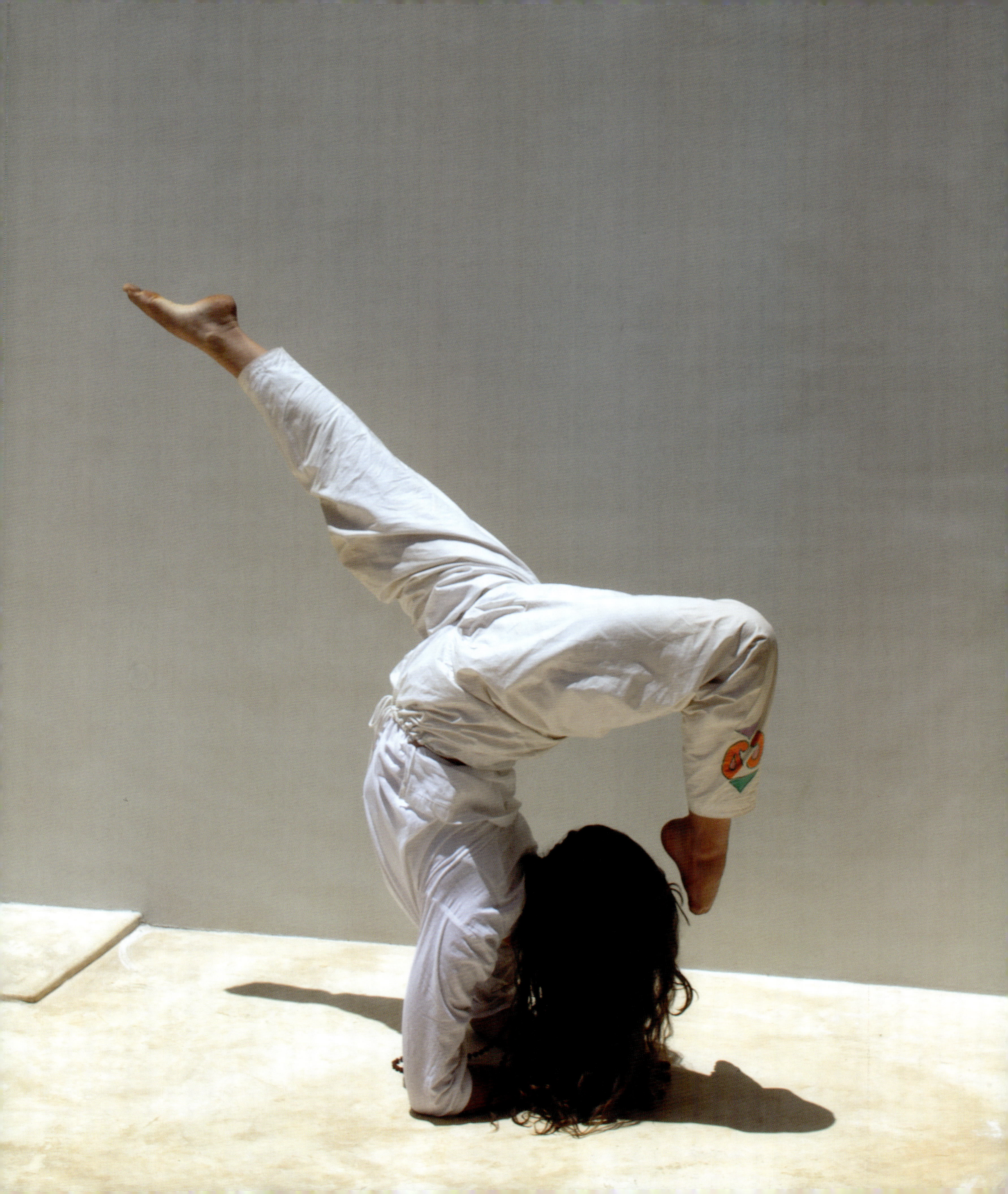

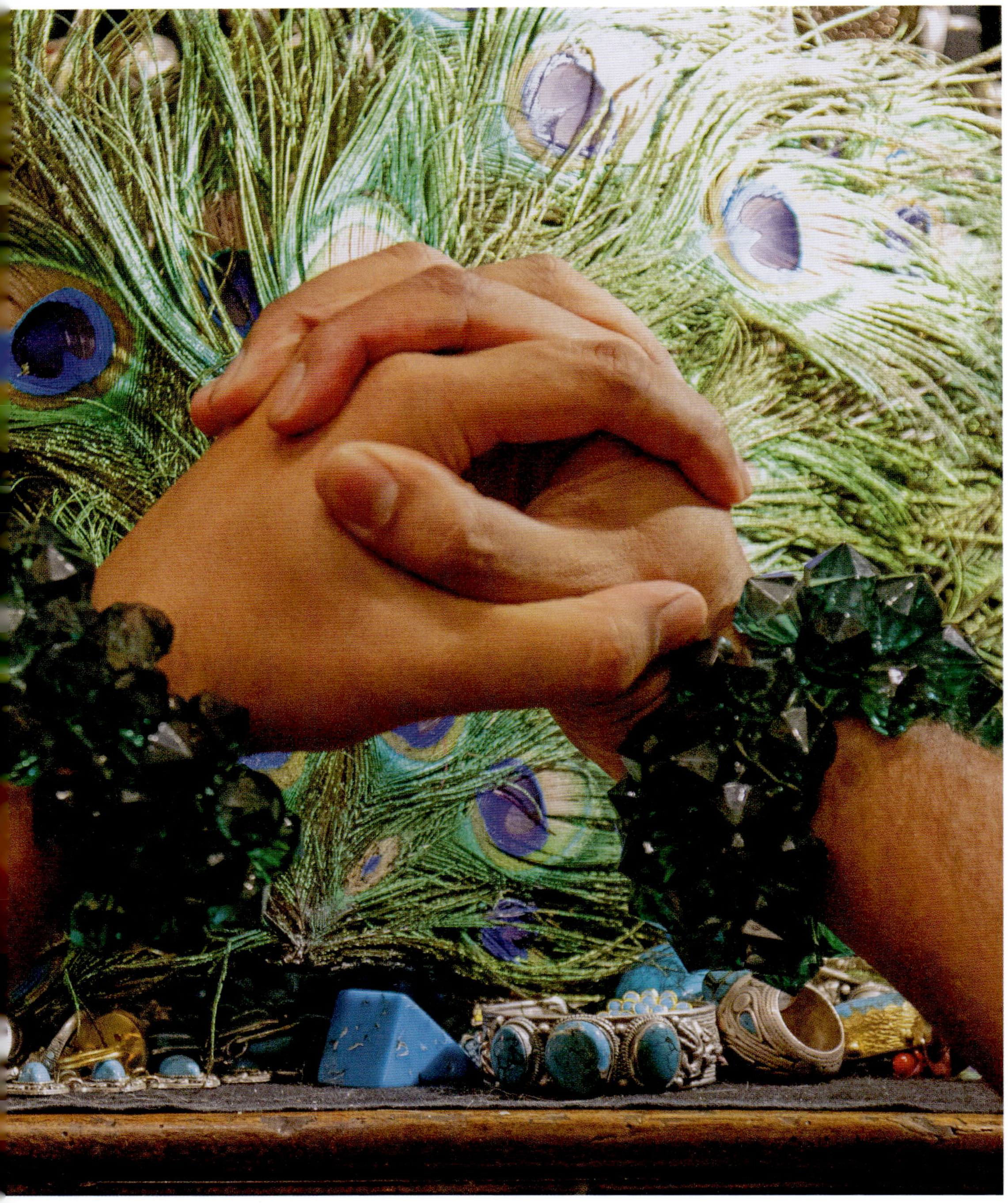

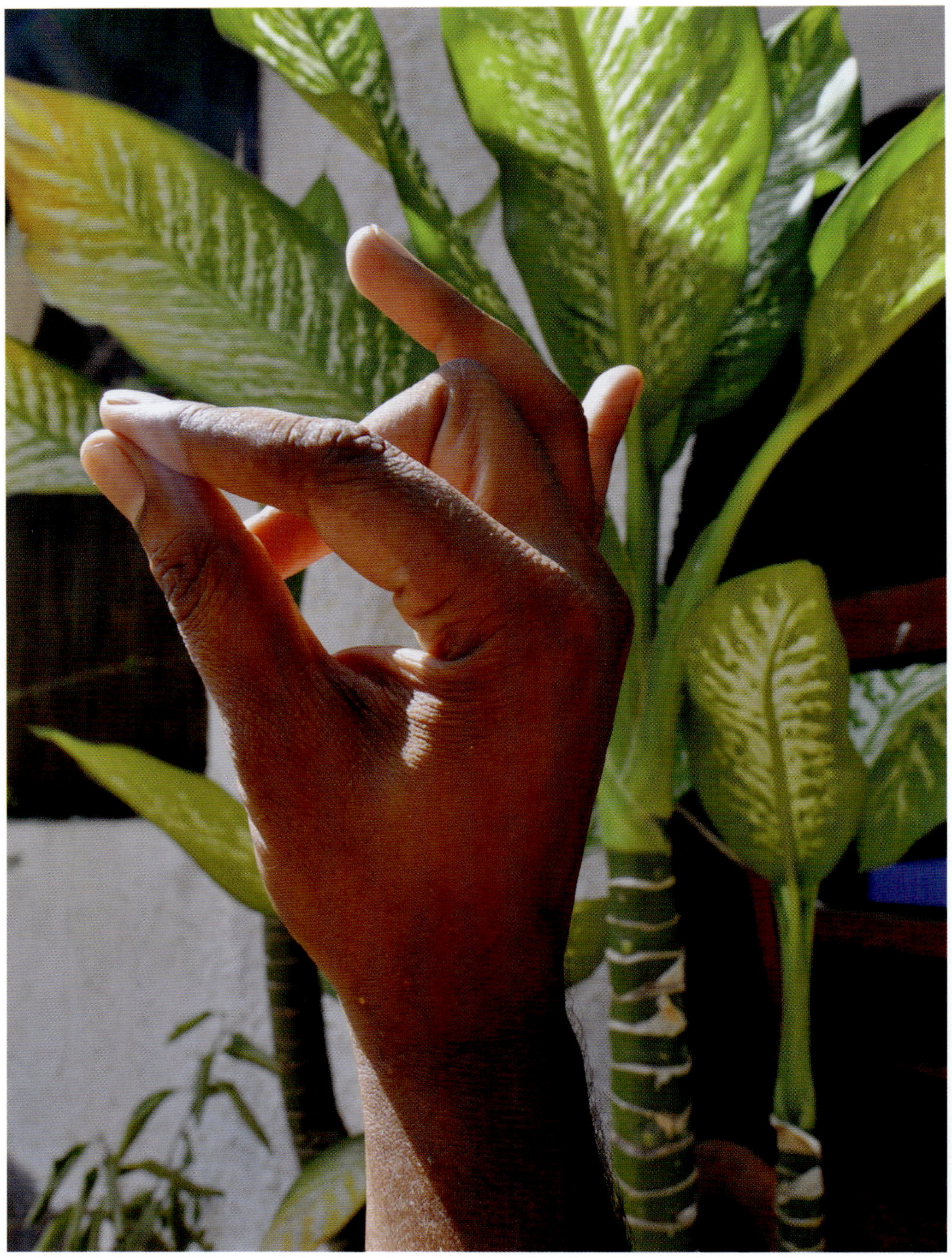

▲ **USHASMUDRA** · Productivity *(left)* **VYANAMUDRA** · Expansion *(right)*

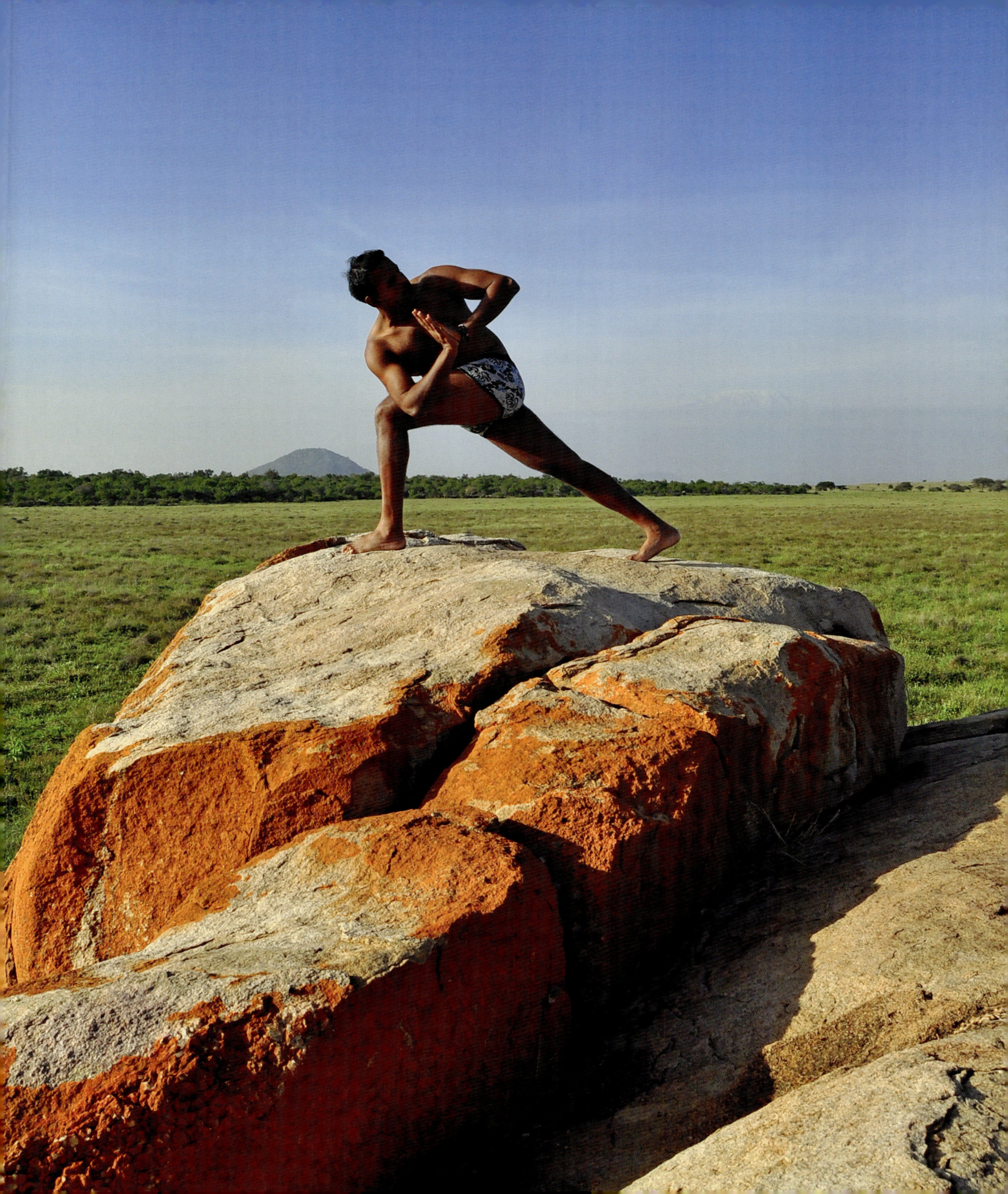

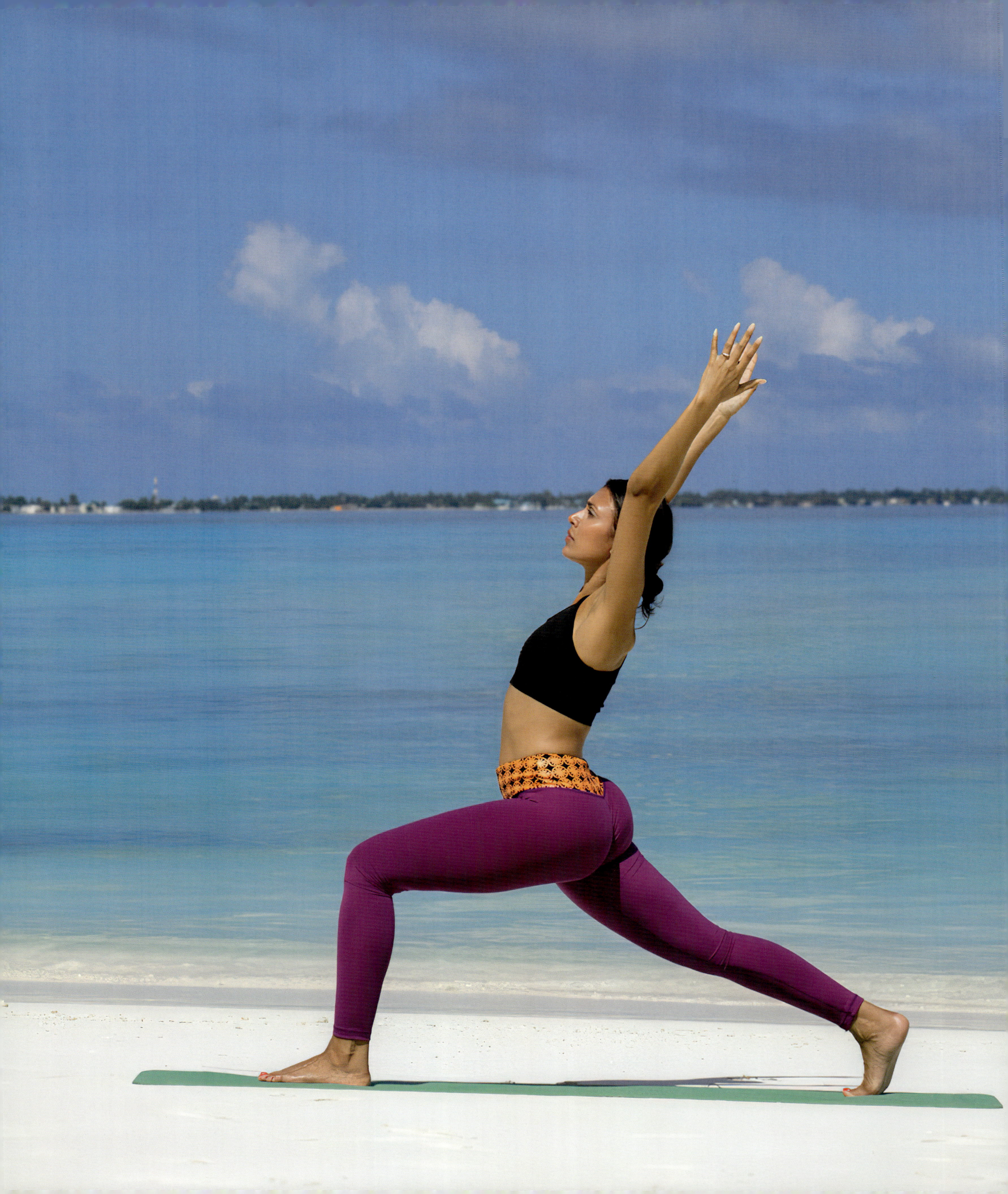

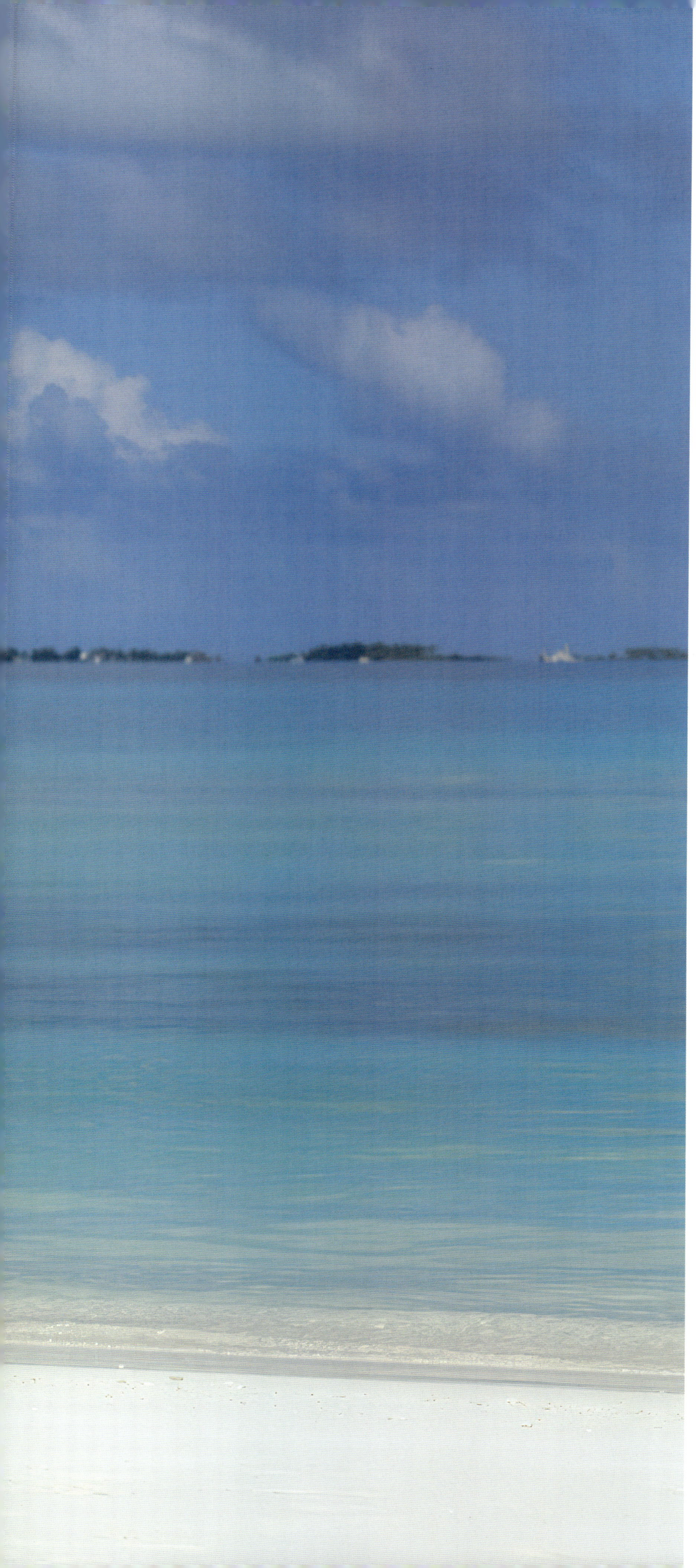

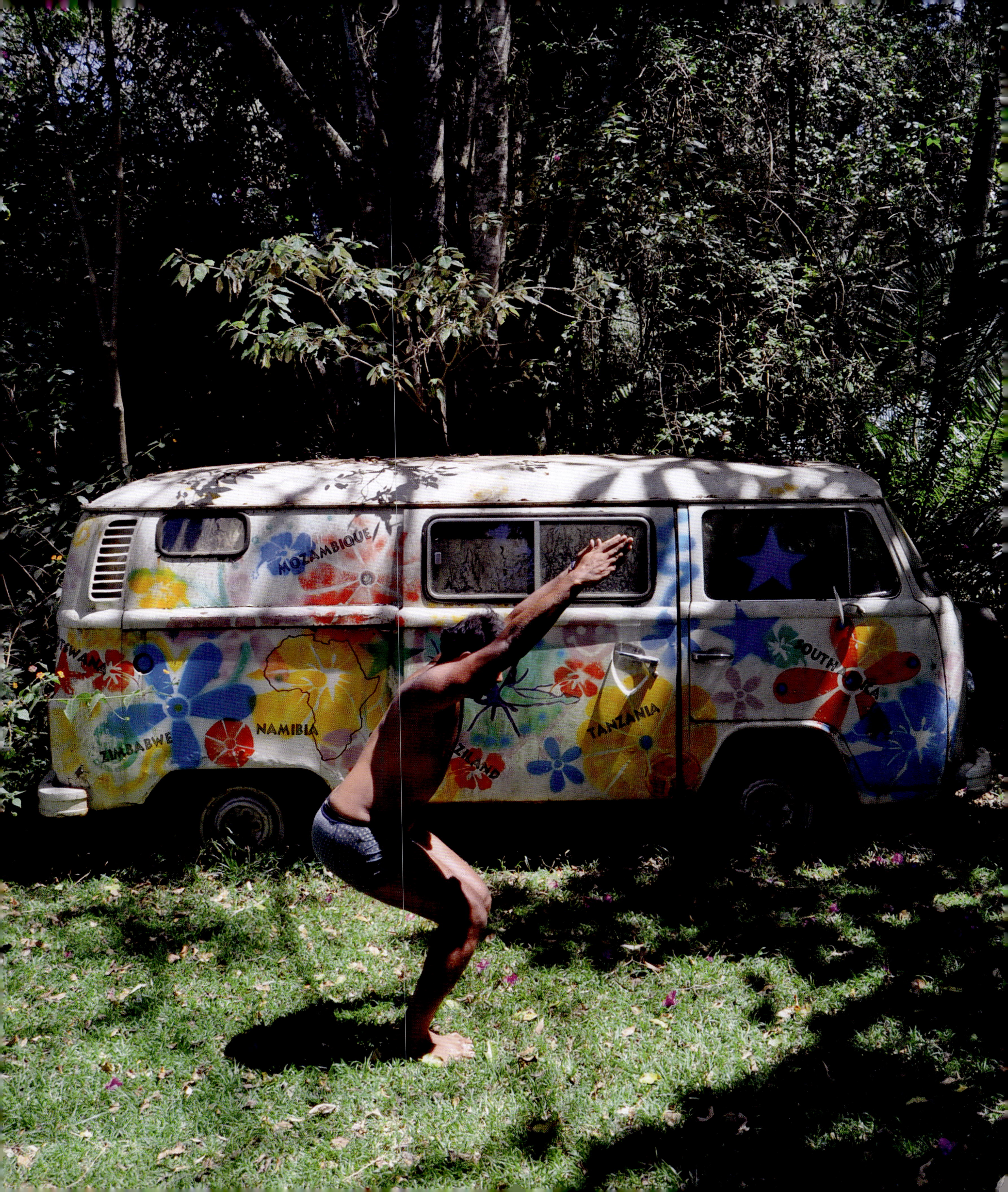
MOZAMBIQUE
NAMIBIA
ZIMBABWE
TANZANIA
SOUTH

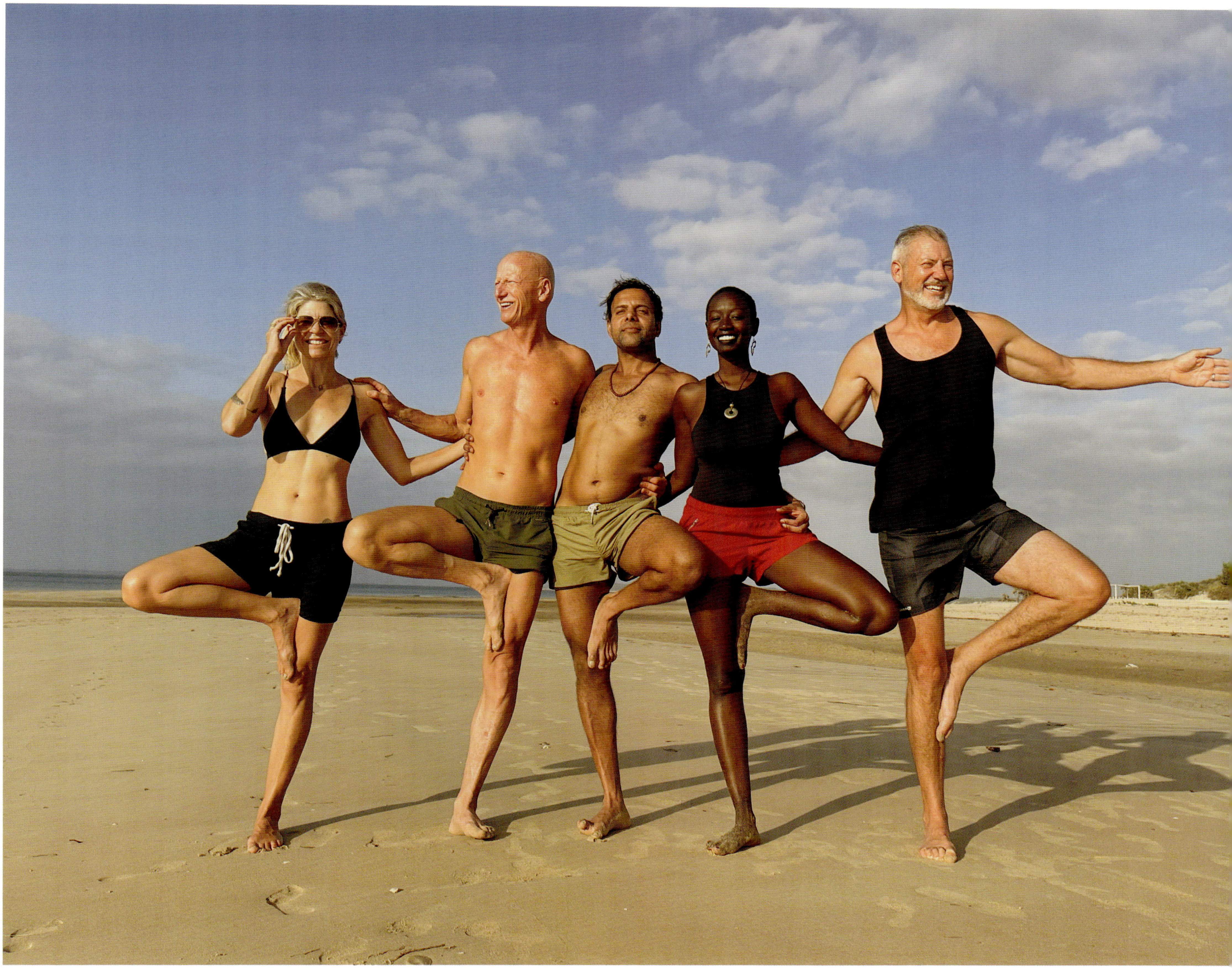

▲ SANGA PED · Gathering Trees

Reconnect to the source of all energy

by going off the grid.

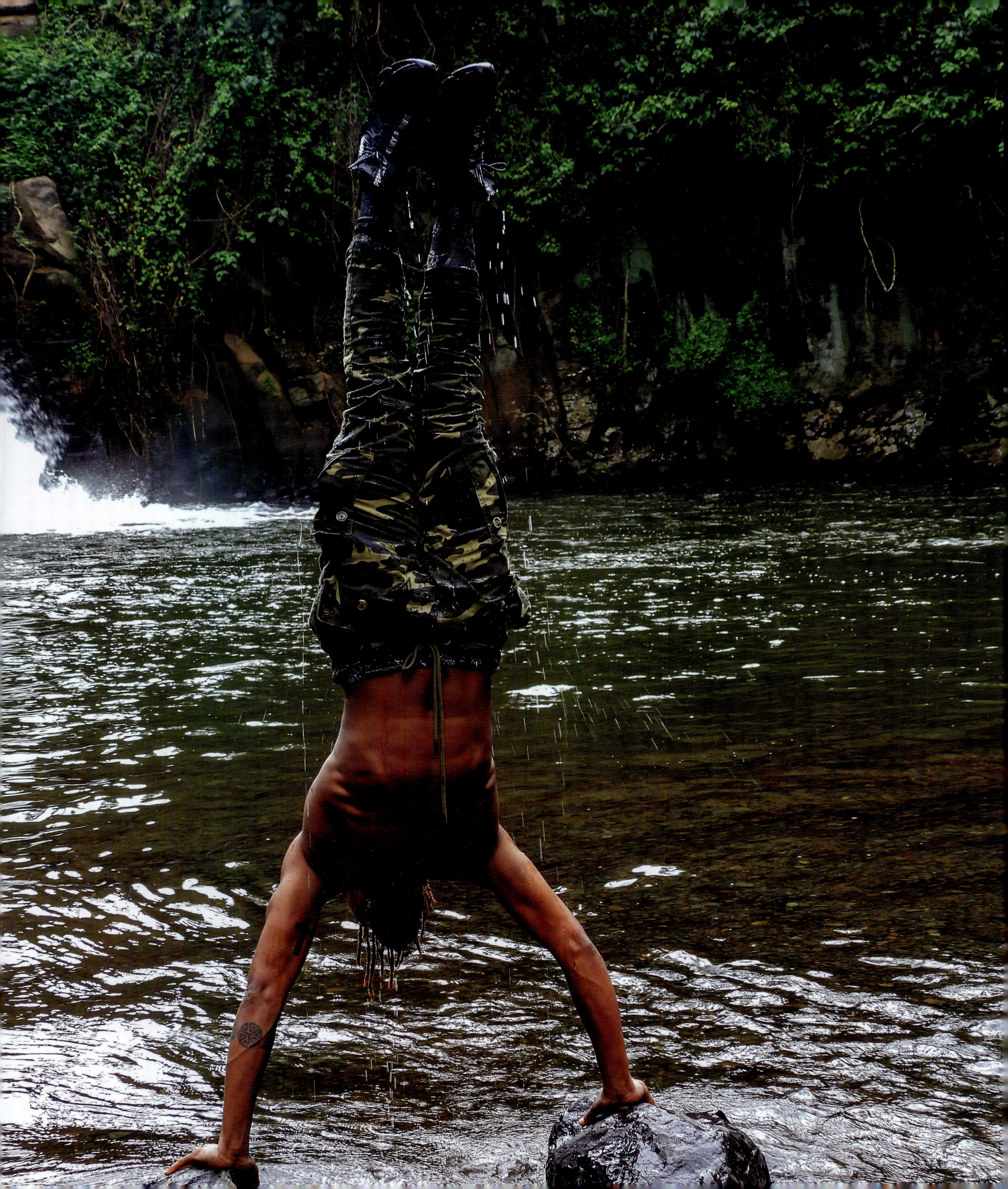

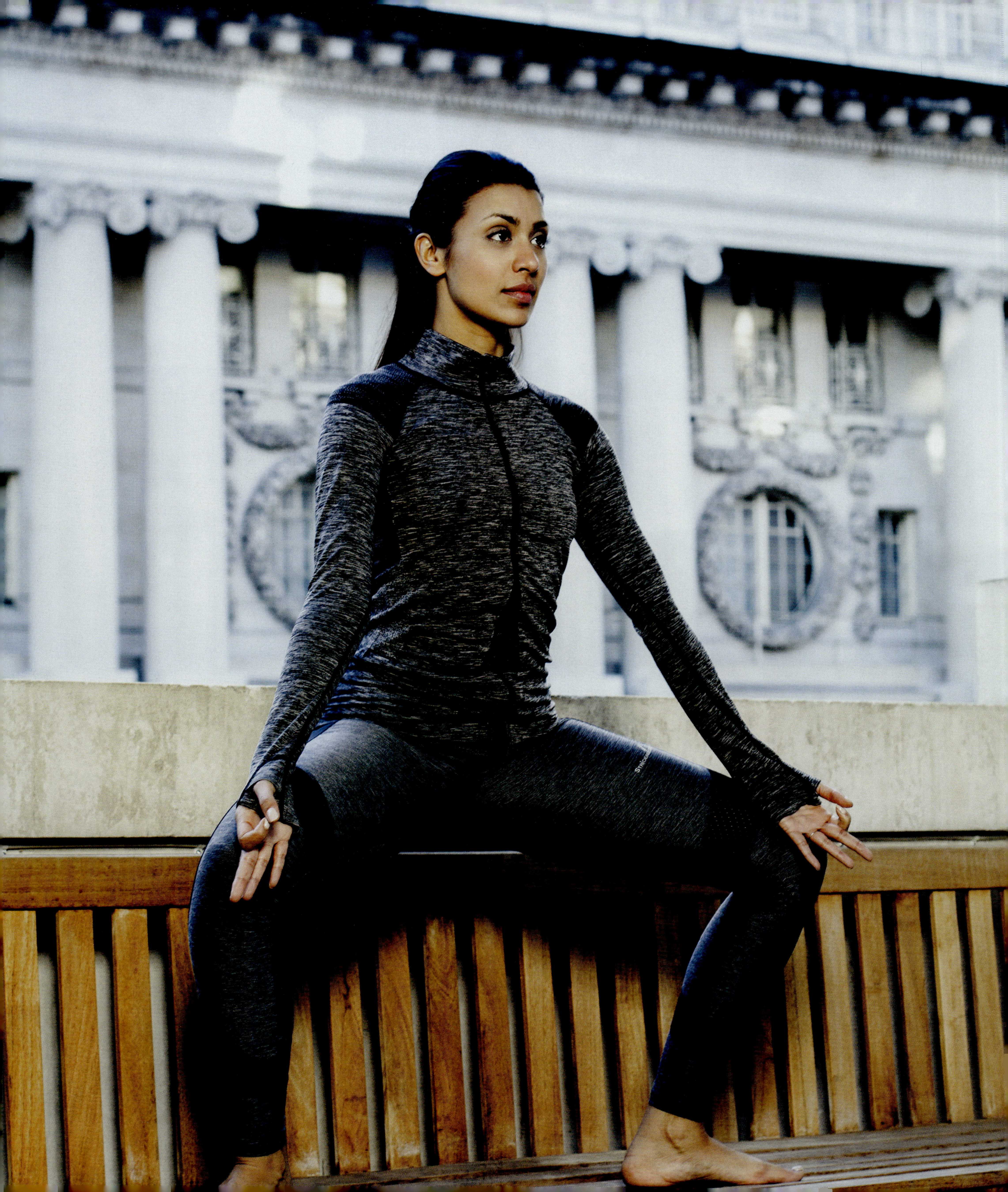

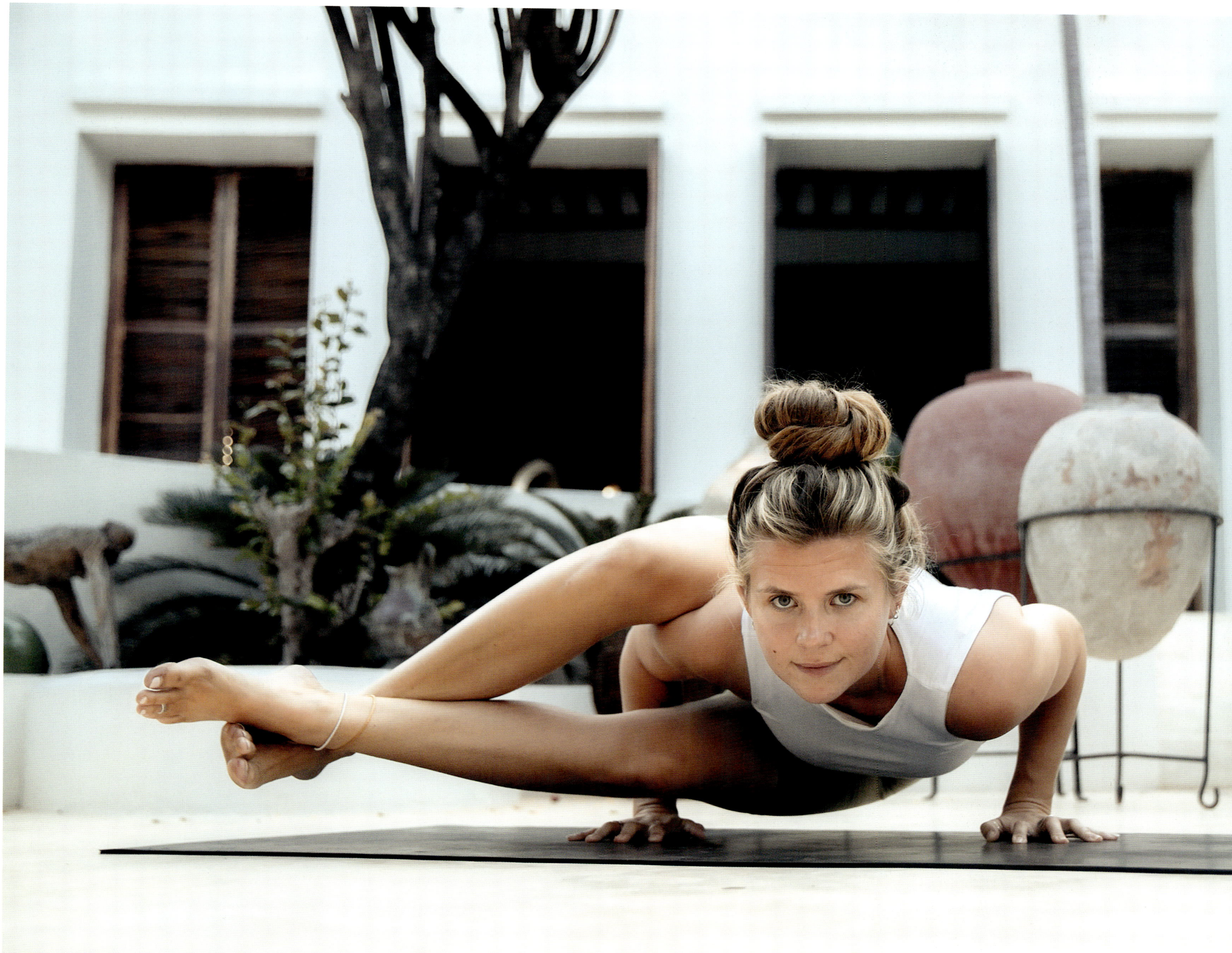

UTKATA KONASANA · Goddess

▲ ASTAVAKRASANA · Eight Angle

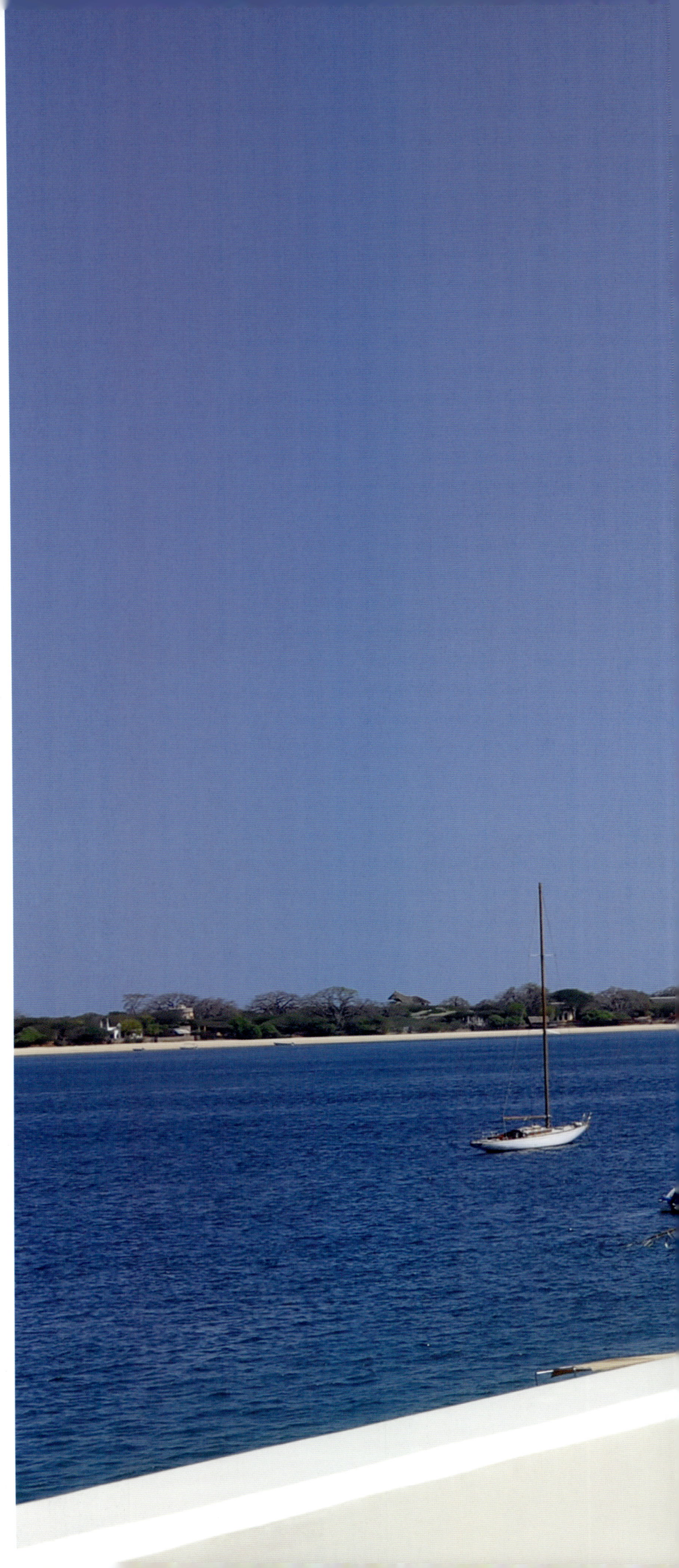

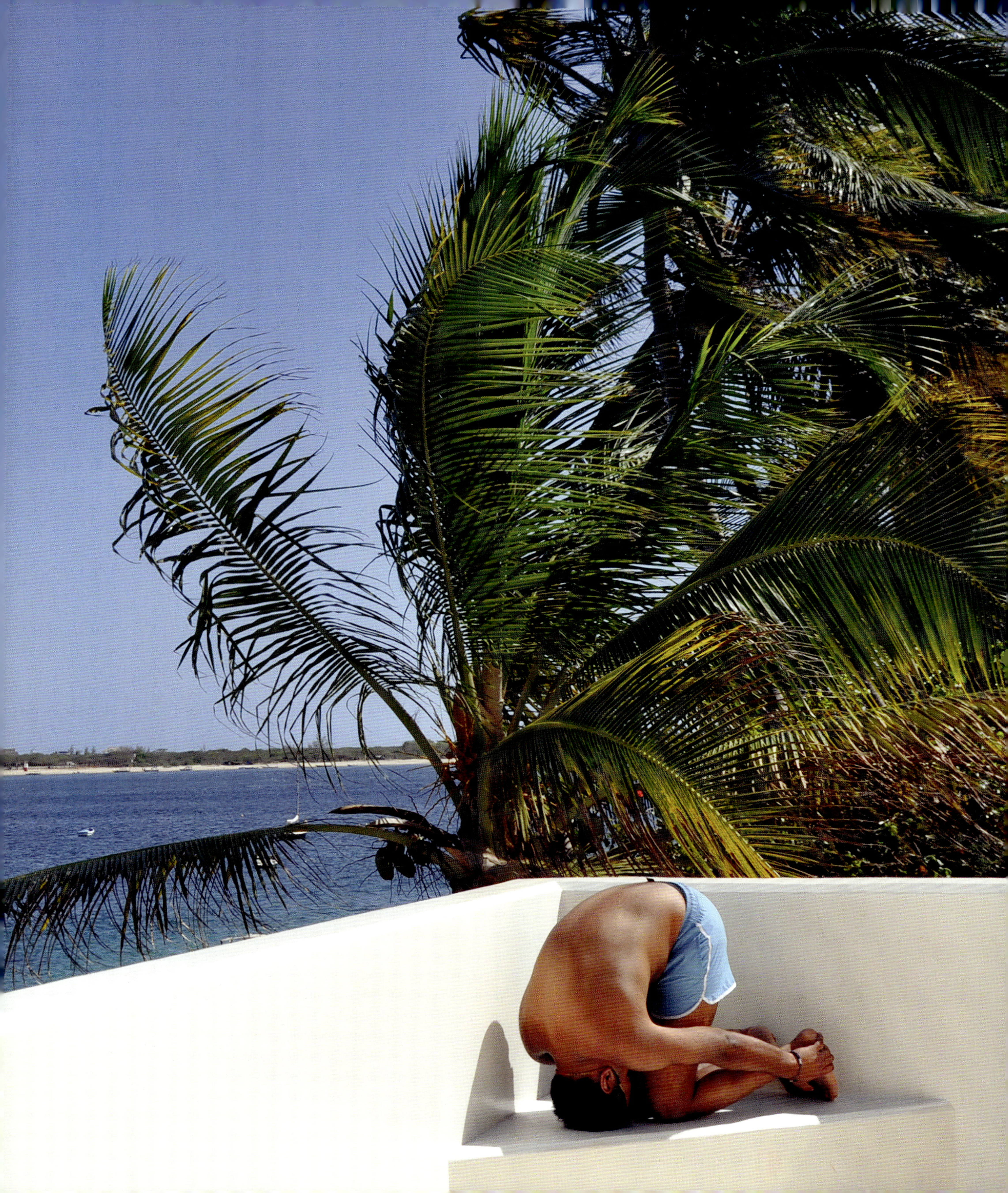

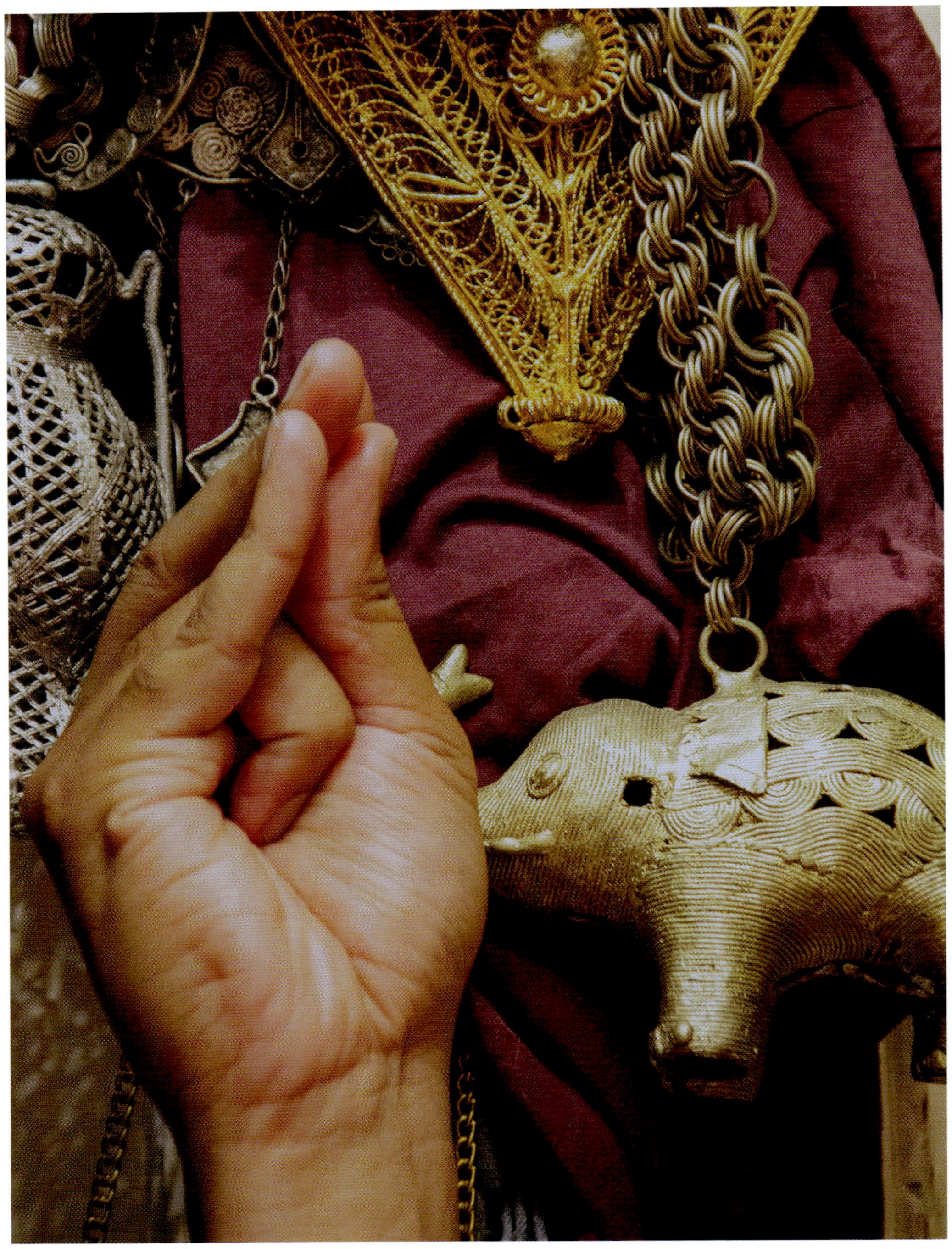

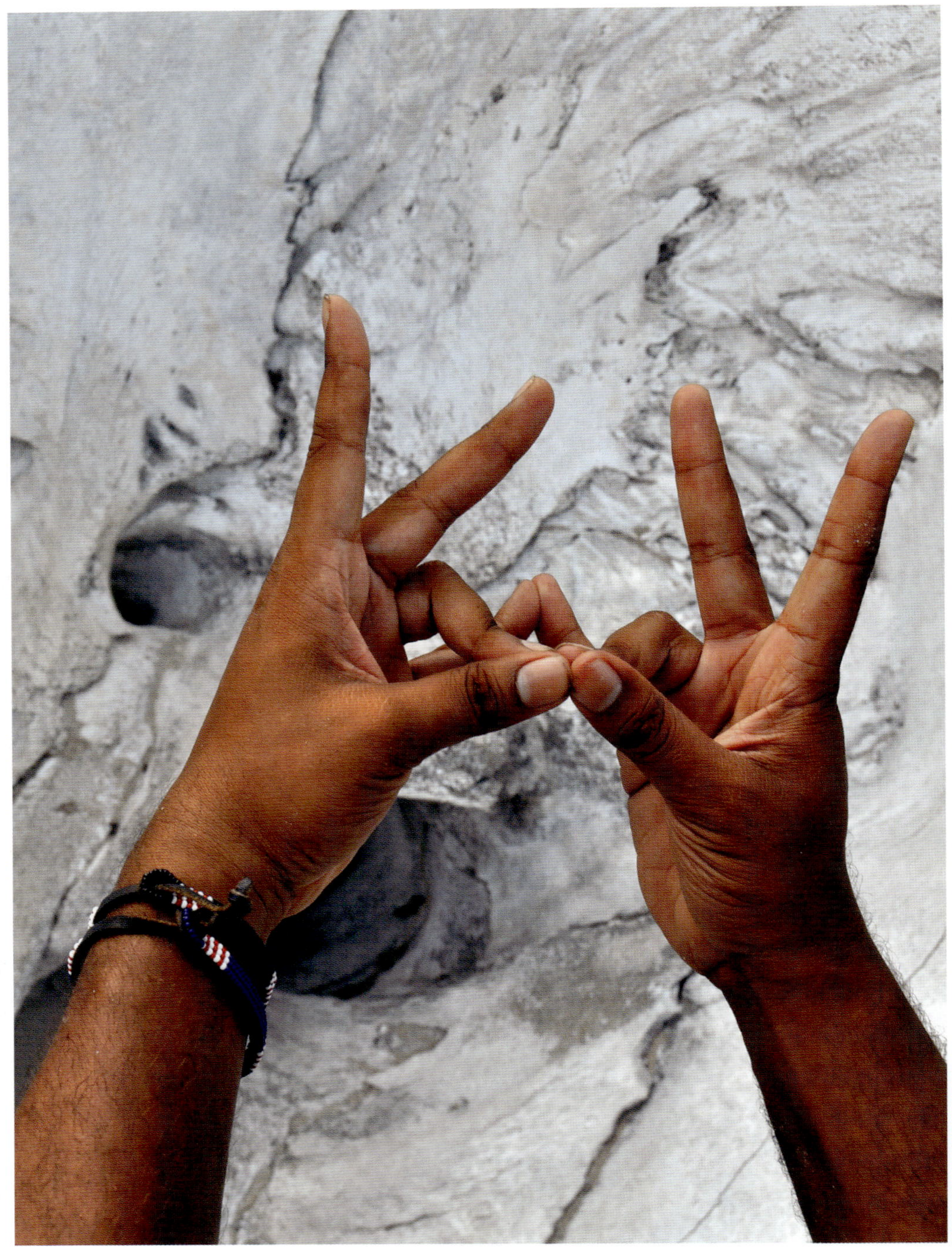

▲ **KANGULAMUDRA** · Potential *(left)* **MAHATRIKAMUDRA** · Fluidity *(right)*

SUKHASANA & KAPITTHAMUDRA · Easy Seated & Creativity

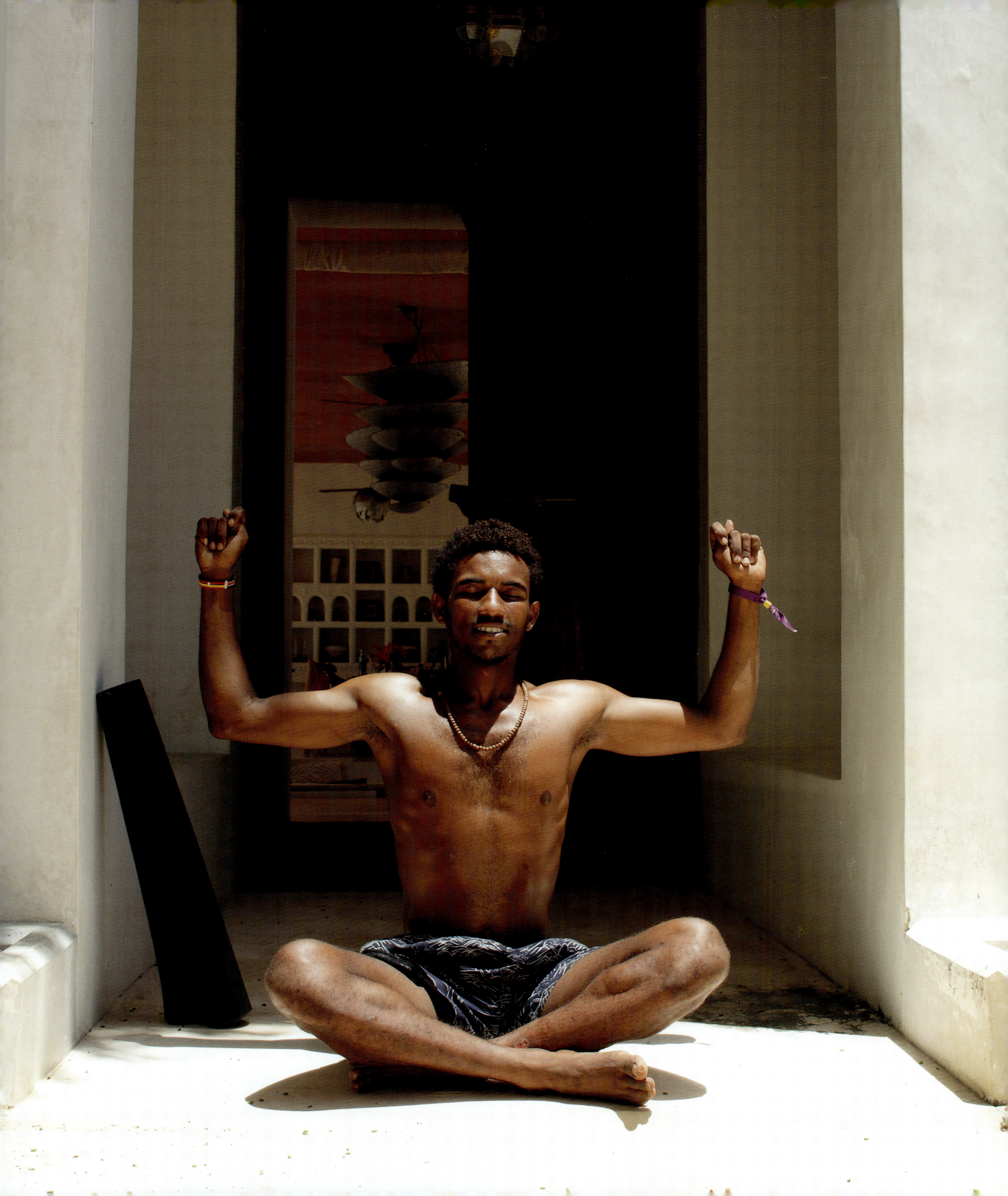

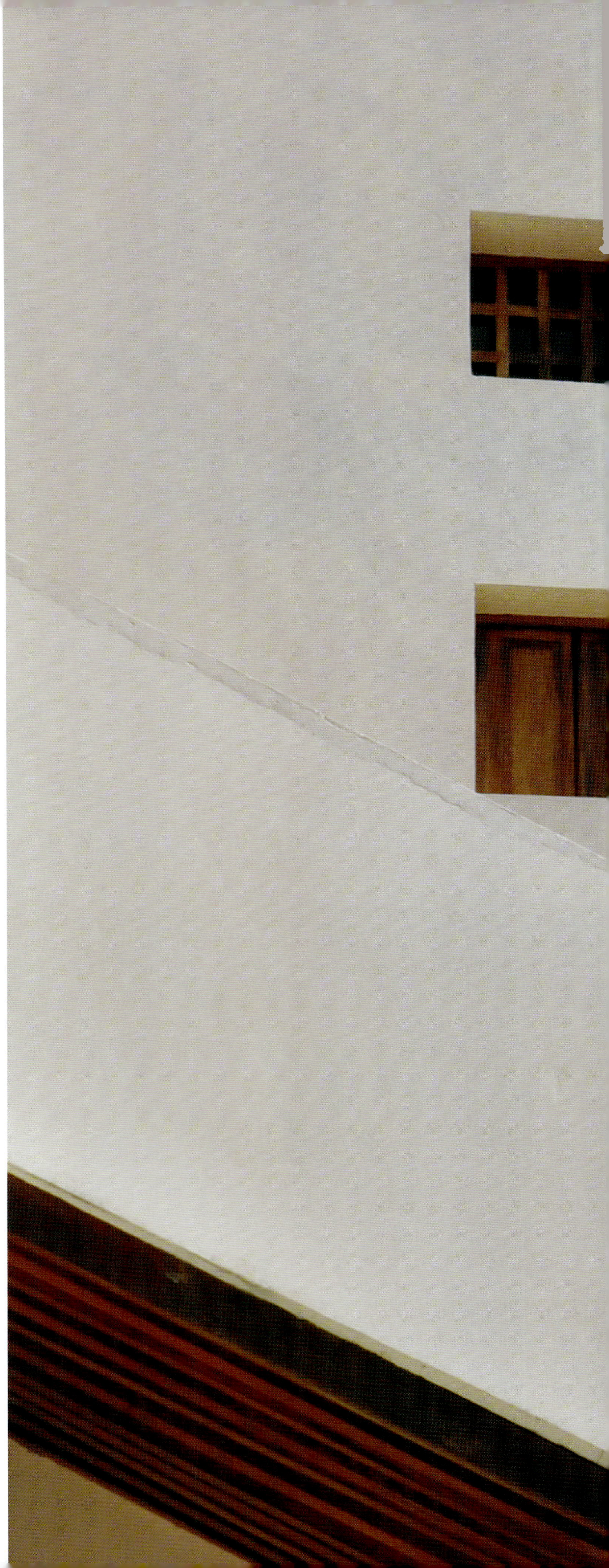

SALABHASANA · Grasshopper

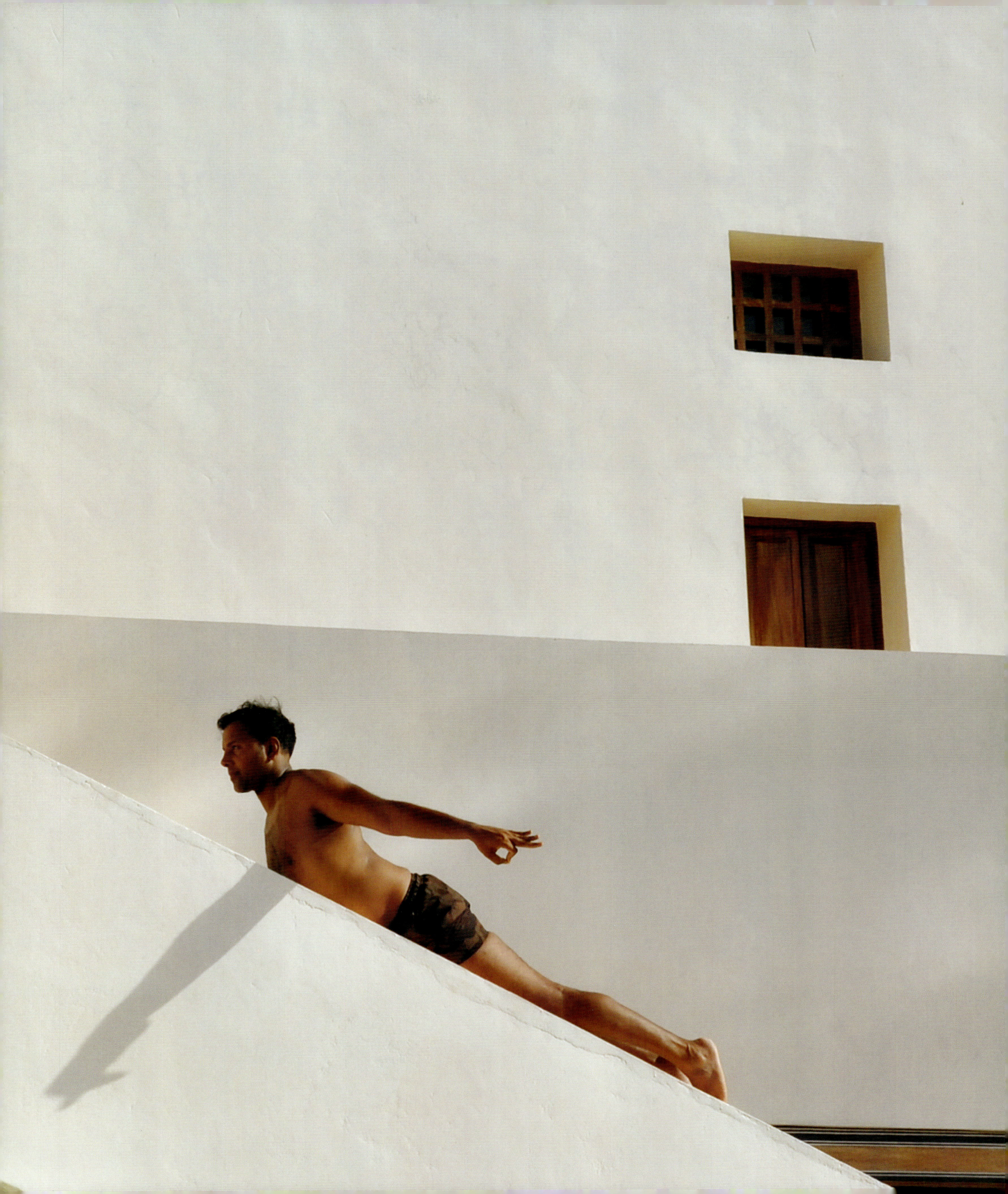

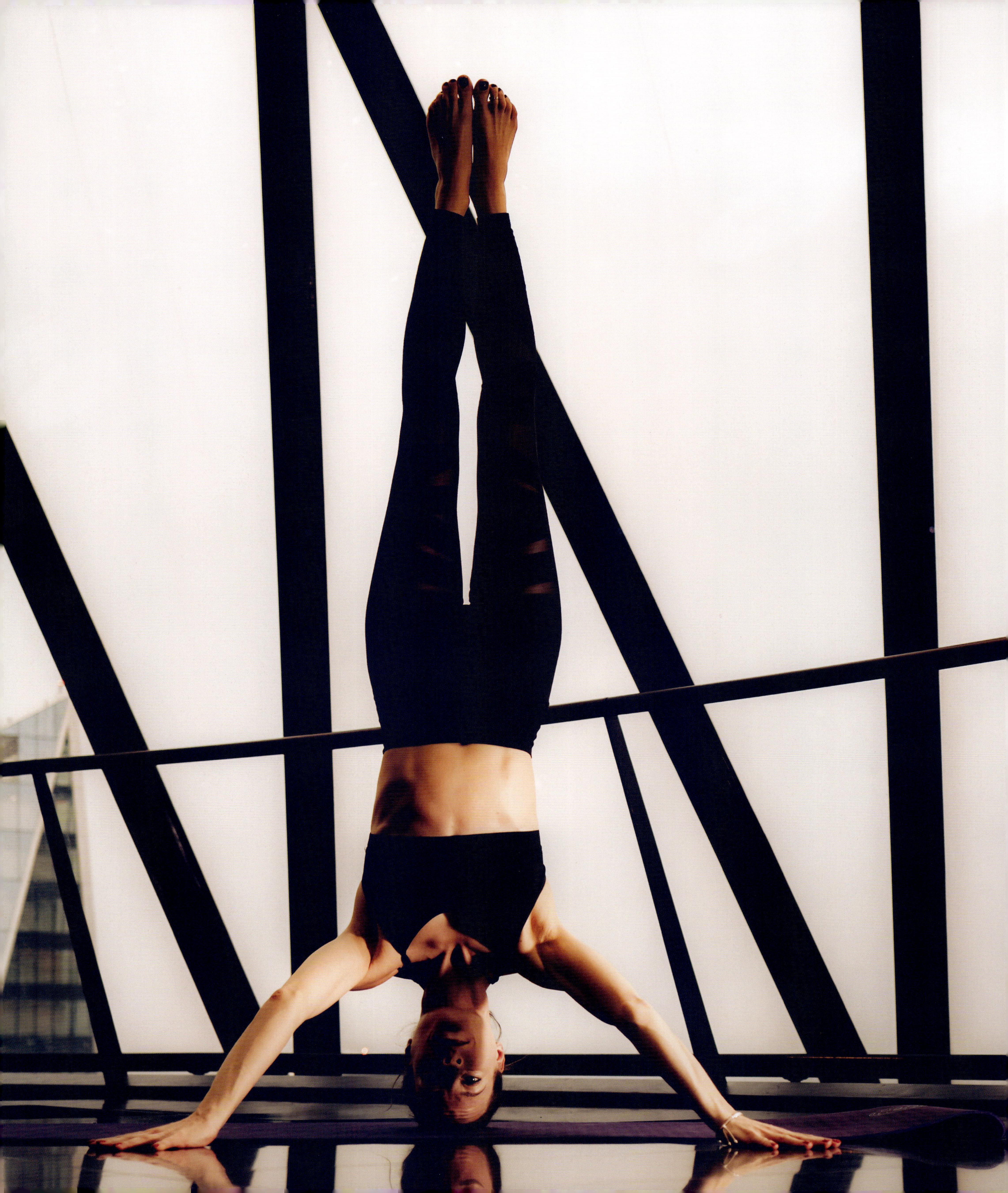

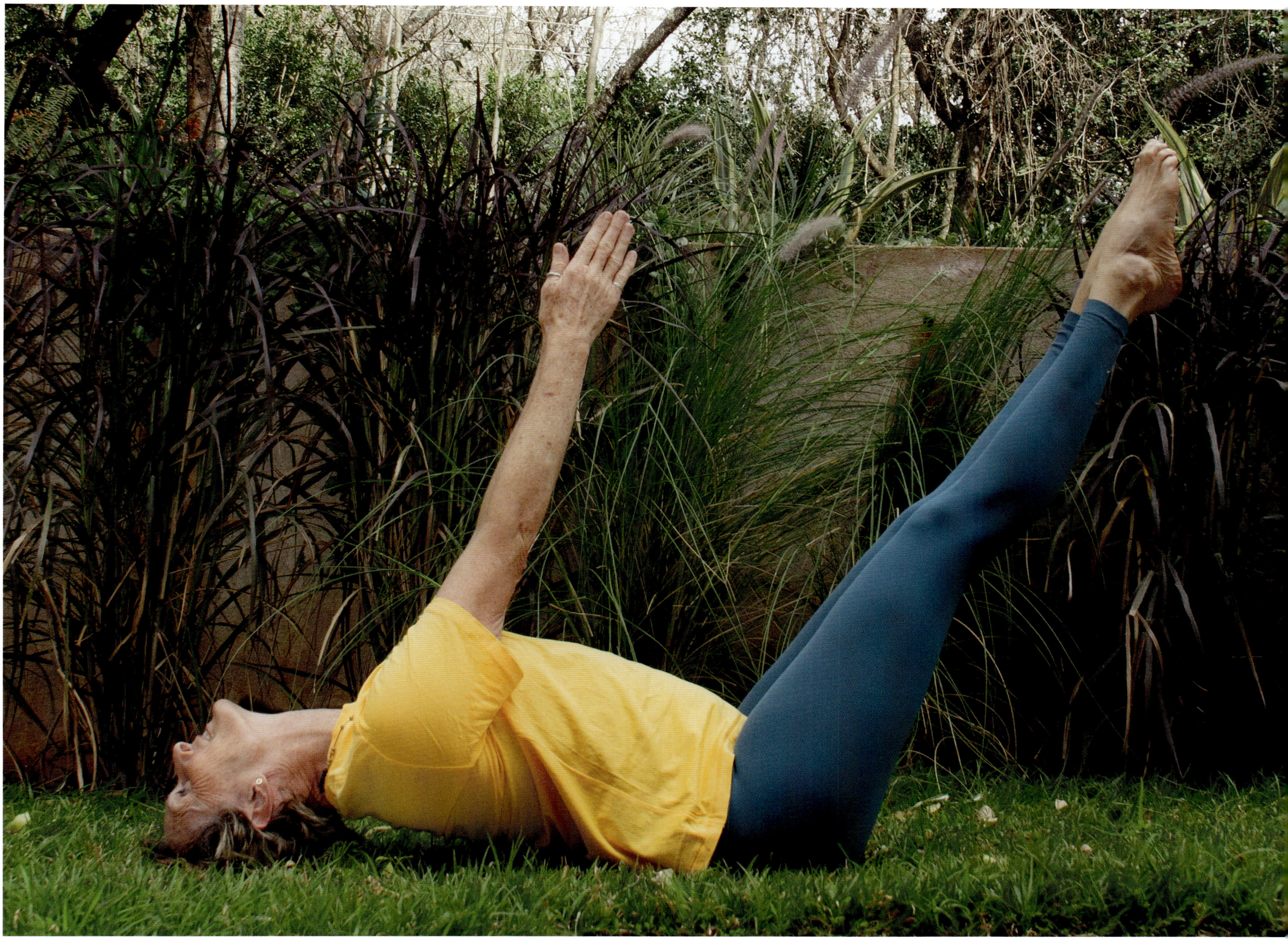

▲ UTTANA HASTA PADASANA · Raised Limbs

If you simply change direction
when there are shadows,
you will always find light.

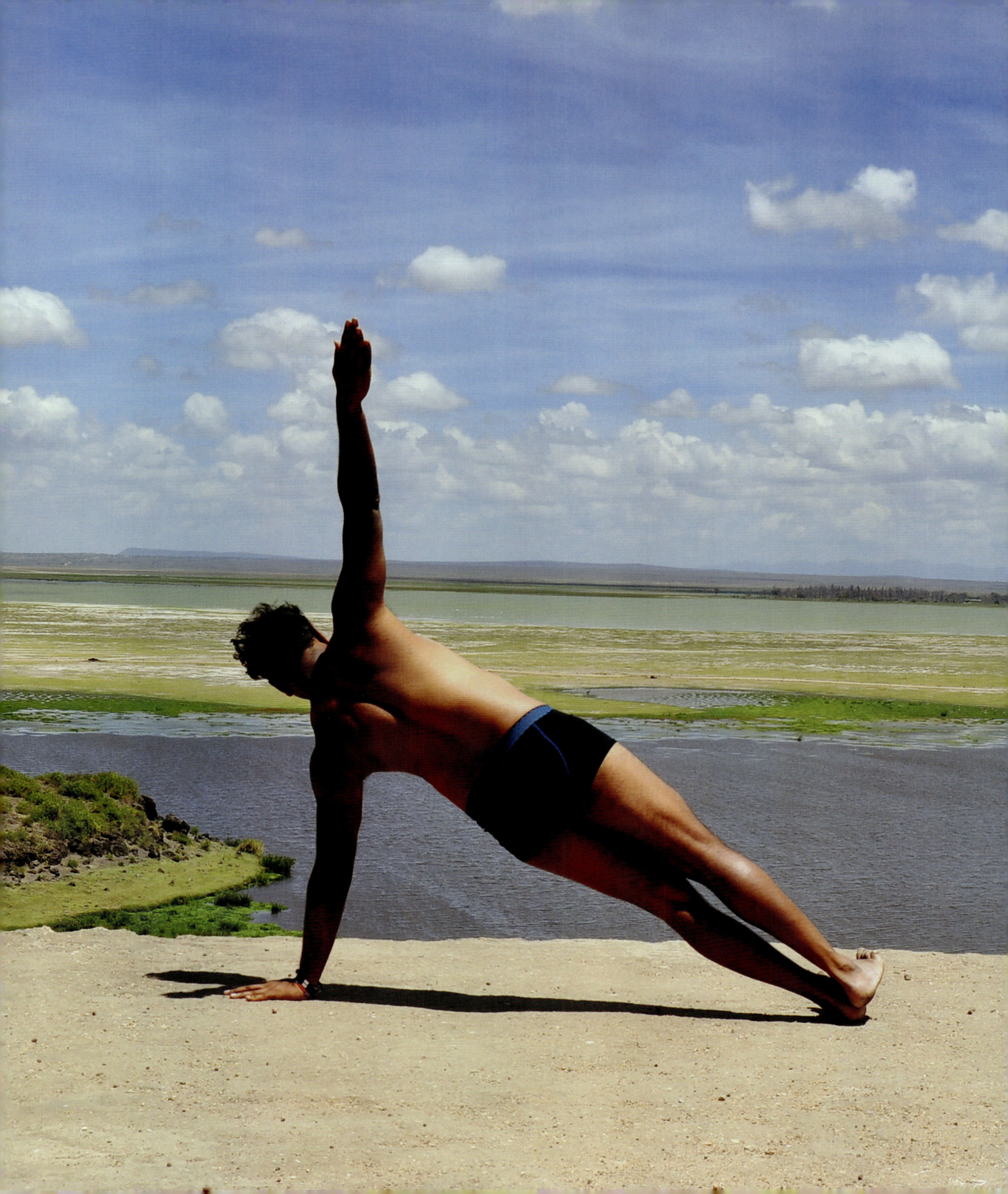

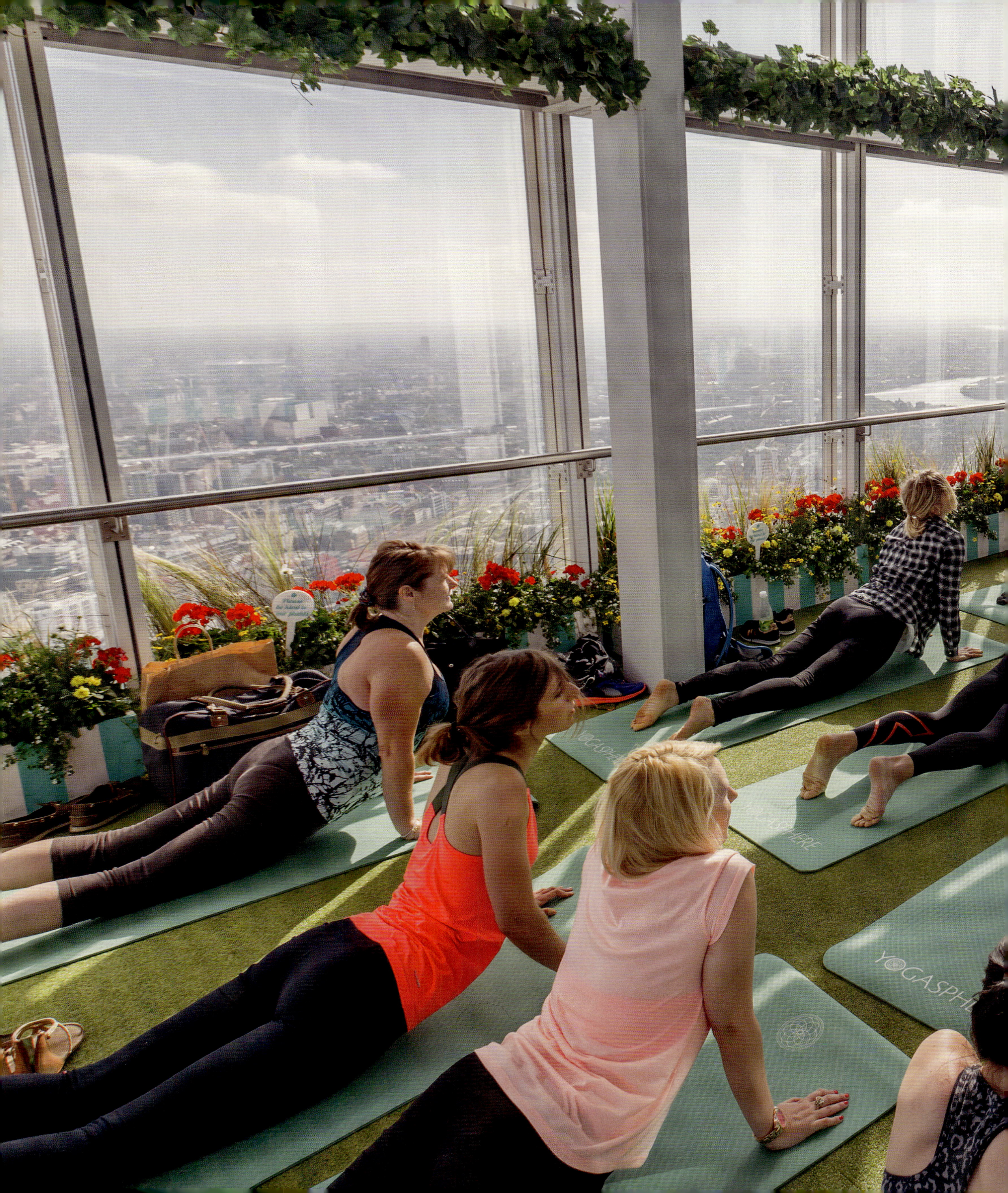
YOGASPHERE

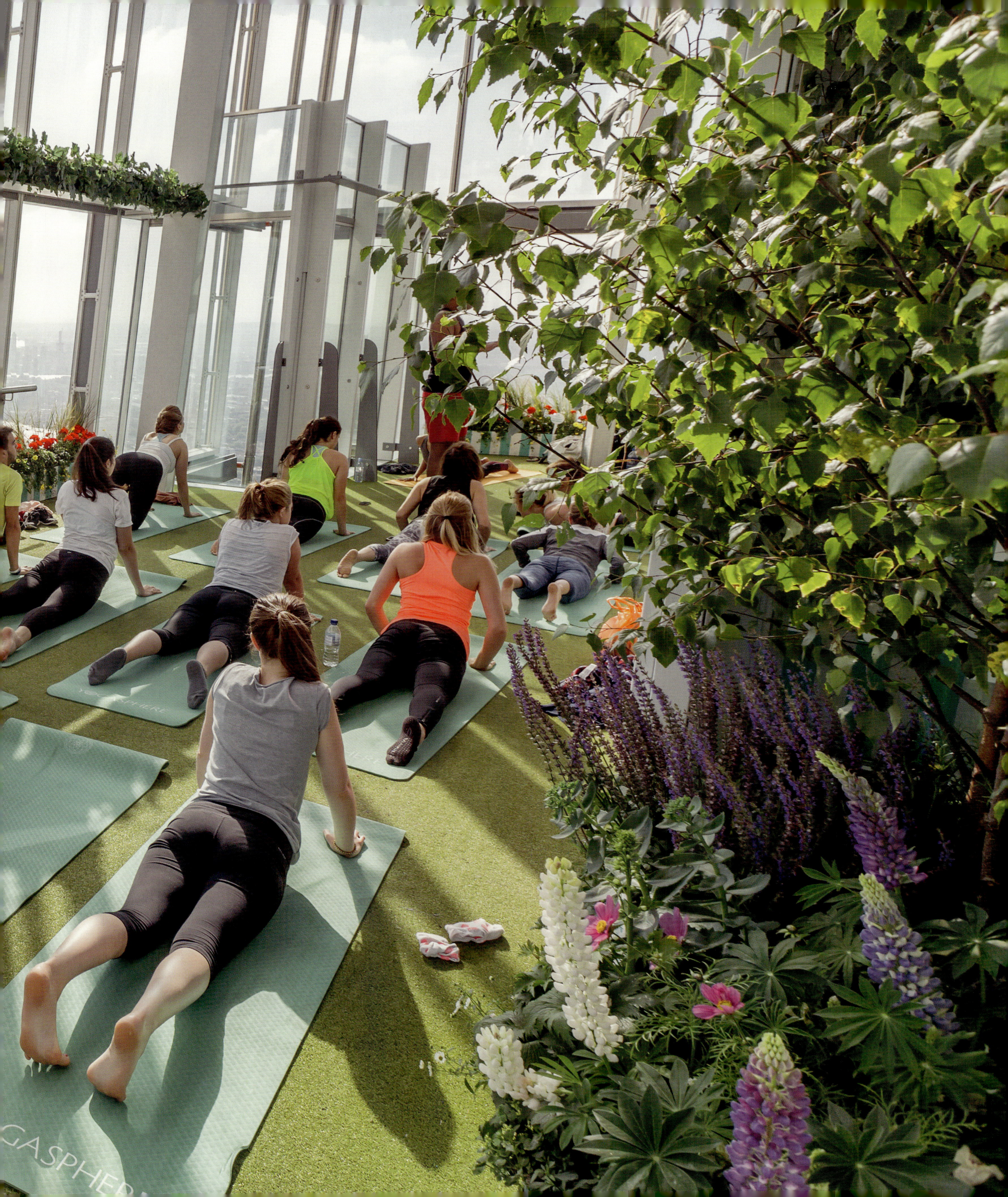

BRAHMA TULA • Libra

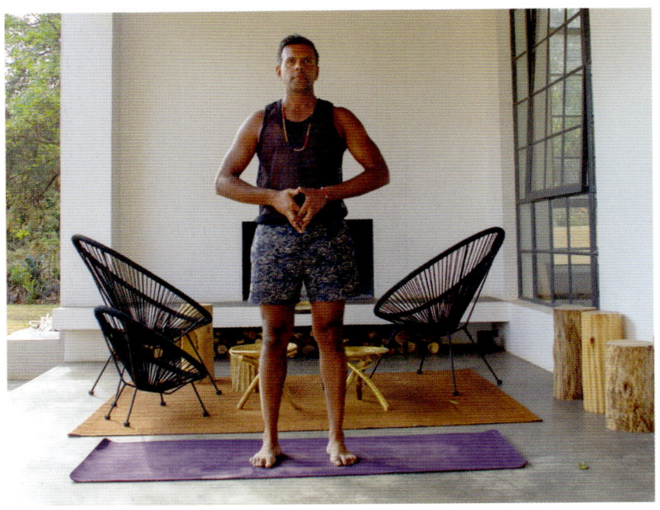

TADASANA & MANIPURACHAKRAMUDRA
Mountain & Willpower

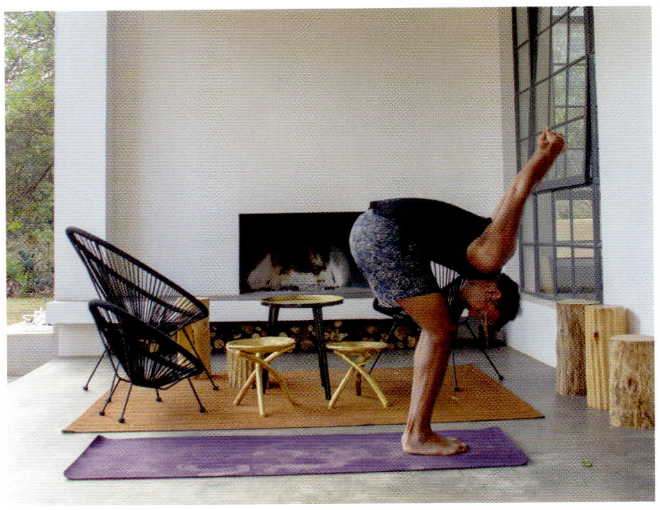

GAINDASANA
Rhino

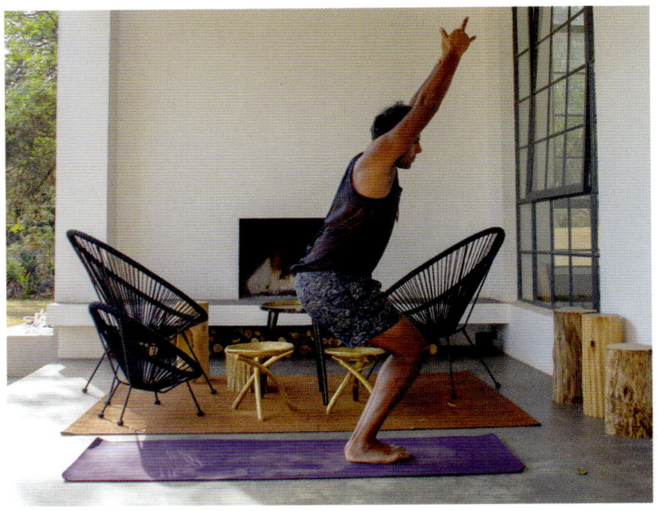

UTKATASANA KAPALABHATI PRANAYAMA & KALESVARAMUDRA
Chair Fire Breath & Opportunity

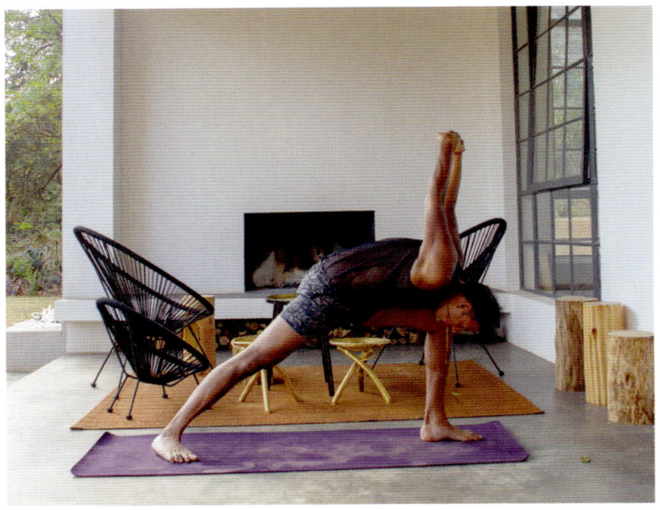

RISHI VIRABHADRASANA
Mystical Warrior

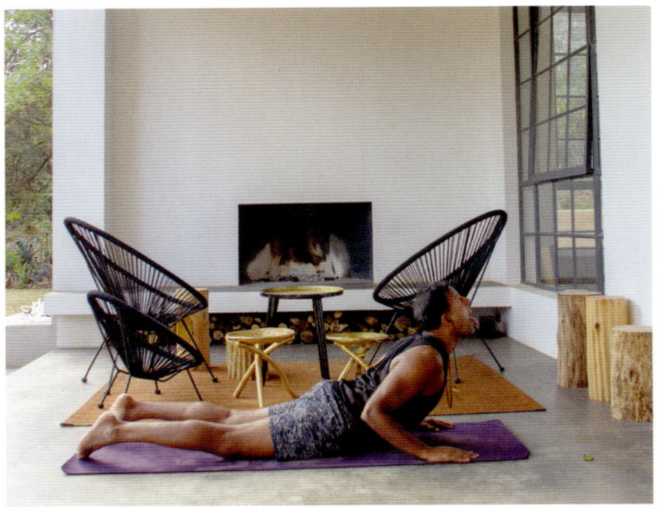

BHUJANGASANA SIMHASANA PRANAYAMA
Cobra Lion's Breath

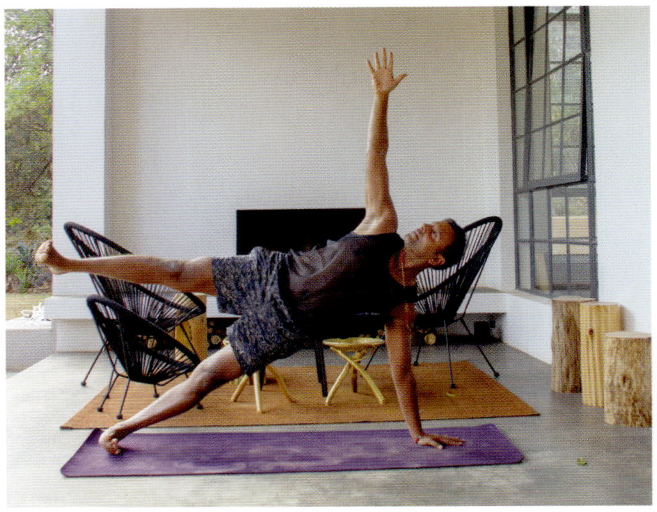

SHAANTIJHANDASANA
Peace Prayer Flag

In Brahma Tula, we are initiating the season of elemental air. This constellation of asanas is energizing, encourages expression, and brings equanimity to the body. The strident movements of the body aid circulation and lift any tiredness, lethargy, or fatigue. Lion's breath, cleansing pranayama, and fire breath create a vivid sharpness of concentration and a sense of assured renewal. The mudras release your personal willpower and give an experiential opportunity for you to sense the expansion of the human energy field. Increased precision of focus provides fluidity in the body and transformation to a higher state of consciousness.

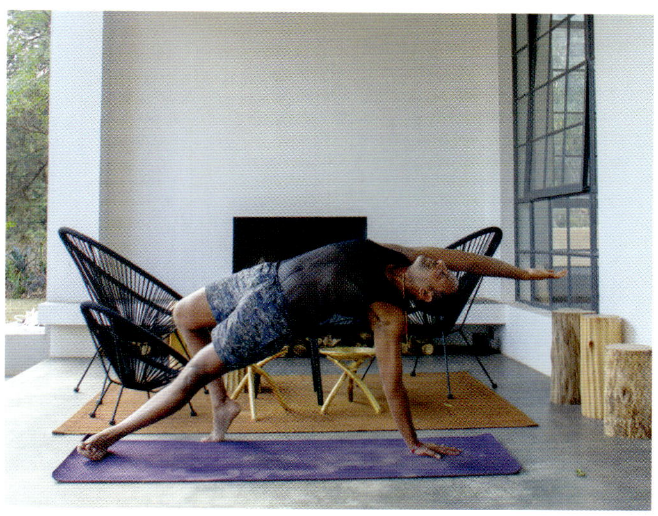

CAMATKARASANA
Enraptured Heart

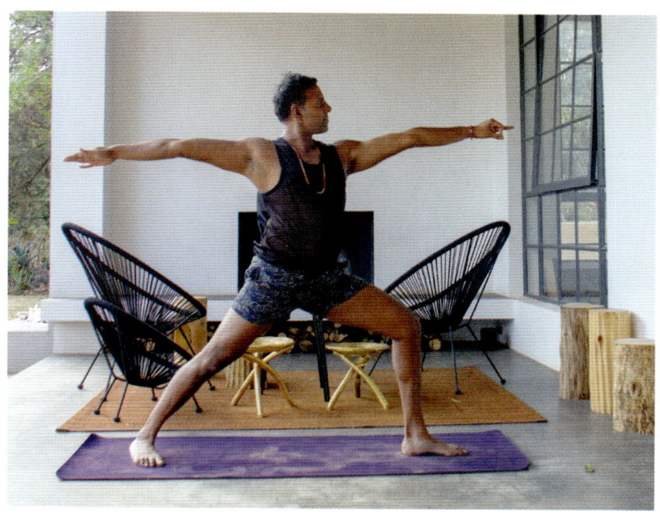

VIRABHADRASANA DVE & VYANAMUDRA
Warrior II & Expansion

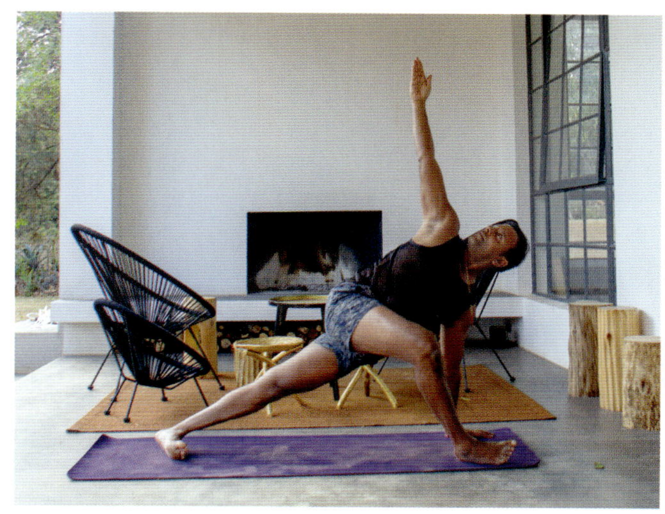

UTTHAN PRISTHASANA
Dragon Lizard

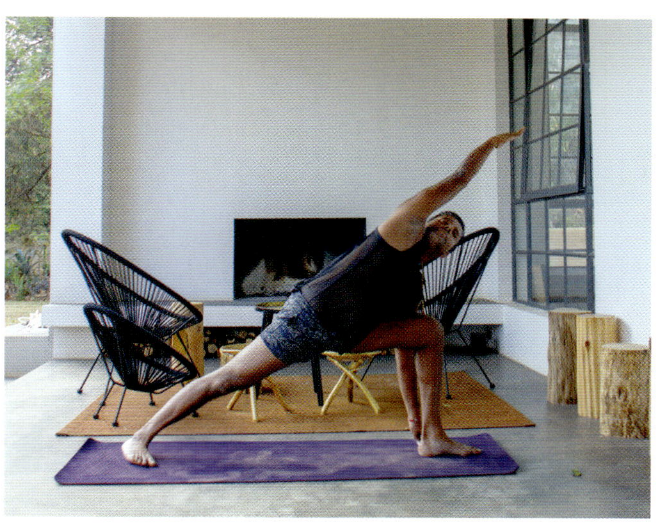

UTTHITA PARSVAKONASANA
Extended Side Angle

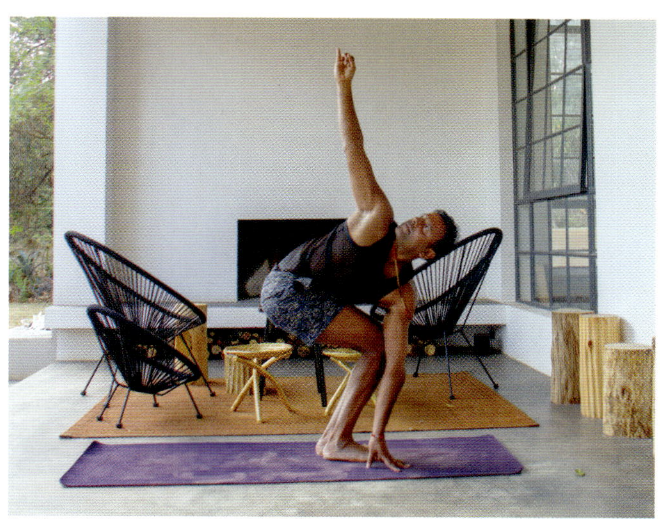

UTTHITA PARIVRTTA UTKATASANA & BANAMUDRA
Revolving Chair & Precision

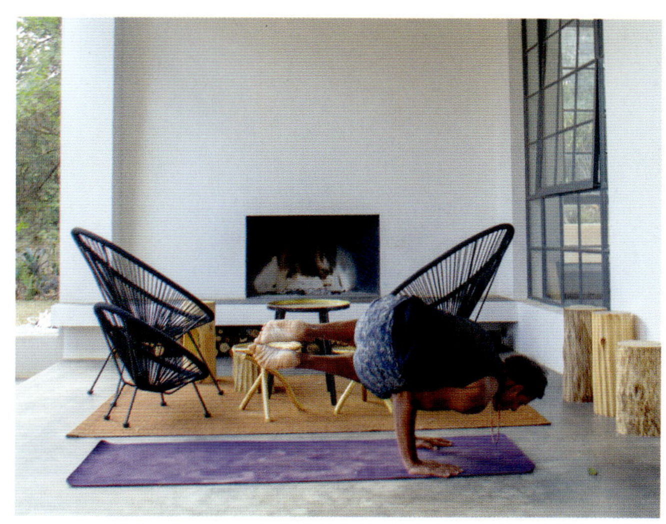

PARSVA BAKASANA
Side Crow

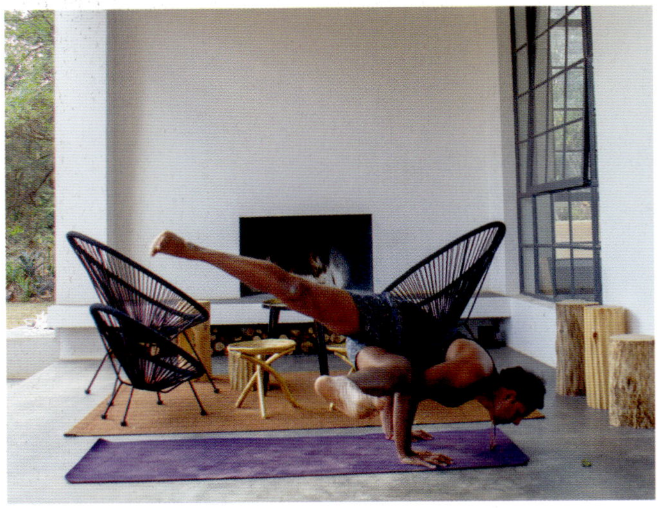

EKA PADA KOUNDINYASANA
Flying Splits

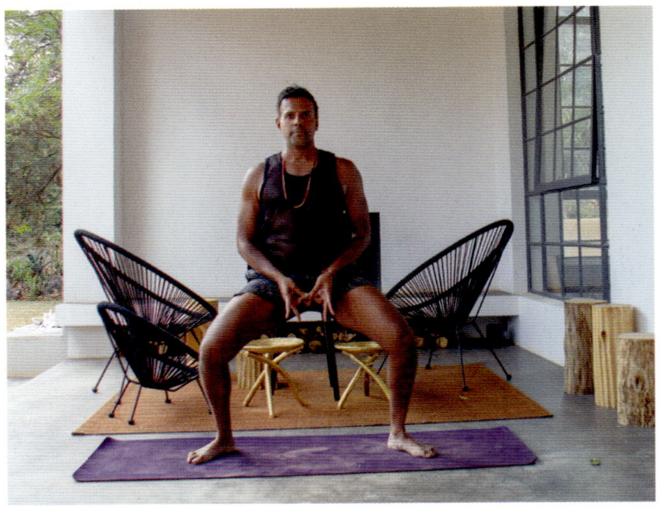

UTKATA KONASANA & MAHATRIKAMUDRA
Goddess & Fluidity

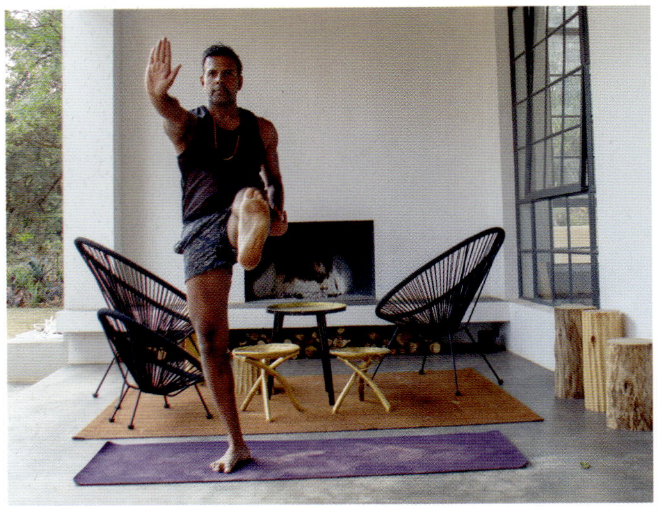

UTTHAN UTKATA KONASANA BHASTRIKA PURAKA PRANAYAMA
Flying Goddess Cleansing Inhale Breath

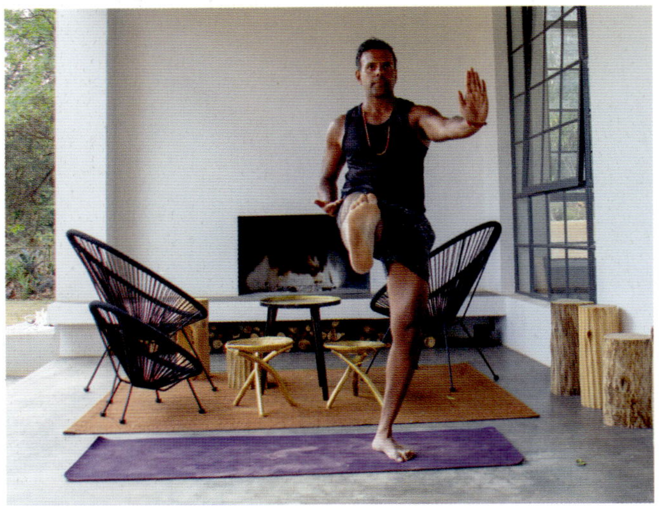

UTTHAN UTKATA KONASANA BHASTRIKA RECHAKA PRANAYAMA
Flying Goddess Releasing Exhale Breath

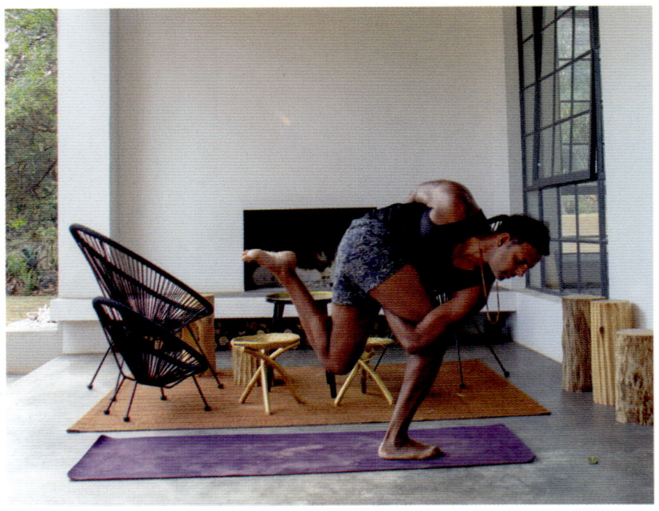

MARAALASANA
Flamingo

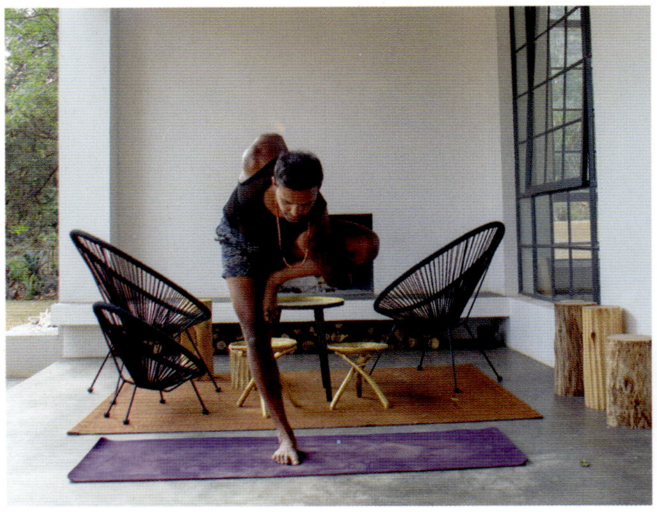

ULLOOASANA
Owl

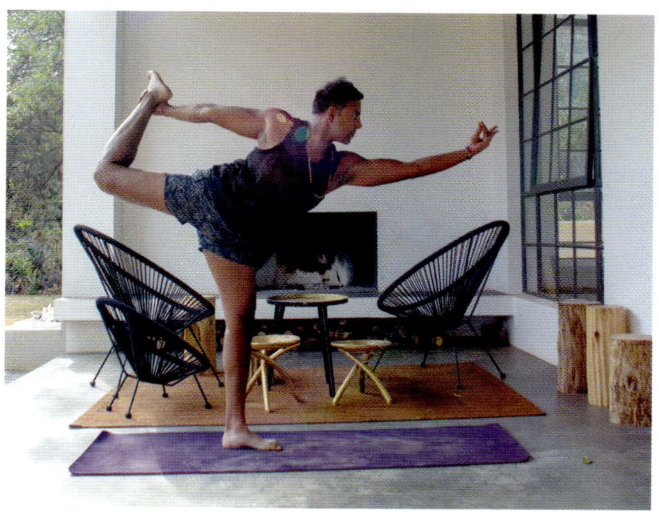

NATARAJASANA & RUDRAMUDRA
Dancer & Transformation

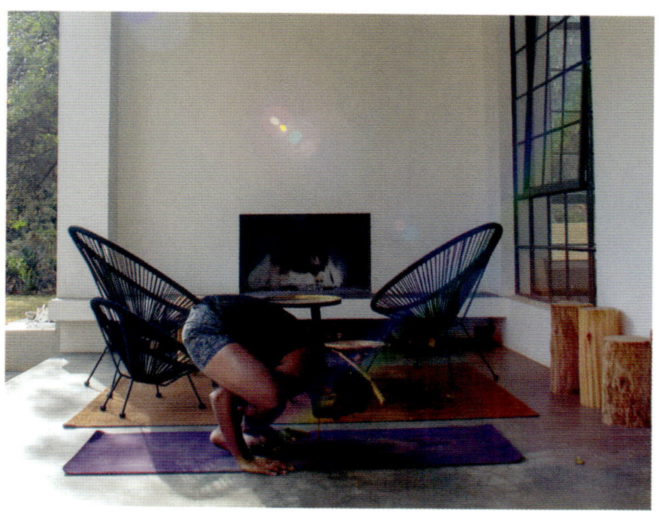

BHUJAPIDASANA
Nightingale

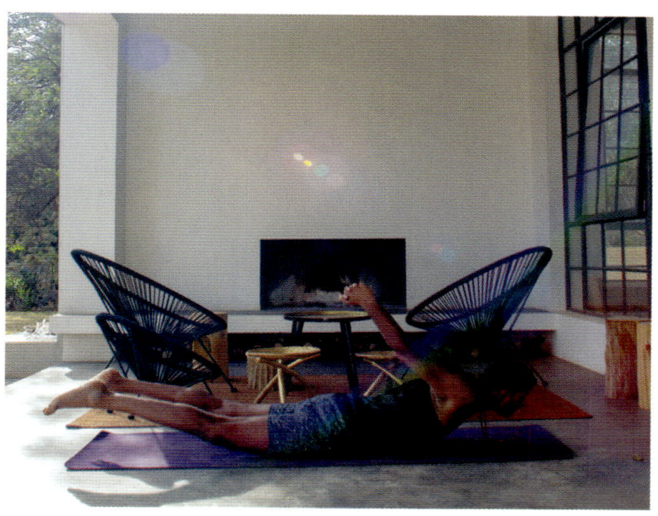

SALABHASANA
Grasshopper

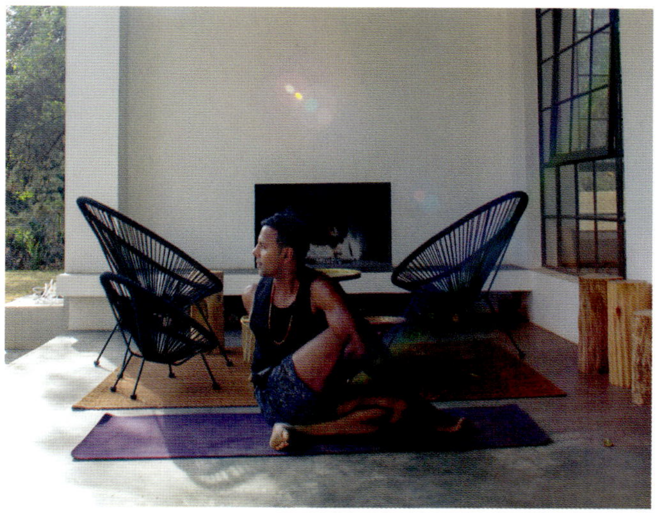

BADDHA ARDHA MATSYENDRASANA
Seated Bound Twist

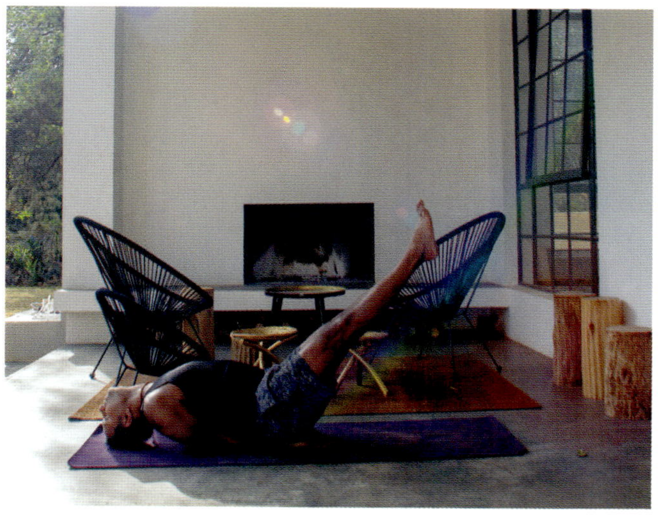

UTPATA MATSYASANA
Flying Fish

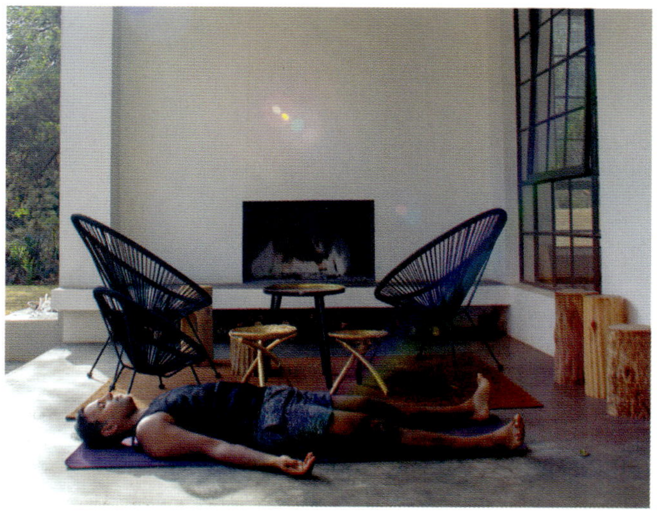

SAVASANA
Resting

BRAHMA VRISHCHIKA • Scorpio

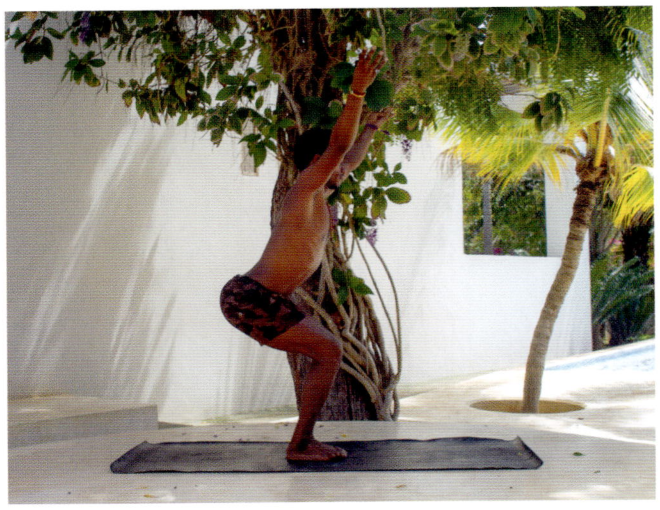

VIDYUTASANA
Lightning

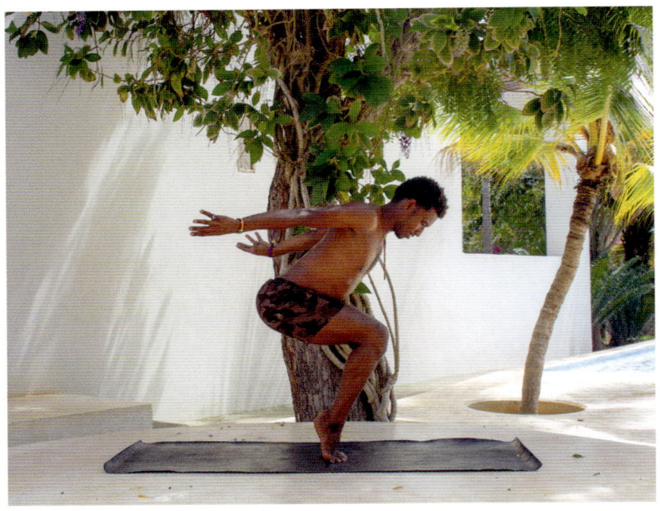

INDRADHANUSHASANA & AVAHANAMUDRA
Rainbow & Connection

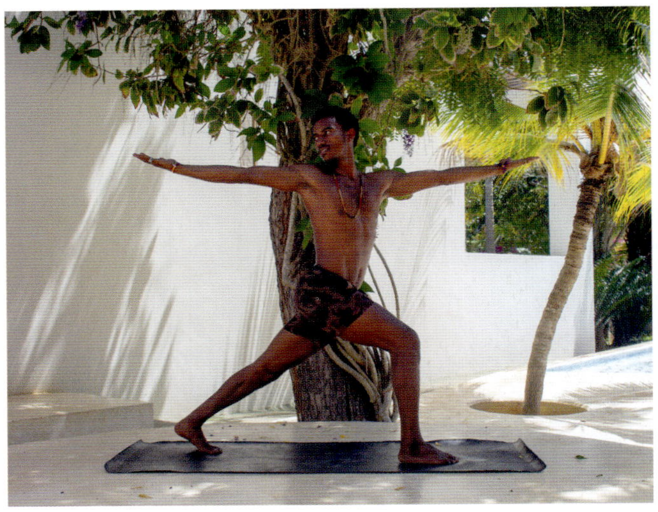

PARIVRTTA VIPARITA VIRABHADRASANA
Twisted Reverse Warrior

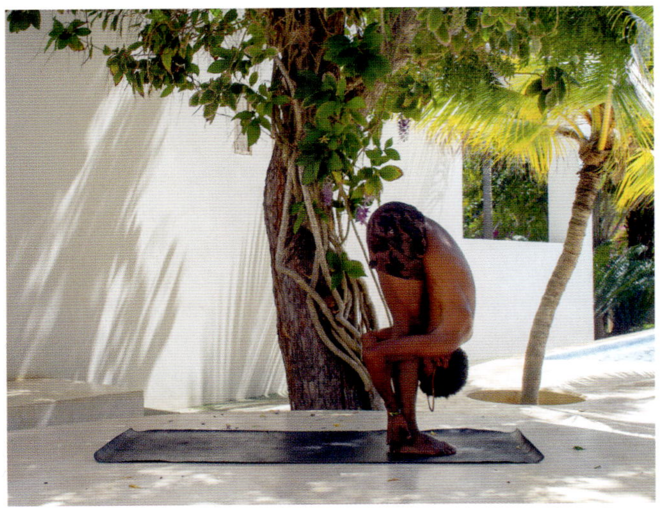

UTTANASANA
Standing Forward Fold

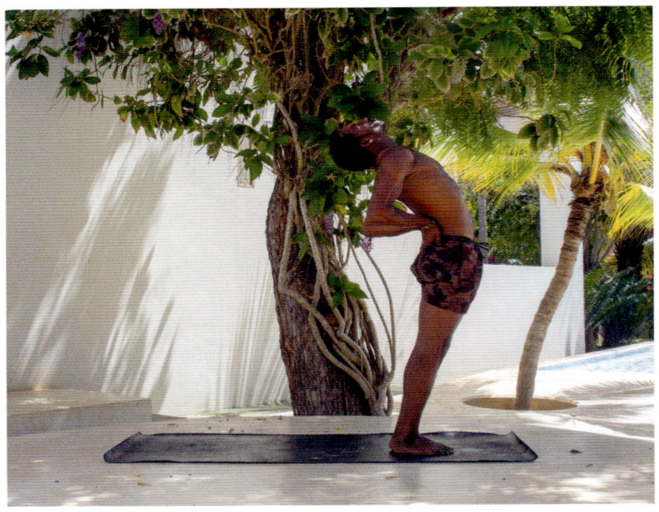

ARDHA ANUVITTASANA
Half Standing Backbend

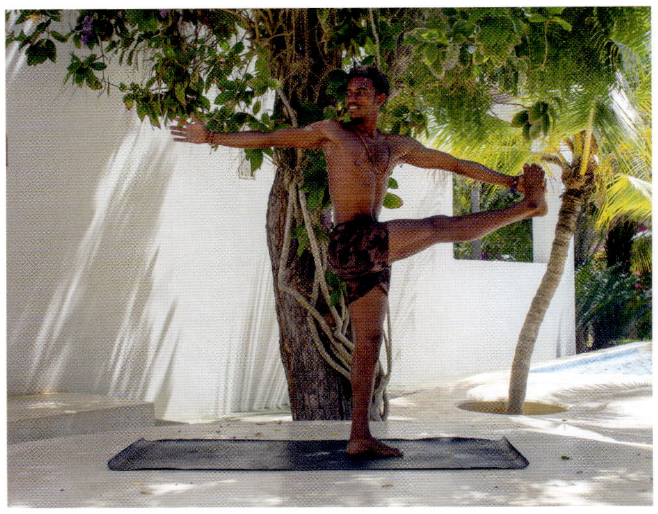

PARIVRTTA HASTA PADANGUSTHASANA
Revolved Hand-to-Big Toe

In Brahma Vrishchika, we are in the settled season of elemental water. This constellation of asanas draws inspiration from when species fearlessly emerged from water. By resourcefully performing forward bends, backbends, twists, side bends, swaying, inversions, lateral movements, rotation, and moderate guided hyperextension, we take the spine through its full range of motion. By raising our energy, we can probe mysterious and complex balances with determination. The mudras activate the connection of emotions to encourage productivity and the prosperity that results from striving to realize our potential. This is an intense and passionate practice that brings inspiration and creativity.

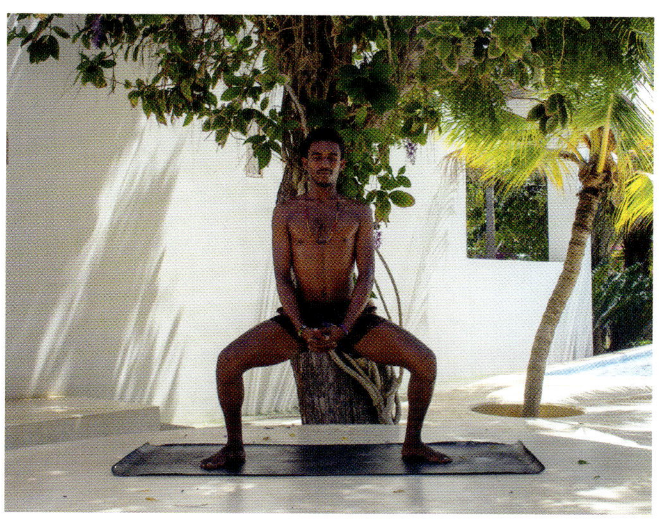

UTKATA KONASANA & USHASMUDRA
Goddess & Productivity

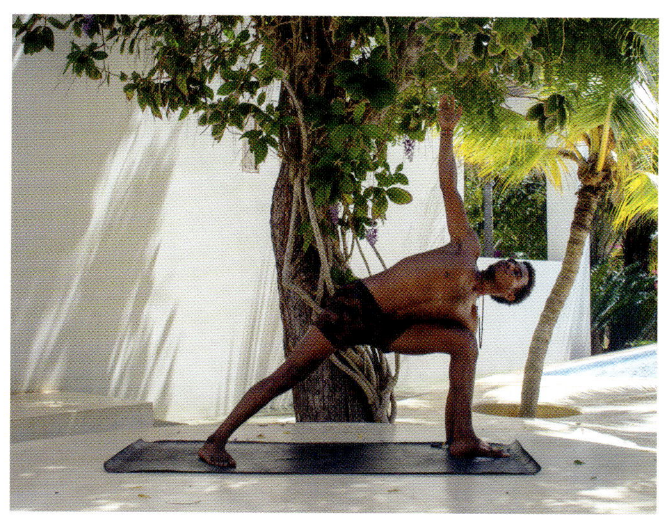

UTTHITA PARSHVAKONASANA
Extended Side Angle

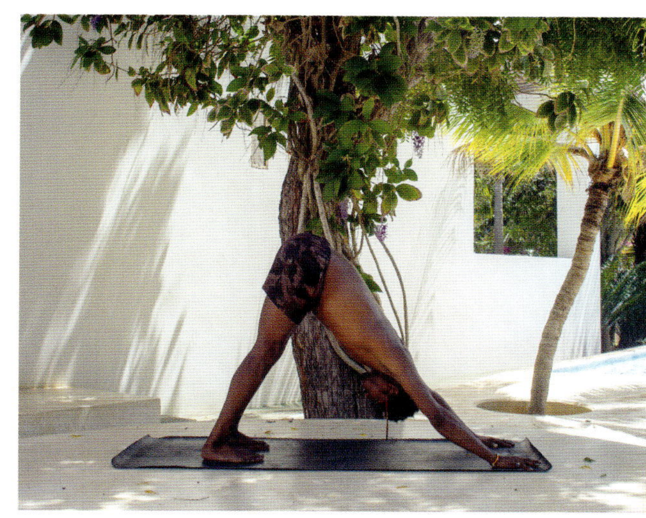

ADHO MUKHA SVANASANA
Downward-Facing Dog

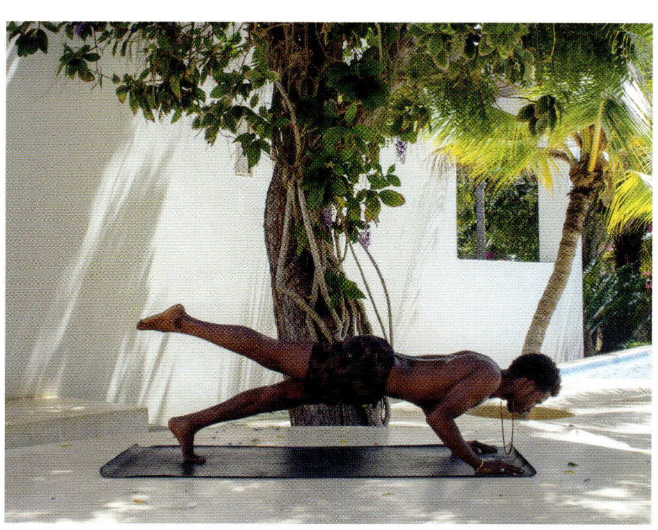

TRINI CHATURANGA DANDASANA
Three-Limbed Staff

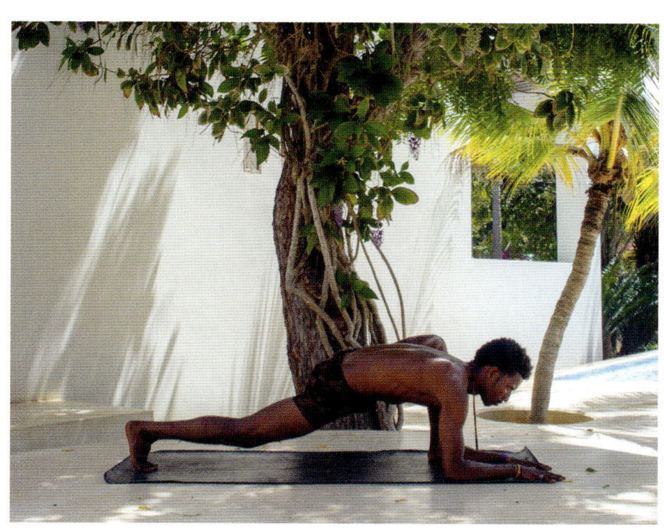

UTTHAN PRISTHASANA
Dragon Lizard

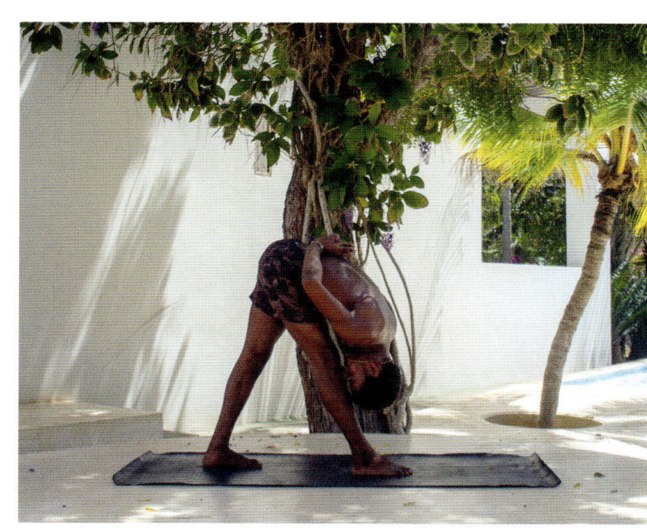

AUNDHA PARSVOTTANASANA & VARUNAMUDRA
Reverse Pyramid & Prosperity

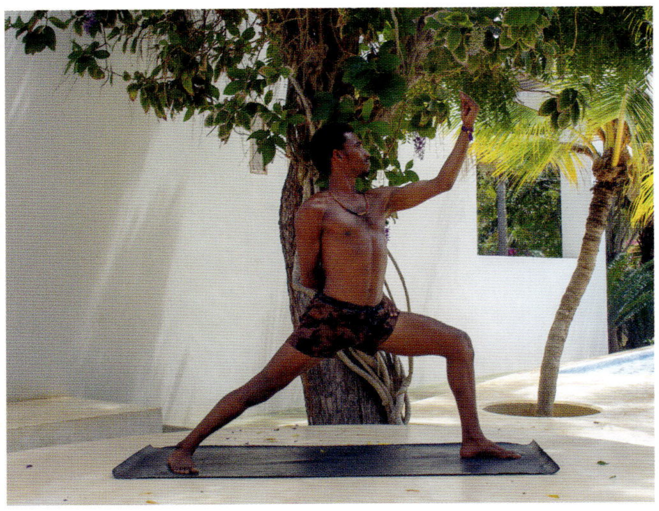

VIRABHADRASANA EKAM & KANGULAMUDRA
Warrior I & Potential

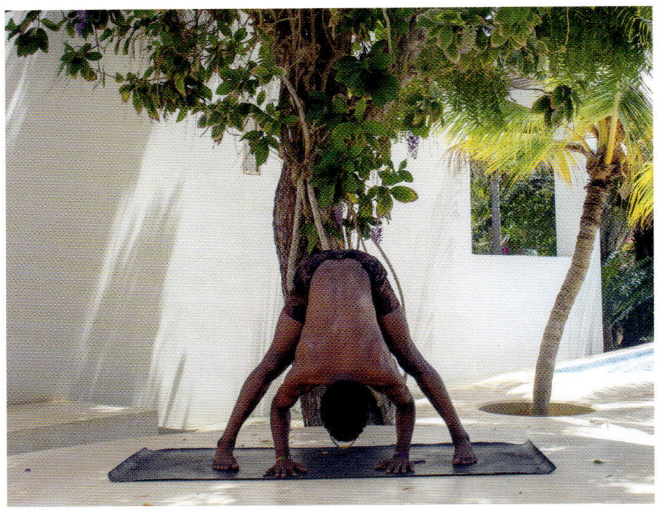

PRASARITA PADOTTANASANA EKAM
Wide-Legged Standing Forward Bend I

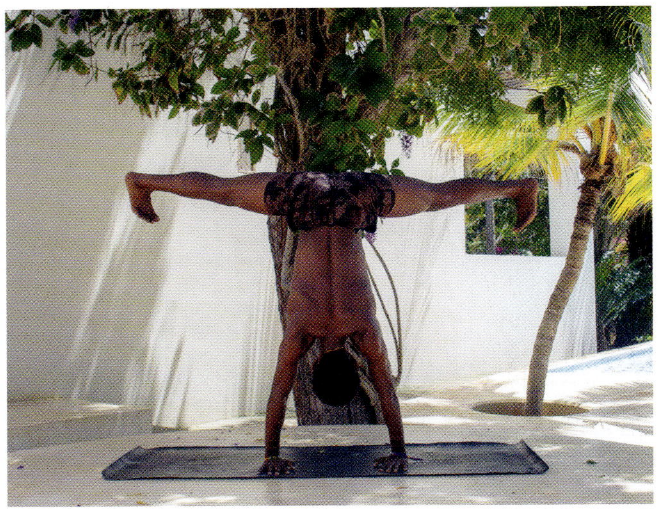

ARDHA ADHO MUKHA VRKSASANA
Half Downward-Facing Tree

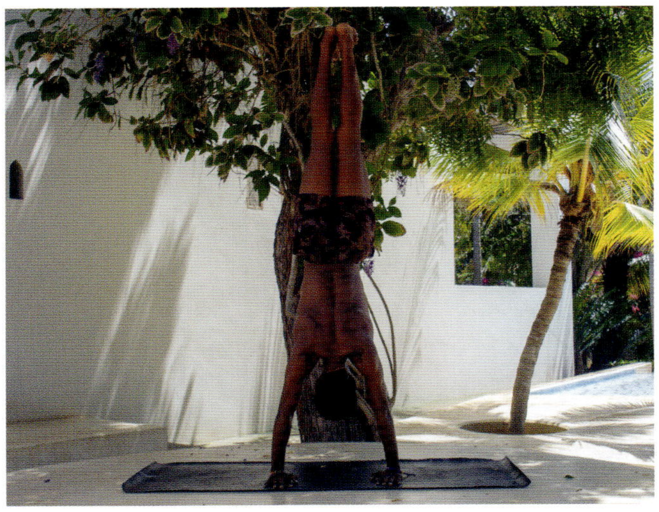

ADHO MUKHA VRKSASANA
Downward-Facing Tree

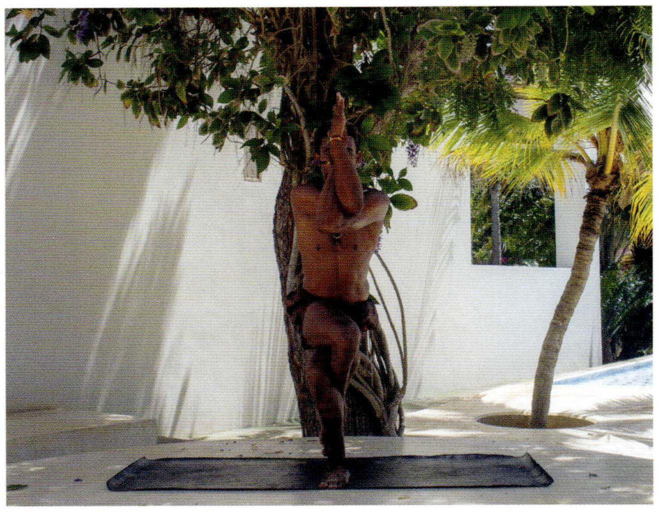

GARUDASANA
Eagle

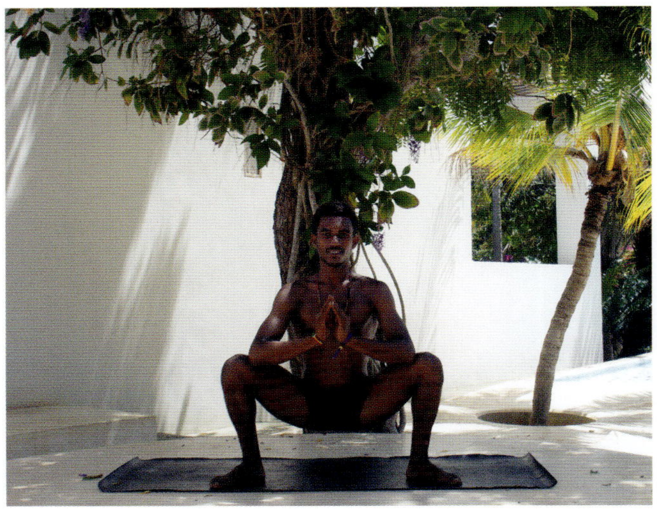

MALASANA & SHAKTIMUDRA
Garland Squat & Inspiration

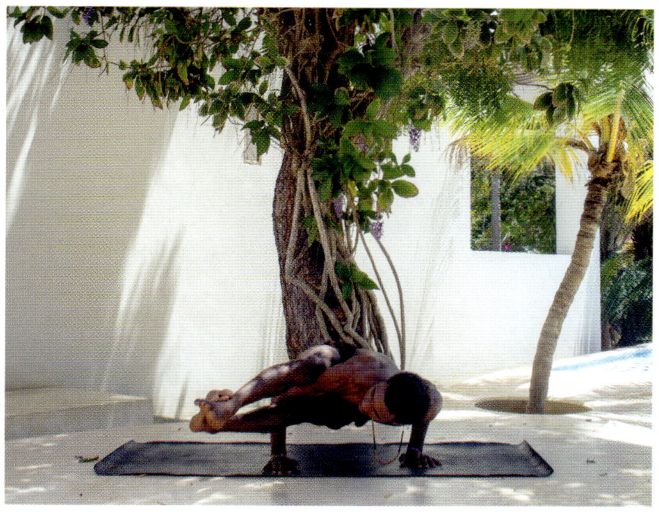

ASTAVAKRASANA
Eight Angle

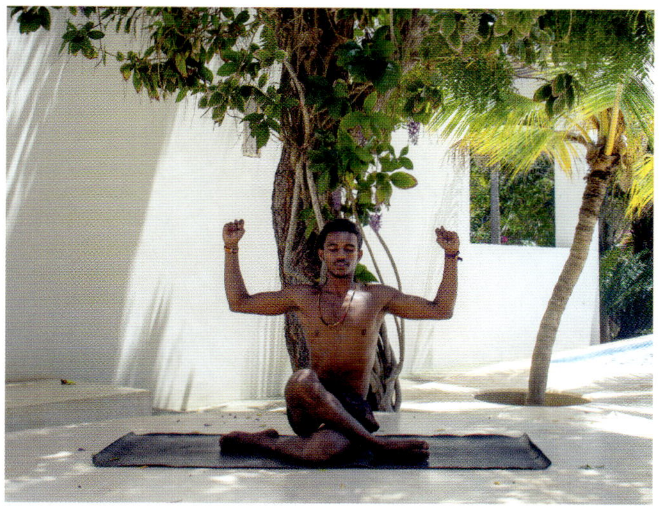

GOMUKHASANA & KAPITTHAMUDRA
Cow Face & Creativity

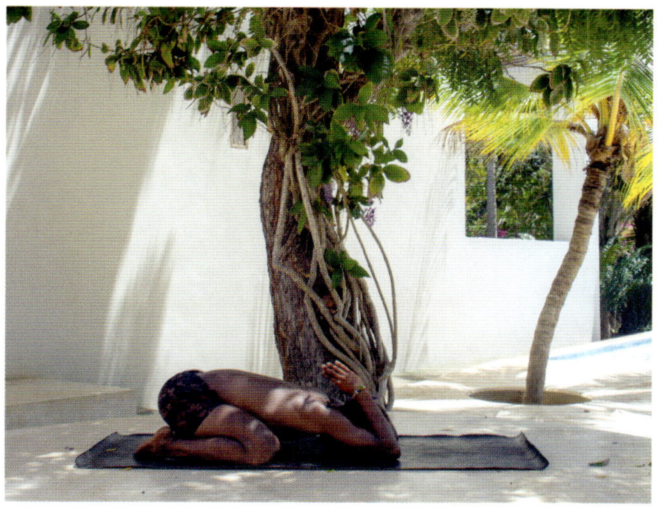

VAJRABALASANA
Thunderchild

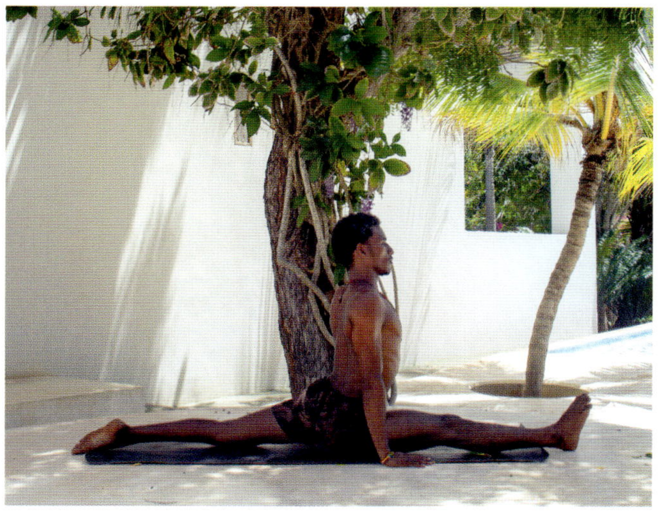

HANUMANASANA
Splits

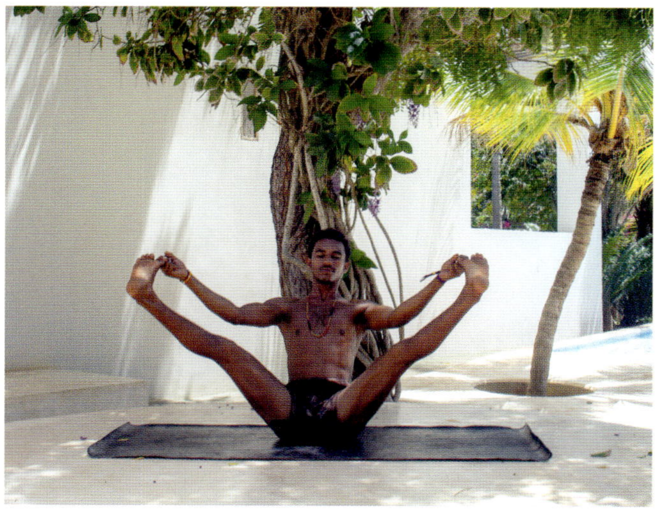

URDHVA UPAVISTHA KONASANA
Upward-Facing Wide-Angle Seated

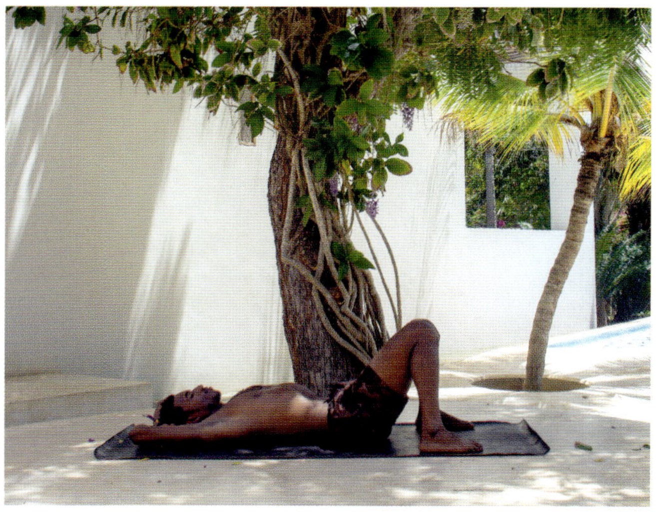

SANTULAN SAVASANA
Balancing Resting

MINDFULNESS & REALIZATION

In Brahma Dhanus / Sagittarius, we are in the shifting season of fire, which corresponds to the power to transmute. We use the energy of fire to release, letting go of all the things that bind us and hold us back from our true selves. In Brahma Makara / Capricorn, we are initiating the season of earth, giving us the courage to make great changes. Through realization, we can fortify our minds. A higher mind is not easily susceptible to outside influence or upheaval.

This chapter focuses on the power of using awareness to resolve deep-seated challenges. The asanas within it lead us to experience mindfulness, a state reached by focusing our awareness on the present moment. In this state, we can calmly recognize and accept feelings, bodily sensations, and thought forms. Training our behaviors brings a deeper understanding of our relationship with our surroundings, including the impact we have on both others and ourselves. Mindfulness uncovers a greater sense of clarity, peace, and well-being.

Practicing mindfulness through Brahma Yoga brings us into a state of heightened awareness to focus on the preciousness of each moment. Since many modern mindfulness techniques are appropriated from ancient spiritual traditions, at times they can be a little reductive. Mindfulness-based stress reduction, for example, has been proven to offer great benefits, but it has removed any trace of spirituality and consciousness. Surely practicing mindfulness holds more meaning than just de-stressing so you can be a better-functioning cog in the grand machine of modernity. By exploring mindfulness while moving the body, we are encouraging a deepened connection between our mind and body.

Attaining a state of self-realization and enlightenment is an ultimate goal of yoga practice. Realization can bring profound insight as part of the process of reflection and self-discovery. By noticing deep-rooted patterns that have contributed to our feelings of anxiety, worry, or depression, we can transmute those experiences into great wisdom. The asanas here offer us an experiential way to reach these realizations so we can bring new perspectives and reframe our thoughts to change our behaviors. We are building great neuroplasticity in our brain by forming new neural connections. Brahma Yoga is helpful in this process because the asanas increase blood flow to the brain, help release hormones that grow new brain cells, and enhance the connections between neurons.

Although they do include meditation, the asanas in this chapter offer psychological benefits that surpass doing only meditation. Regular yoga practice can increase oxygen flow and the release of feel-good chemicals in the brain. As we move, we allow the chemical messengers to travel through our entire body while letting go of negative thoughts. The asanas included also help with the lymphatic drainage of the body.

We are engaging the mind to create new stories with a section of laughter yoga, where we combine intentional laughter with physical movements, kriyas, and breath work. This creates a playfulness that lightens the mood and gives us immediate relief. Laughter is one of the most natural forms of stress relief and is great for regulating emotions and improving mental health. Laughing for no reason is one of the best lessons in nonattachment. Brahma Yoga wants you to feel great and experience the bliss that you deserve rather than letting hardship continue to hold you down.

BRAHMA YOGA SUTRAS

BRAHMA DHANUS • Sagittarius

- By centering myself, I develop the conscious practice of moving more into stillness.
- I value authenticity, and I choose love, not attachment.
- I enjoy good communication and cherish the relationship I have with myself and others.
- I release and regulate my emotions by giving myself time to reflect and regenerate.
- What is the point of running, if I feel like I have never arrived? When I am in a state of realization, I can be here now.
- There does not need to be any specific reason in order for me to be happy.
- I am mindful in meditation of what I pay attention to.
- I will love in any form I wish, as I know that love, or the absence of it, ultimately becomes my life story.
- I invent my future when I reconcile my past. I suffer the outcomes if I ignore my origins, so I keep choosing to have faith in myself.

BRAHMA MAKARA • Capricorn

- I have courage to know that it does not matter how far I go; it matters how near I am.
- My goals are like magnets being easily drawn to me through the divination of both nature and the universe.
- By understanding all our needs in entirety, our options and desires naturally change.
- I acknowledge the interdependence of all relationships, and I am willing to be responsible in order to claim the freedom that is available to me.
- I have patience and discipline, and I no longer try to preempt setbacks, as that simply causes more obstacles.
- Even though at times I may face challenges, I completely love and accept myself. Each day I am becoming more of me.
- Love and hate are equal passions simply facing the opposite direction. I respect cooperation, and I can be tender without being vulnerable.
- I am self-sufficient by living from the cause and not the effect and by understanding the universal principles of karma.
- Brahma Yoga shows me a way to not be afraid of failure when I am excited about opportunities in life.

Meditation is not escapism.

Be present and release whatever comes up

to reconnect to a deep sense of oneness.

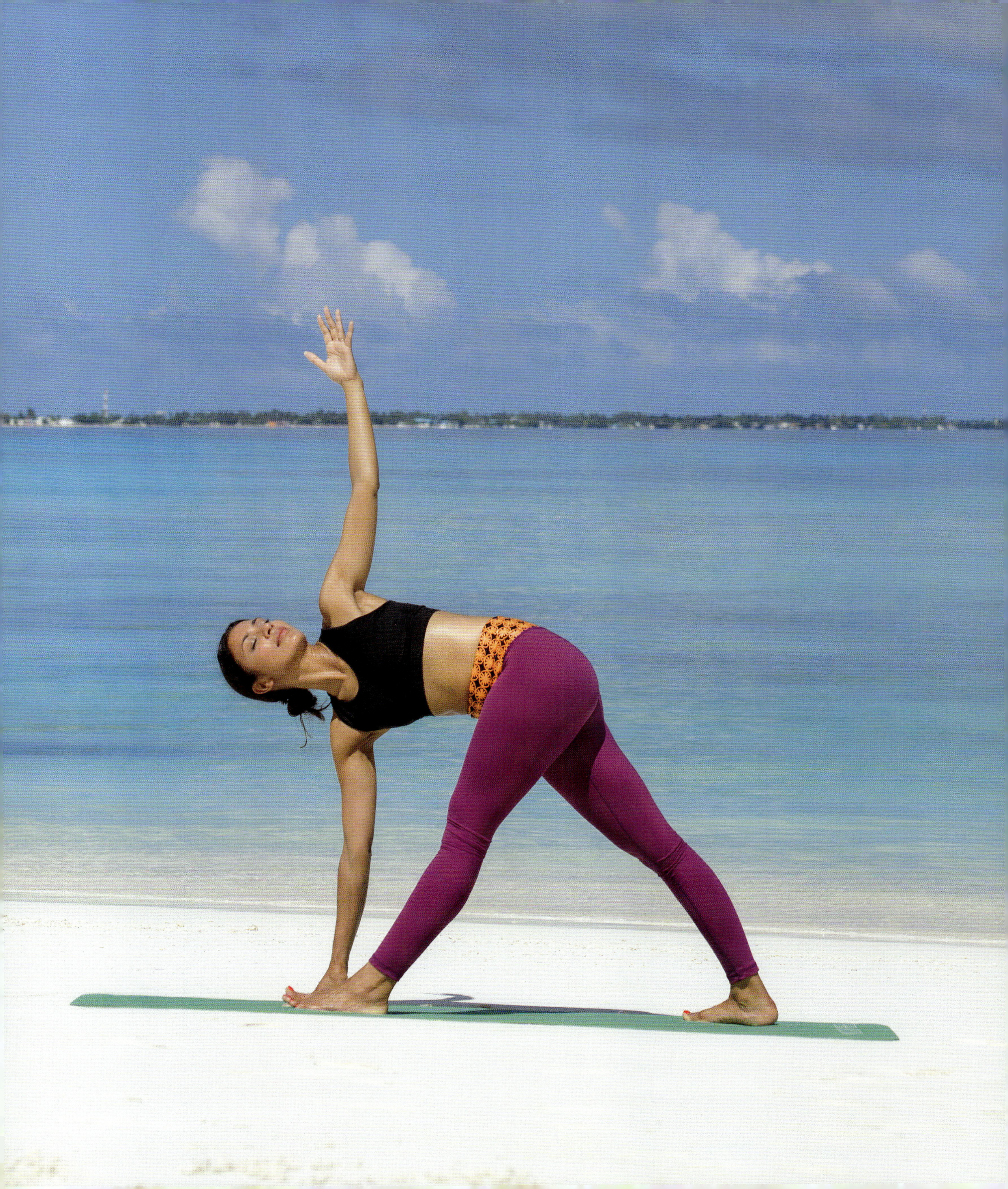

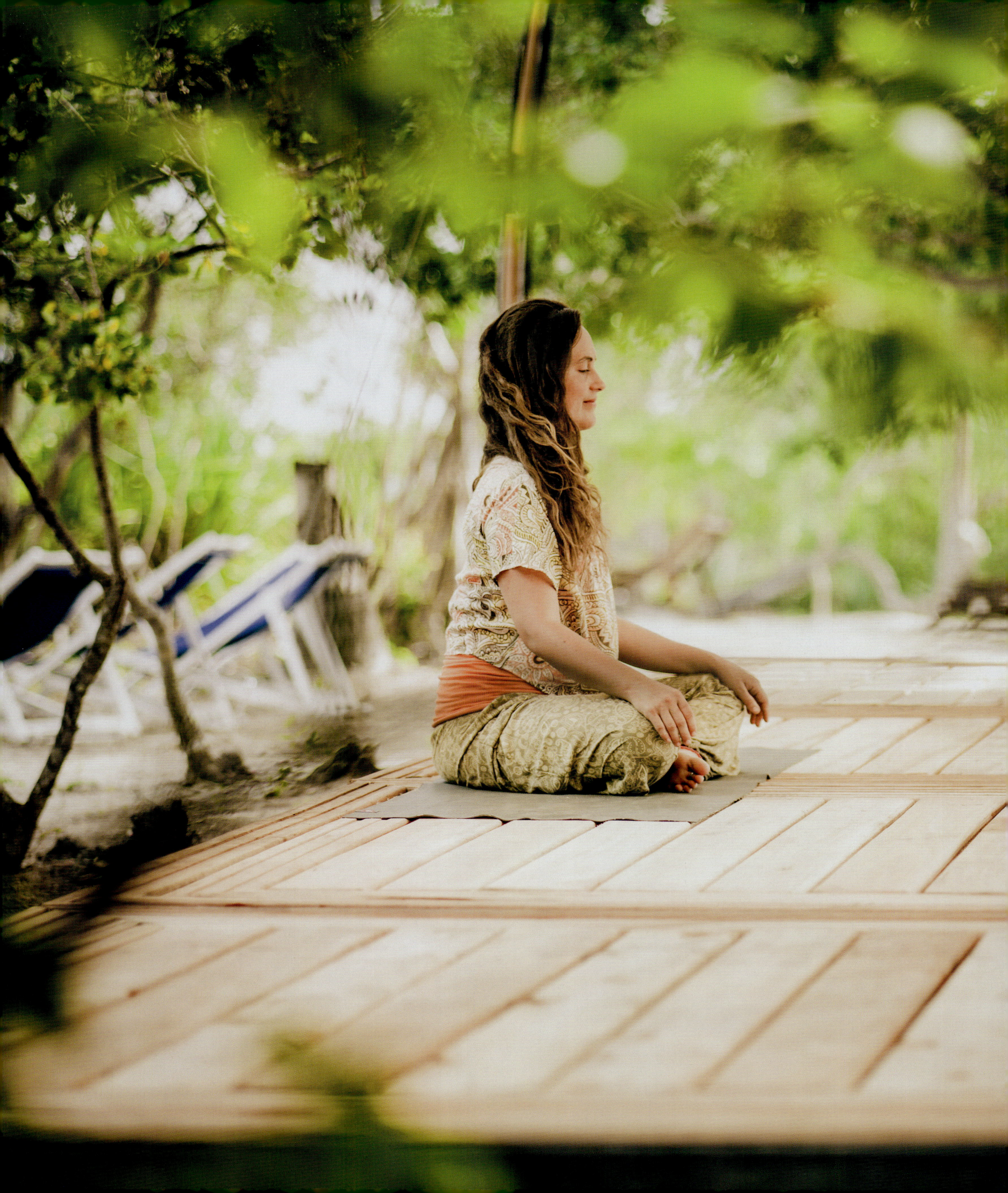

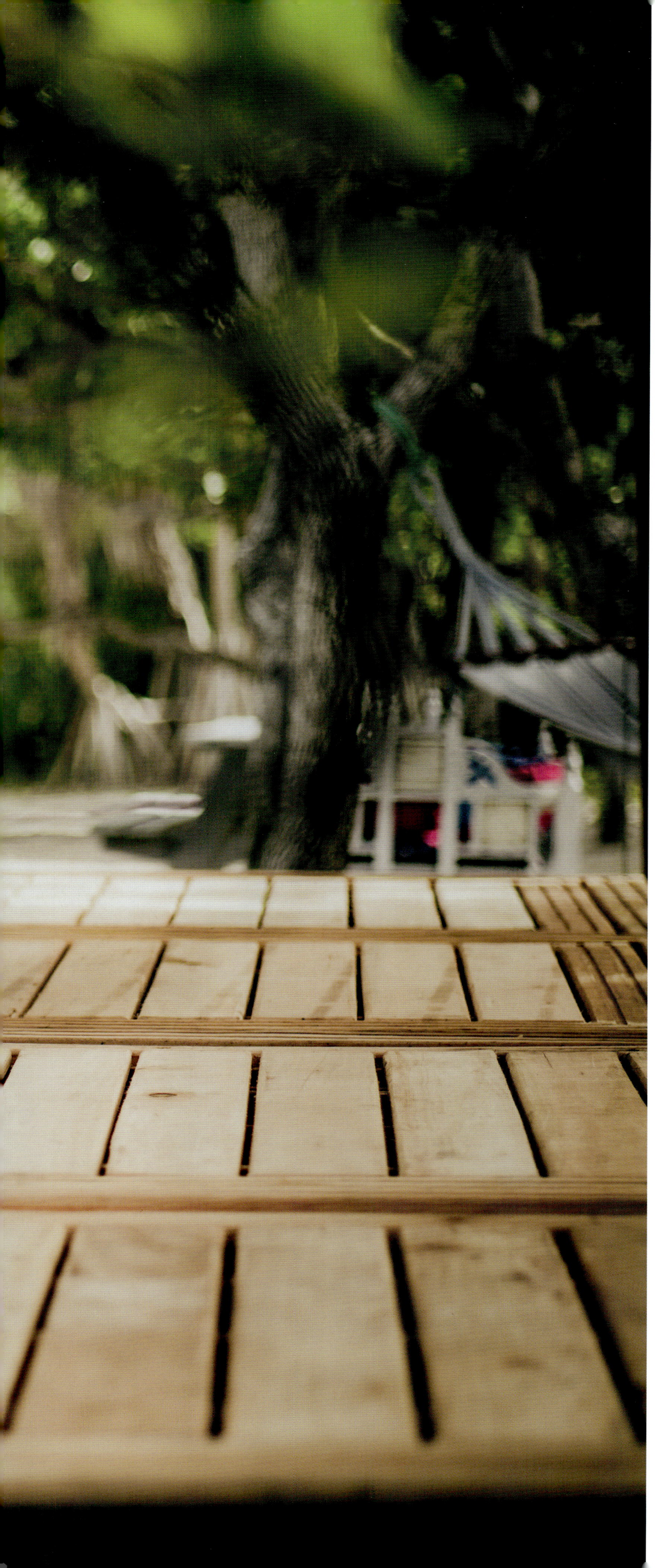

Never delay
until tomorrow
what you
can resolve
indefinitely today.

Your moods change like the weather, but your consciousness remains constant like the sky.

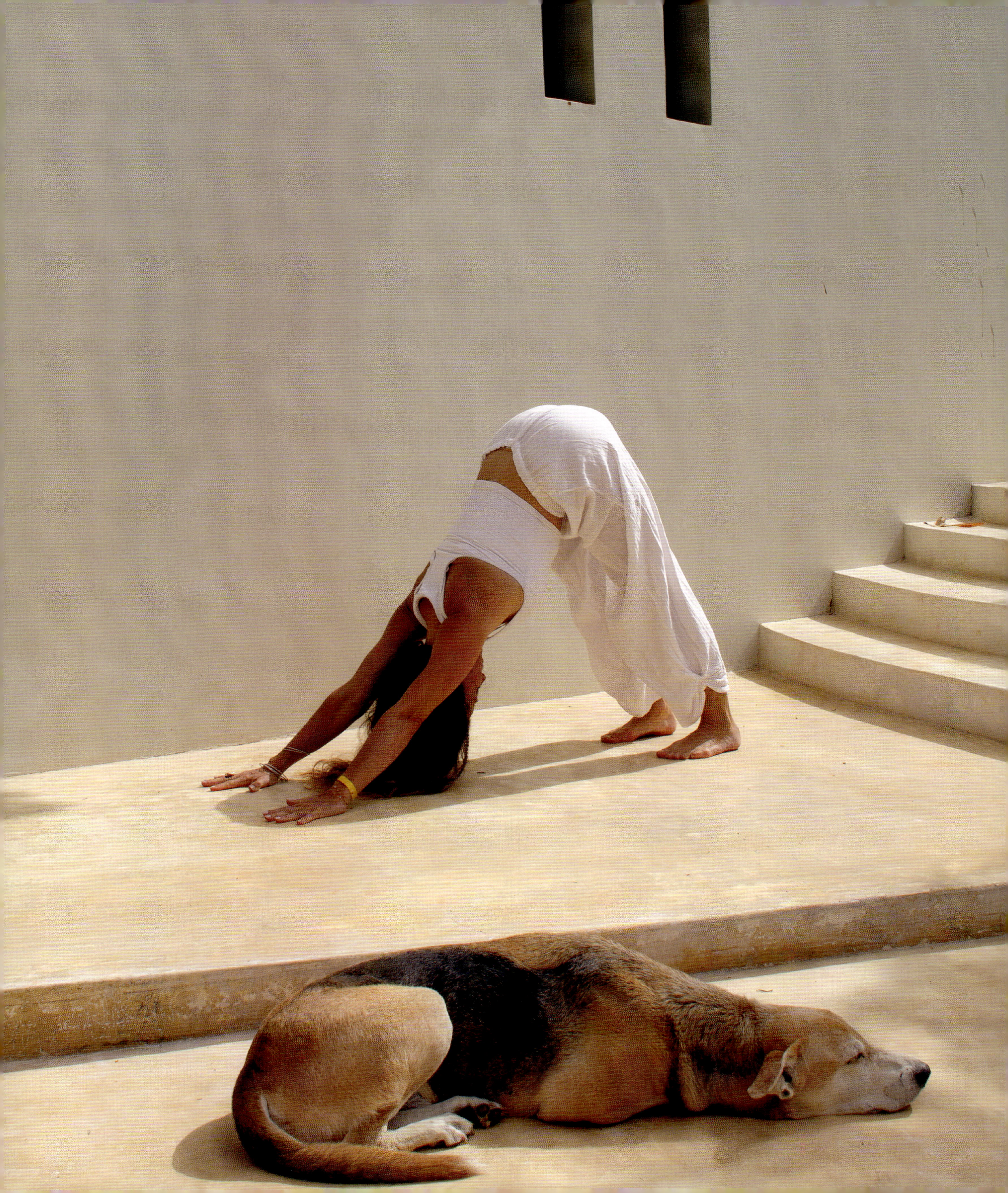

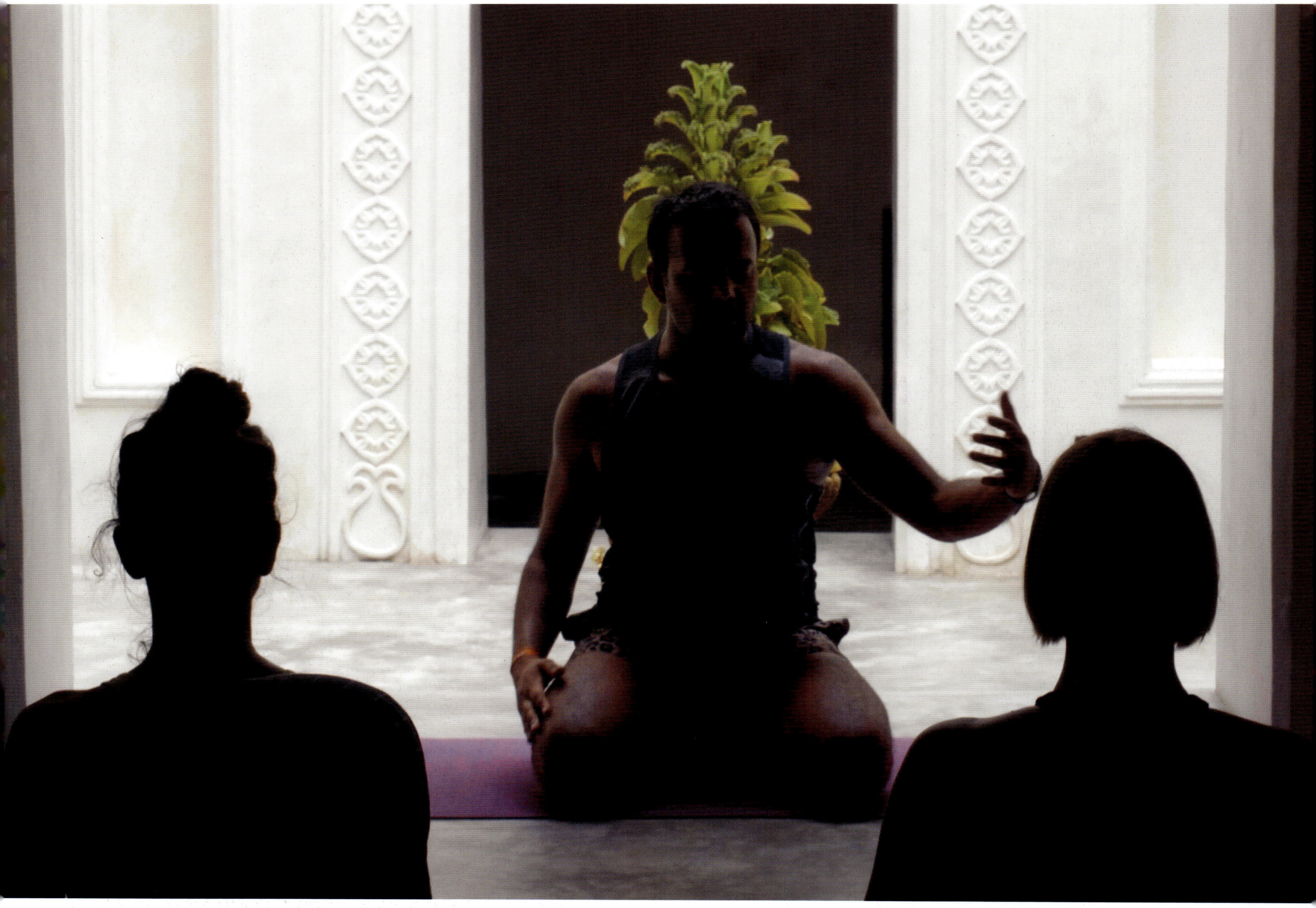

▲ SUNANA · Listening

PADMASANA · Lotus

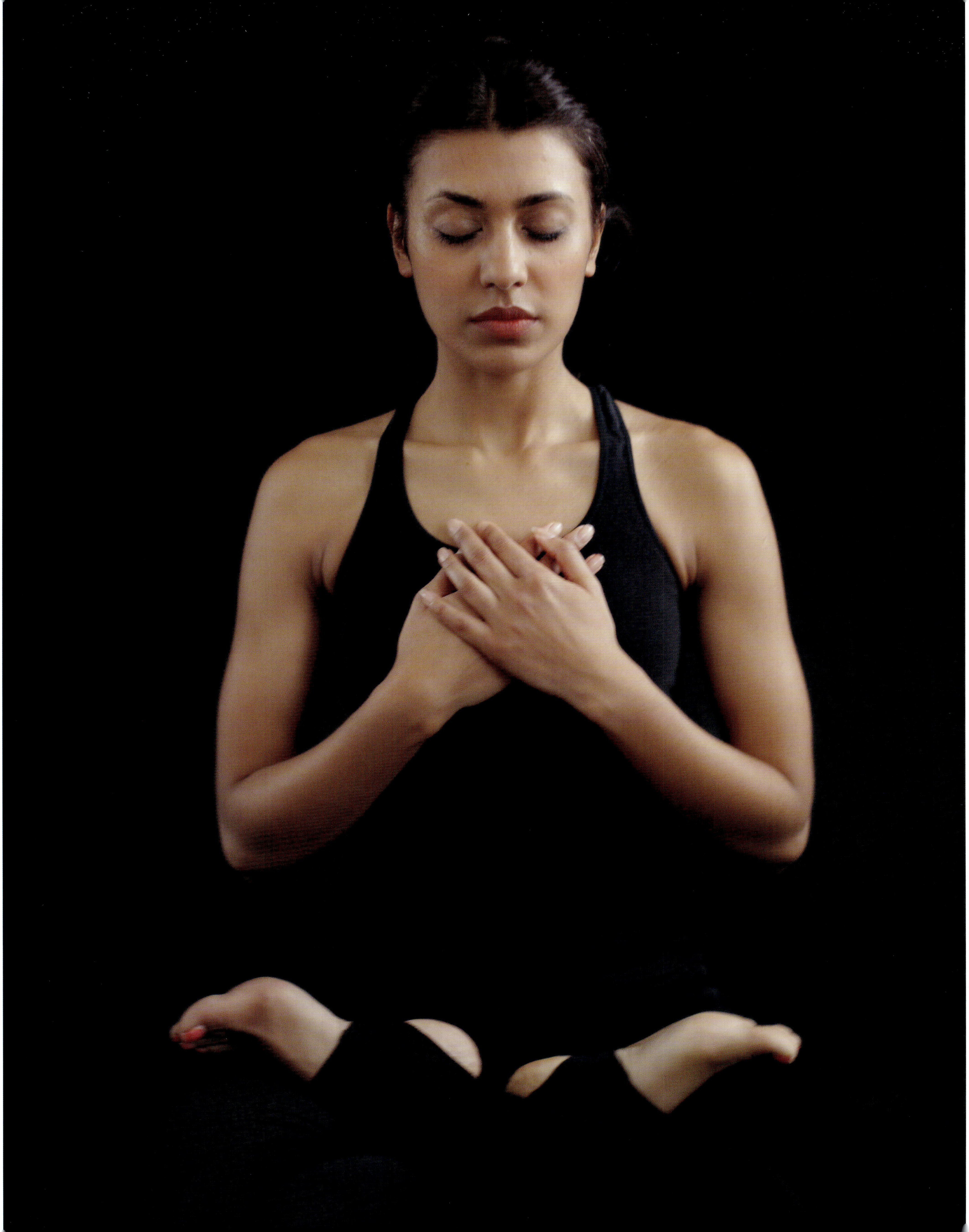

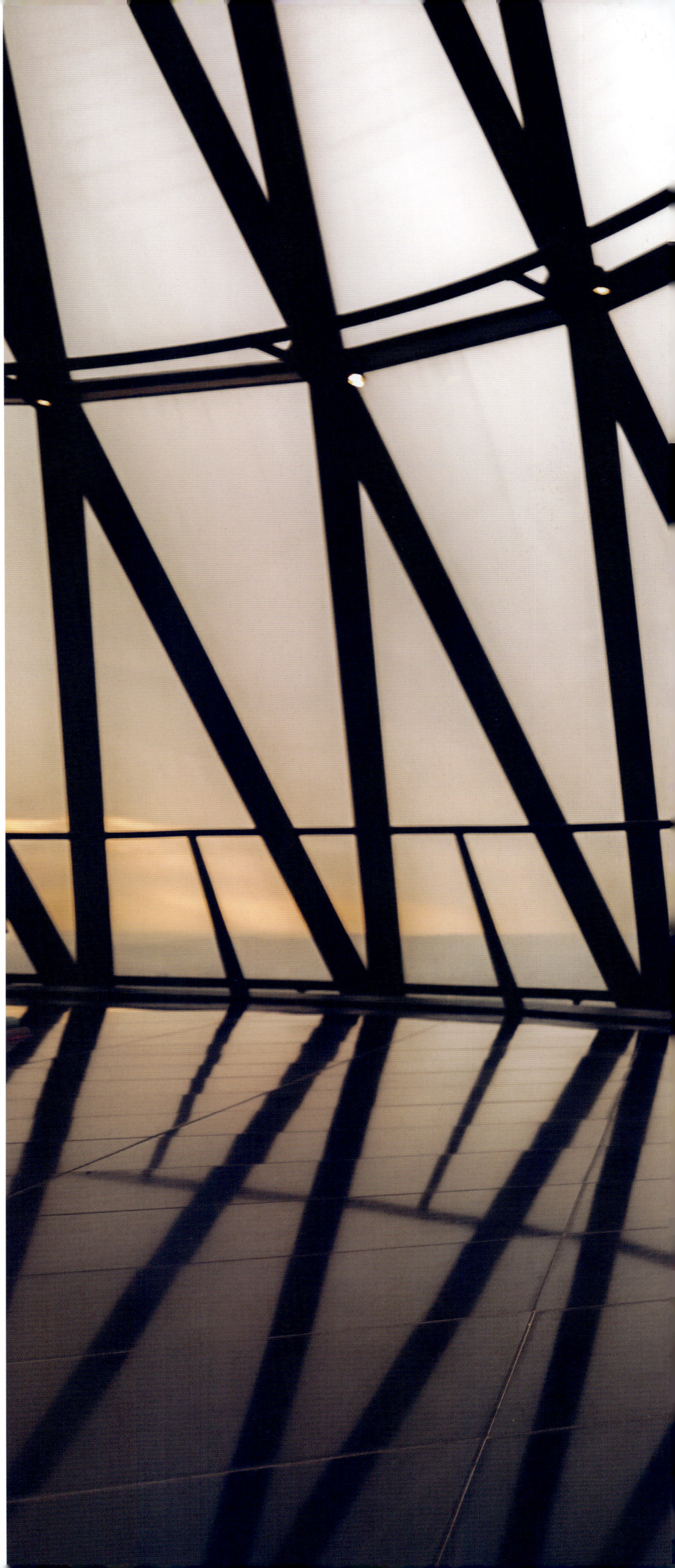

TRI PADA ADHO MUKHA SVANASANA · Three-Legged Downward-Facing Dog

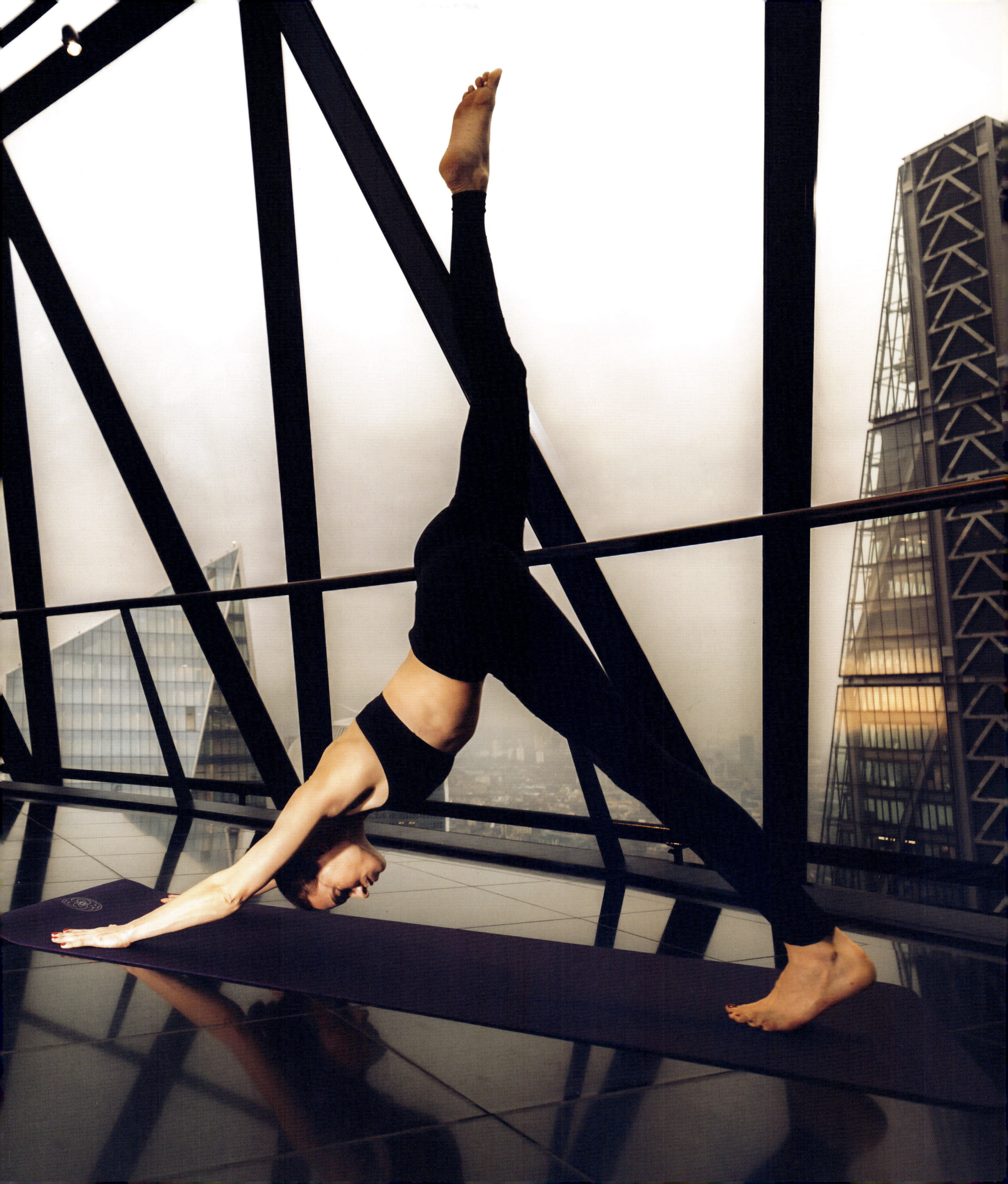

Being well is not the absence of worries.
It is the capability to overcome them repeatedly.

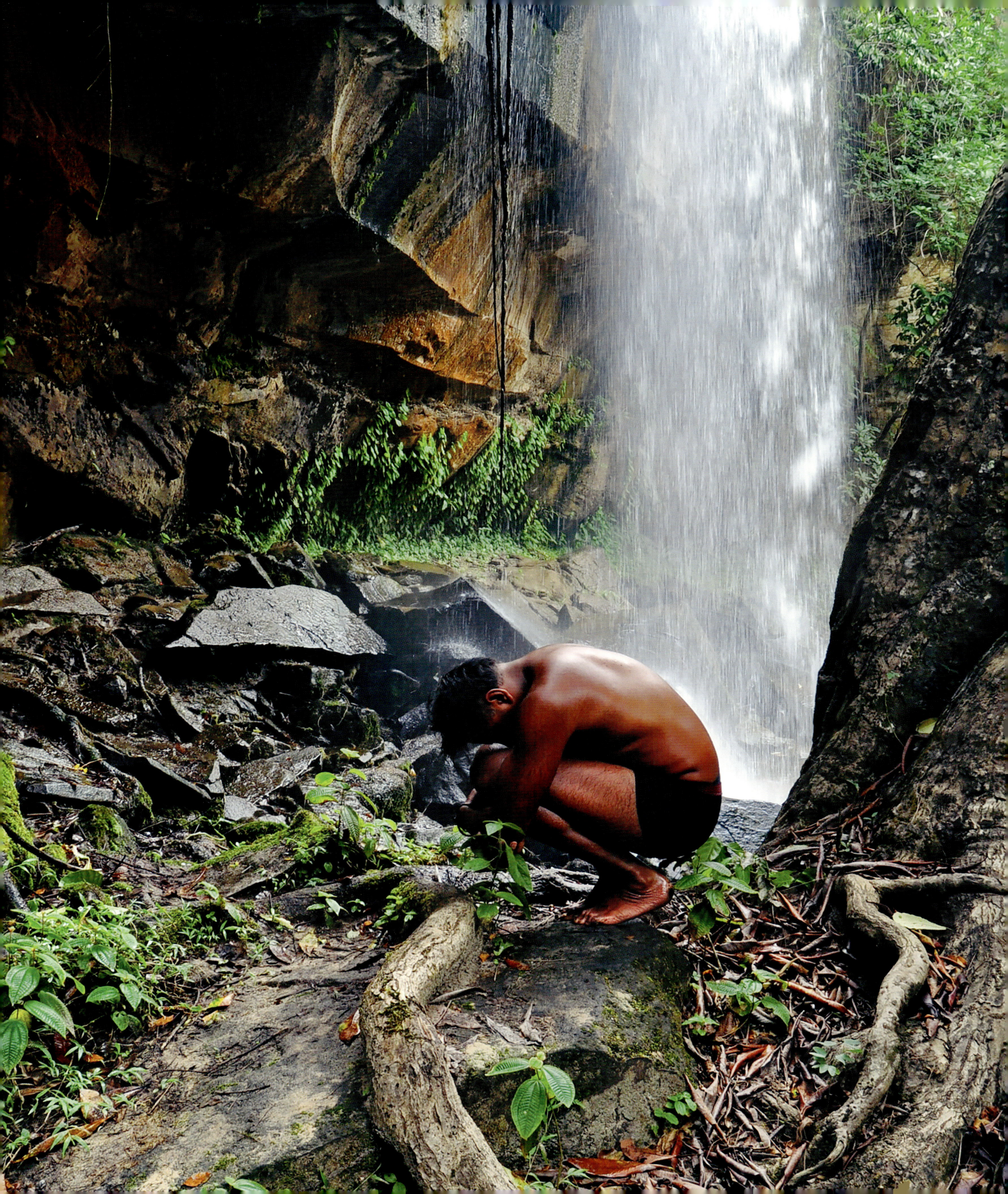

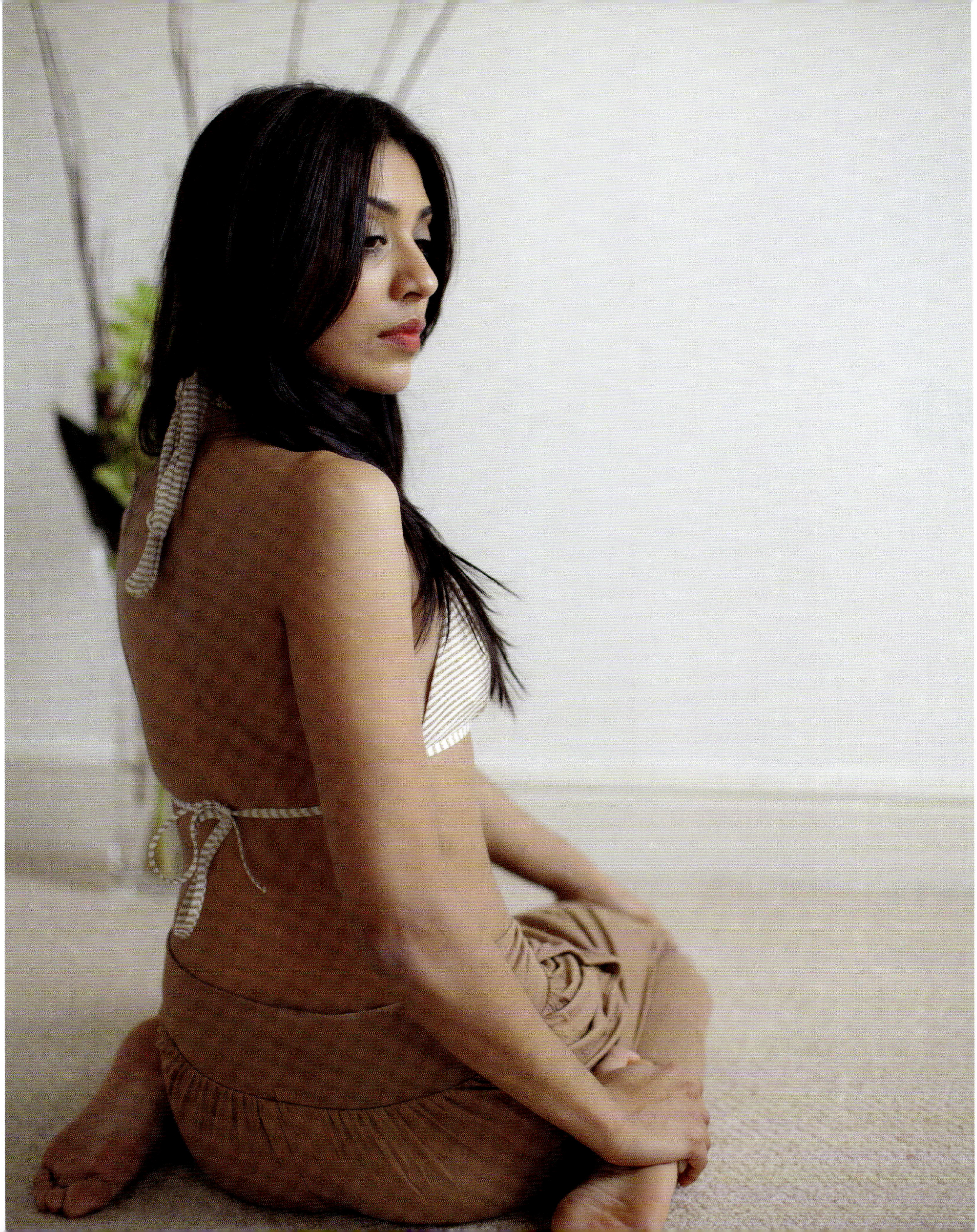

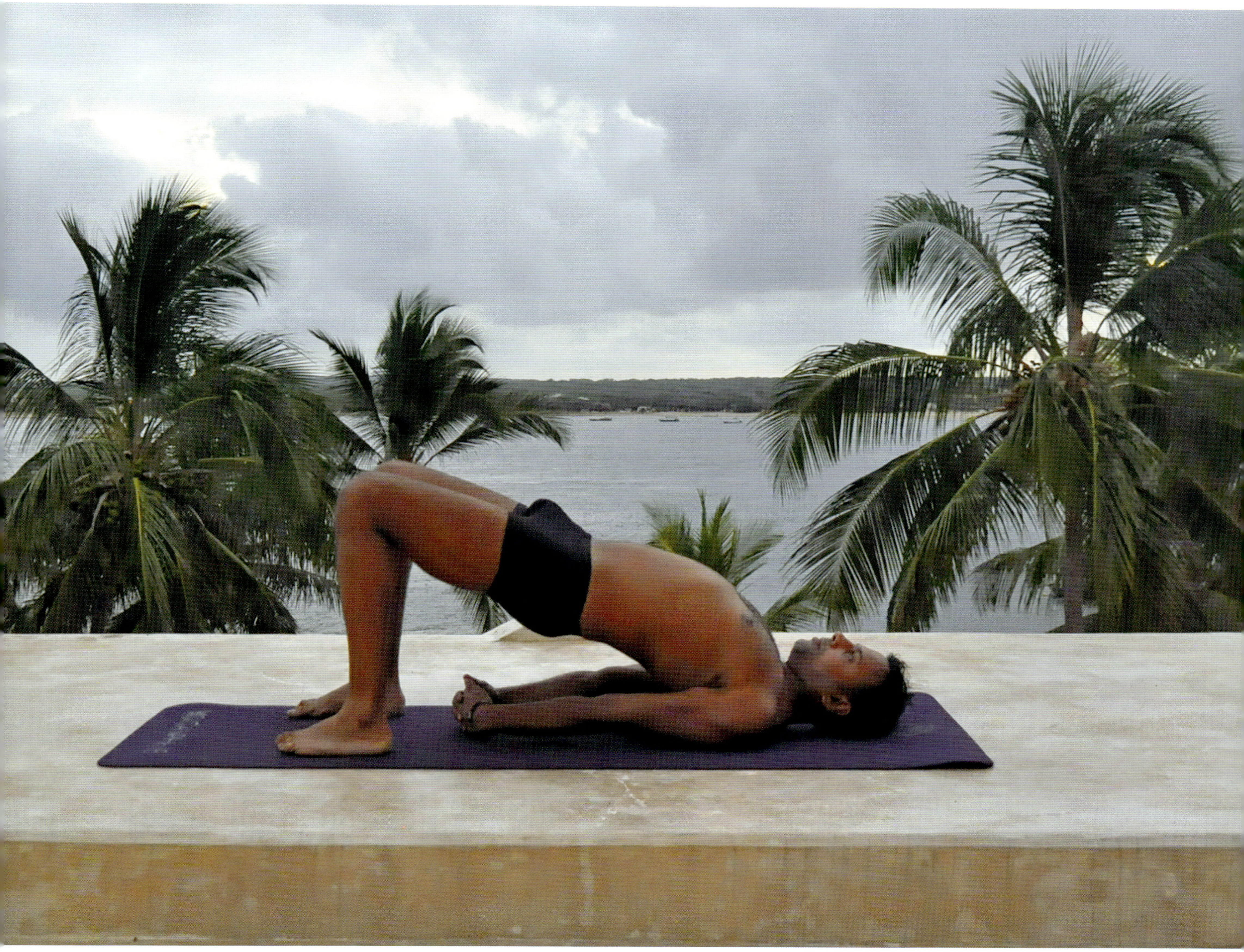

PARIVRTTA VAJRASANA • Twisted Thunderbolt

▲ SETU BANDHA SARVANGASANA • Bridge

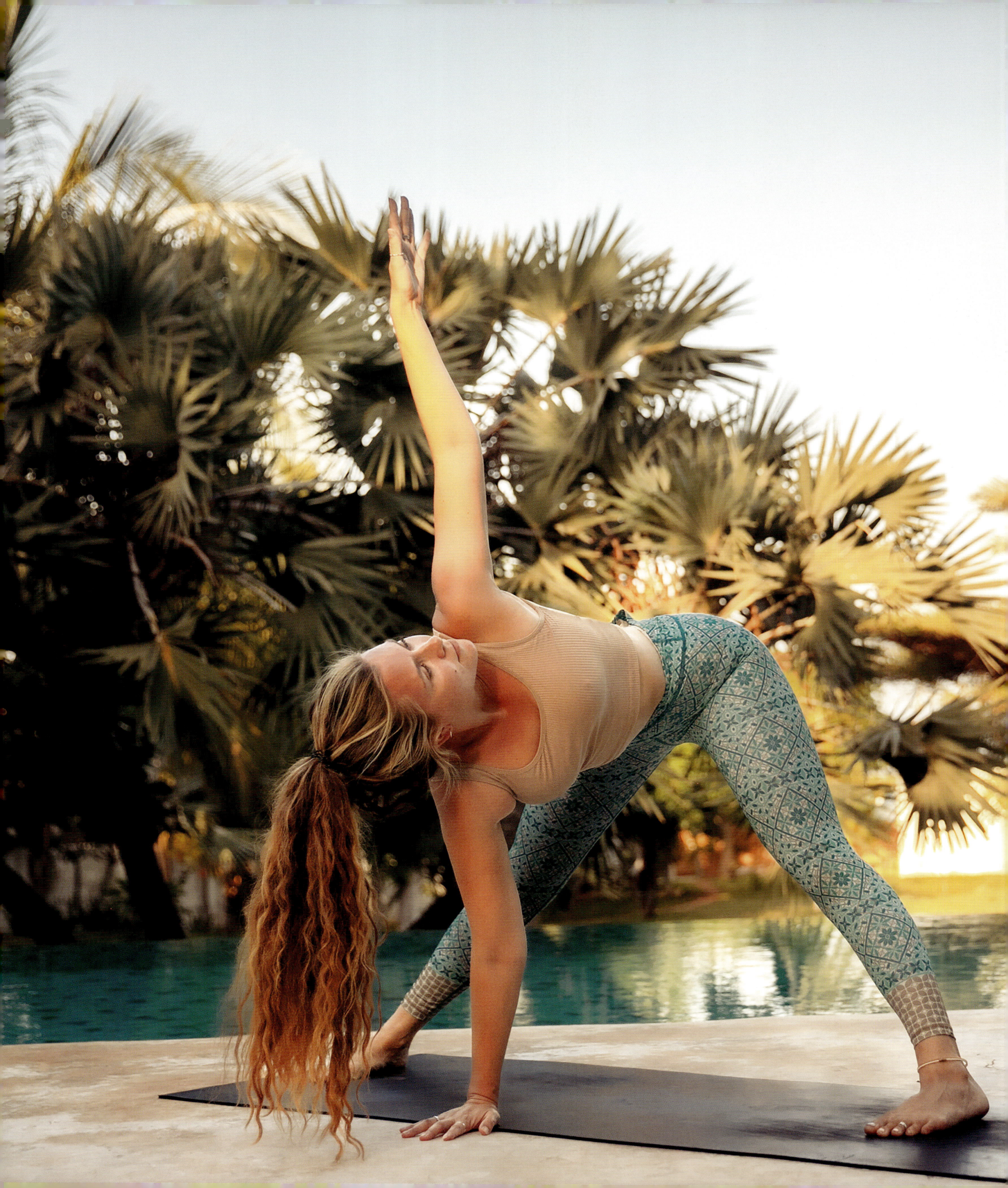

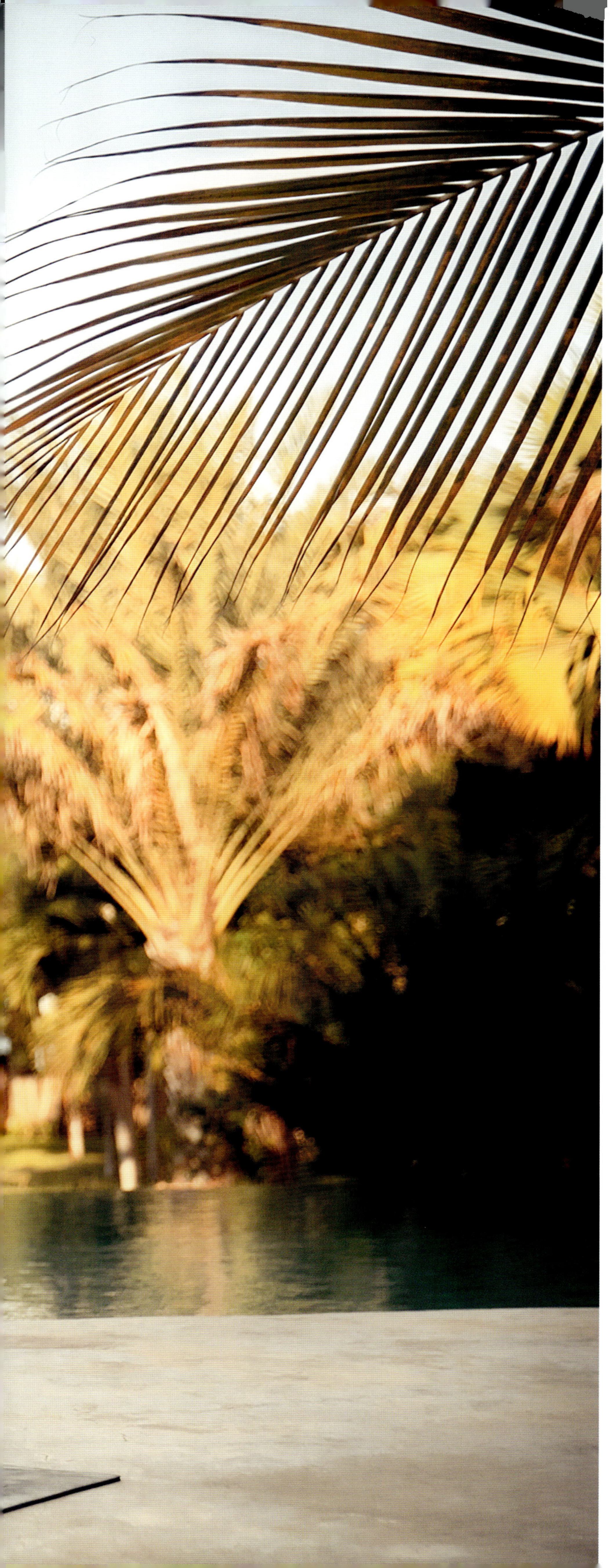

PARIVRTTA PRASARITA PADOTTANASANA • Wide-Legged Standing Twisted Forward Bend

When we imagine fear as curiosity,

we broaden our horizons.

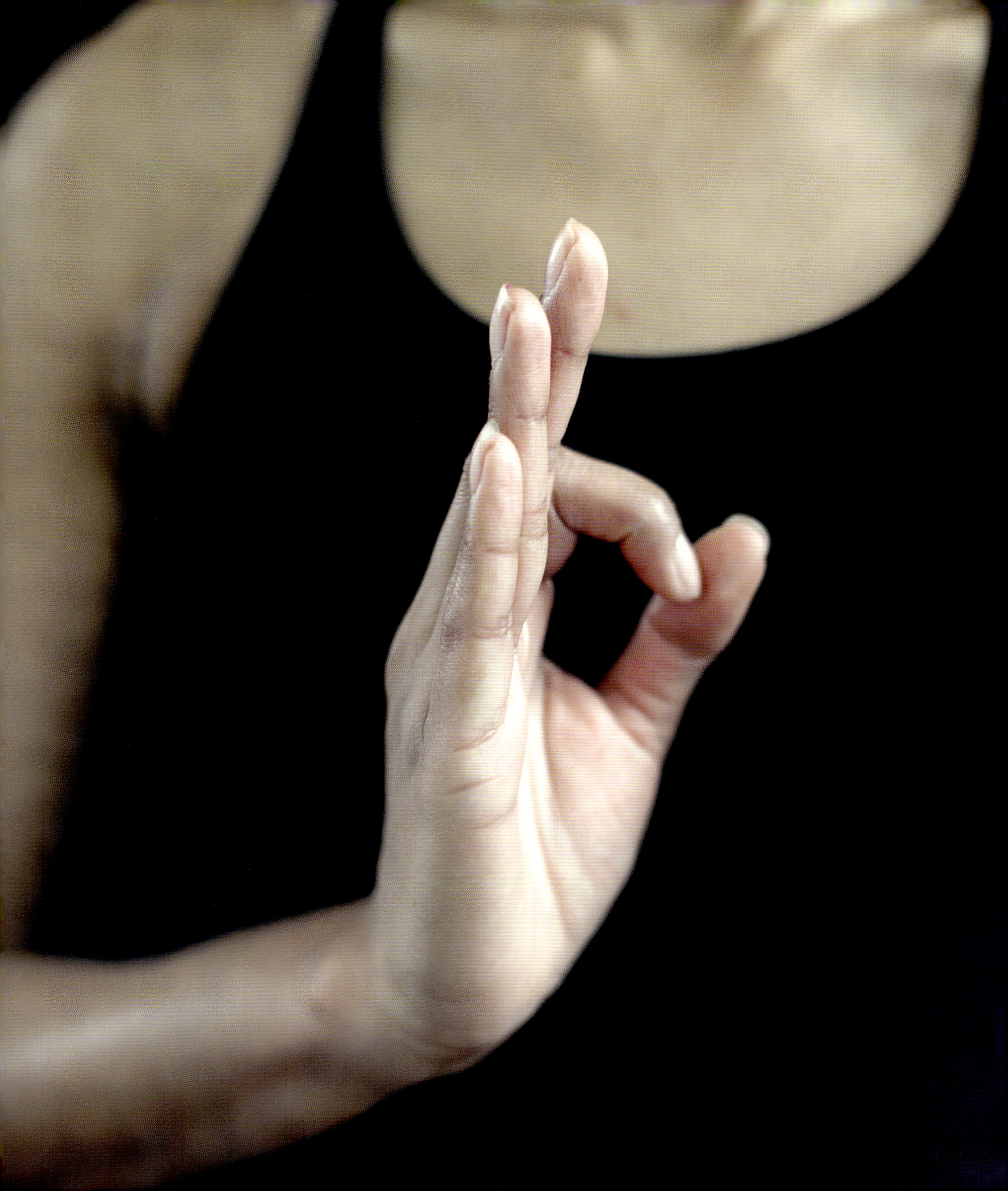

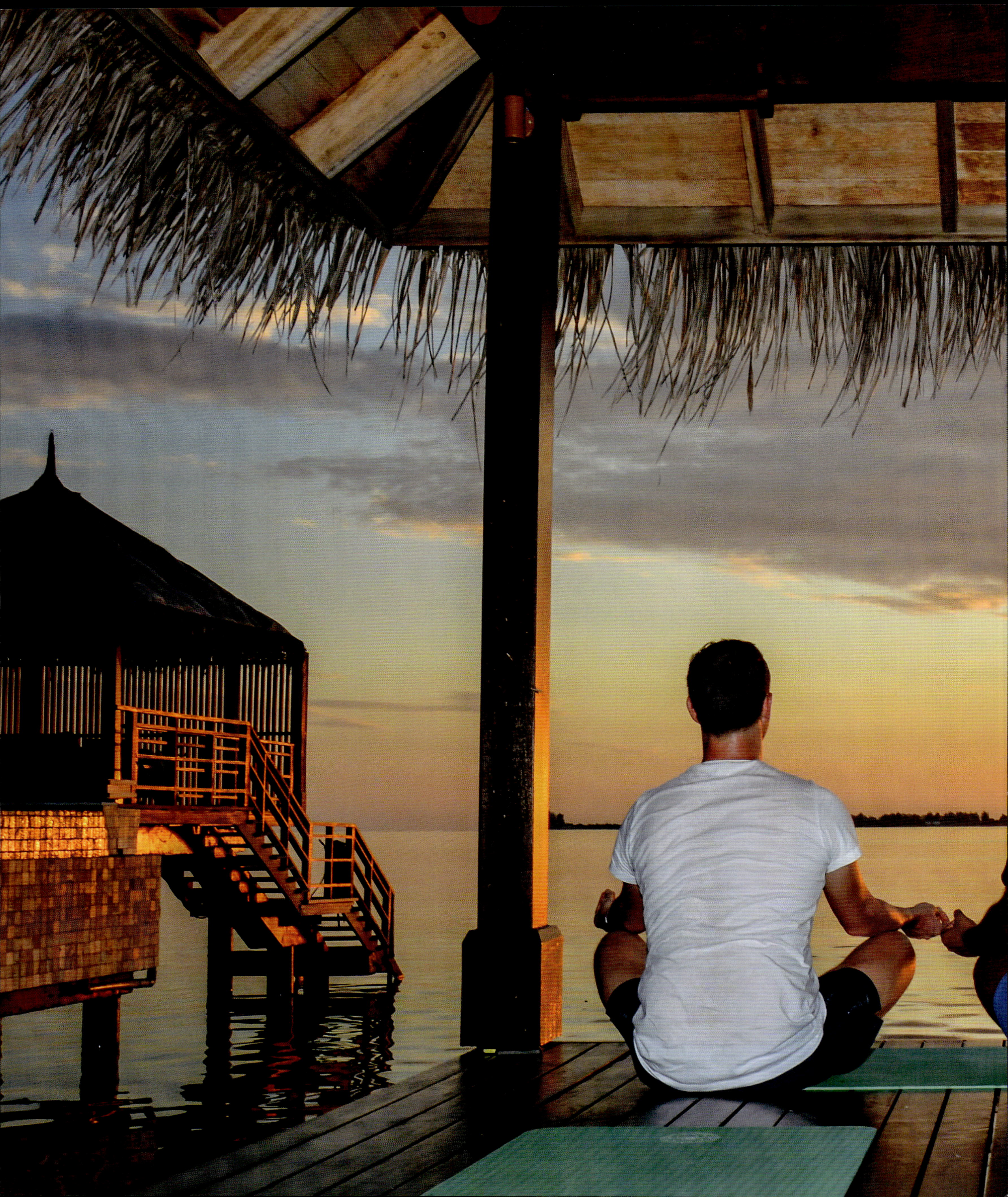

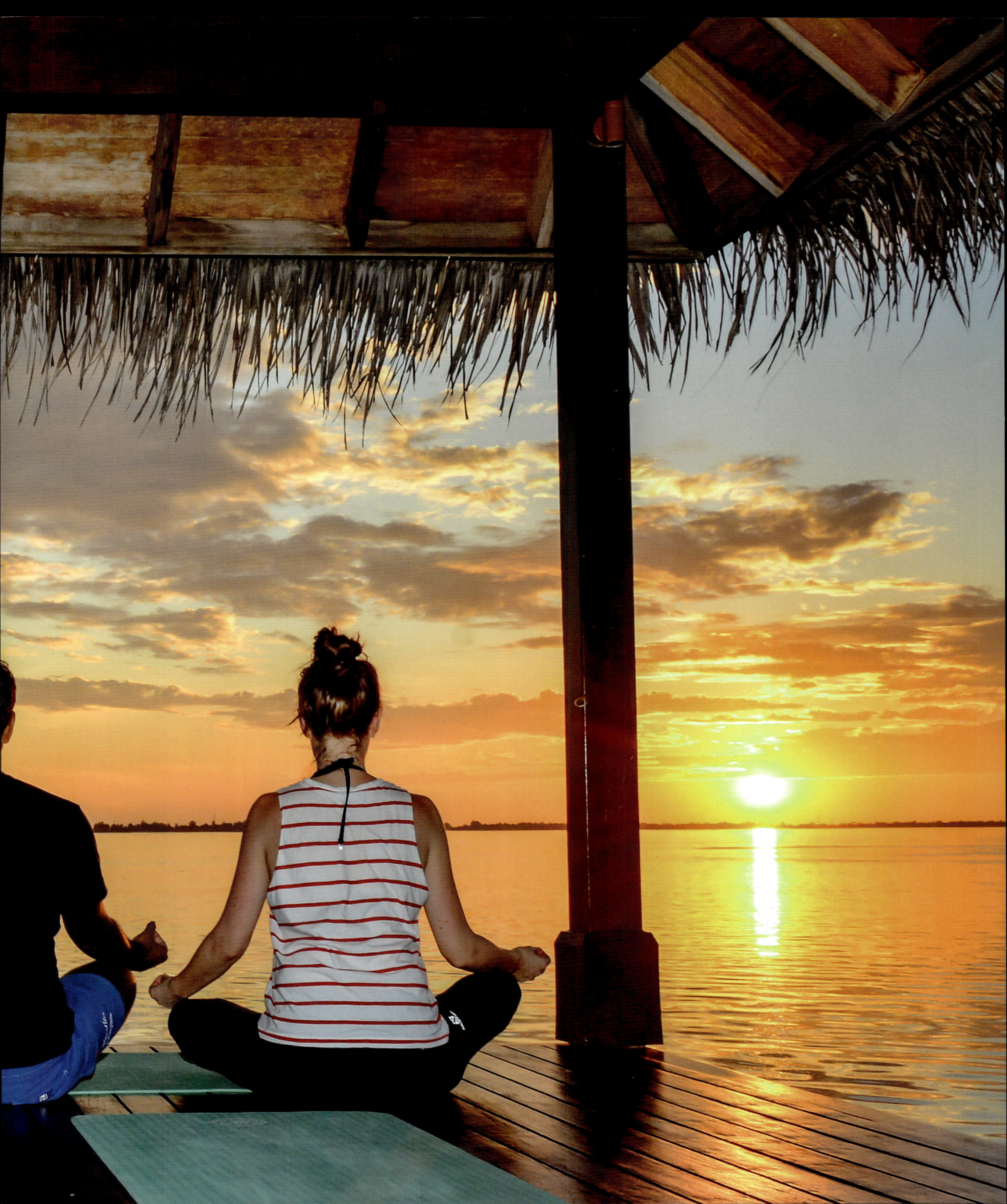

There are four parts to each breath cycle—
the inhale, the exhale,
and the spaces in between.

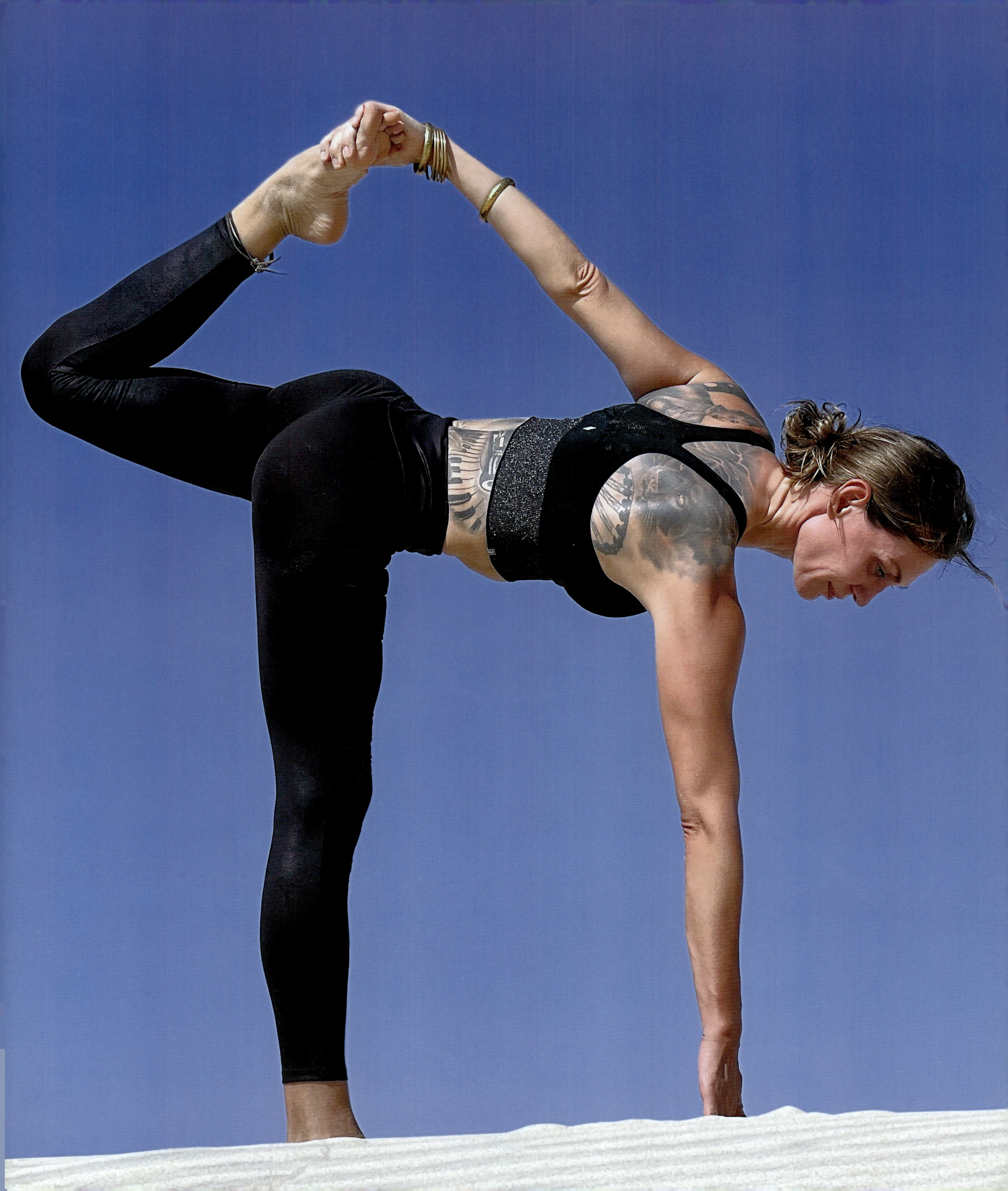

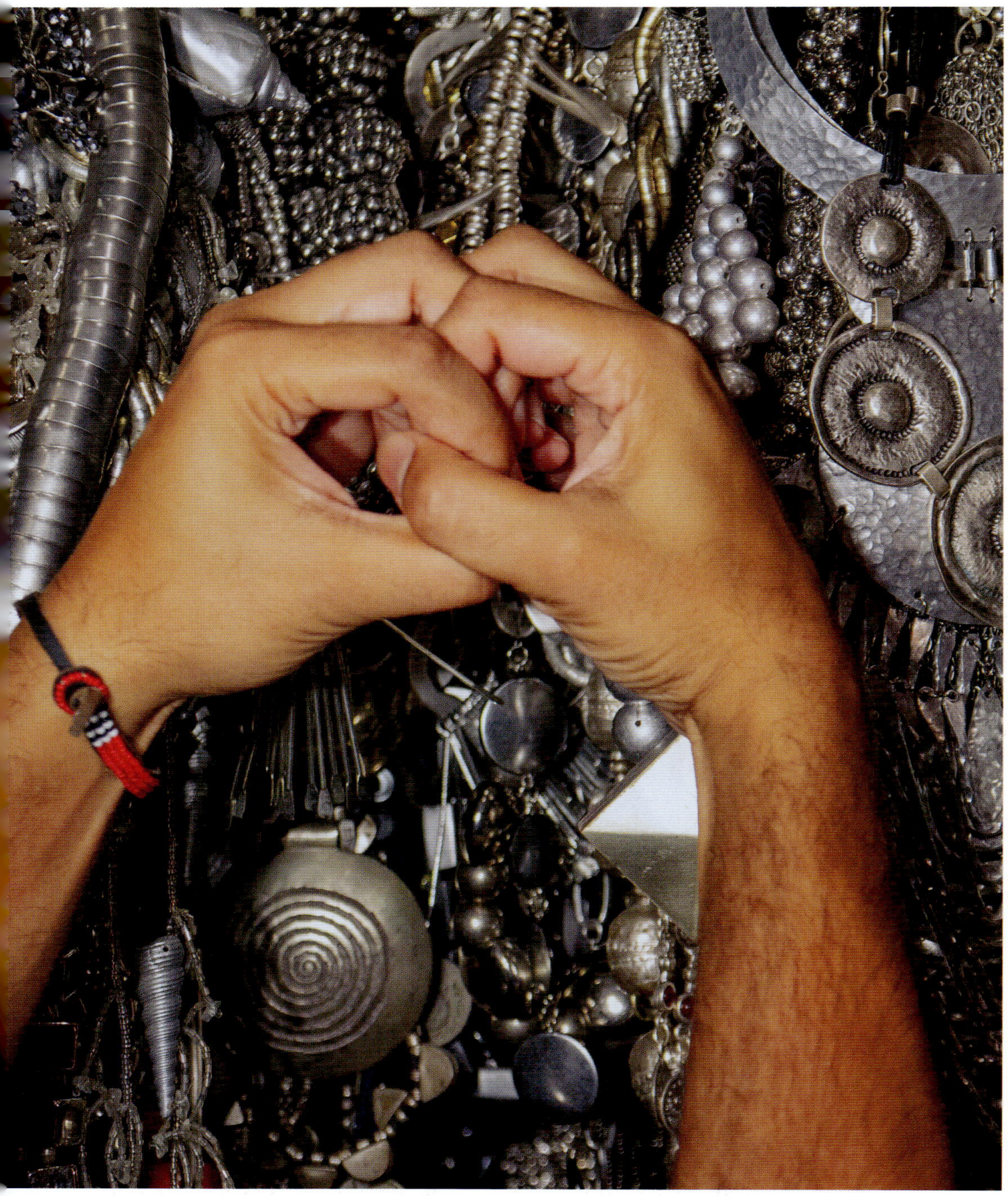

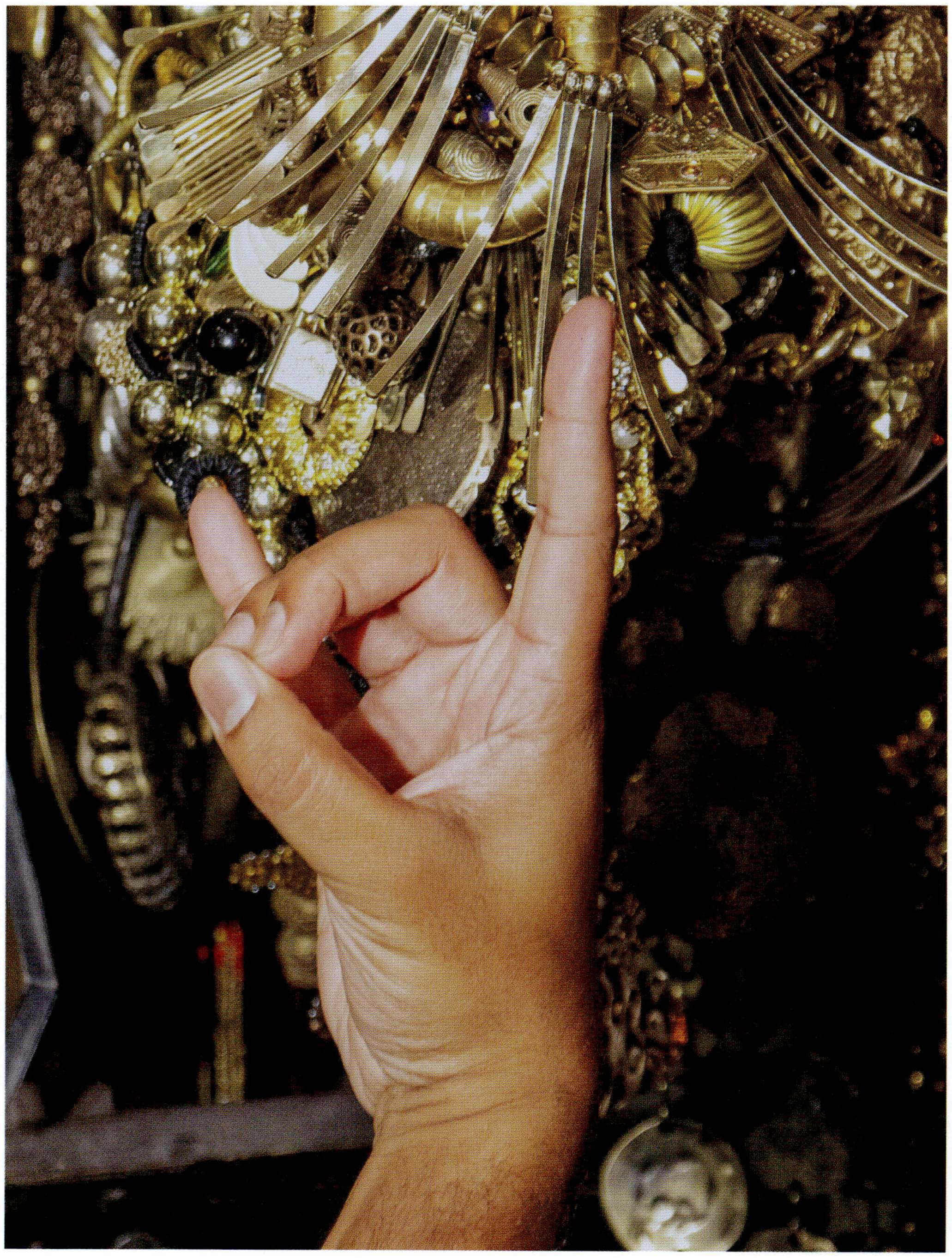

▲ **VISHUDDHACHAKRAMUDRA** · Communication *(left)* **APANAMUDRA** · Release *(right)*

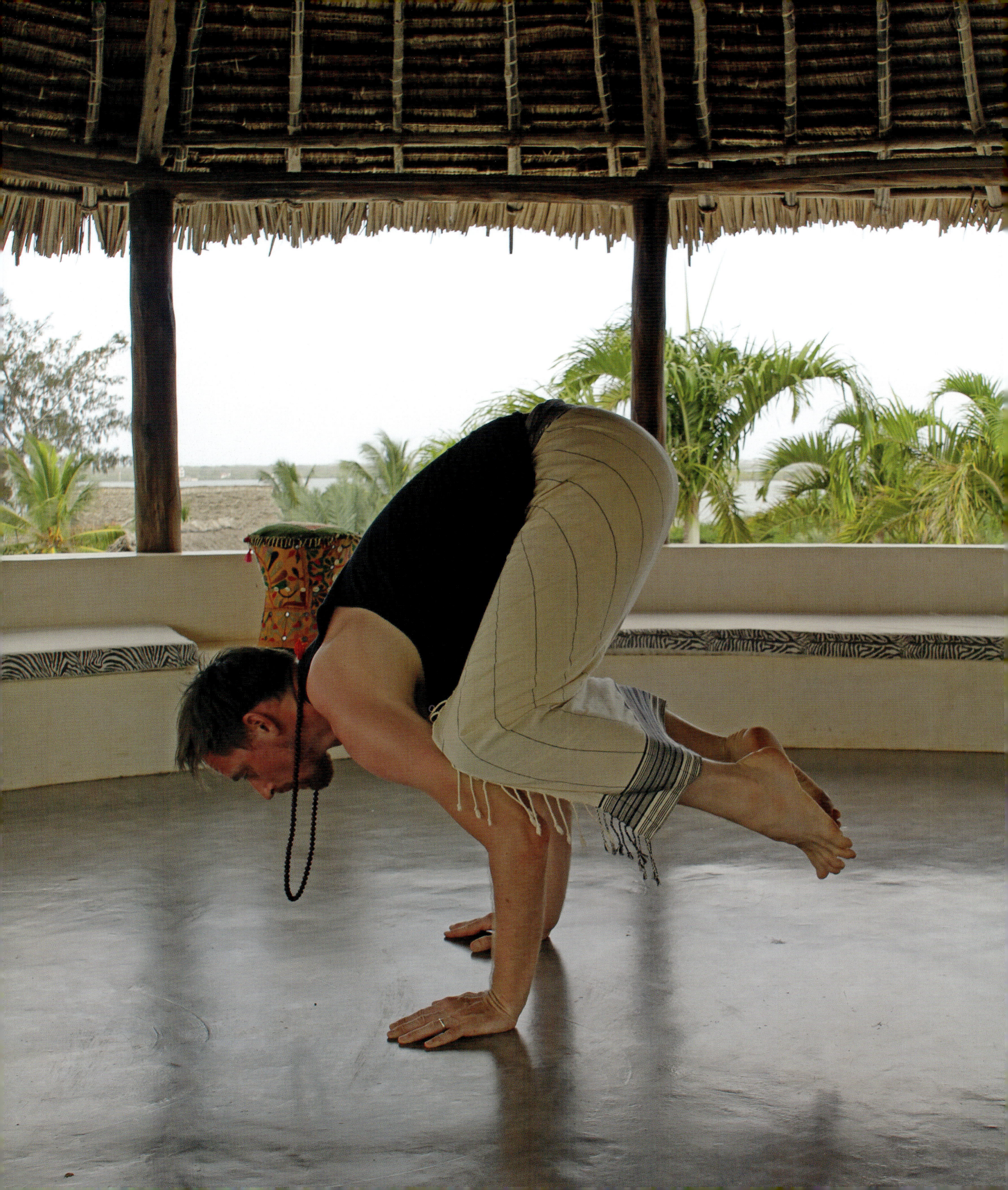

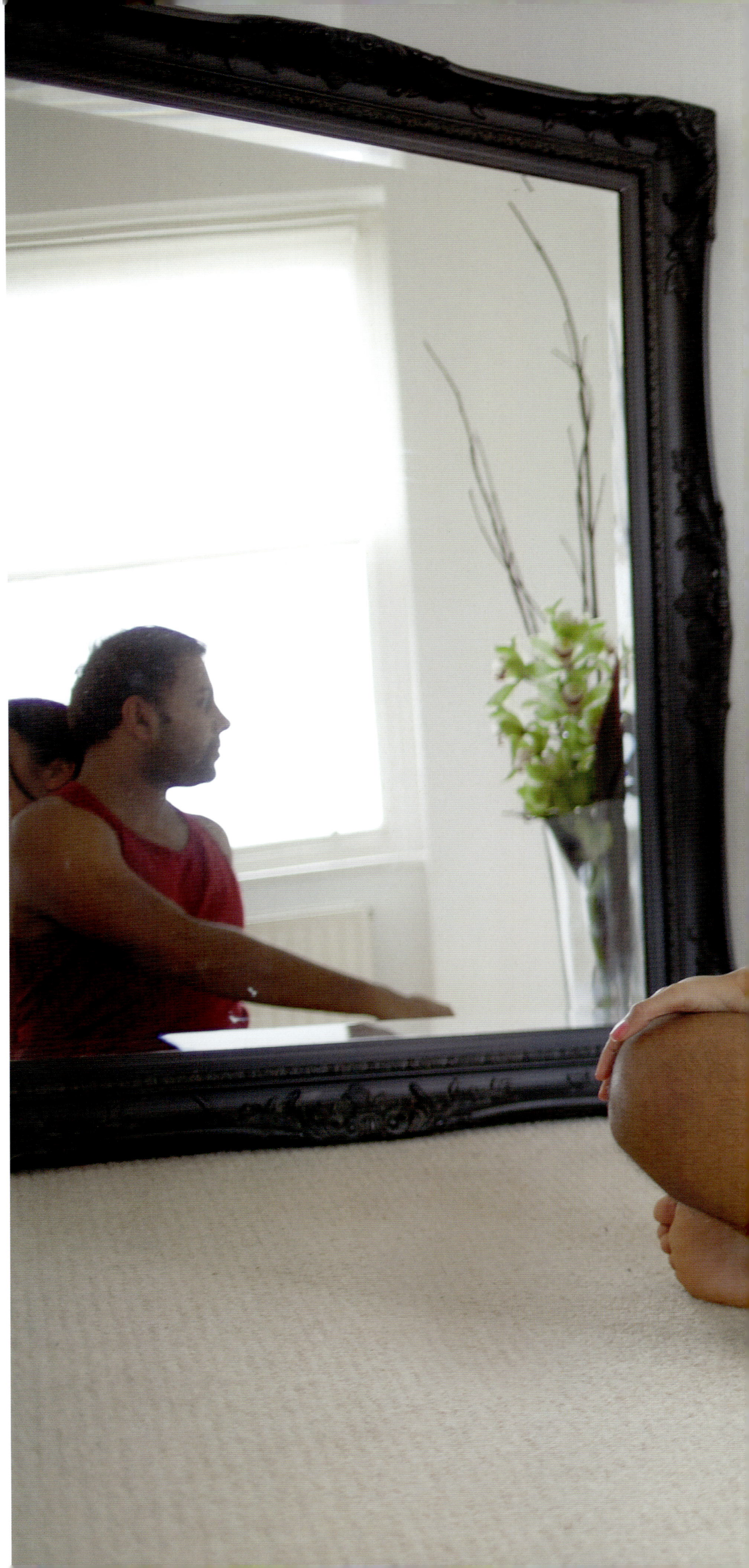

DARPAN PARIVRTTA SUKHASANA • Easy Seated Mirror Twist

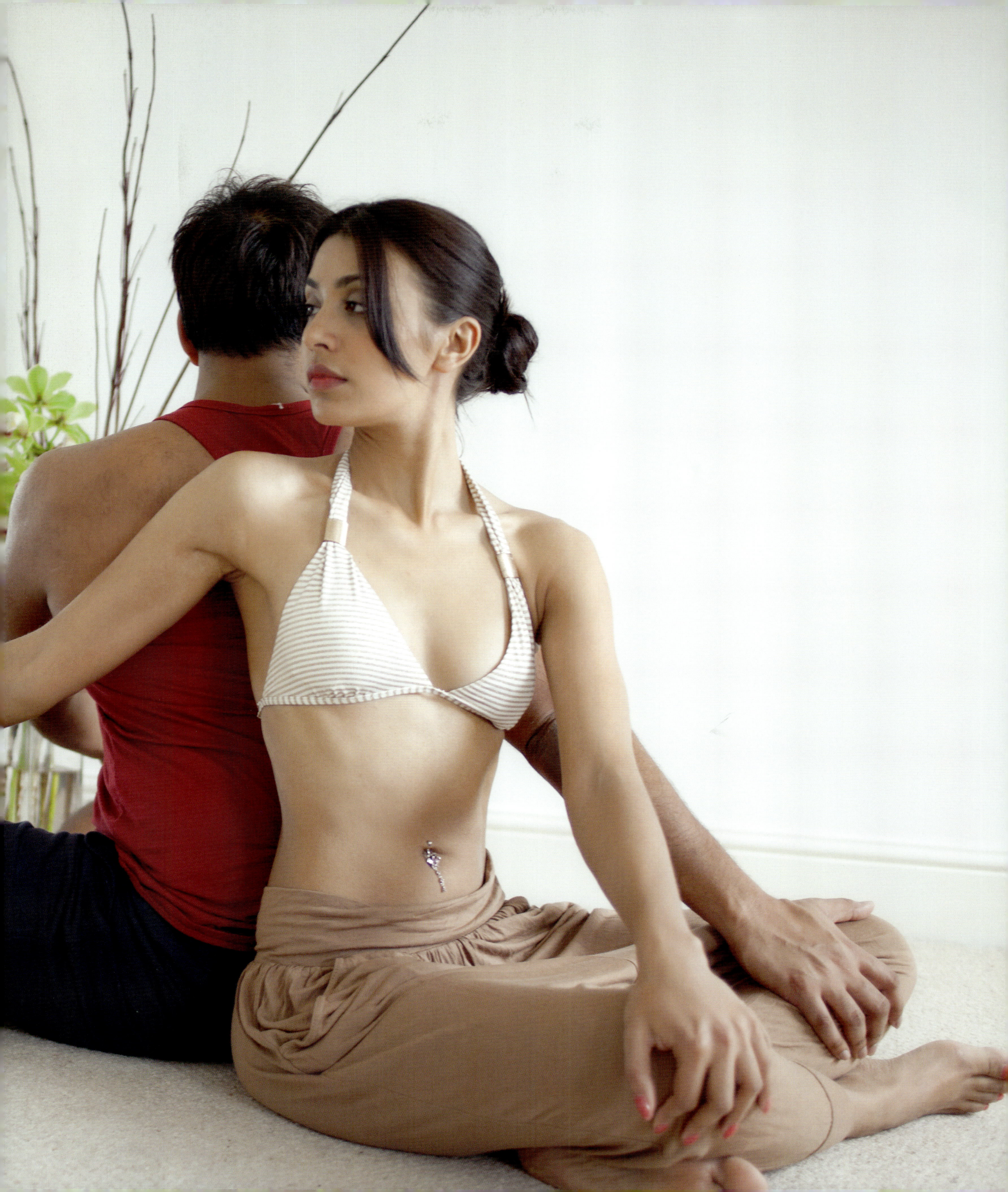

Often the lens needs adjusting, not the landscape.

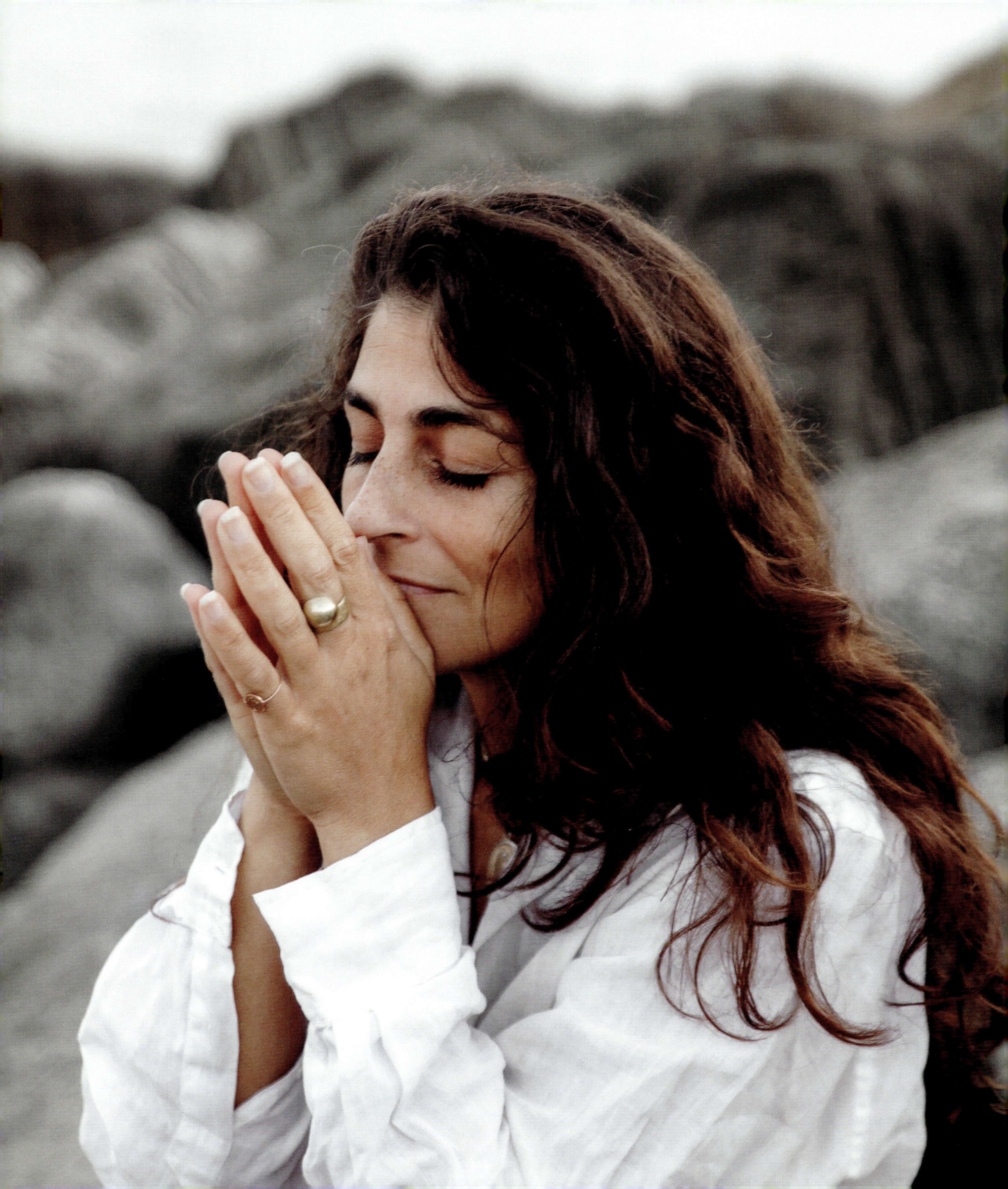

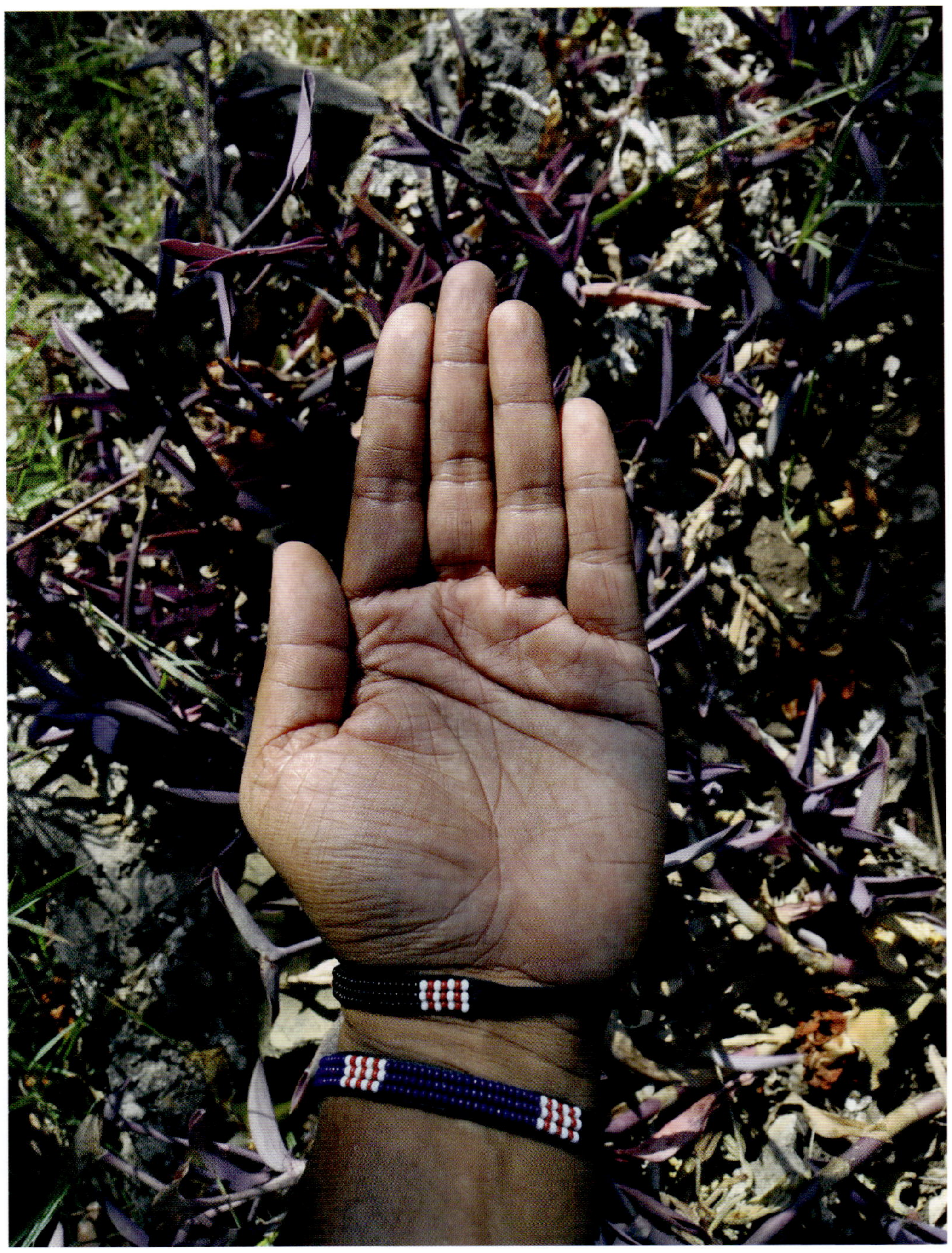

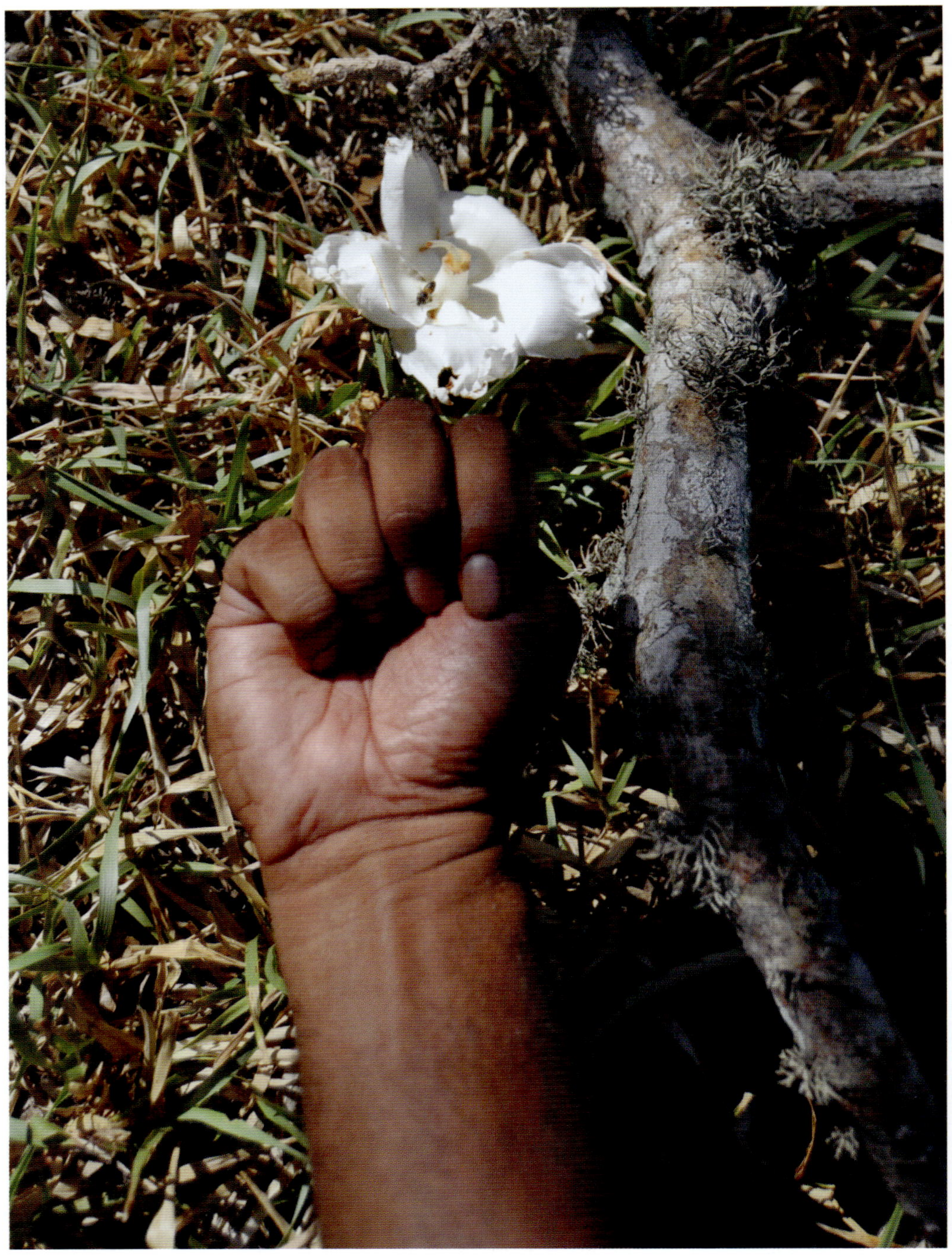

▲ **ABHAYAMUDRA** · Courage *(left)* **MUSHTIMUDRA** · Centering *(right)*

ARCHAKAMUDRA · Divination

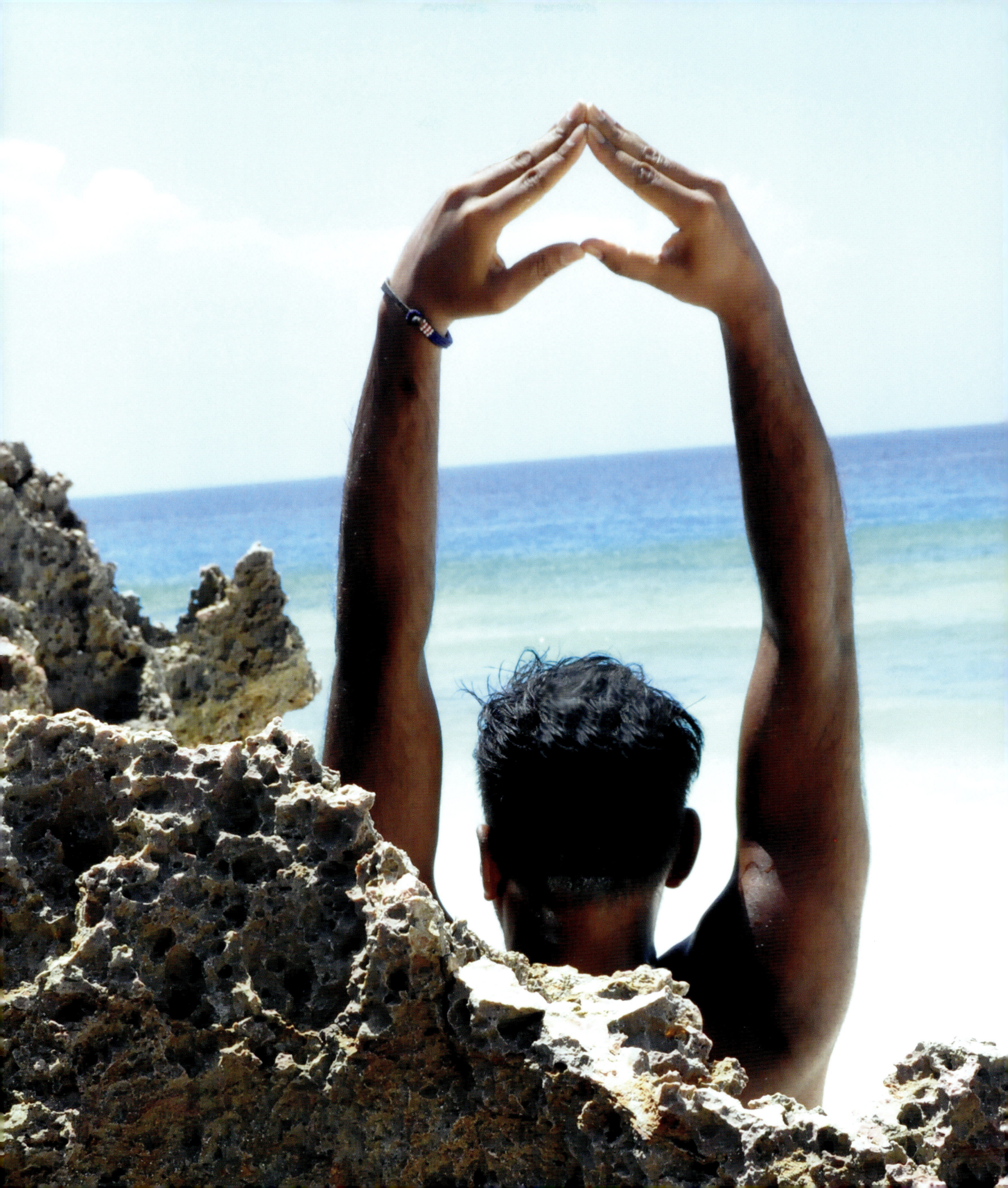

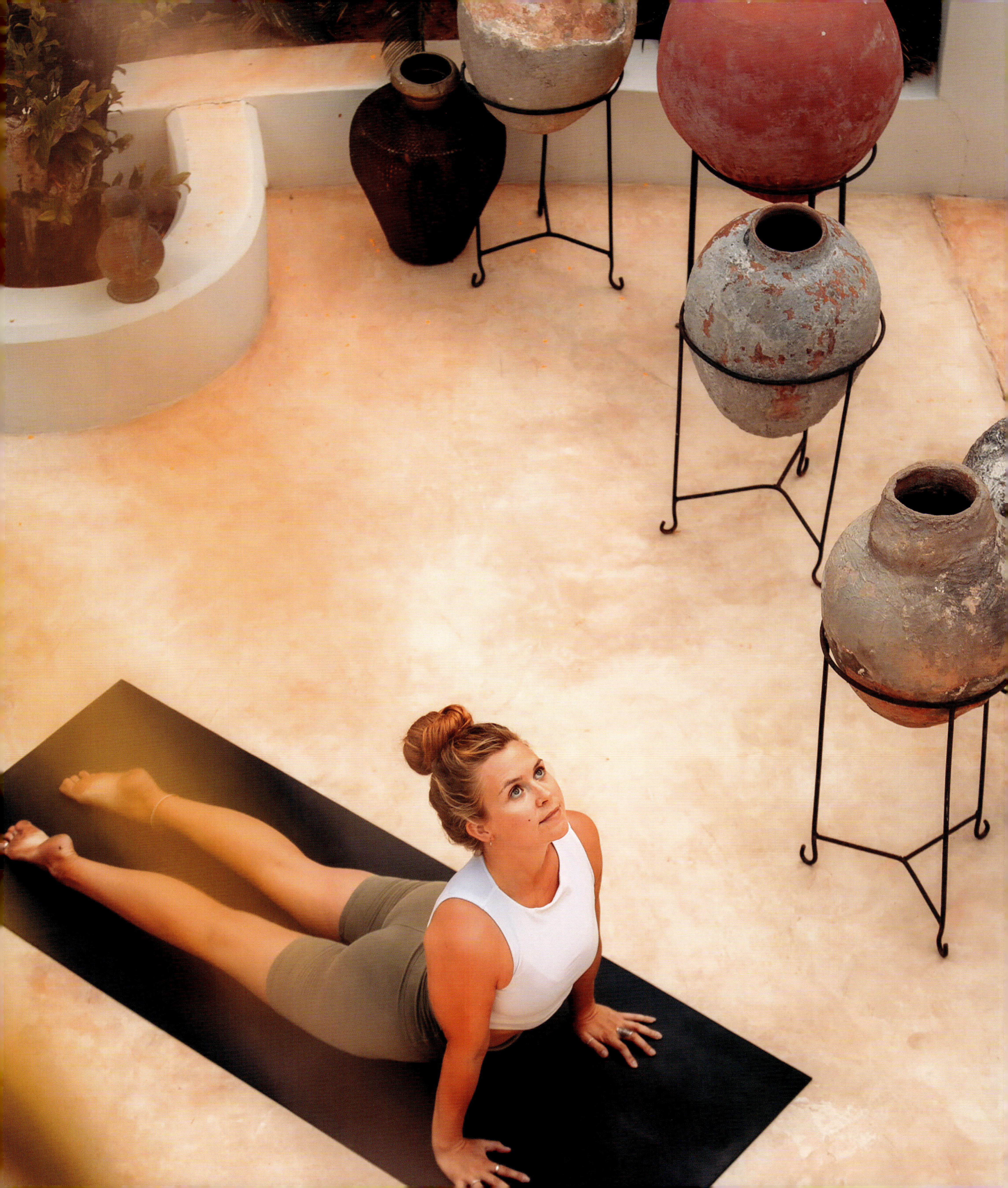

Stress is not the consequence of problems. It is simply a signal that should not be ignored. Take ownership, take action, and transform your life.

BRAHMA DHANUS • Sagittarius

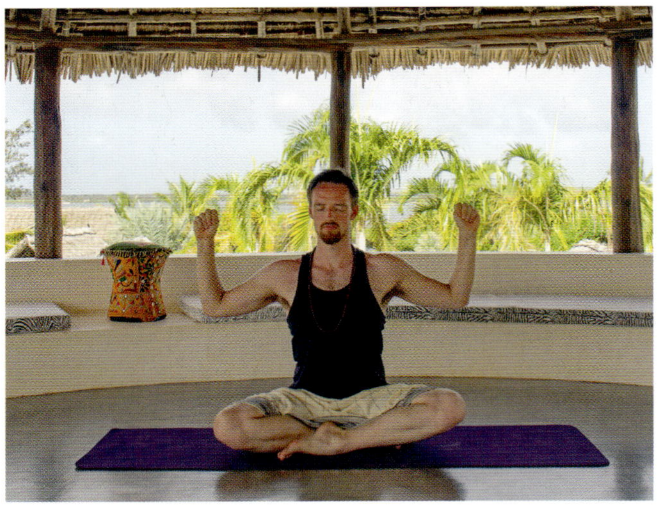

SIDDHASANA & MUSHTIMUDRA
Seated Accomplished & Centering

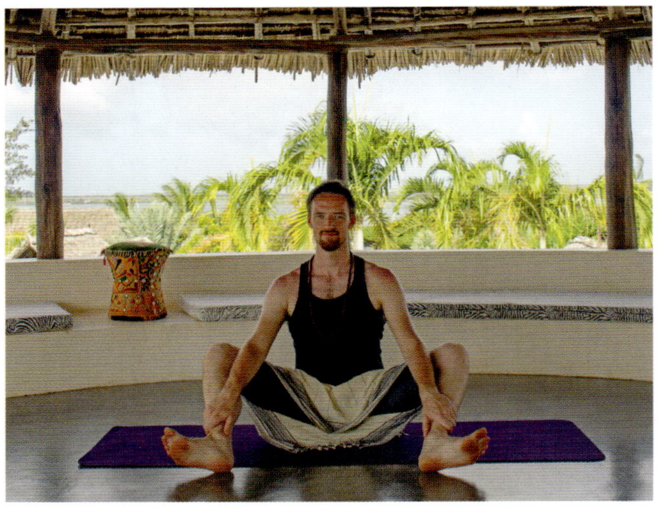

TITALIASANA
Wide-Winged Butterfly

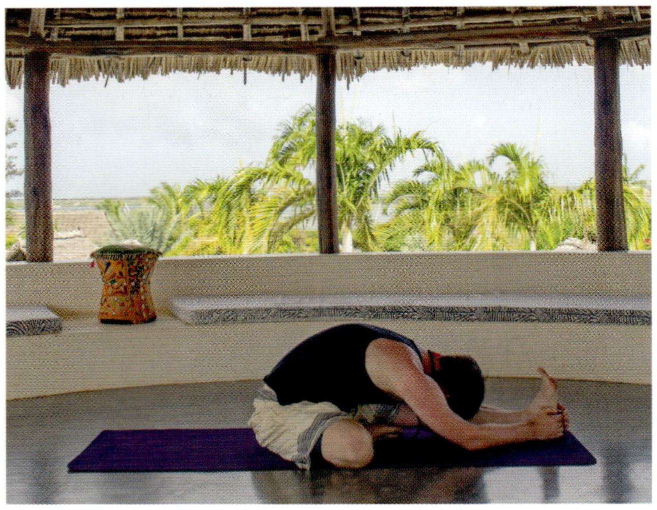

JANUSIRSASANA
Head-to-Knee Forward Bend

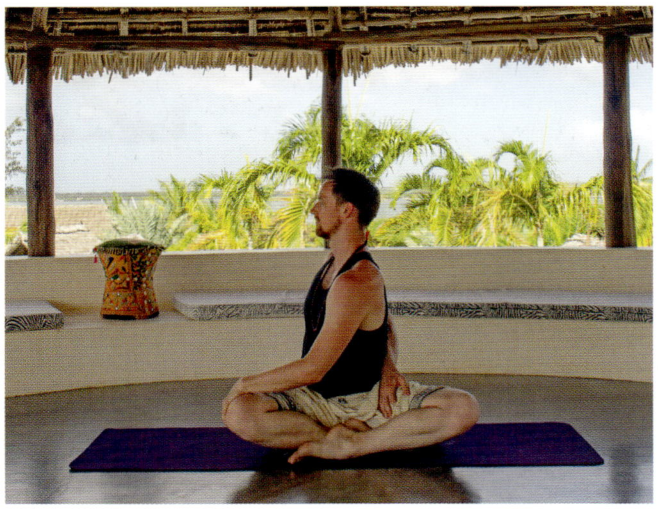

PARIVRTTA SUKHASANA
Easy Seated Twist

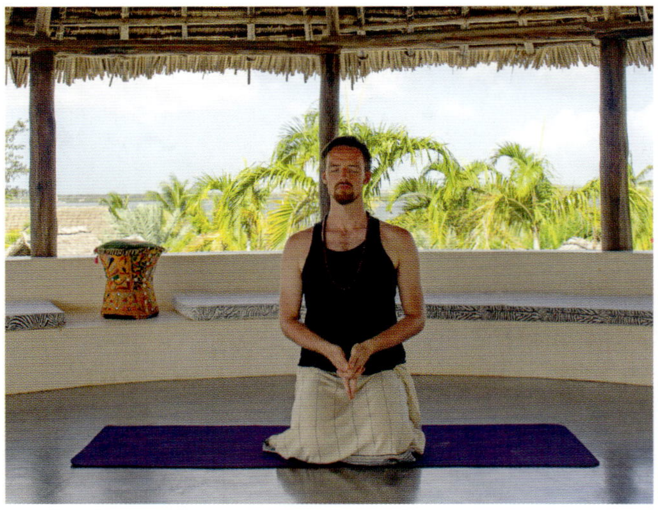

VAJRASANA & MATANGIMUDRA
Thunderbolt & Authenticity

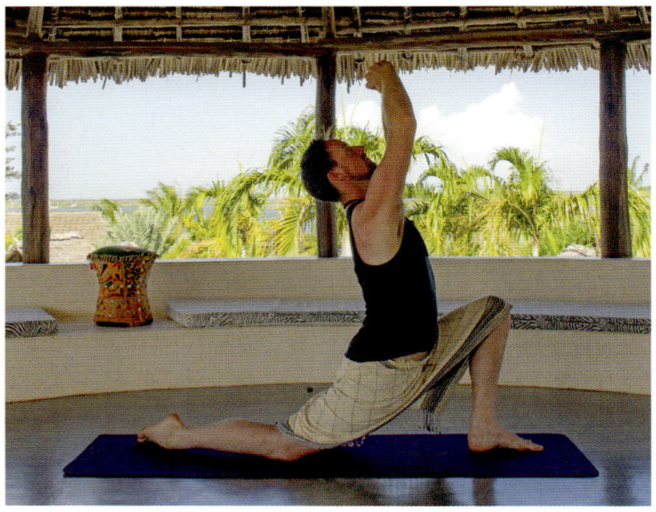

ANJANEYASANA & VISHUDDHACHAKRAMUDRA
Crescent Lunge & Communication

In Brahma Dhanus, we are in the shifting season of elemental fire. This constellation of asanas encourages the essence of free-spirited movement, leaving you feeling good. Applying the philosophical aspects of yoga inspires a wakeful rest that makes us feel optimistic and open-minded when exploring a broad range of holds. The mudras bring centering to slow down the restless mind, encouraging authenticity in expression and a greater experience of intrapersonal communication. This provides release, realization, and 60 seconds of blissful laughter therapy, which spontaneously brings a deep state of meditation.

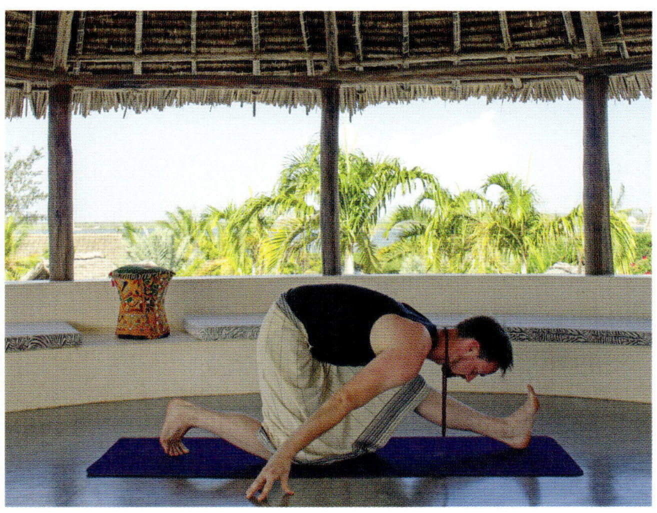

GAURAKHARASANA
Wild Donkey

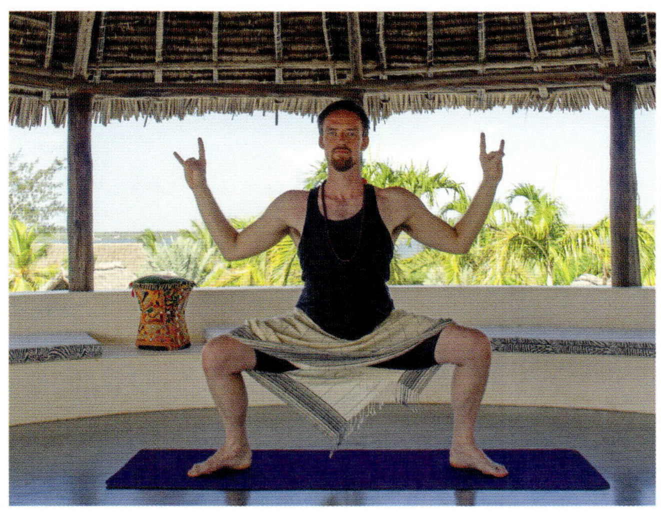

UTKATA KONASANA & APANAMUDRA
Goddess & Release

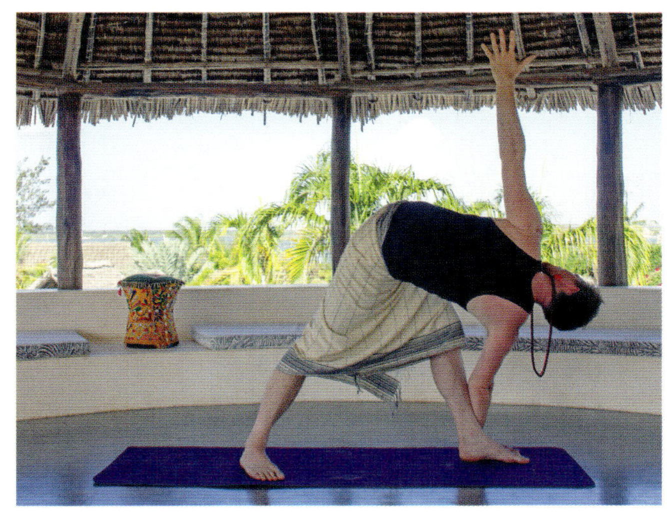

PARIVRTTA TRIKONASANA
Revolved Triangle

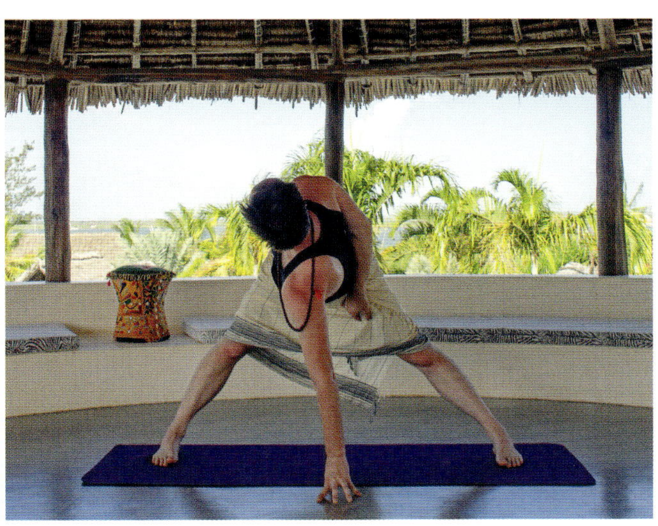

PARIVRTTA PRASARITA PADOTTANASANA
Wide-Legged Standing Twisted Forward Bend

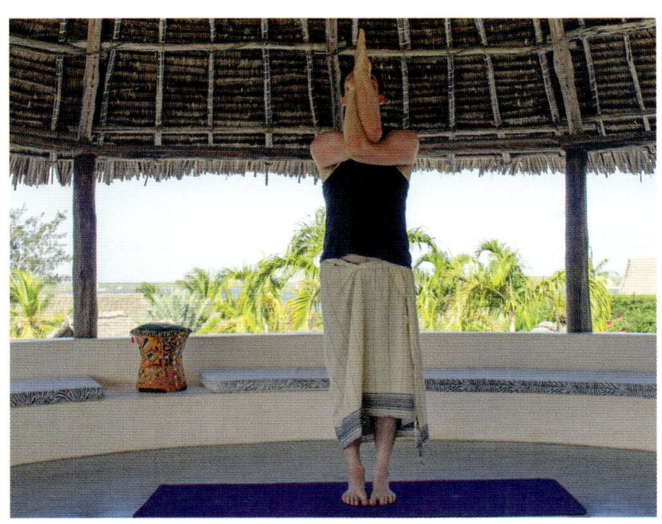

GARUTADASANA
Perched Eagle

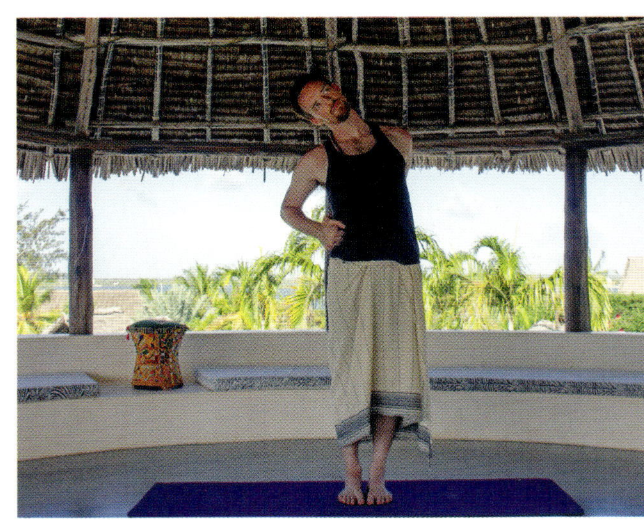

KANTAKASANA
Bamboo

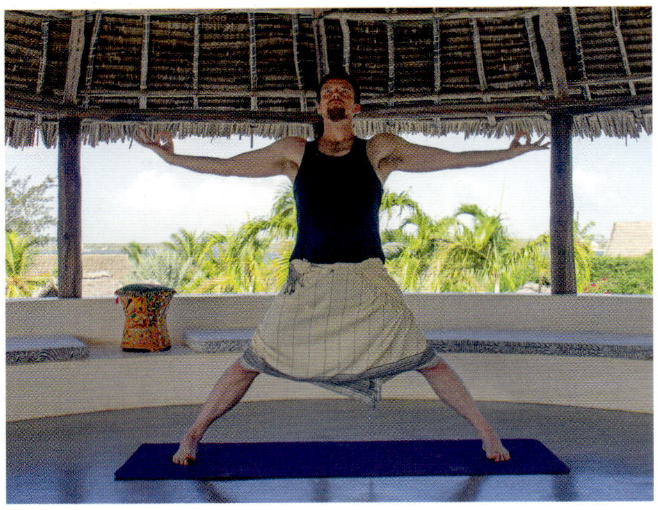

PRASARITA & JNANAMUDRA
Wide Standing & Realization

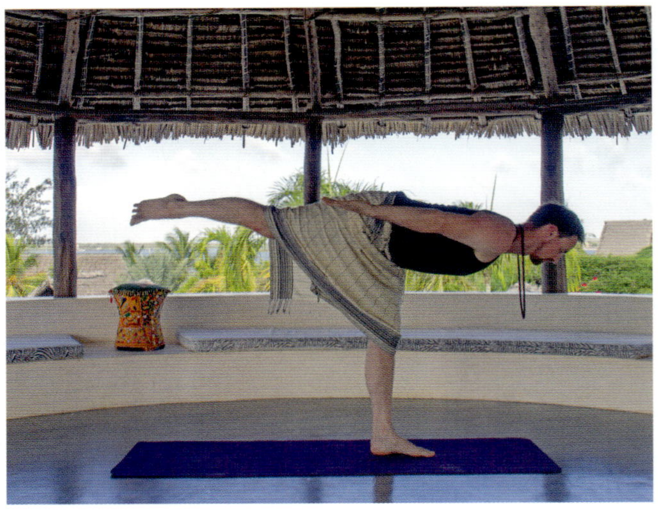

JATAPAKSA VIRABHADRASANA
Winged Warrior

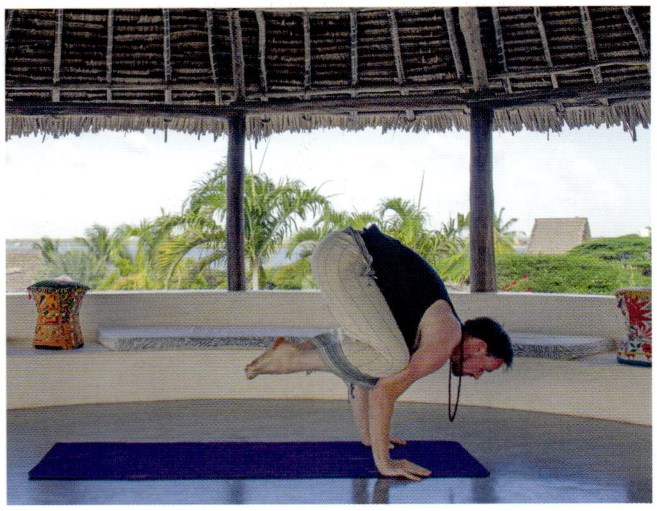

BAKASANA
Crow

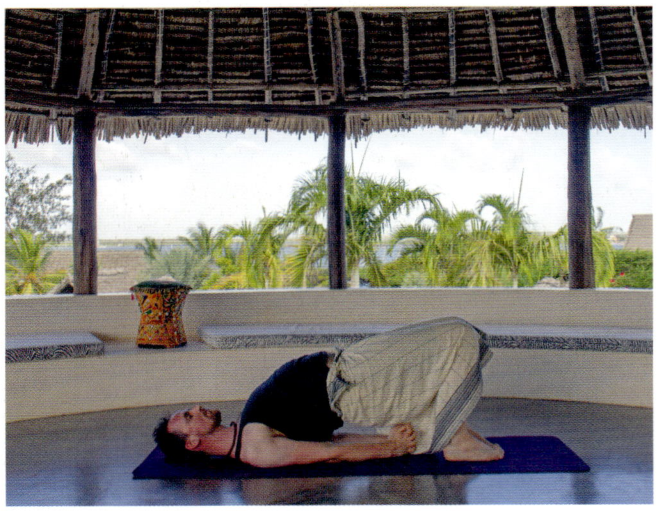

SETU BANDHA SARVANGASANA
Bridge

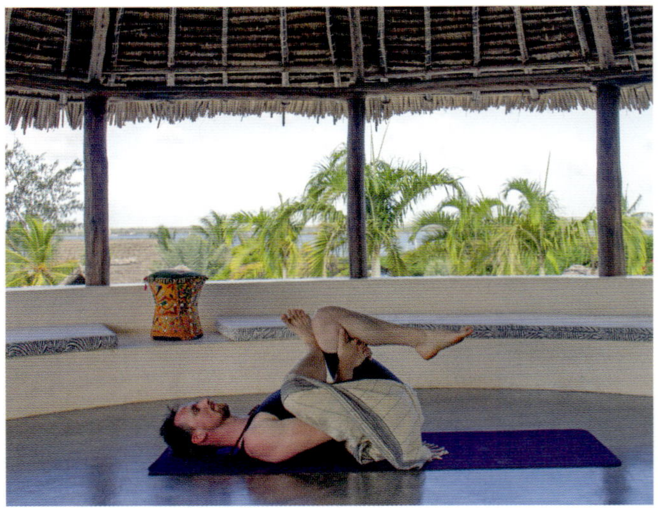

SUPTA KAPOTASANA
Reclining Pigeon

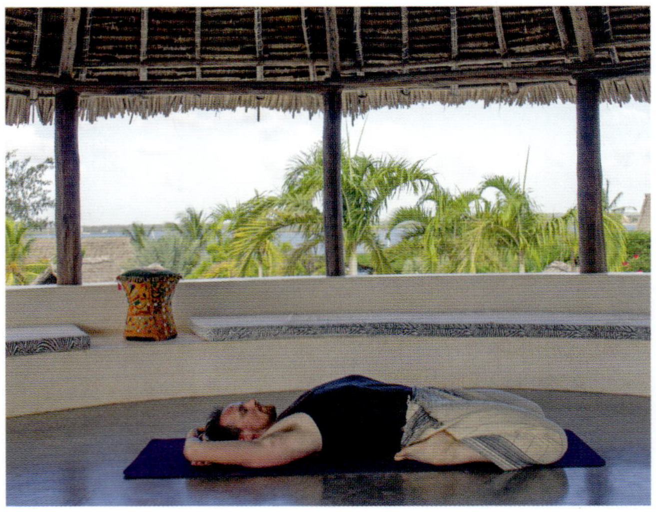

SUPTA VIRASANA
Reclining Hero

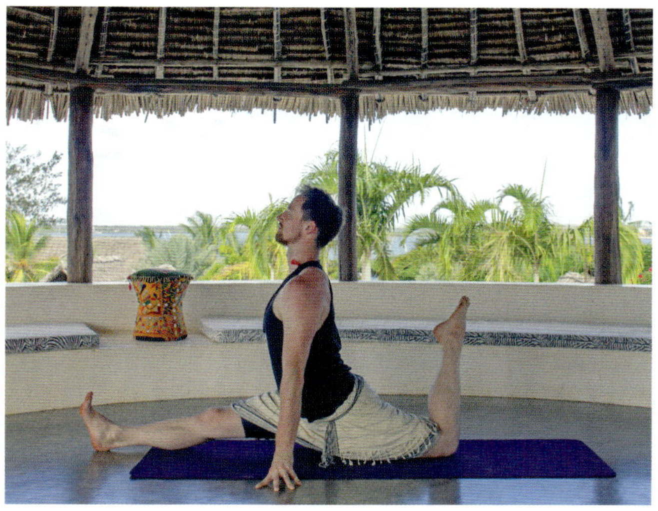

EKA PADA HANUMANASANA
Monkeytail Splits

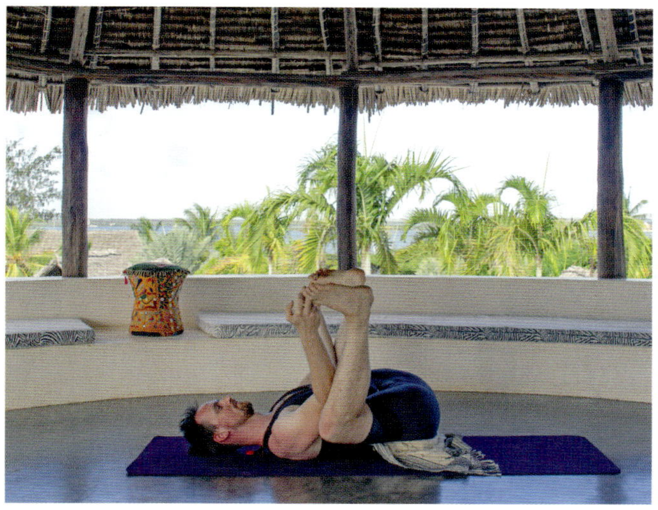

ANANDA BALASANA
Happy Baby

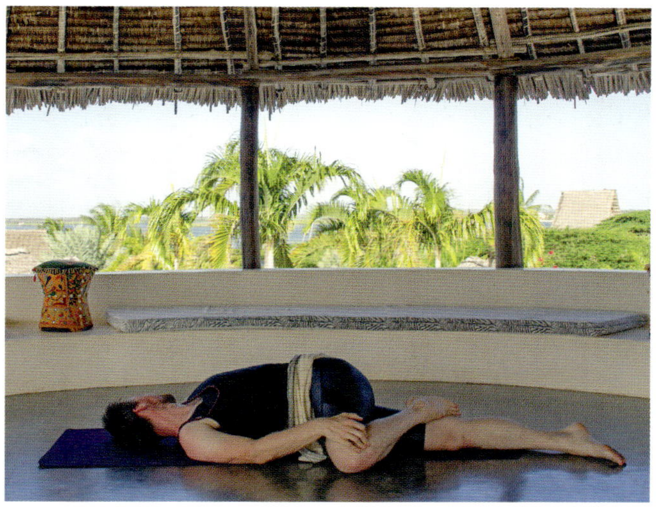

SUPTA MATSYENDRASANA
Supine Spinal Twist

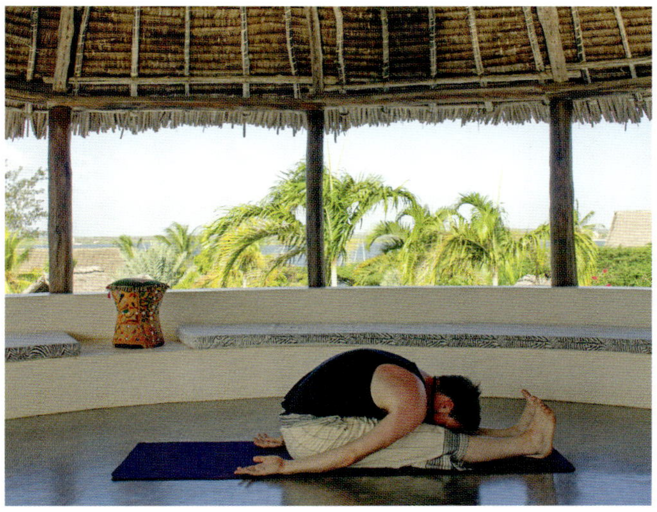

AVAYA PASCHIMOTTANASANA
Yielding Seated Forward Bend

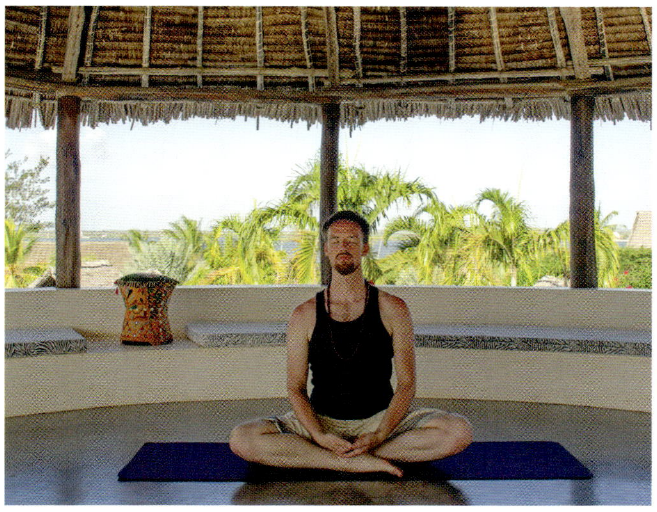

SIDDHASANA & DHYANAMUDRA
Seated Accomplished & Meditation

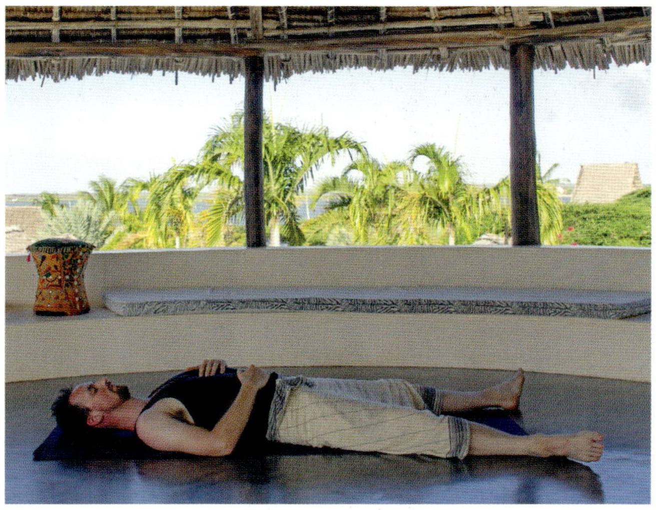

SAVASANA
Resting

BRAHMA MAKARA • Capricorn

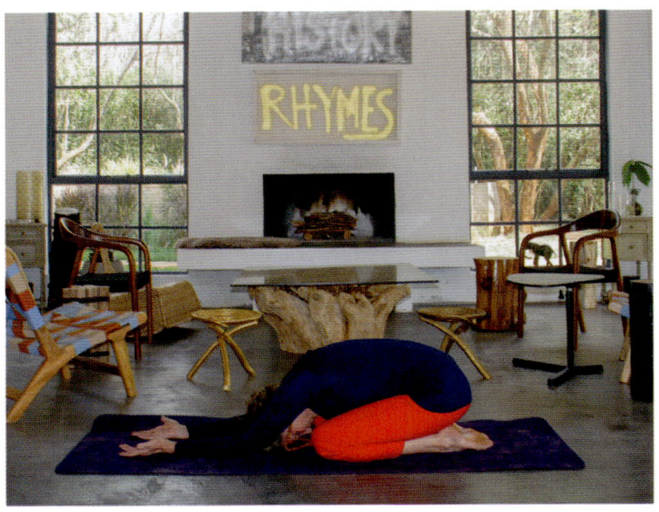

BALASANA & ABHAYAMUDRA
Child's & Courage

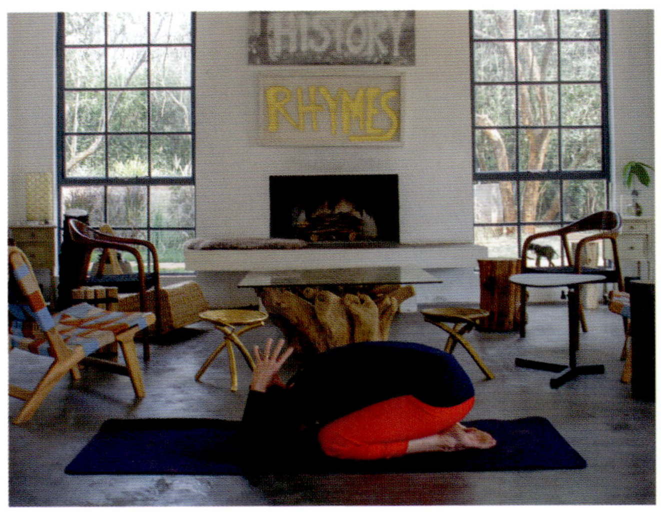

BALASANA & ARCHAKAMUDRA
Child's & Divination

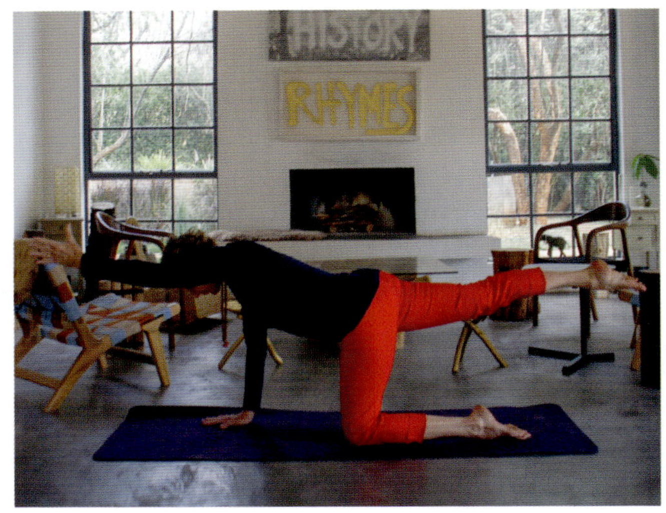

PARSVA BALASANA & ARDHACHANDRAMUDRA
Crawling Child's & Entirety

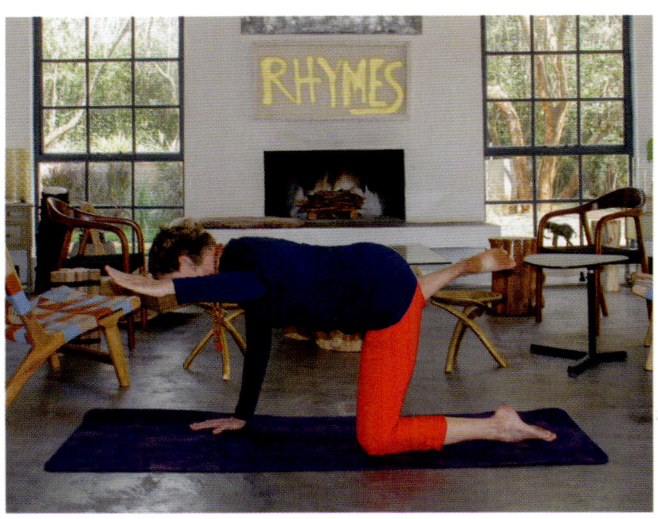

DEVASANA
Angel

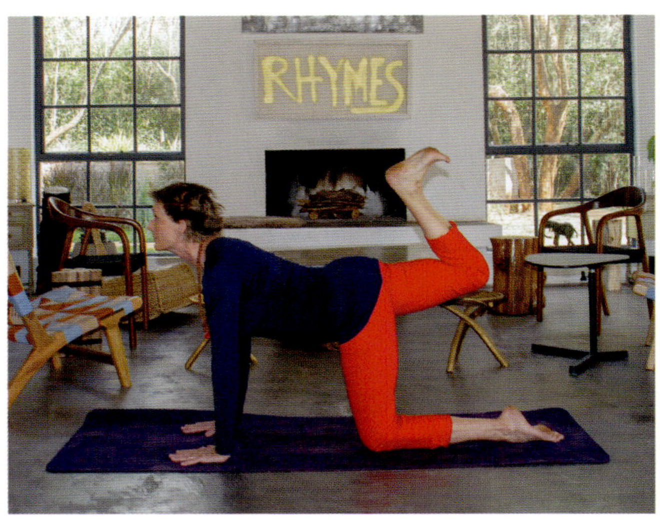

EKA PADA BITILASANA
Rising Cow

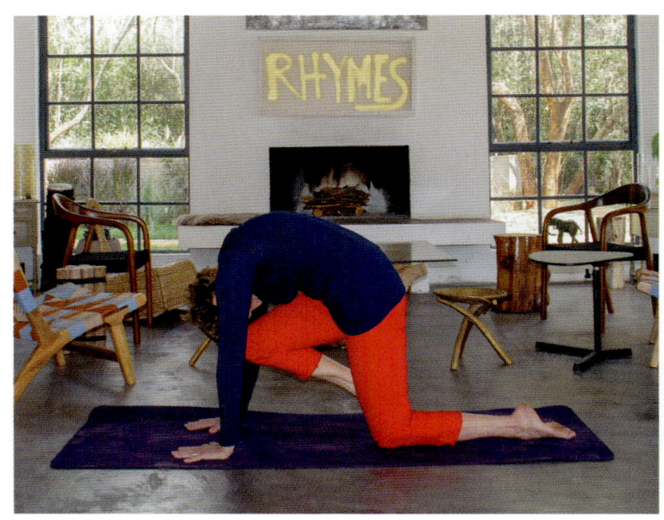

MARJARIASANA
Cat

In Brahma Makara, we are initiating the season of elemental earth. This constellation of asanas supports mindfulness of movement through discipline and taking personal responsibility, and focuses on alternate nostril breathing and a balanced mind. The poses bring a compassionate yet stoic resolve to our practice. The mudras strengthen the courage of our character by focusing on the divination of the mind, body, and spirit. This brings an omniscient awareness of our entirety, merging our inner and outer worlds, and the interdependence that patience, hard work, and cooperation affirm in our lives.

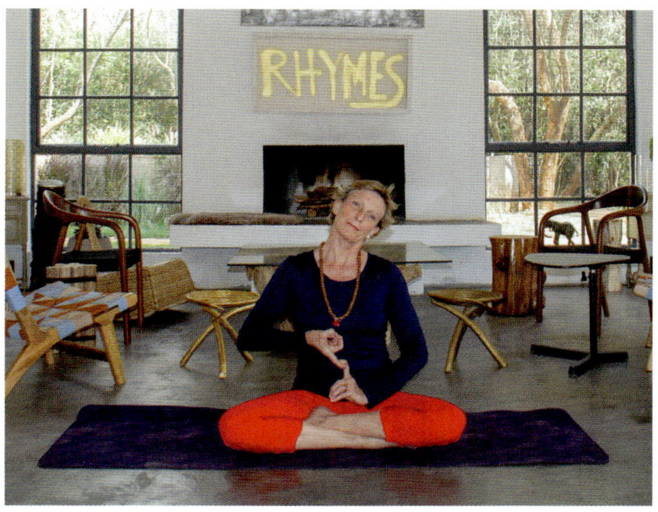

SIDDHASANA & YAMAPASHAMUDRA
Seated Accomplished & Interdependence

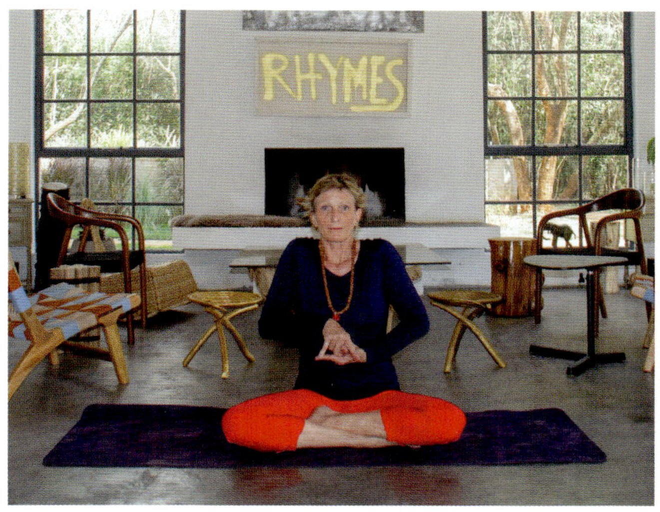

SIDDHASANA & KURMAMUDRA
Seated Accomplished & Patience

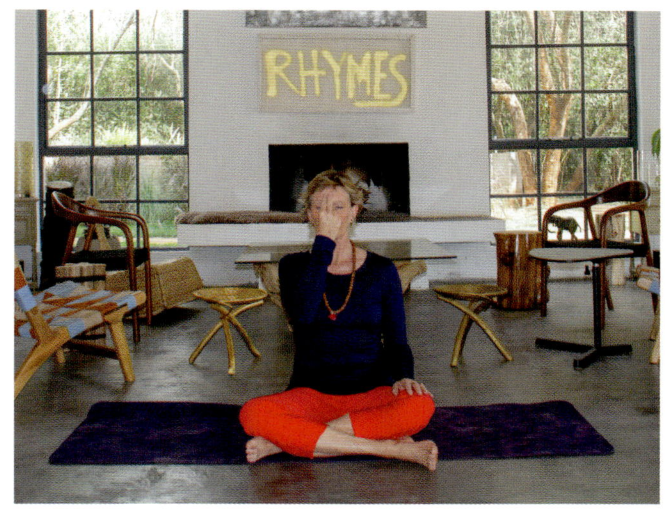

SUKHASANA & NADISHODHANA PRANAYAMA
Easy Seated & Alternate Nostril Breathing

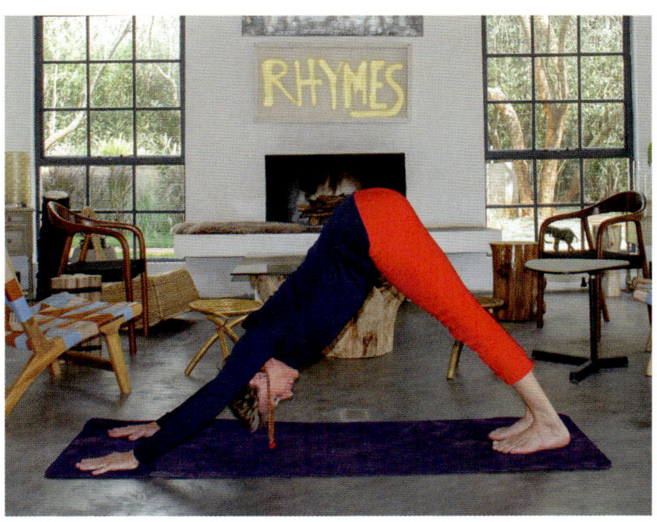

ADHO MUKHA SVANASANA
Downward-Facing Dog

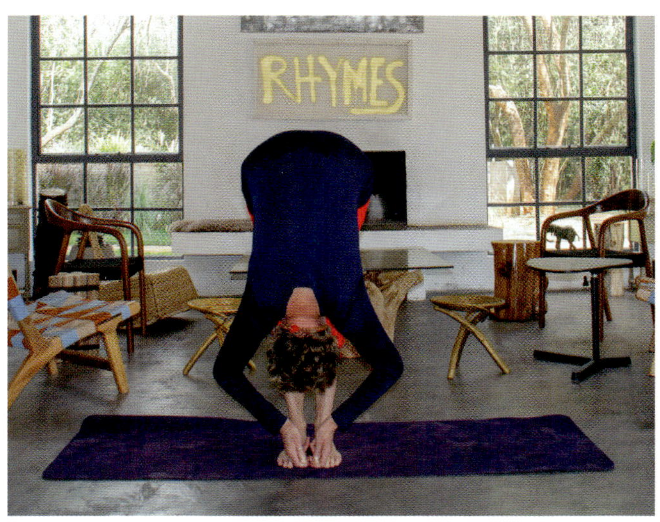

PADANGUSTHASANA
Big Toe Forward Fold

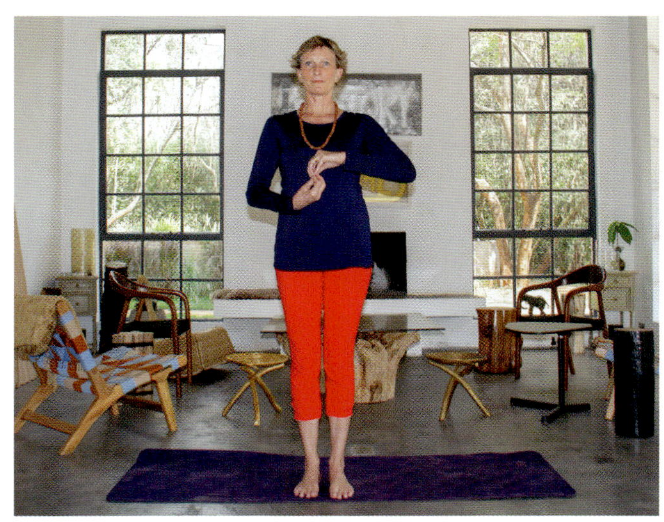

TADASANA & CHONMUKHAMUDRA
Mountain & Cooperation

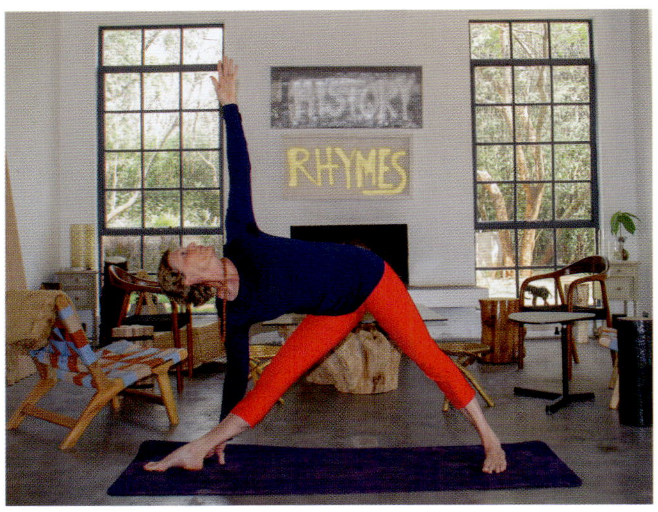

AVANI TRIKONASANA
Ground Triangle

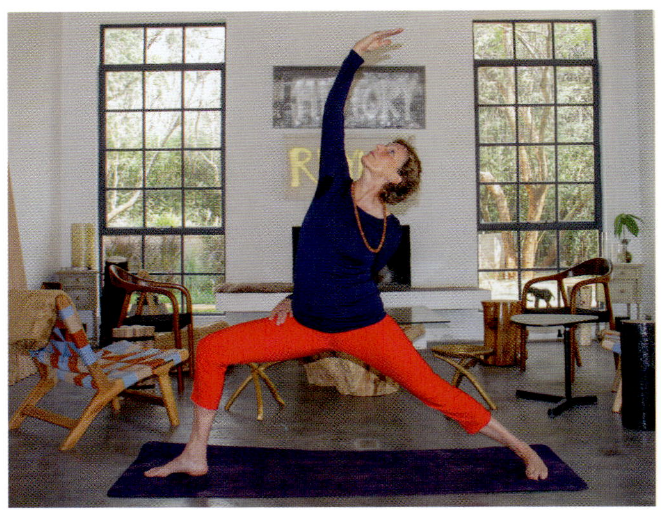

VIPARITA VIRABHADRASANA
Reverse Warrior

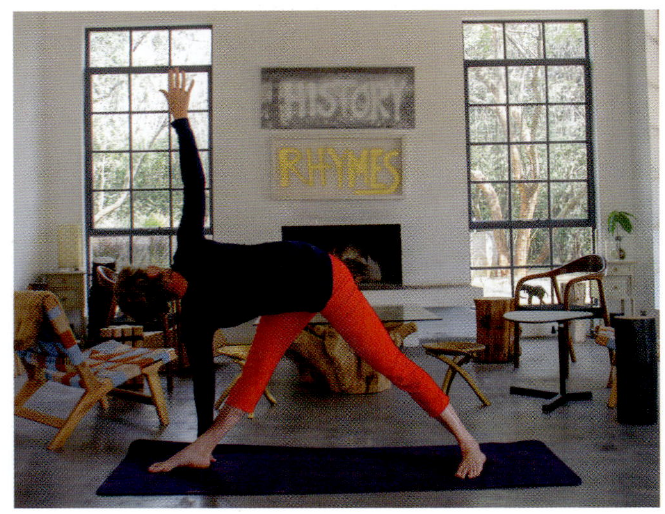

PARIVRTTA TRIKONASANA
Revolved Triangle

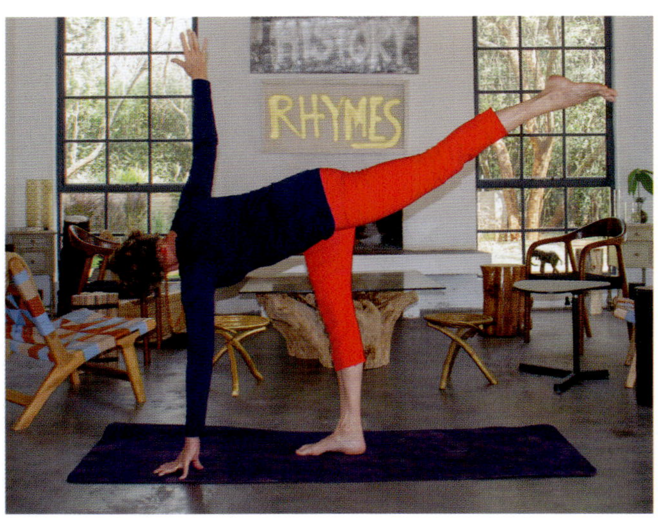

PARIVRTTA ARDHA CHANDRASANA
Twisted Half Moon

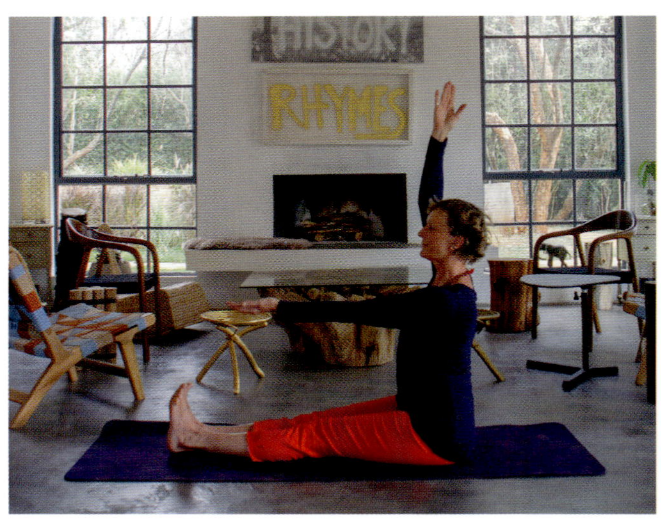

STHIRA SUKHA DANDASANA
Steady Easy Staff

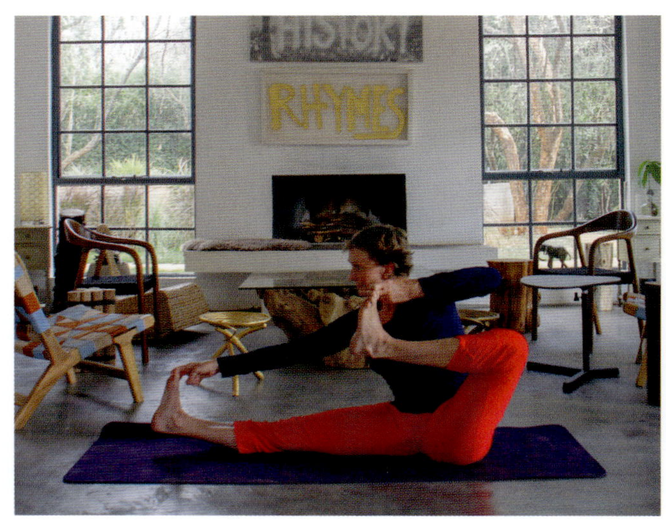

AKARNA DHANURASANA
Archer

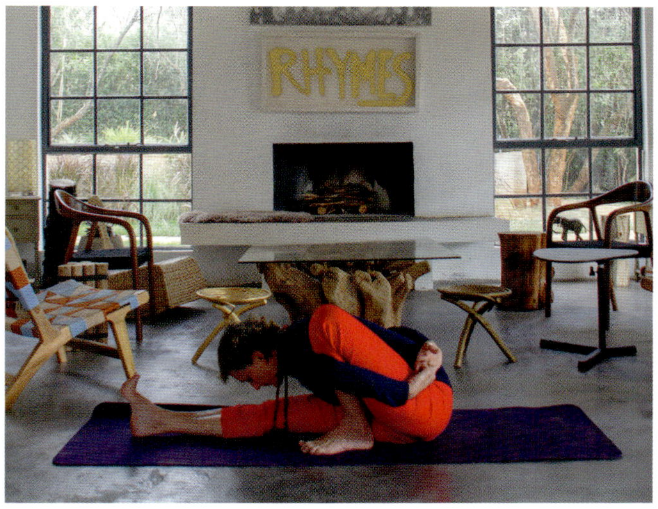

MARICHYASANA
Bowing Sage

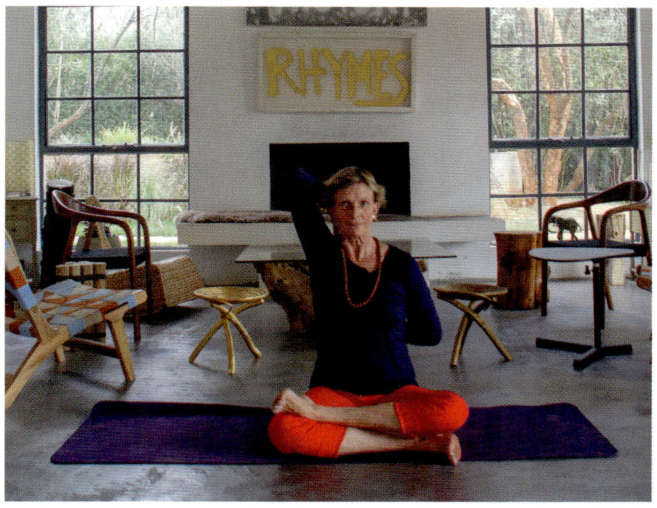

BADDHA AGNISTAMBHASANA
Bound Firelog

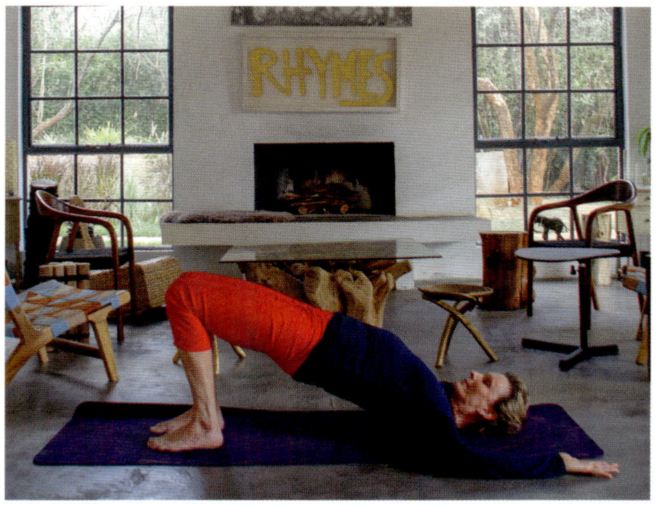

SETU BANDHASANA
Open Bridge

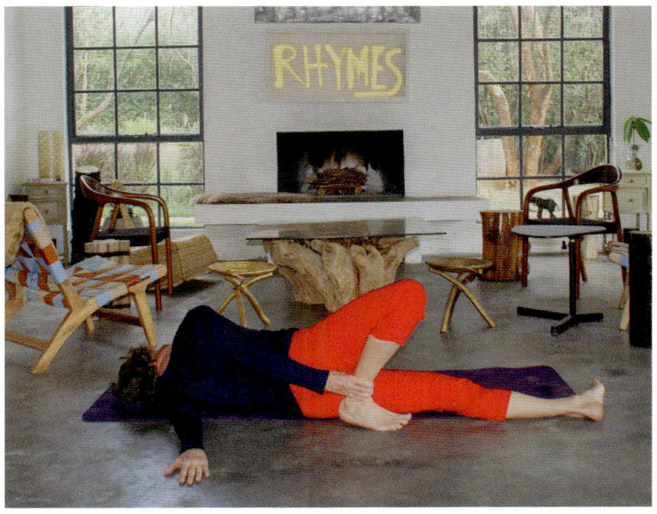

SUPTA VRISCHIKASANA
Sleeping Scorpion

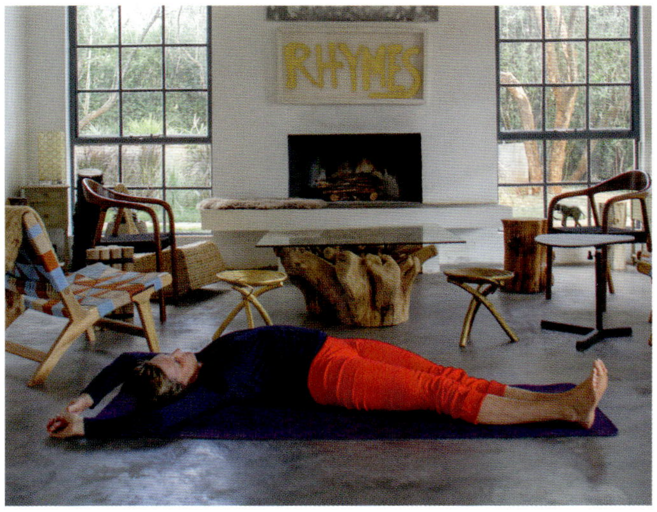

KELASANA
Plantain

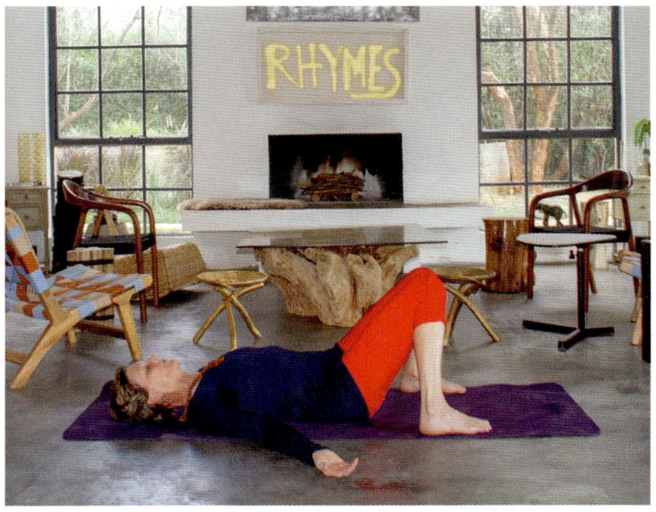

SANTULAN SAVASANA
Balancing Resting

INNER ALIGNMENT

In Brahma Kumbha / Aquarius, we are in the settled season of air, which is the etheric space of unconventional and positive change. From that primordial space all innovation and creation come into existence. Deep inside, you were always a creative spirit brimming with possibility. I am sorry the world we live in now works so hard to help you forget this truth for its own gains. Together, through our practice, we can change this so the freedom you seek can become yours. I have created the sequences of asanas in this chapter to honor humanity and offer the creative tools to overcome great ecological challenges as we heal Gaia together. In Brahma Meena / Pisces, we are in the shifting season of water, which is where the aspect of movement comes in. This chapter is about spiritual liberation and a way to recalibrate our body, which is the compass for our greater purpose.

In the embryonic space of our mother's wombs, we may as well be a glorious creature undulating in the ocean. We are conceived in transcendence. Then we are born into a hard, harsh world of edges and gravity, and the materiality of life forces us into the dogma of whichever civilization we happen to incarnate in. We are taught to grow up, when in fact our best moments come from the openness, imagination, and curiosity we have as children. As the years pass, the joy subsides, and without true guidance it is easy to lose our way. Brahma Yoga brings the mystery back to your awakening and wonder. It reestablishes the crucial bond we had and still depend on with both air and water.

We are mostly made up of water, which is one of the most mystical substances. It shifts and changes its form to solid ice, snow, liquid water, vapor, and steam. Then, through transpiration of plants and respiration of species, the cycle continues. The day that the value of water is more revered than the value of diamonds will be a wonderful period for humanity and its level of consciousness. I hope to live to see that world in my lifetime.

Brahma Yoga offers a framework that I have created, supported by principles of Vedic cosmology, to achieve inner alignment. The asanas in this chapter offer a window directly into elevated consciousness, causing us to be more sensitive and intuitive, live with gratitude, and be adaptable, as well as to connect with all of life on an emotional level, and if desired, a spiritual level.

As we move through the elaborate and beautiful asanas, we start to shift into a more gentle and subtle space to experience our aura and human energy field. We do this by slowing things down to prepare for a state of meditation. We come full circle by a series of dedicated movements, such as prostrating to the earth as a sign of reverence and devotion. When we lean on the ground, it is a way of practicing humility and surrendering to purify ourselves. The Brahma Yoga system concludes with the final asana in the final sequence: padmasana and brahmamudra. The lotus represents the beautiful process of a flower emerging from a murky pond. The mudra connects us to our eternal chord and state of Brahman through infinity.

BRAHMA YOGA SUTRAS

BRAHMA KUMBHA • Aquarius

- As part of my awakening, I am willing to be rebellious. I am prepared to let go of everything I once owned in order to find myself again.
- In my illumination, I am brimming with possibility.
- Existence supports my process, and my essence emerges in wondrous forms.
- By receiving kindness and having appreciation, I can participate and connect to the law of attraction.
- When I observe selflessness, I can love without any need or expectation.
- I know we will all be nostalgic about the past in the future, so I live in the present moment and understand that all time is one.
- I draw the right vibration to me and the exact constellation of people that I need.
- Brahma Yoga reveals methods that help me commit to reaching deeper levels of evolution.
- I am in alignment, and the universe intended me.

BRAHMA MEENA • Pisces

- Whenever I do not have a resolution to a question, I gain a mystery.
- I am pure love and light, and each day, in many ways, I am falling in love with myself.
- Rejection in my life has no effect whatsoever on my self-worth, and I will not be pulled in any direction I do not belong.
- There are several paths to attain enlightenment, one of which is Brahma Yoga.
- Reflecting on my past has no value if it continues to hurt me.
- In my transcendence, I wish nothing more than to be loved fully down to every cell, across all ancestral lines and all incarnations, until my spirit is brimming in delight.
- Freedom comes from knowing that I can heal my life and no longer need to invent a space in myself for others to fill.
- From the omnipresent viewpoint of the universe, both questions and answers know one another and are bonded. They are one.
- I will reach the highest realms of infinity when I grow to feel in experience what I have always held deep in my spirit. I am connected eternally to all of existence.

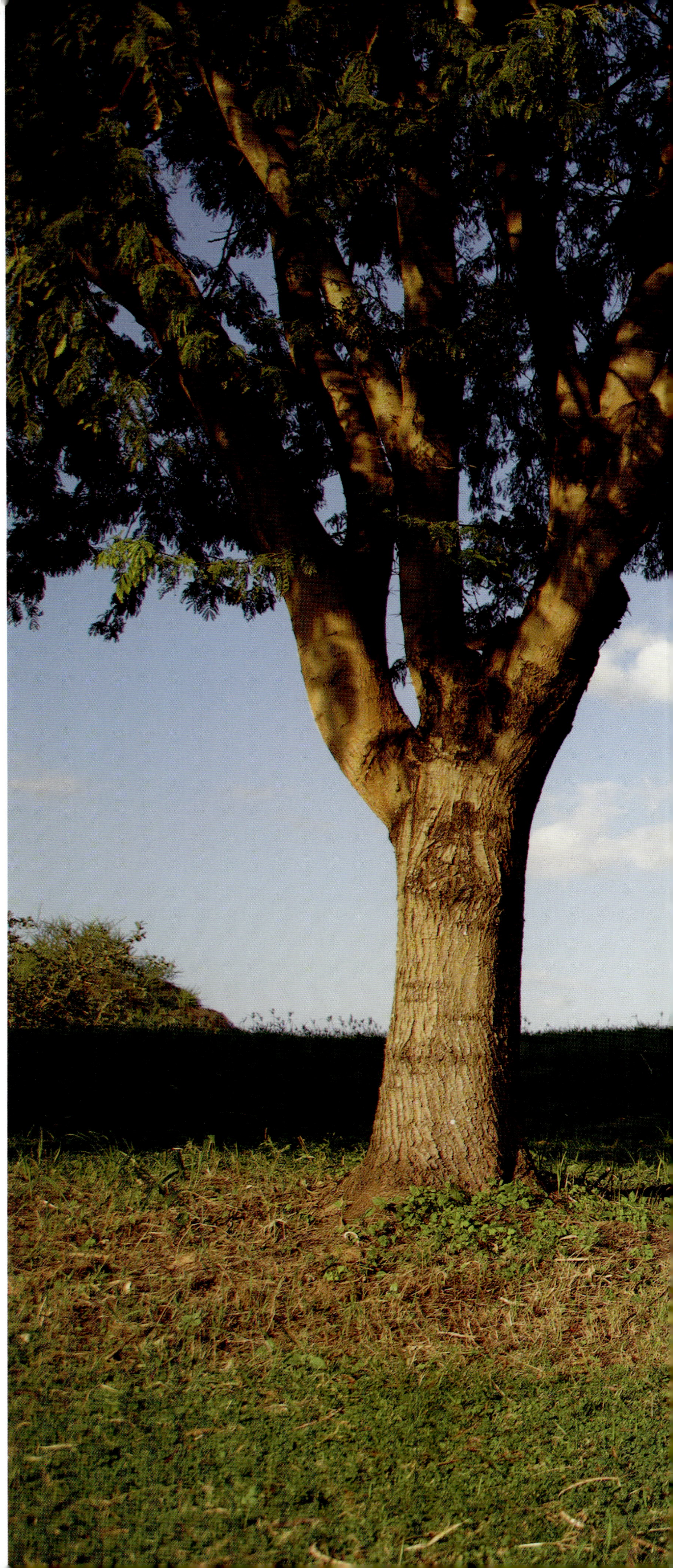

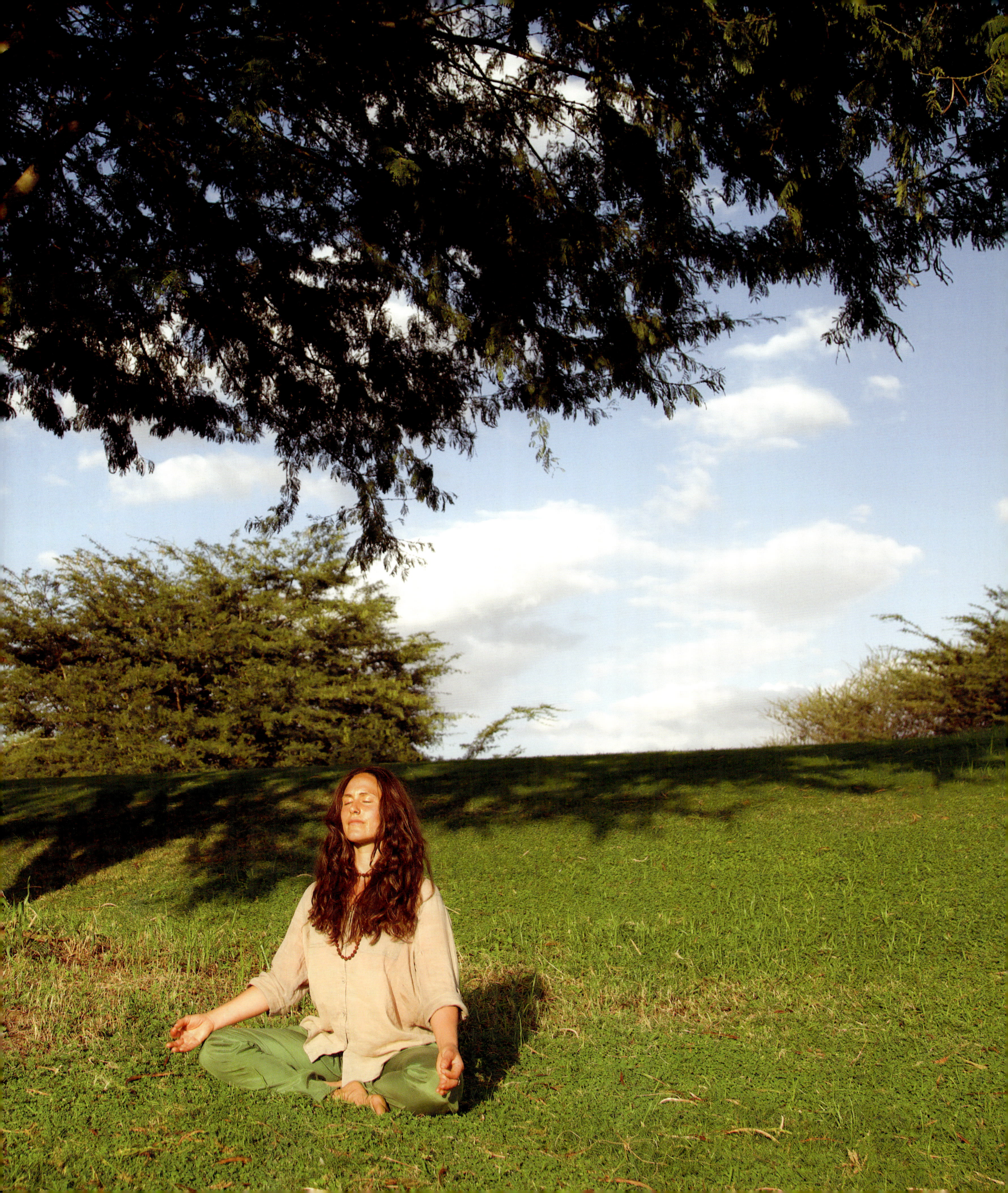

Through Brahma Yoga, you become the
perfect balance of opposites.

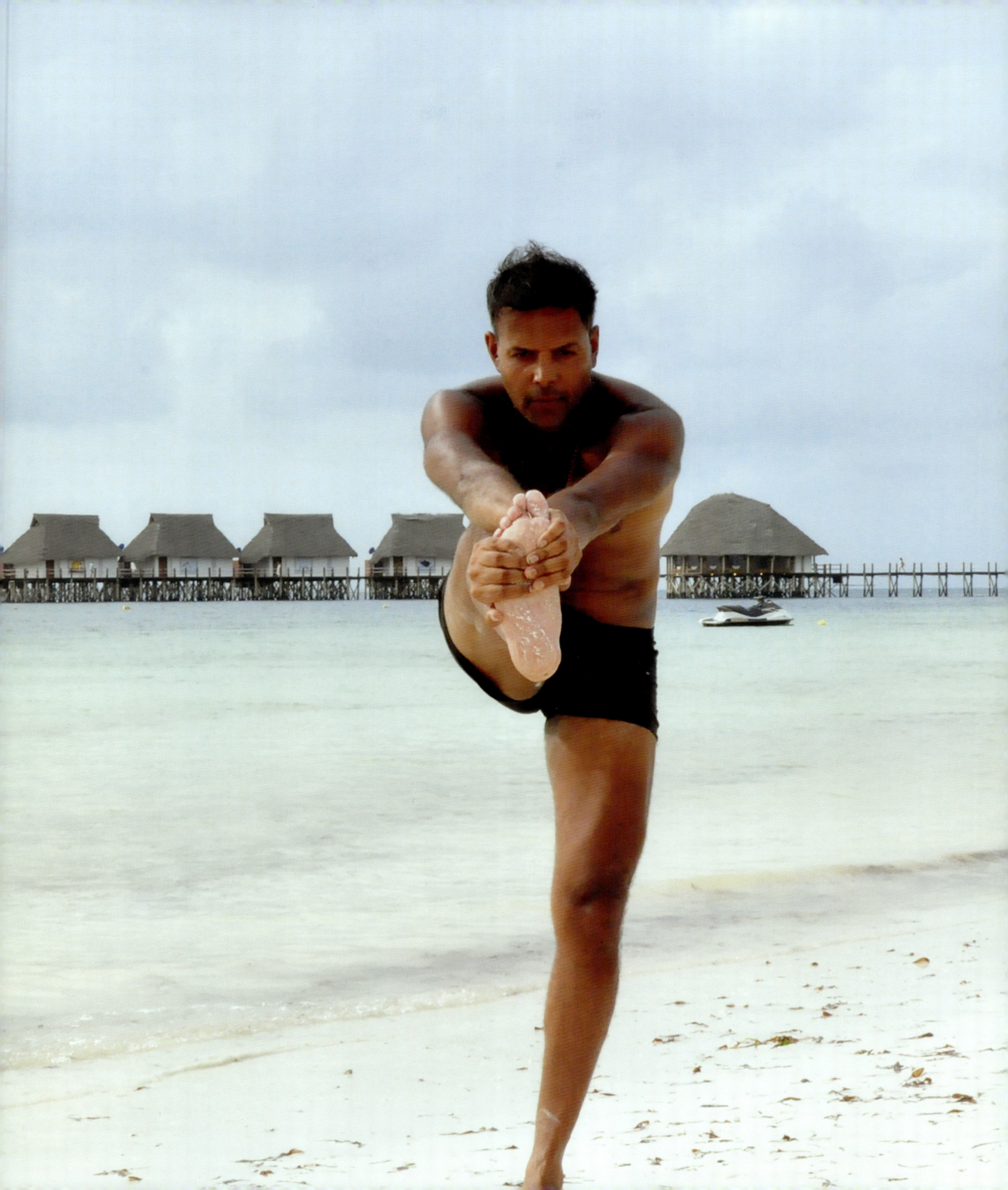

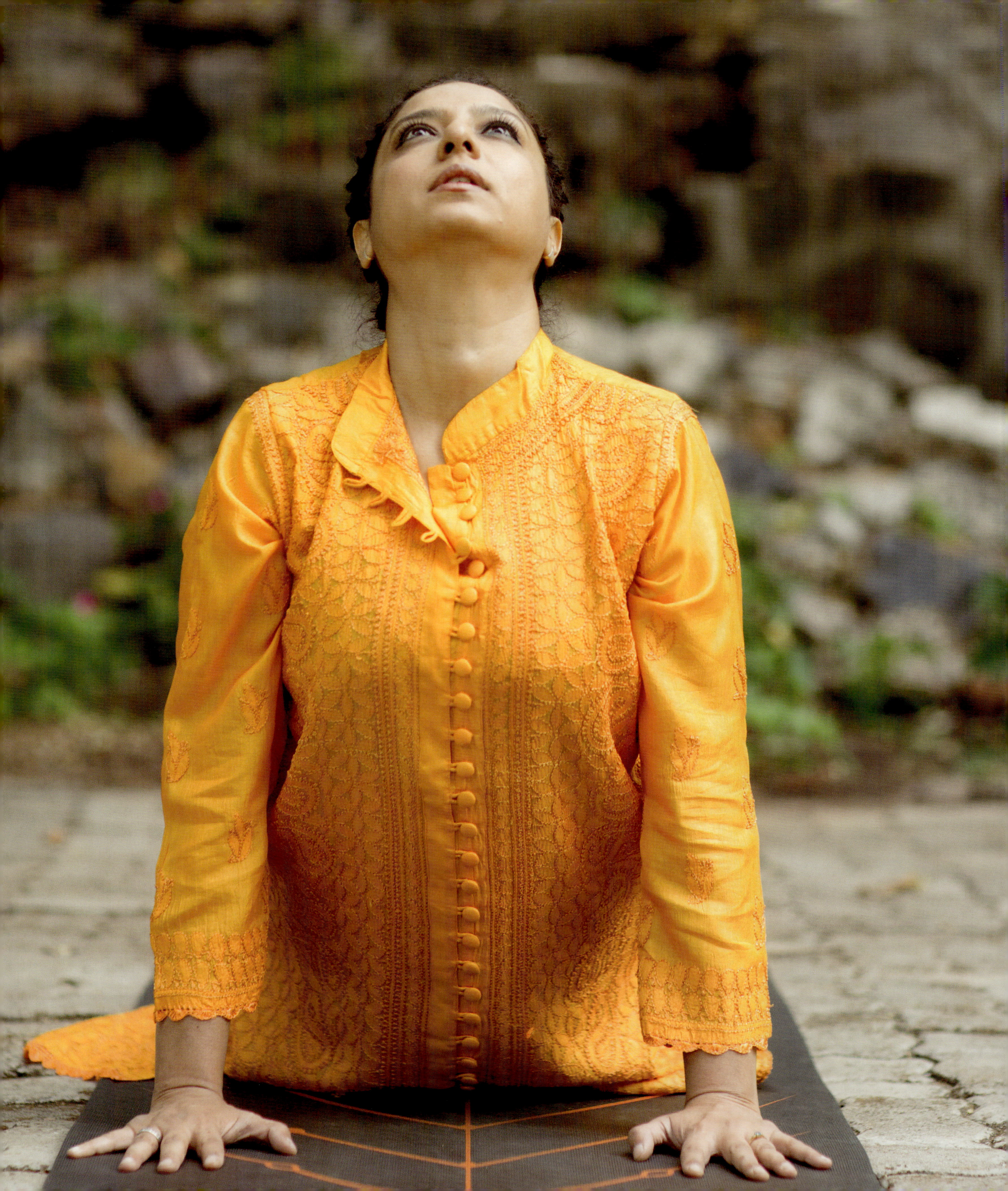

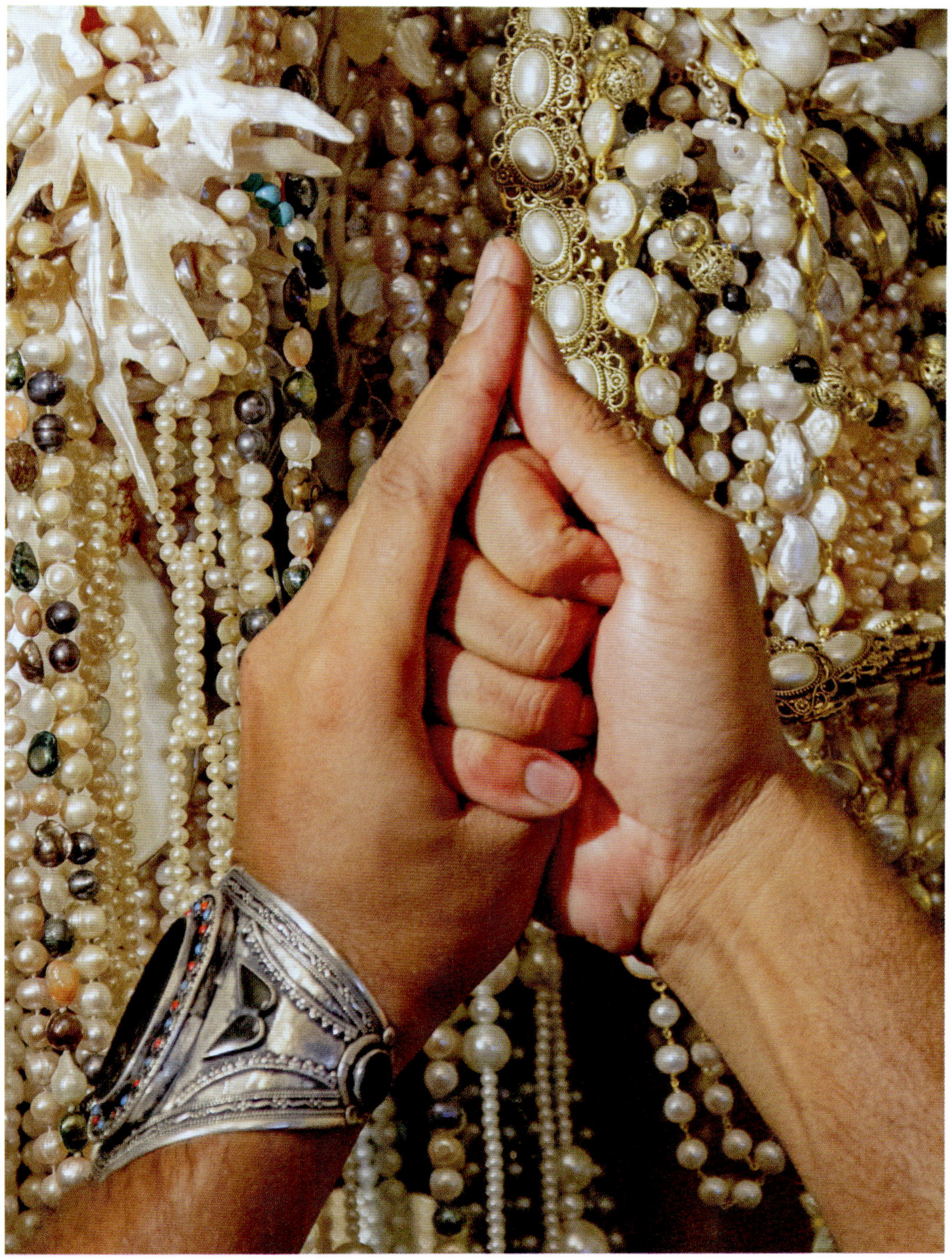

UTTHITA RAANEE NIRAVALASANA • Queen Seal

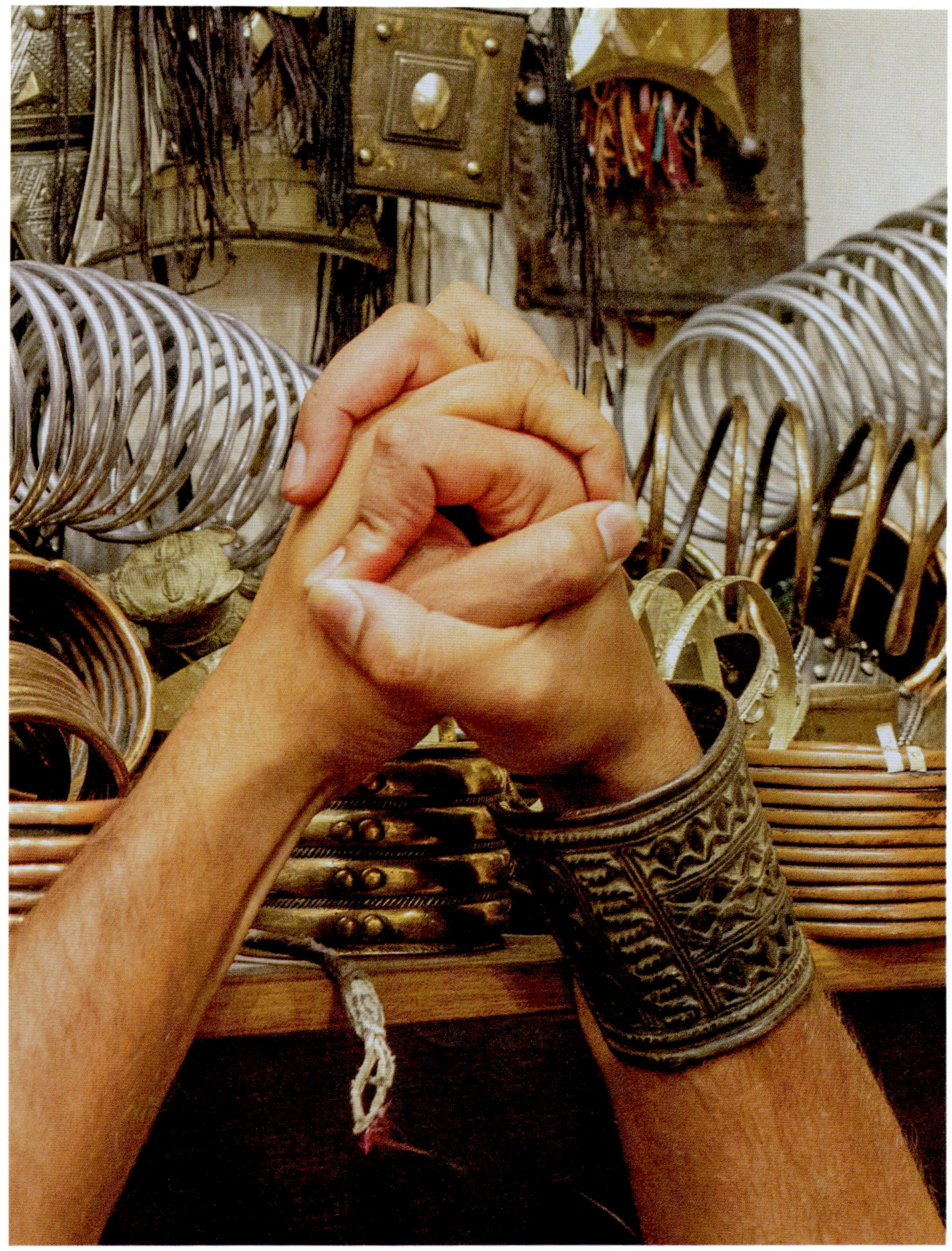

▲ SHANKHMUDRA • Mystery *(left)* GRANTHITAMUDRA • Transcendence *(right)*

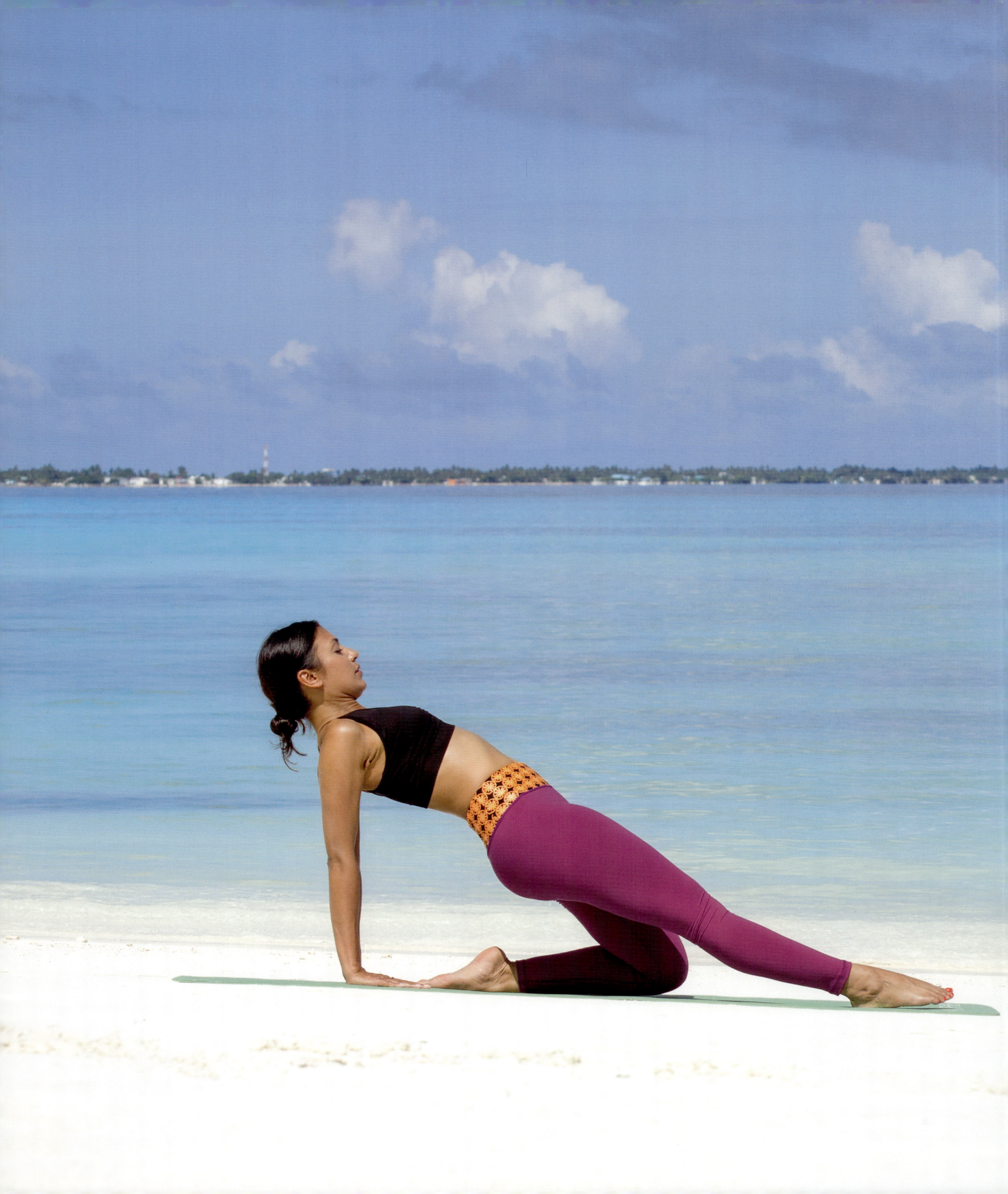

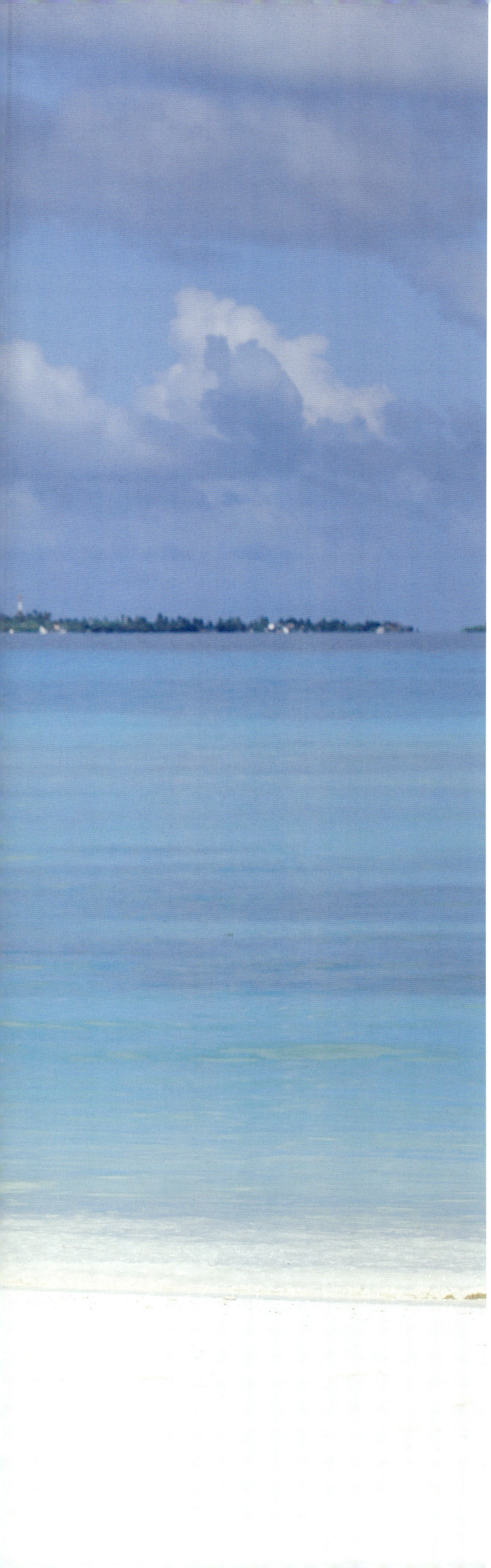

EKA PADA PURVOTTANASANA • One-Legged Upward Plank

When we disconnect from ourselves,

we cannot truly connect with others.

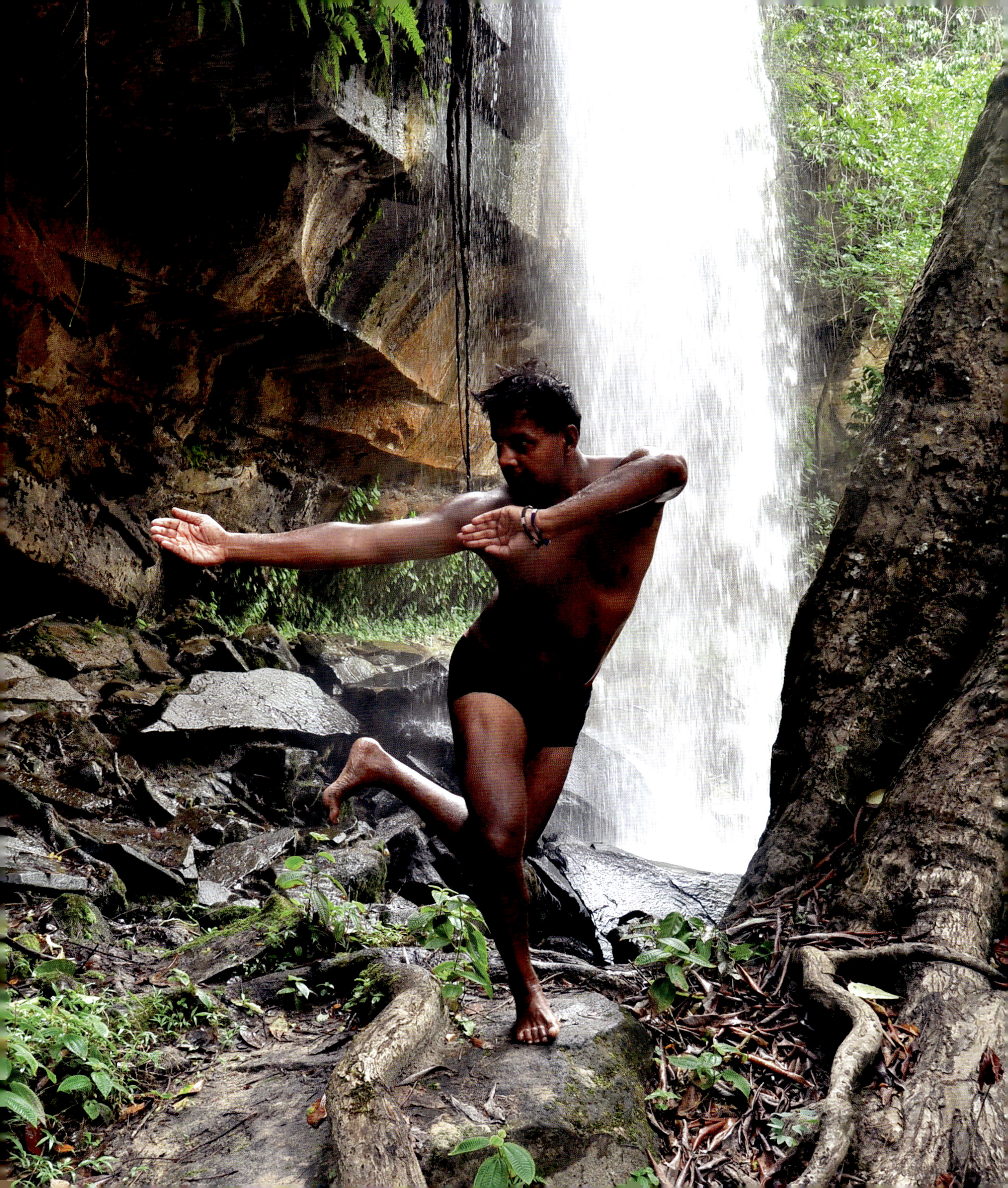

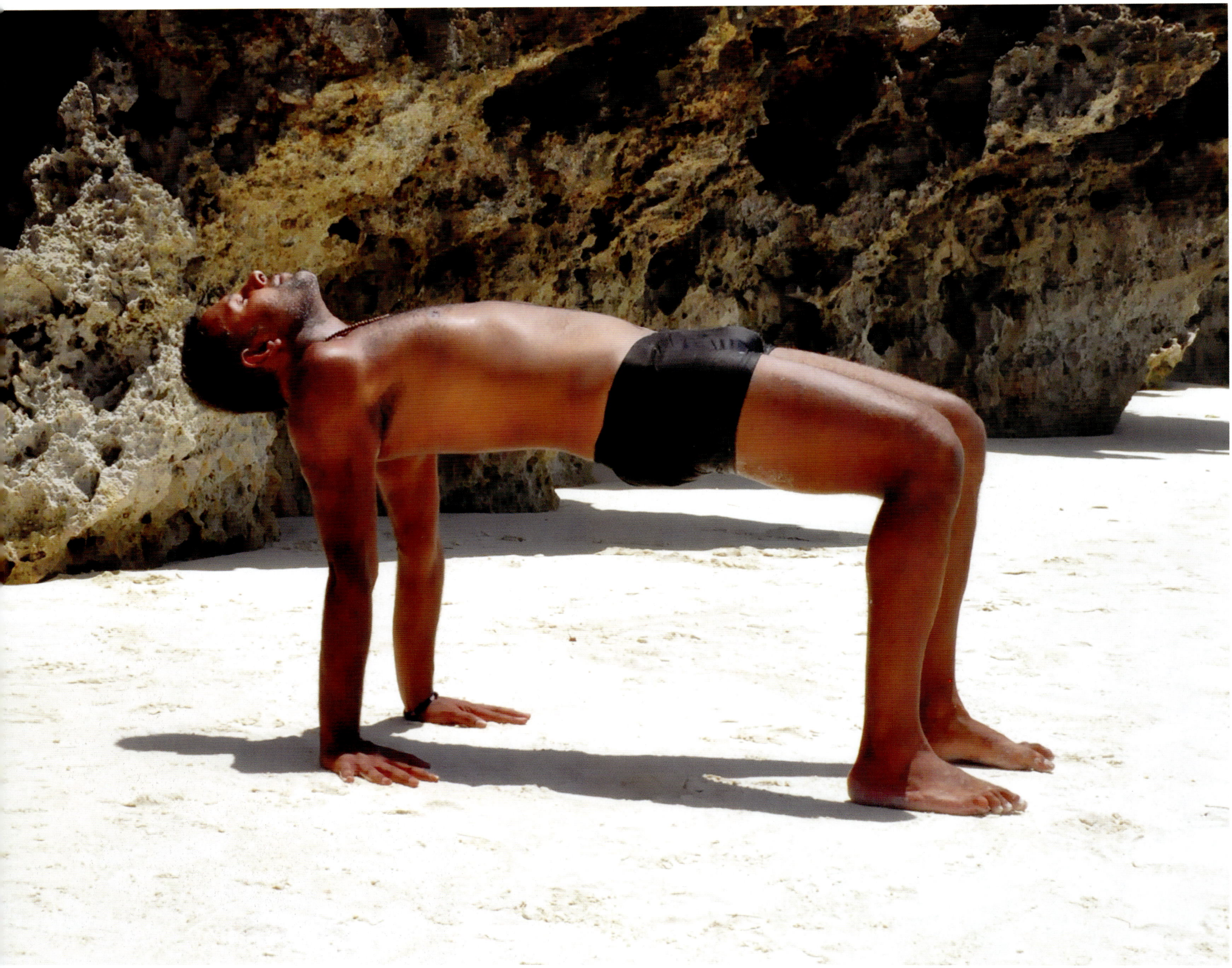

▲ **ARDHA PURVOTTANASANA** · Half-Inclined Plane

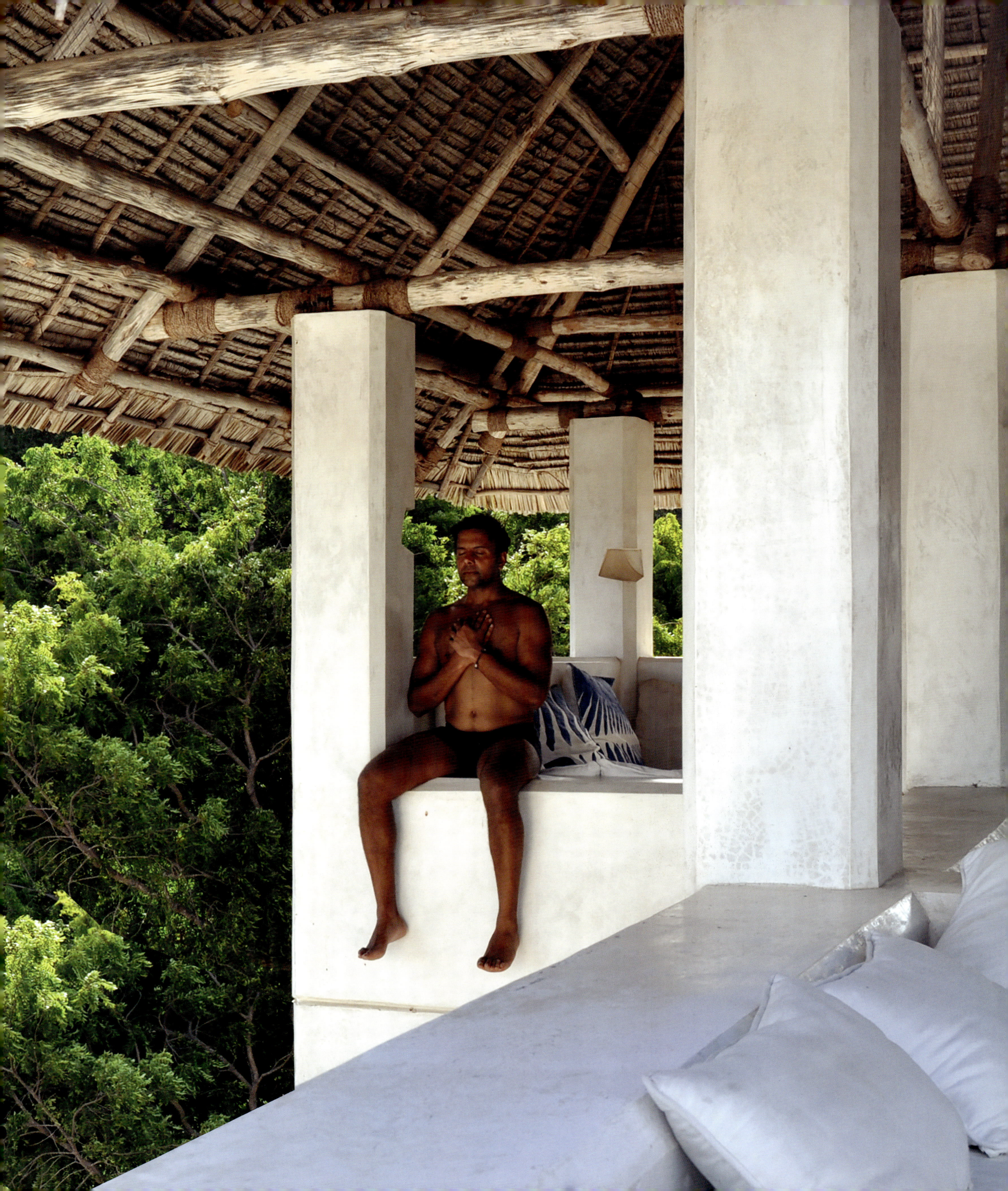

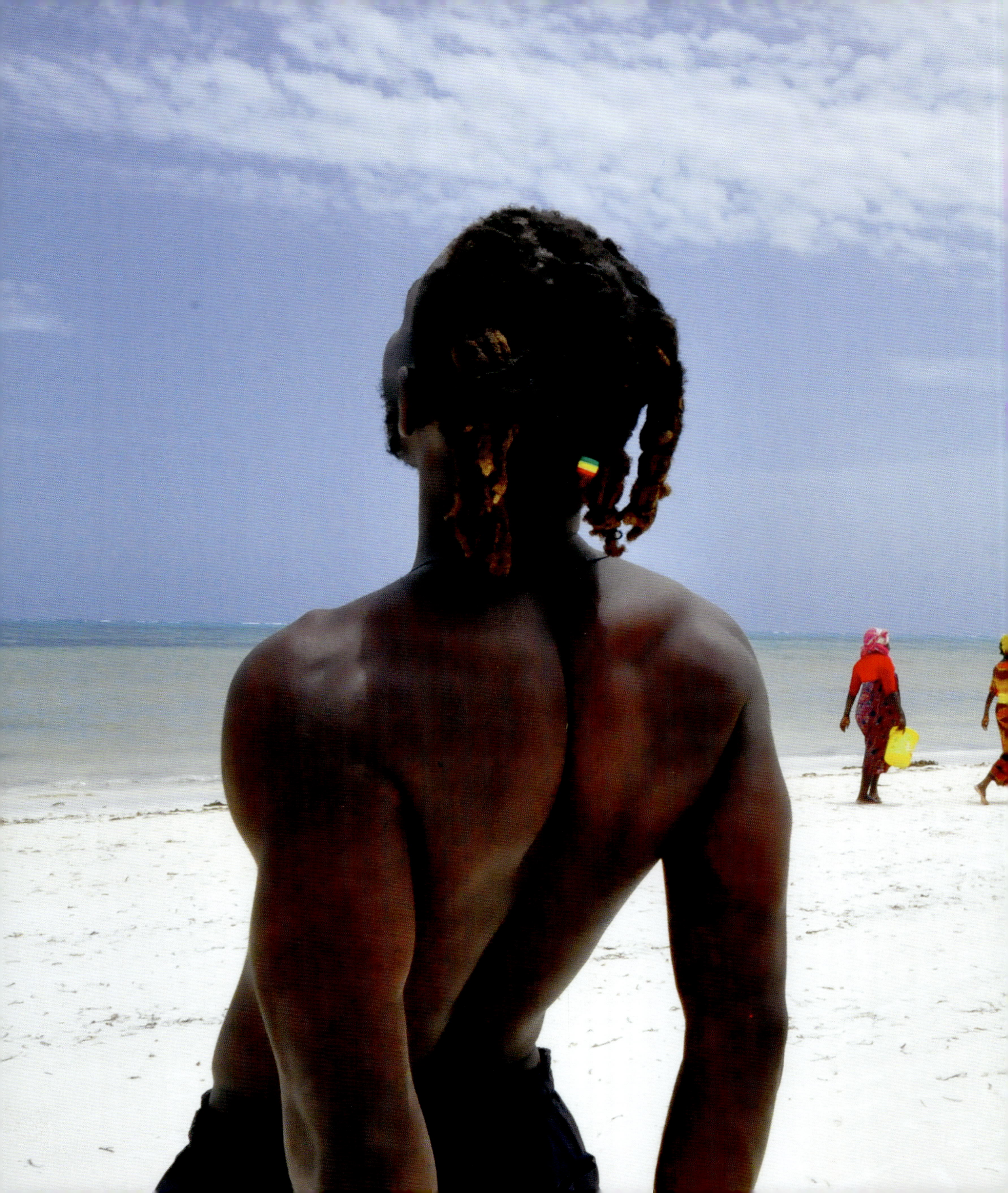

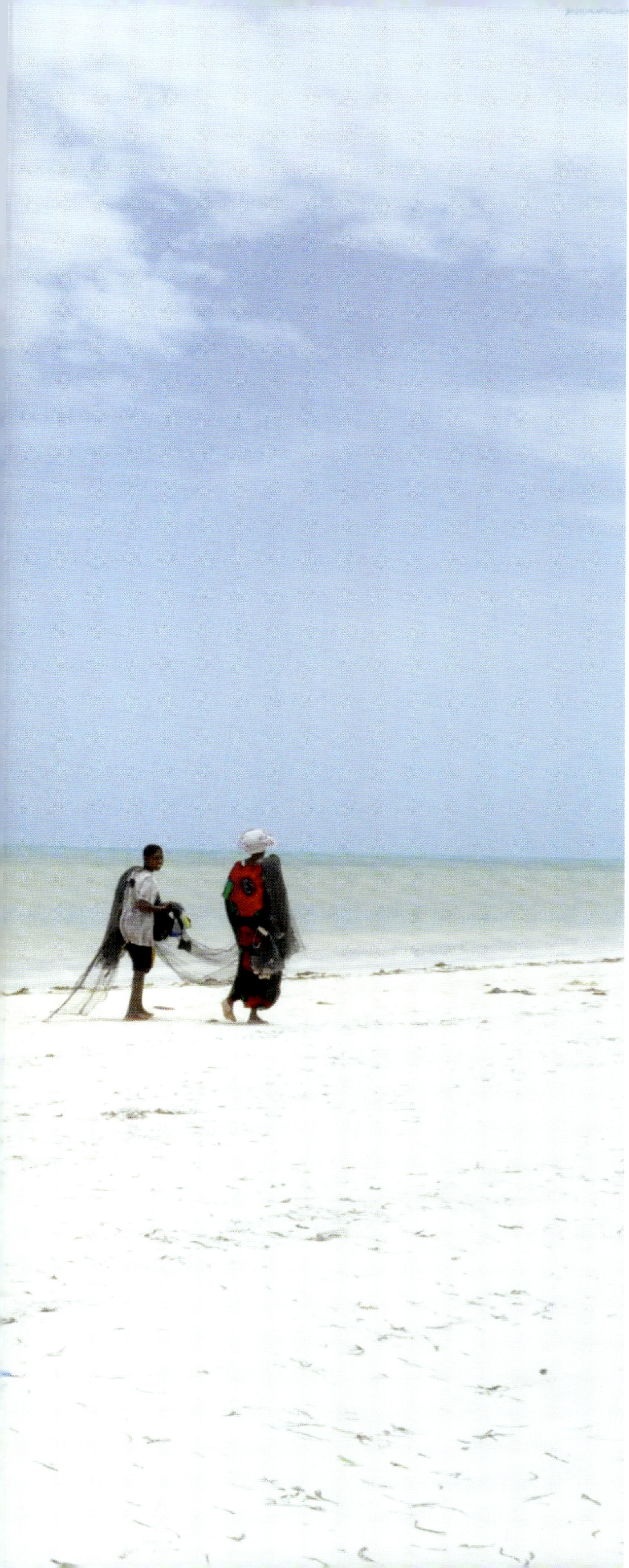

Bliss is boundless.

BADDHA ANUVITTASANA · Bound Standing Backbend

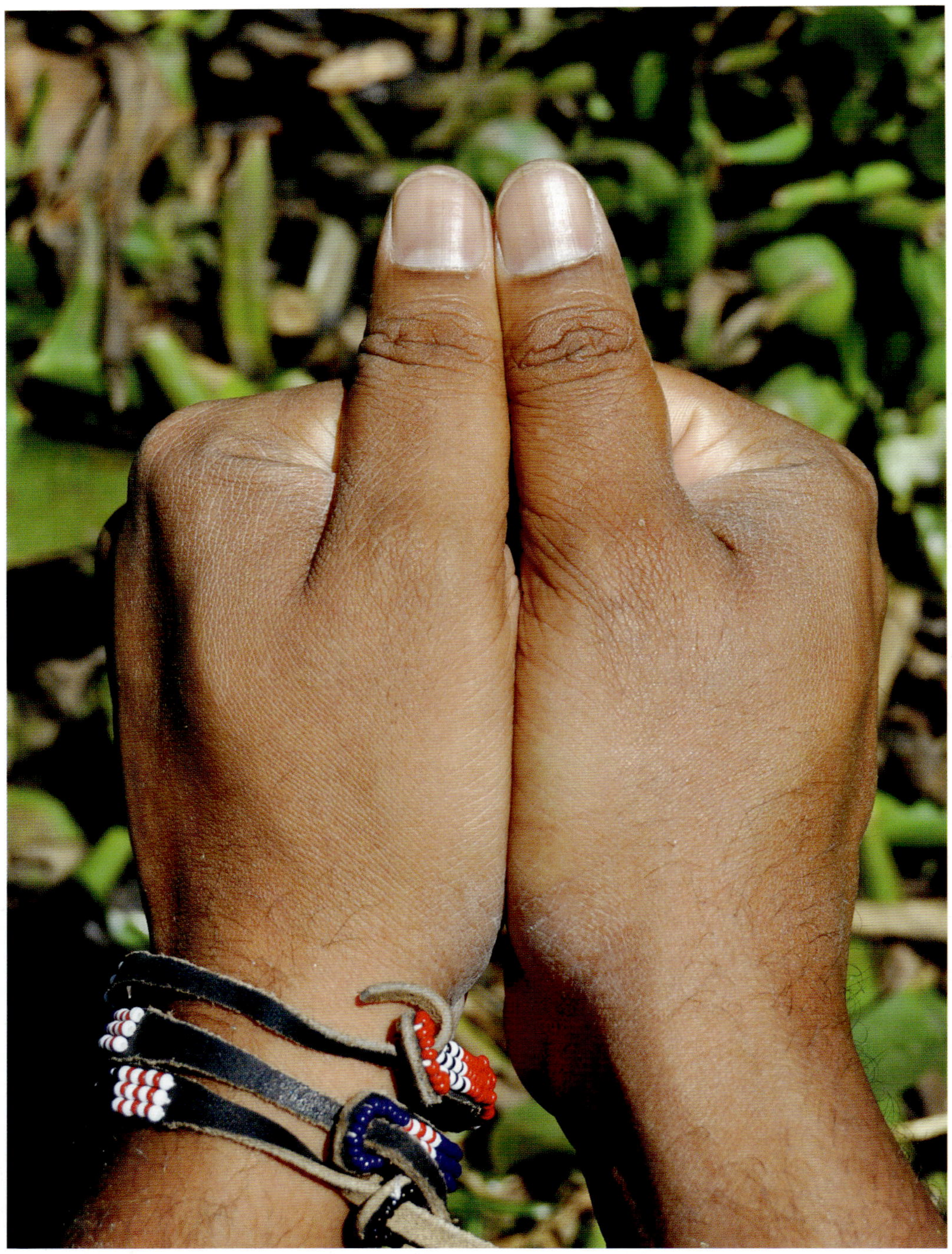

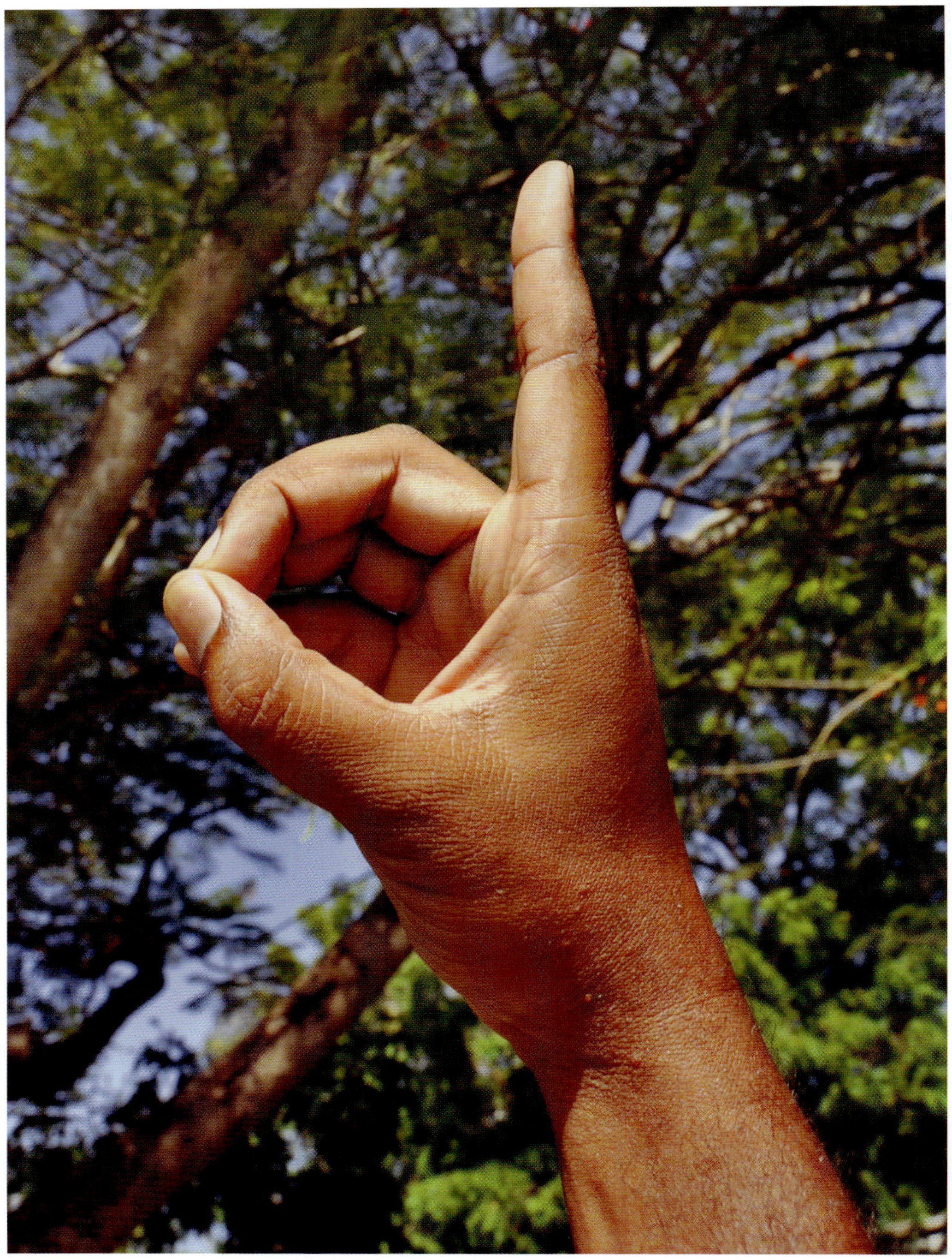

▲ **MUSHTIKAMUDRA** · Selflessness *(left)* **HAMSIMUDRA** · Illumination *(right)*

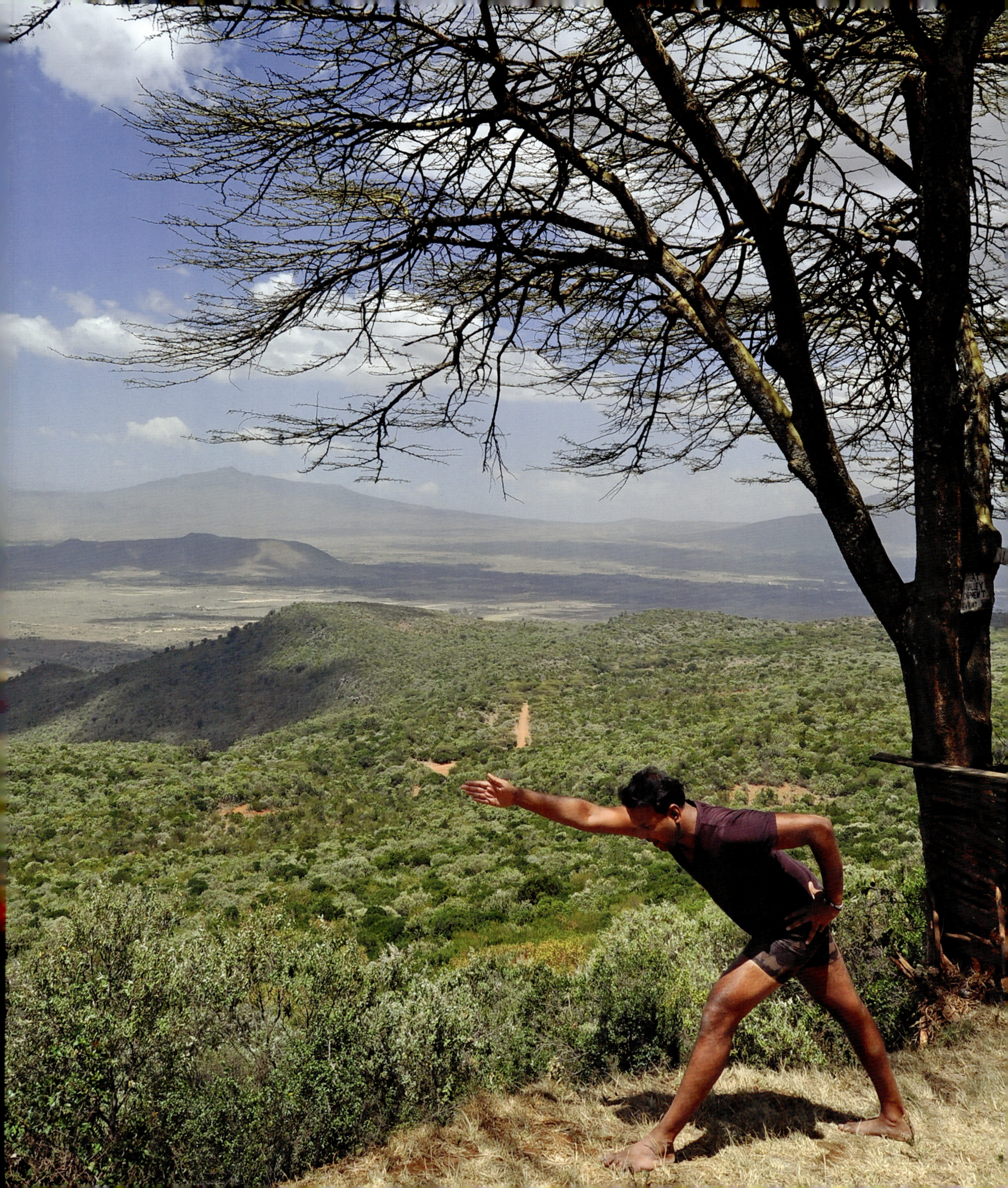

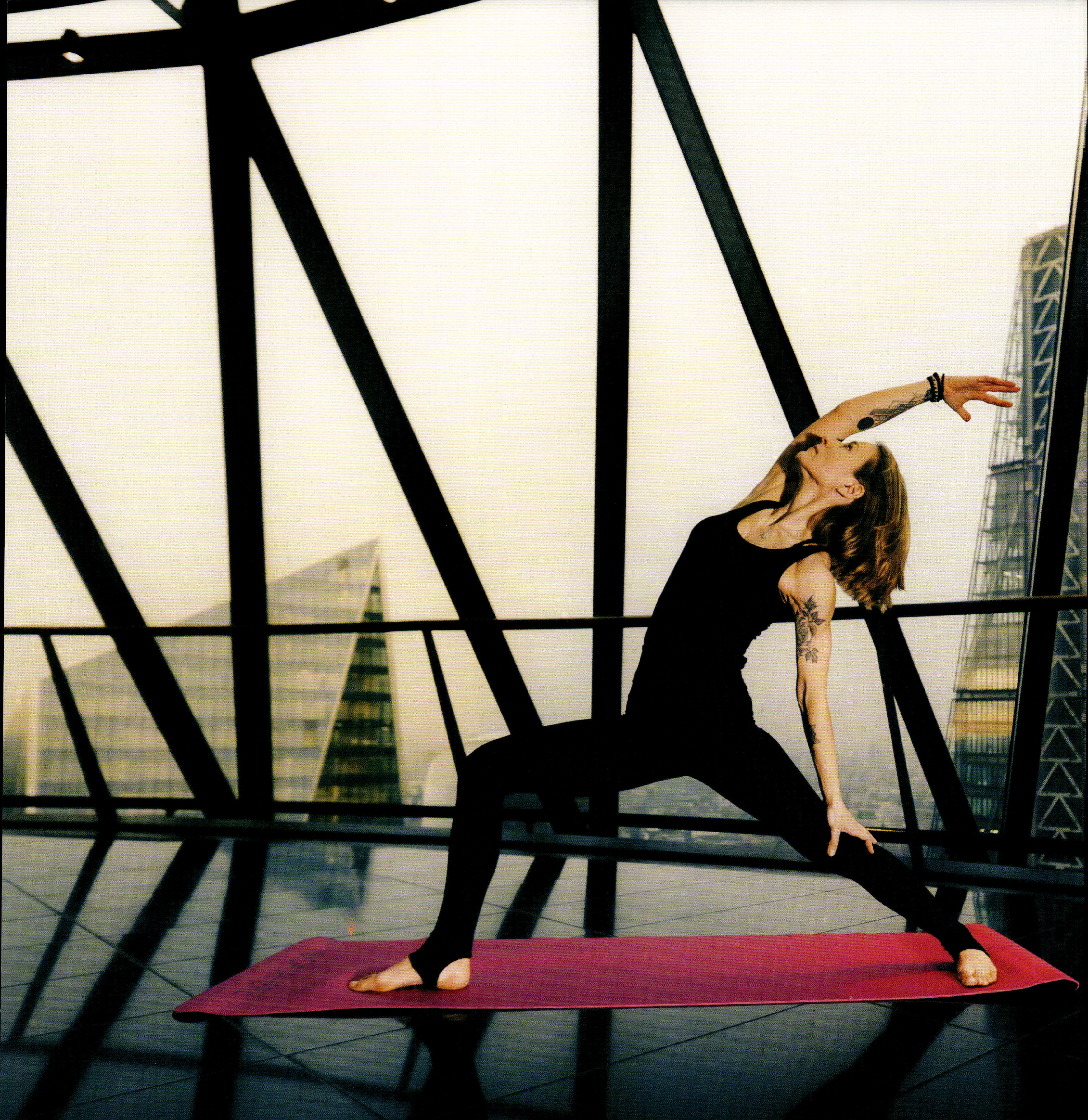

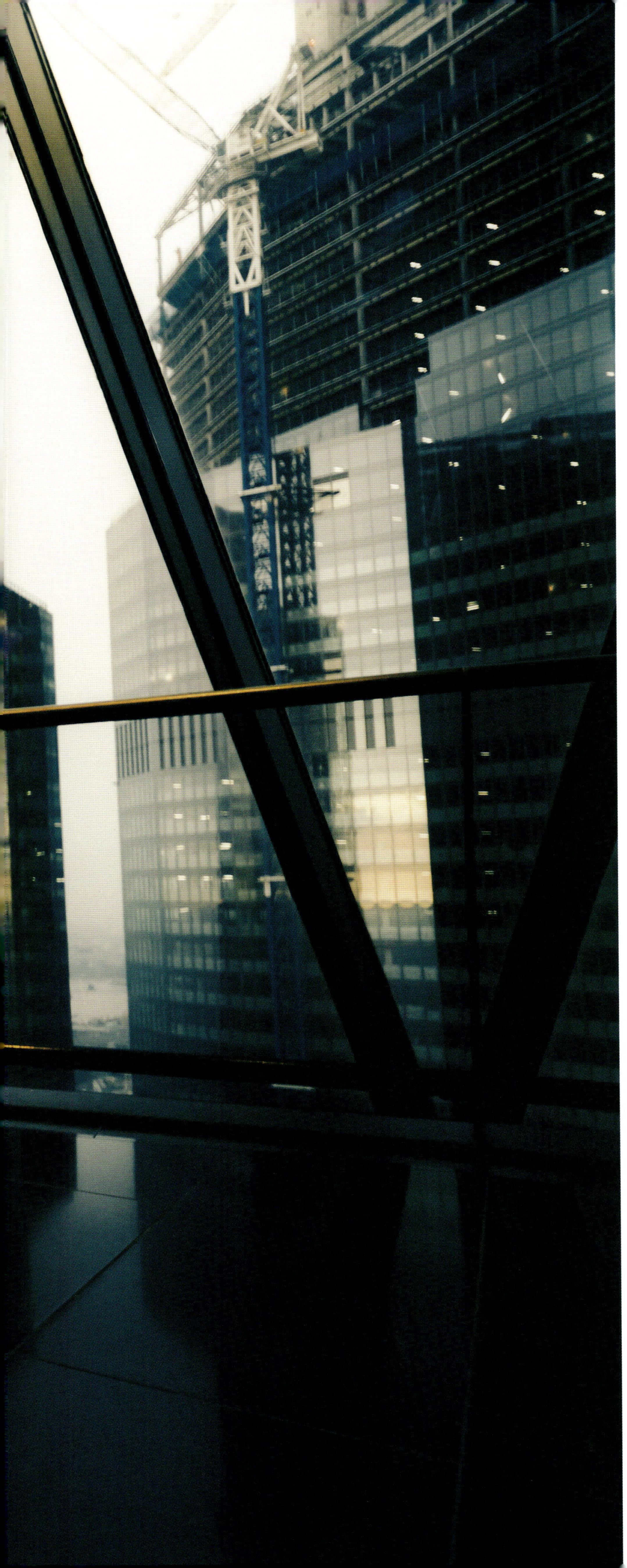

VIPARITA VIRABHADRASANA • Reverse Warrior

You can only live once as yourself in this lifetime.
If you live fully, once is enough.

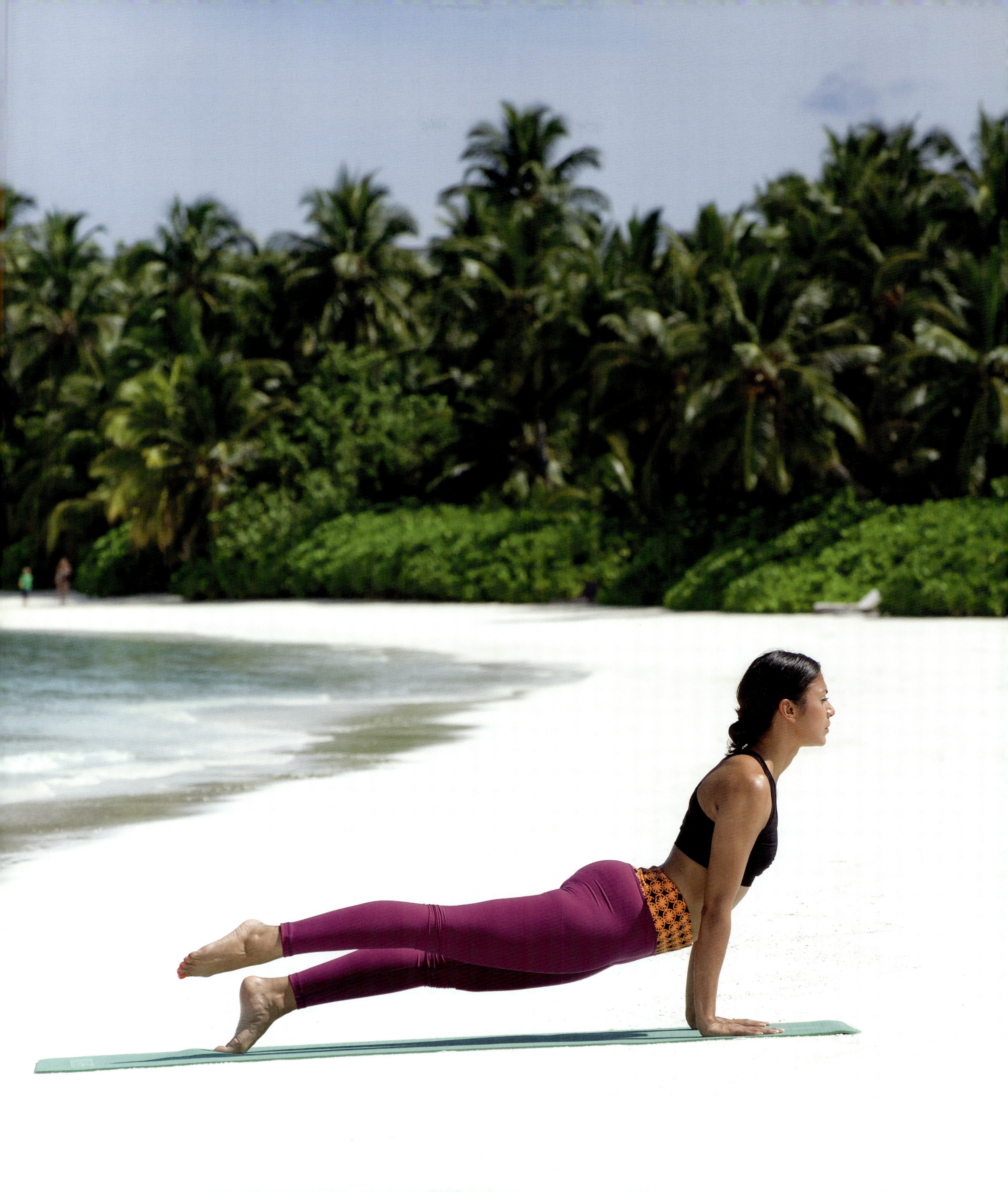

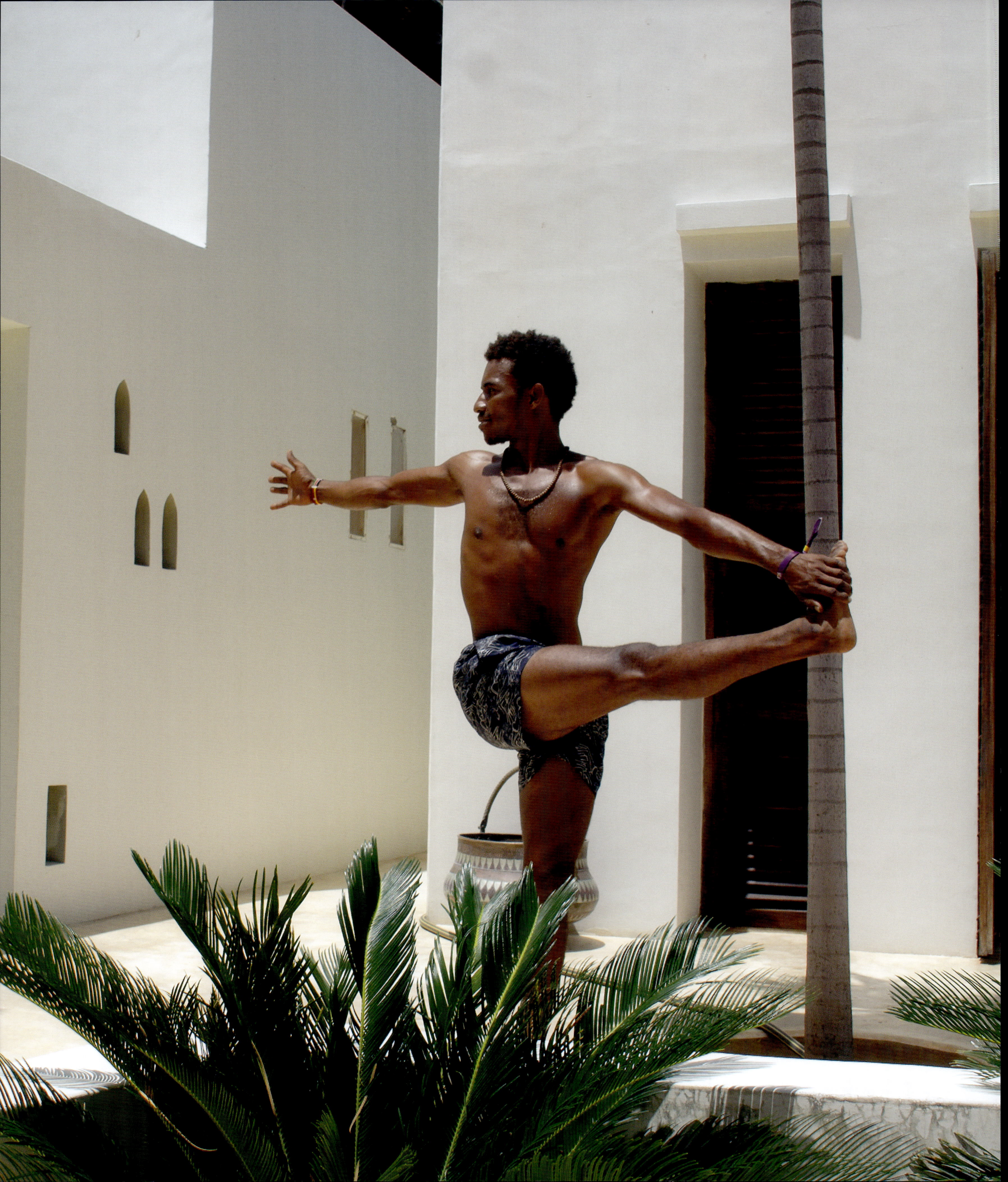

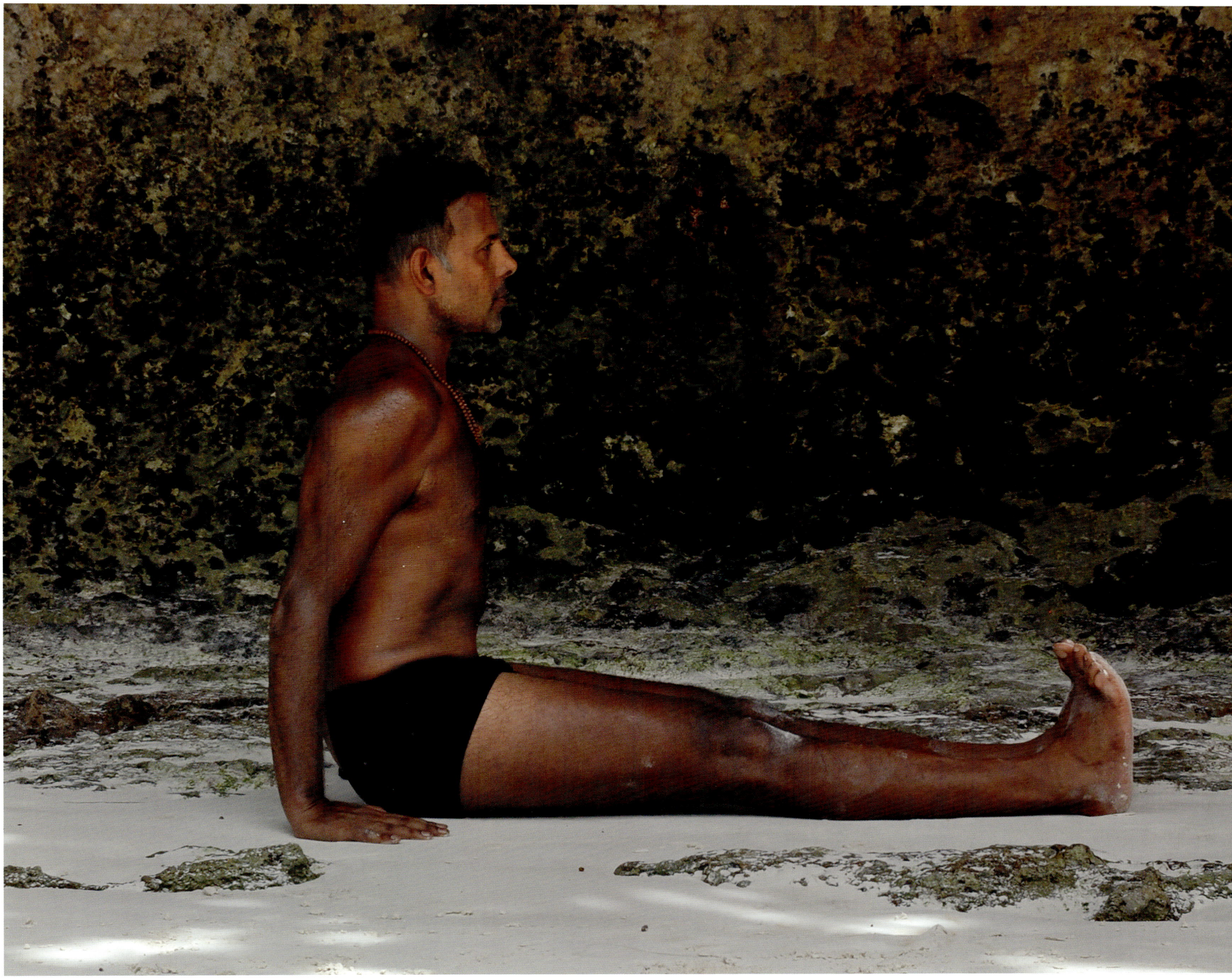

▲ DANDASANA • Staff

While defining the current narrative,
we are missing the dawn of a new paradigm.

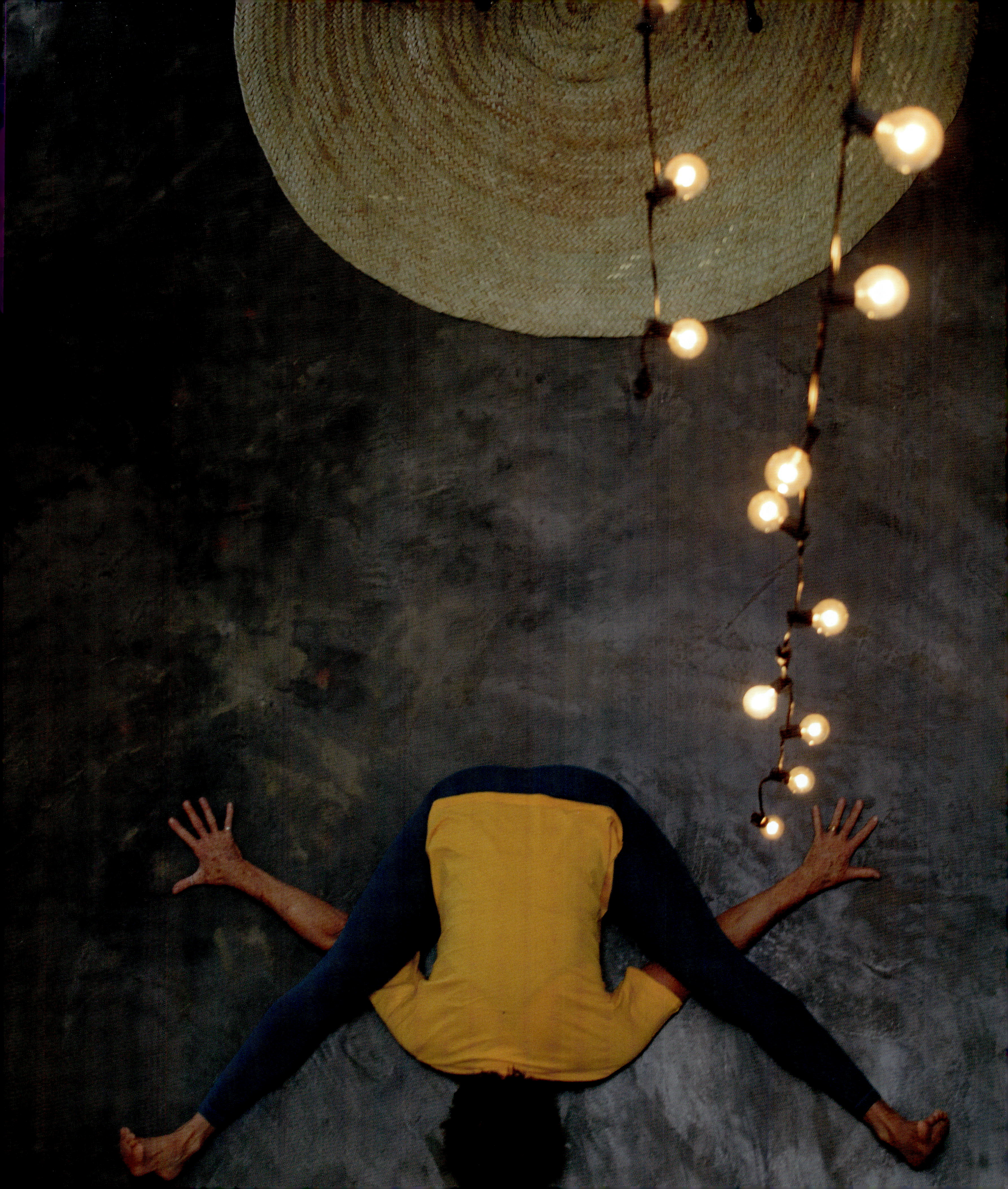

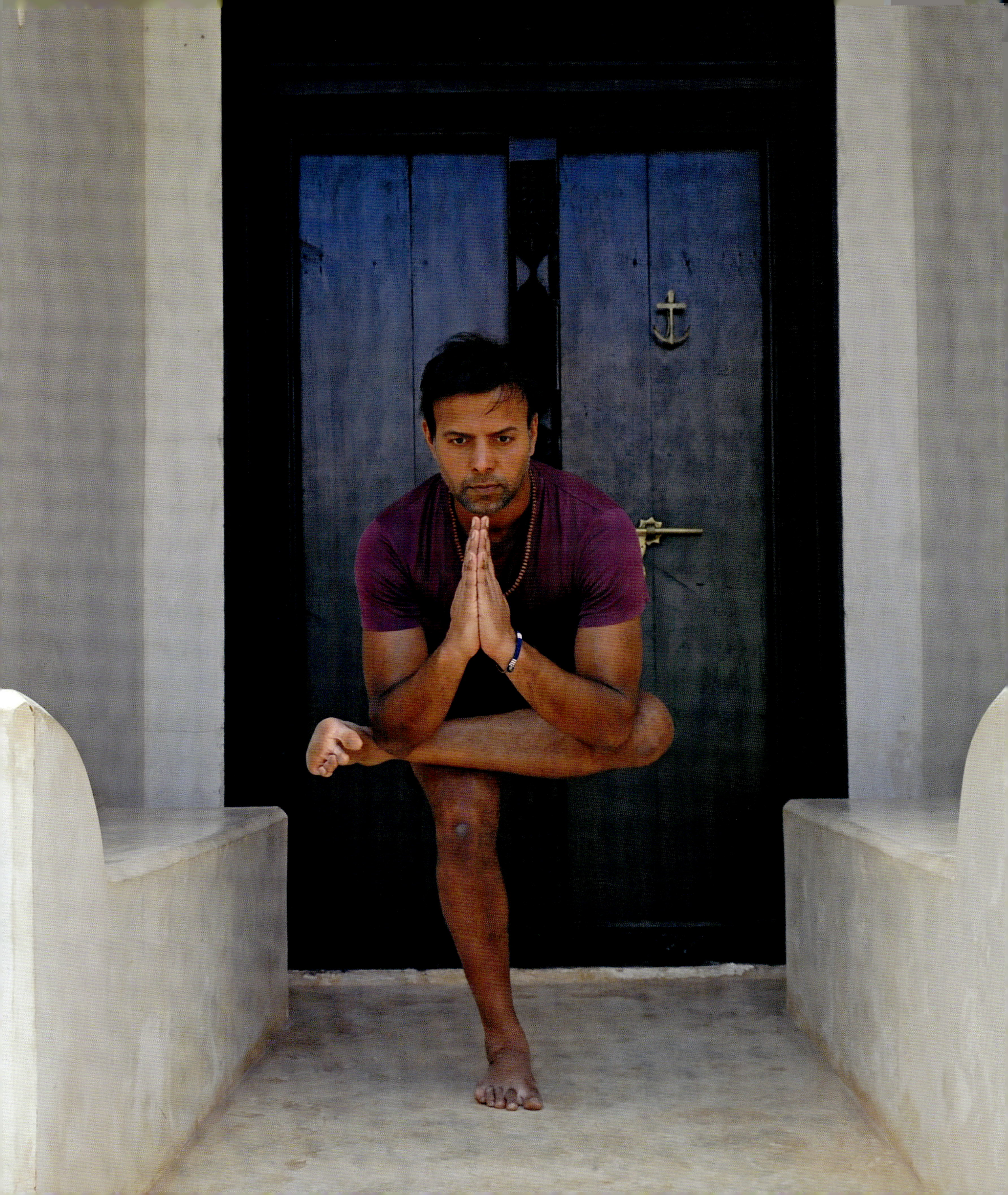

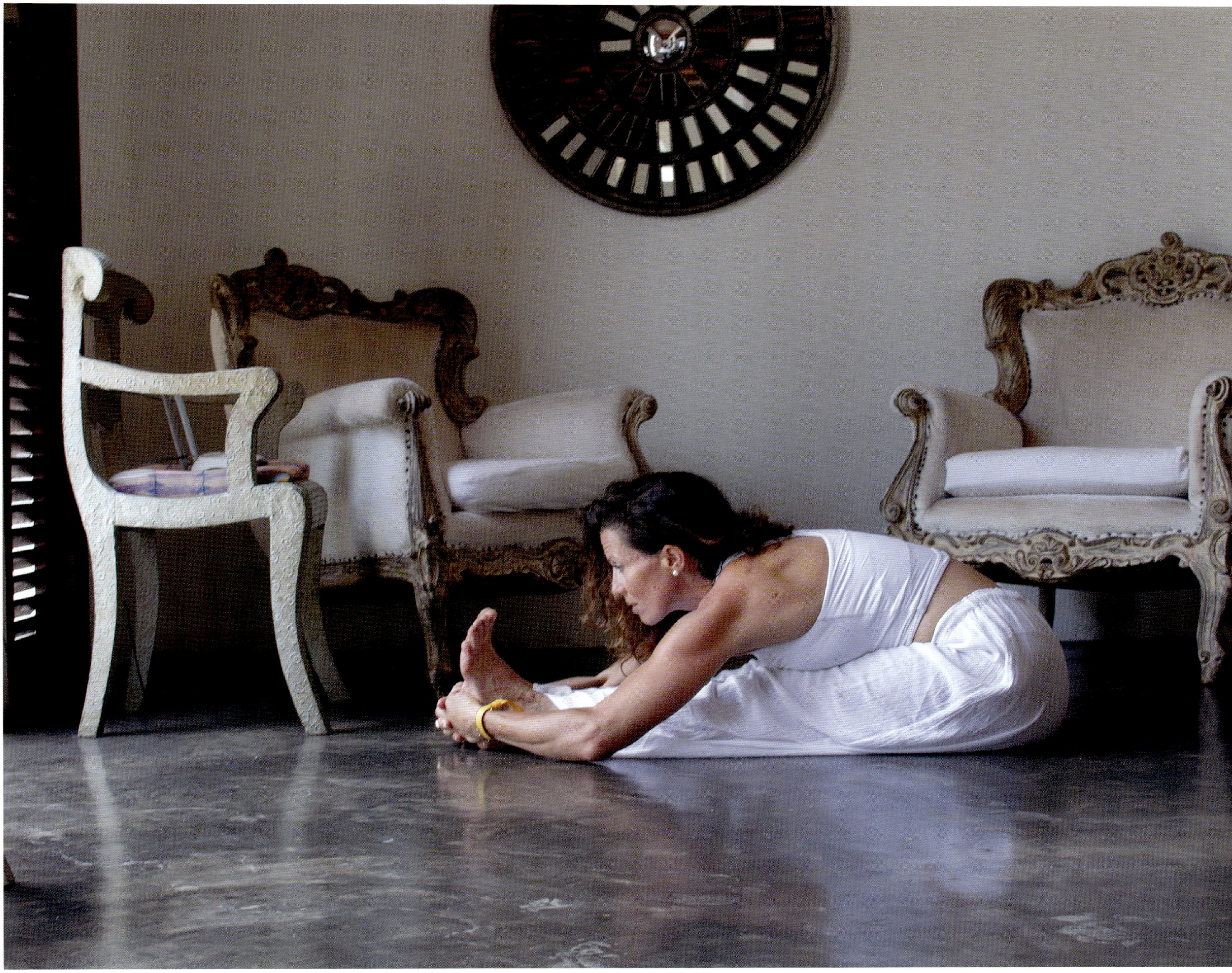

TADA KAPOTASANA • Standing Pigeon

▲ TRATAKA PASCHIMOTTANASANA • Eye Focus Forward Bend

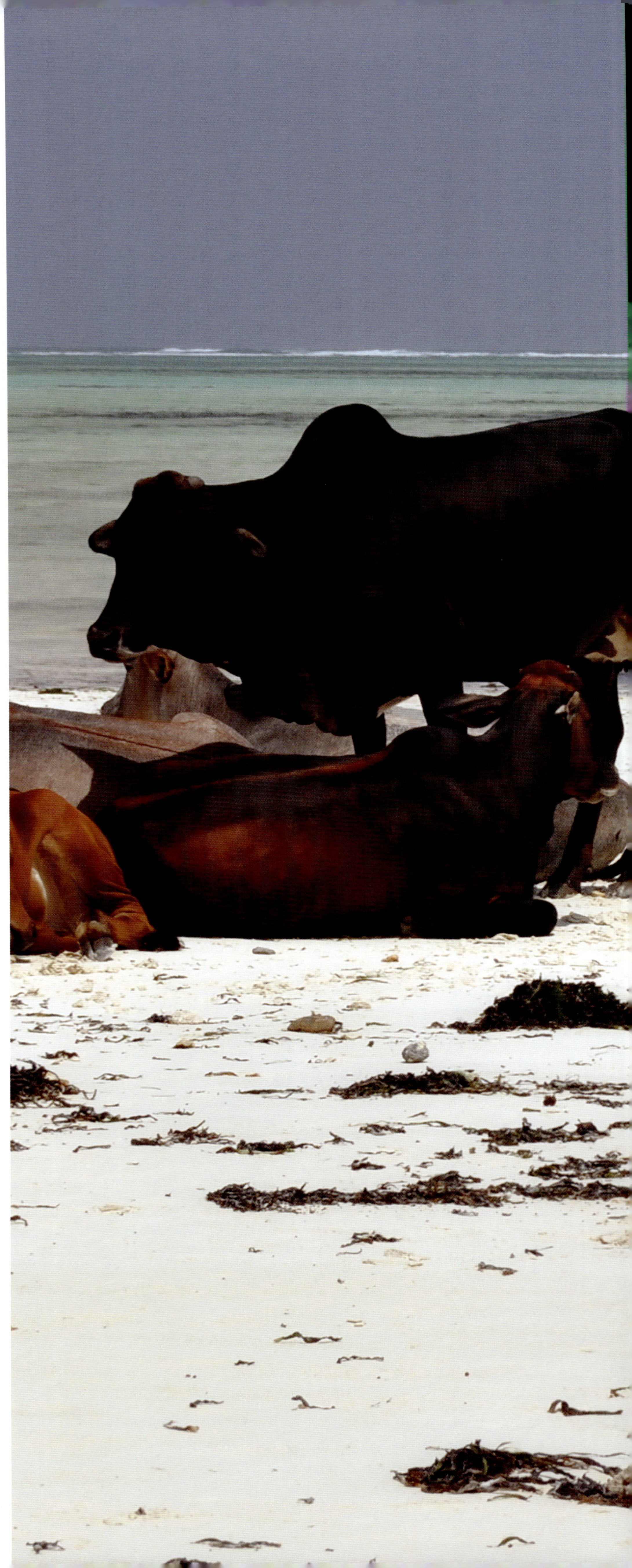

GOMUKHASANA UTTHAN · Cow Face Forward Fold

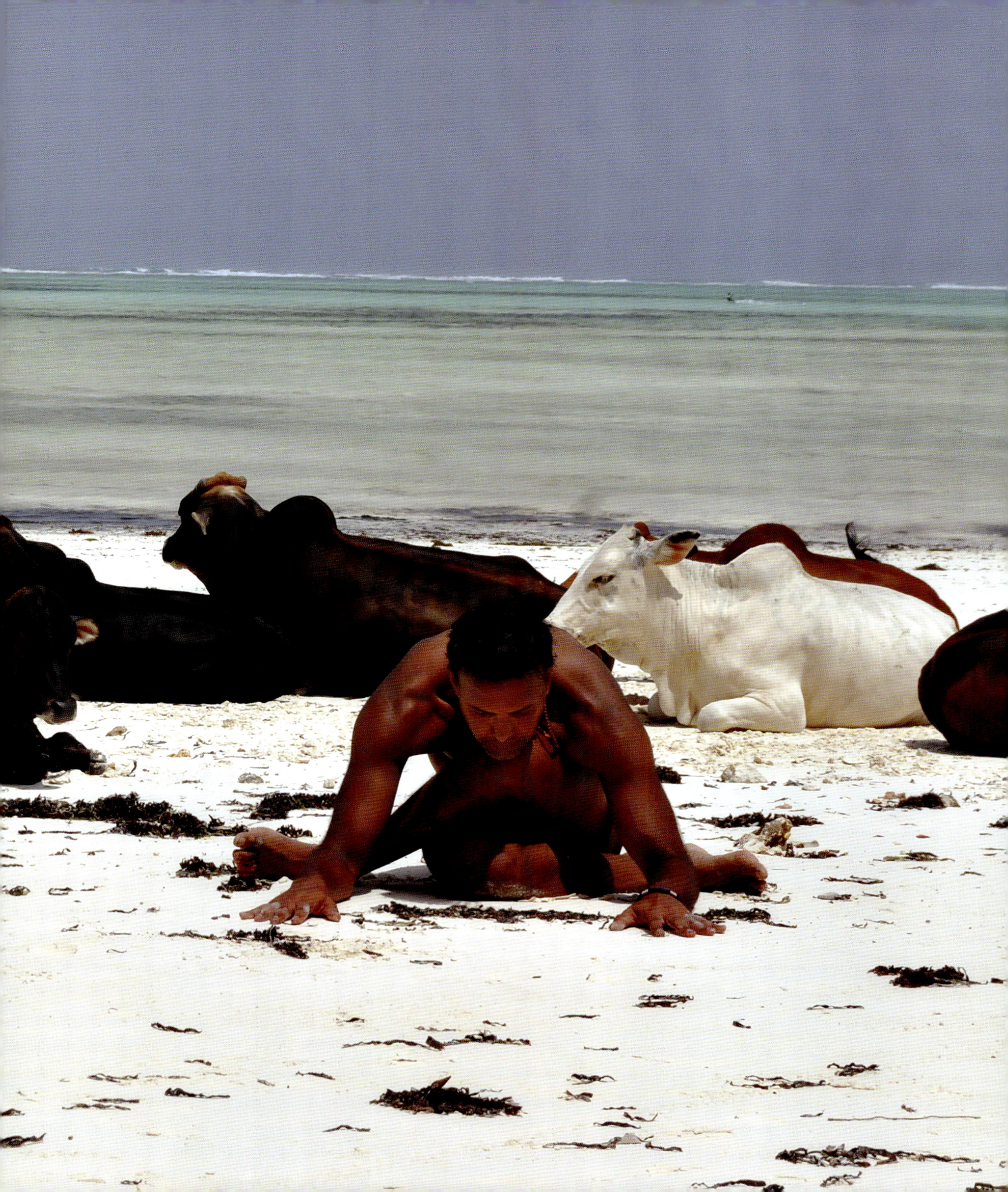

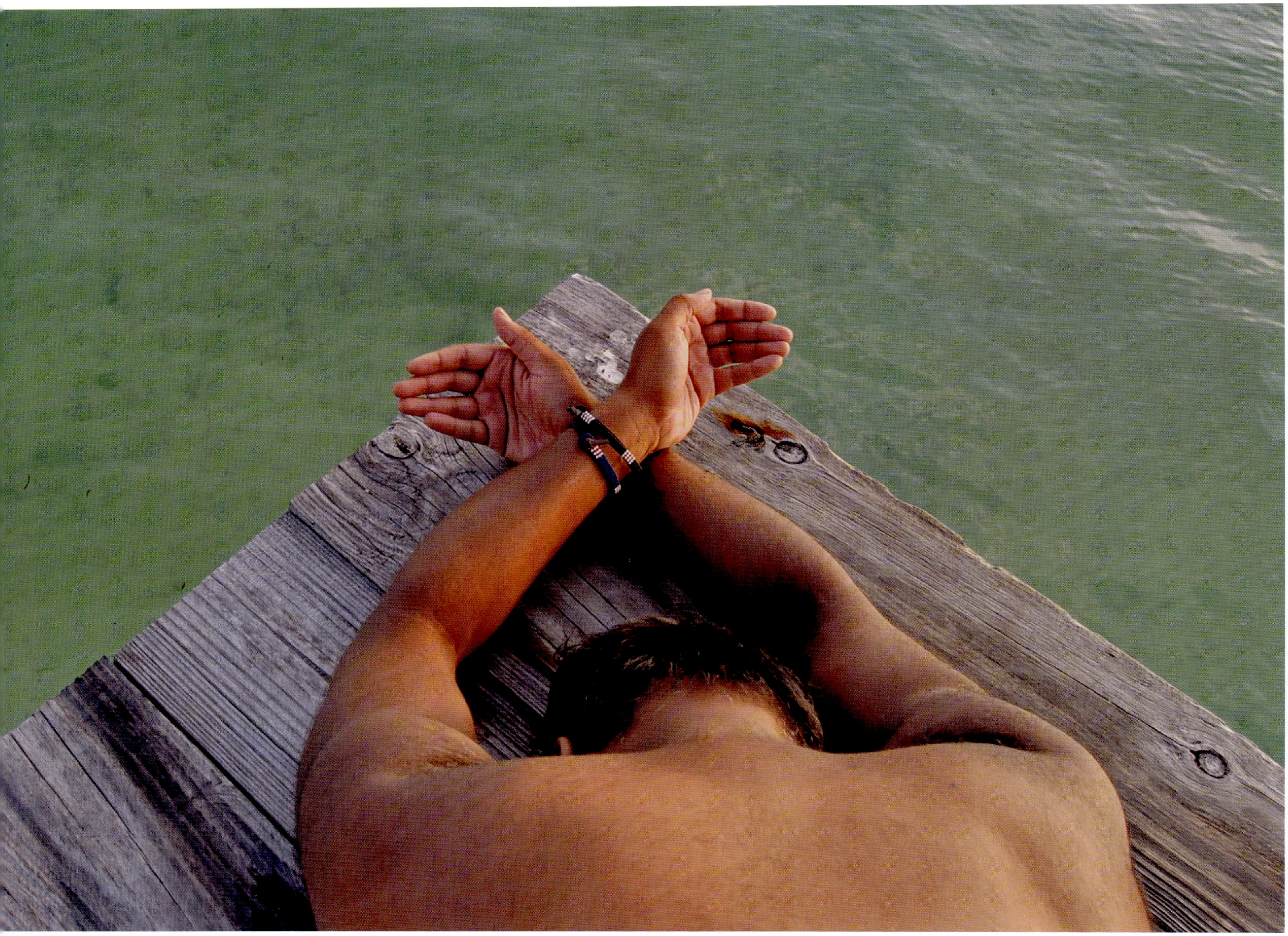

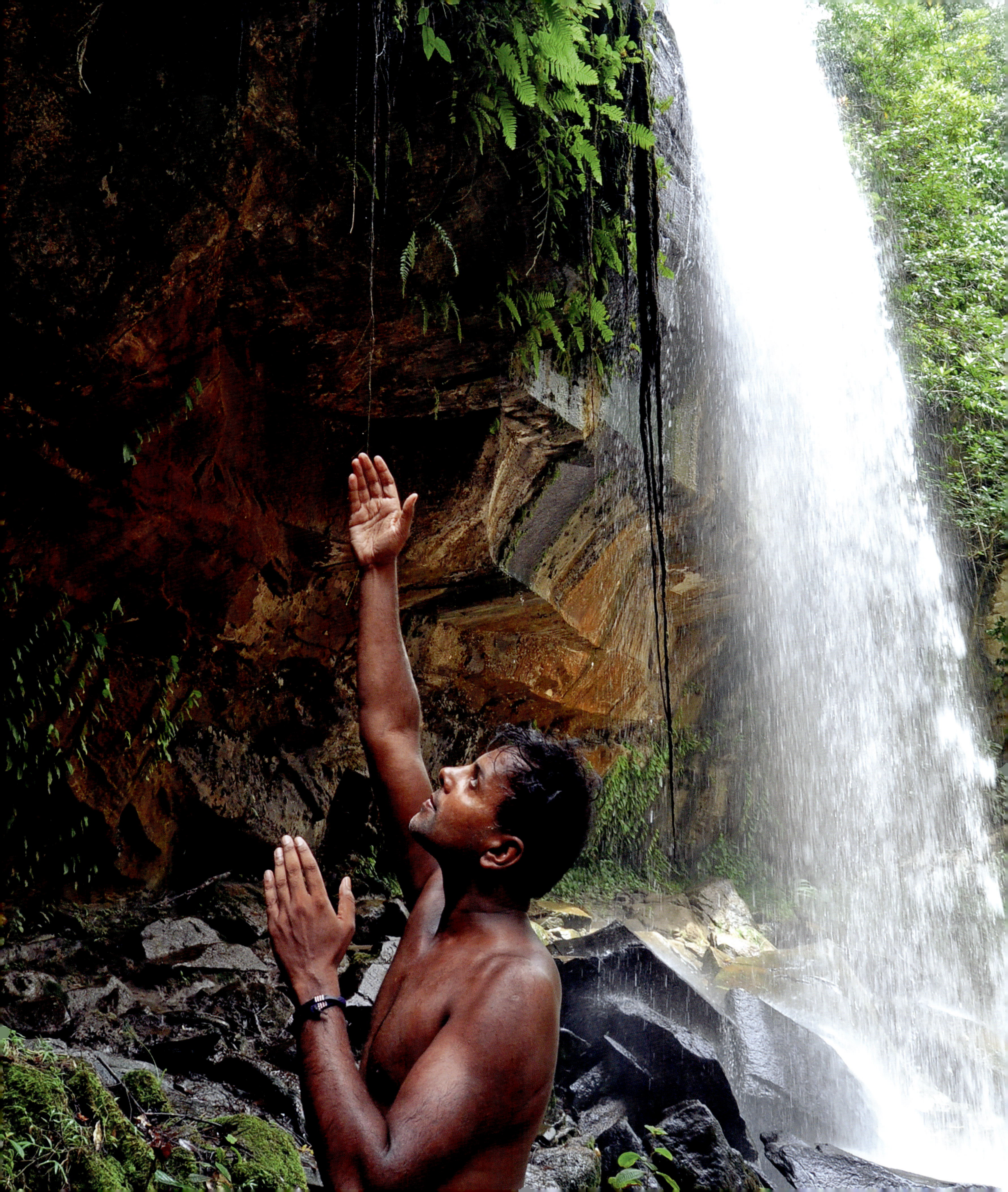

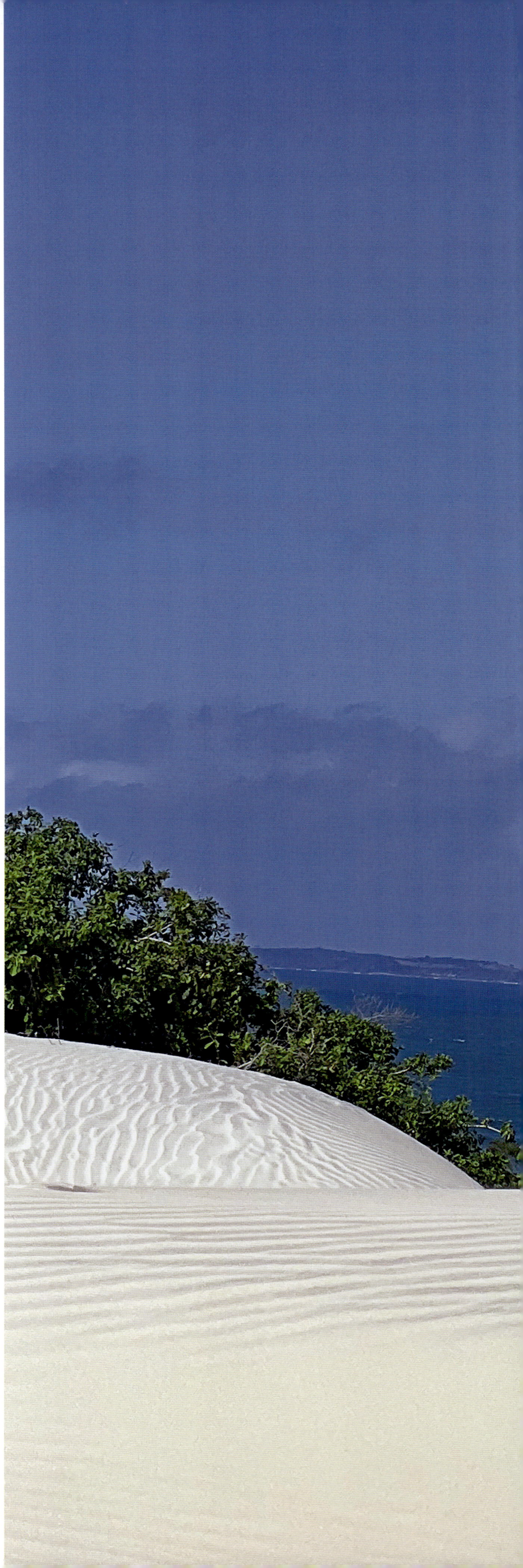

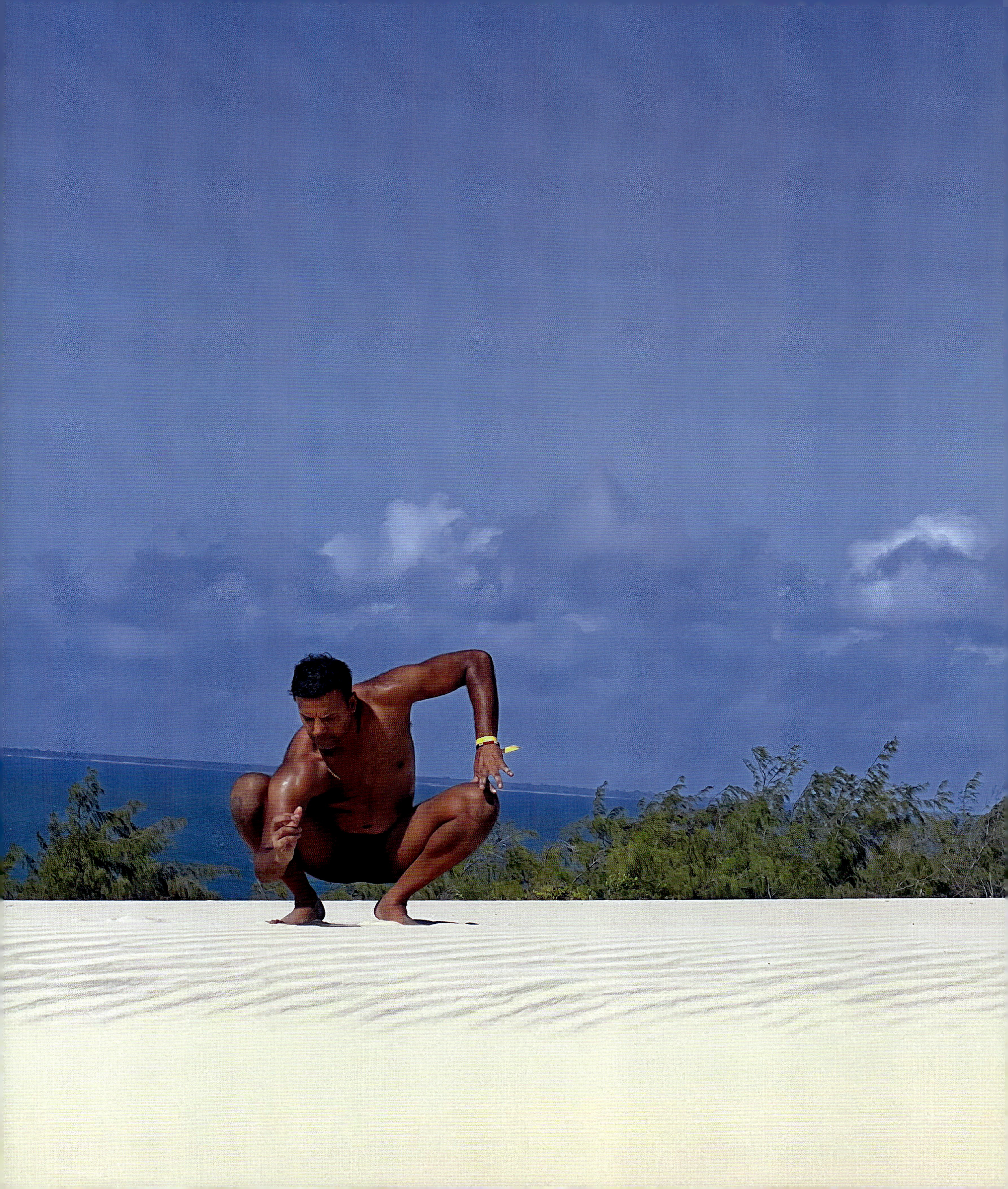

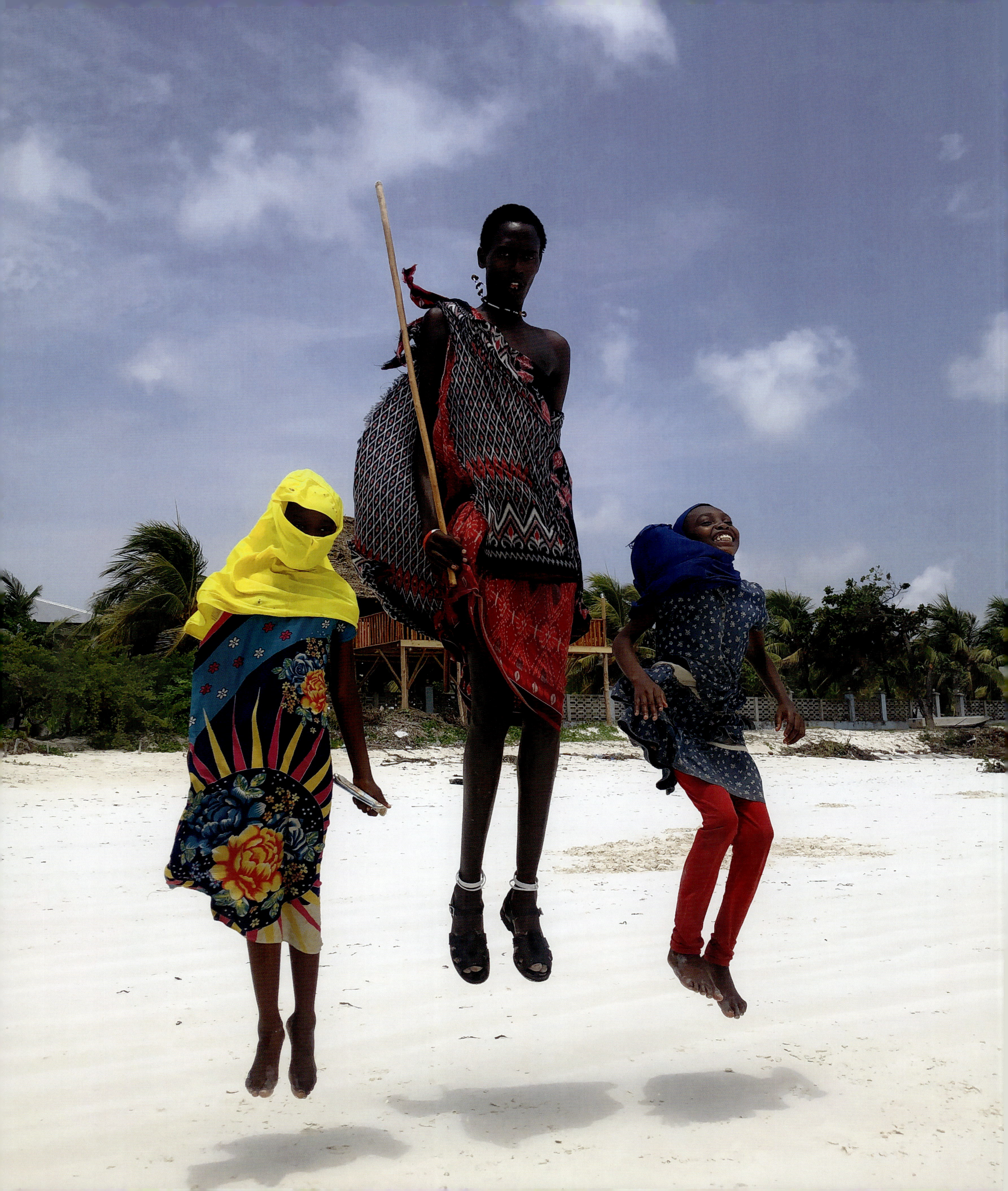

When there is love, even in the absence
of opportunity, there will always be hope.
Then anything is possible.

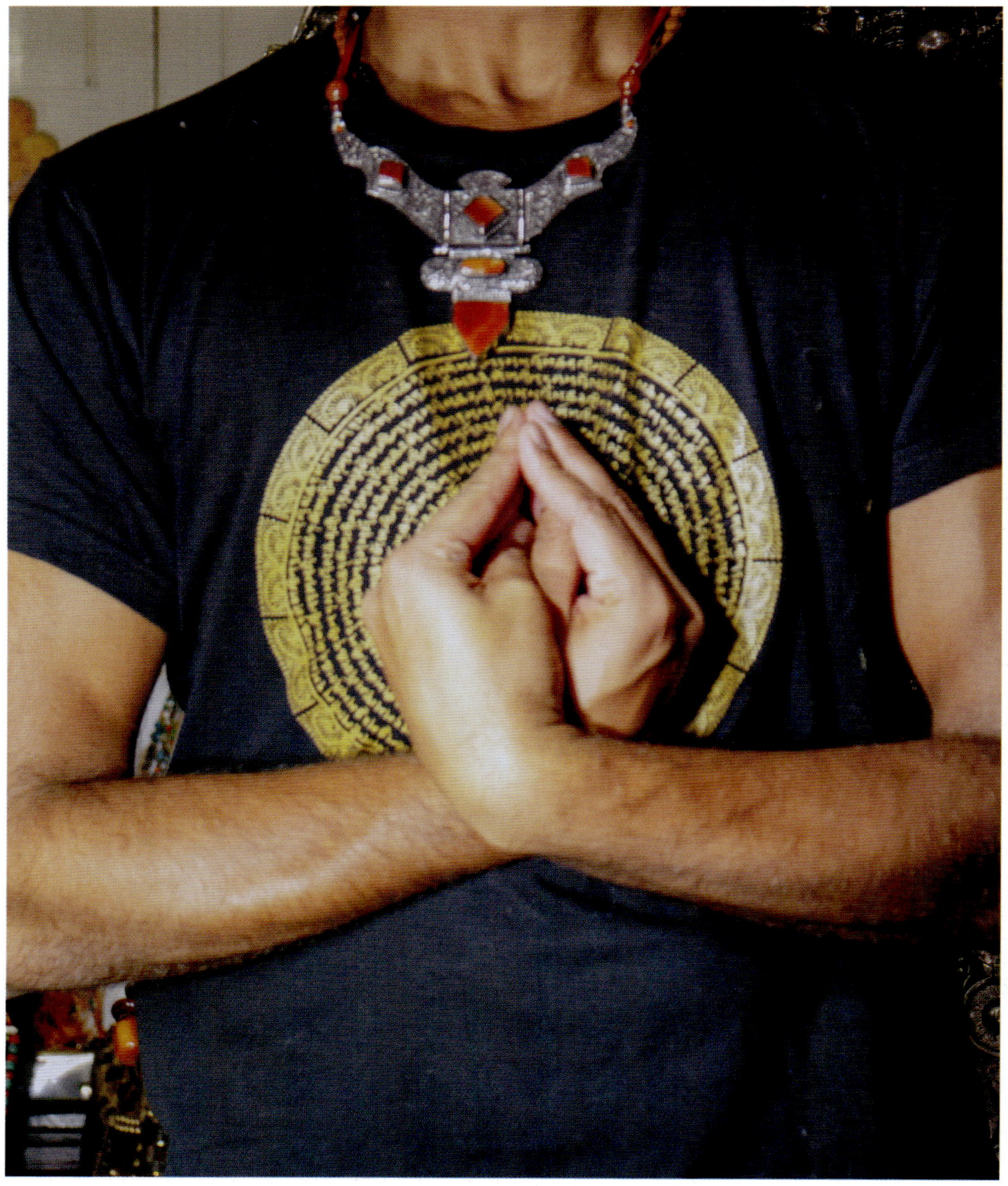

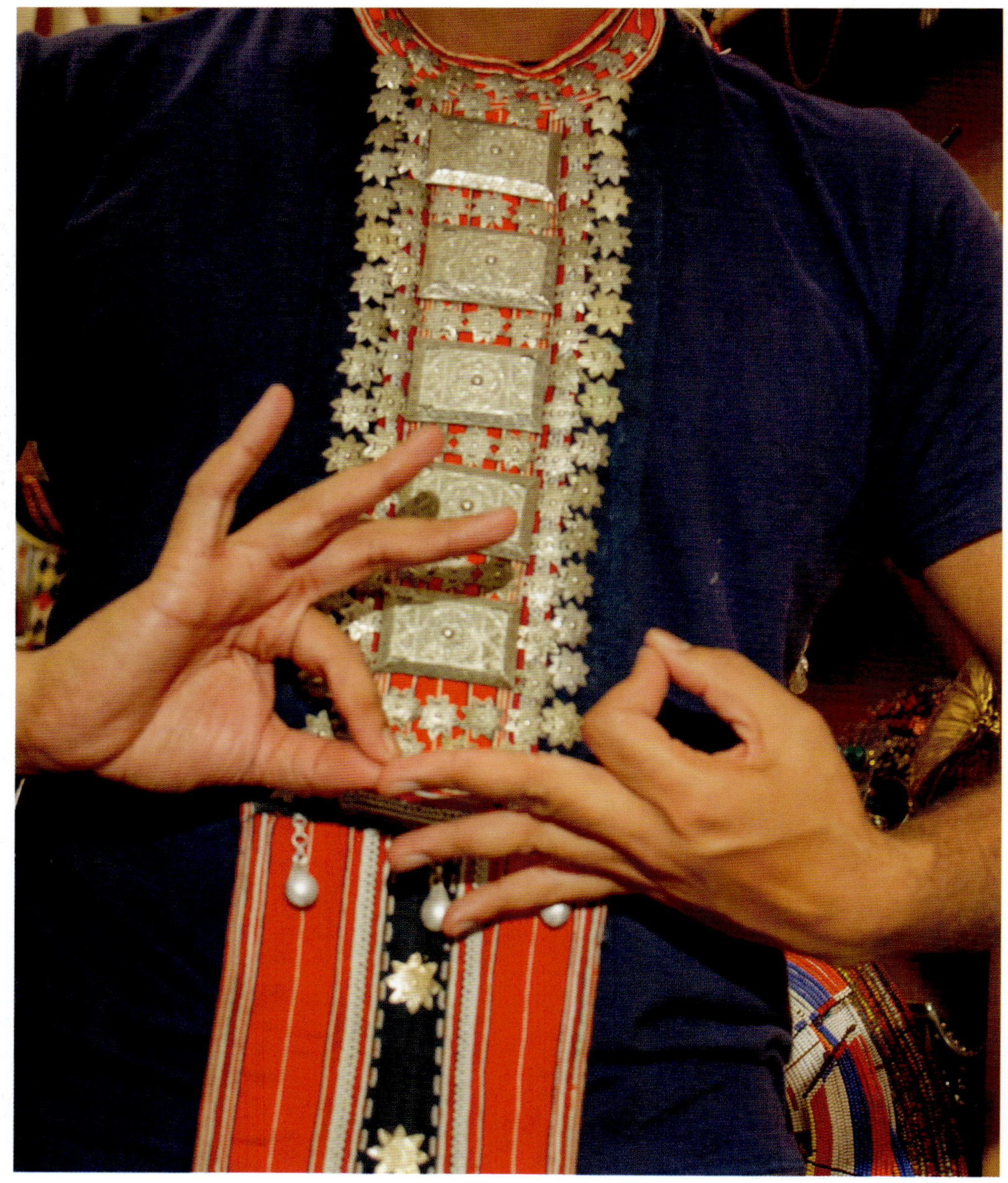

▲ **NIRVANAMUDRA** · Awakening (*left*) **DHARMACHAKRAMUDRA** · Alignment (*right*)

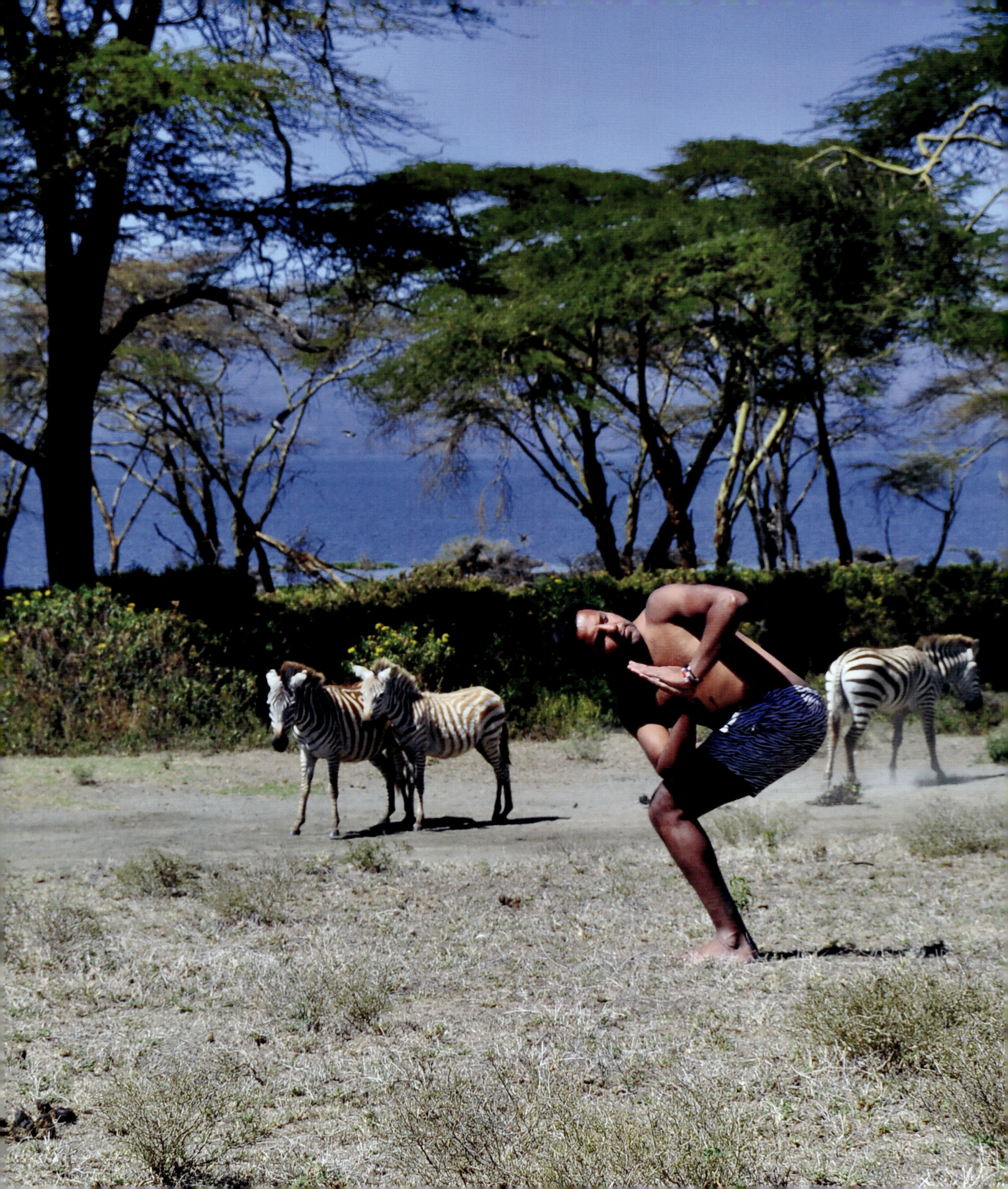

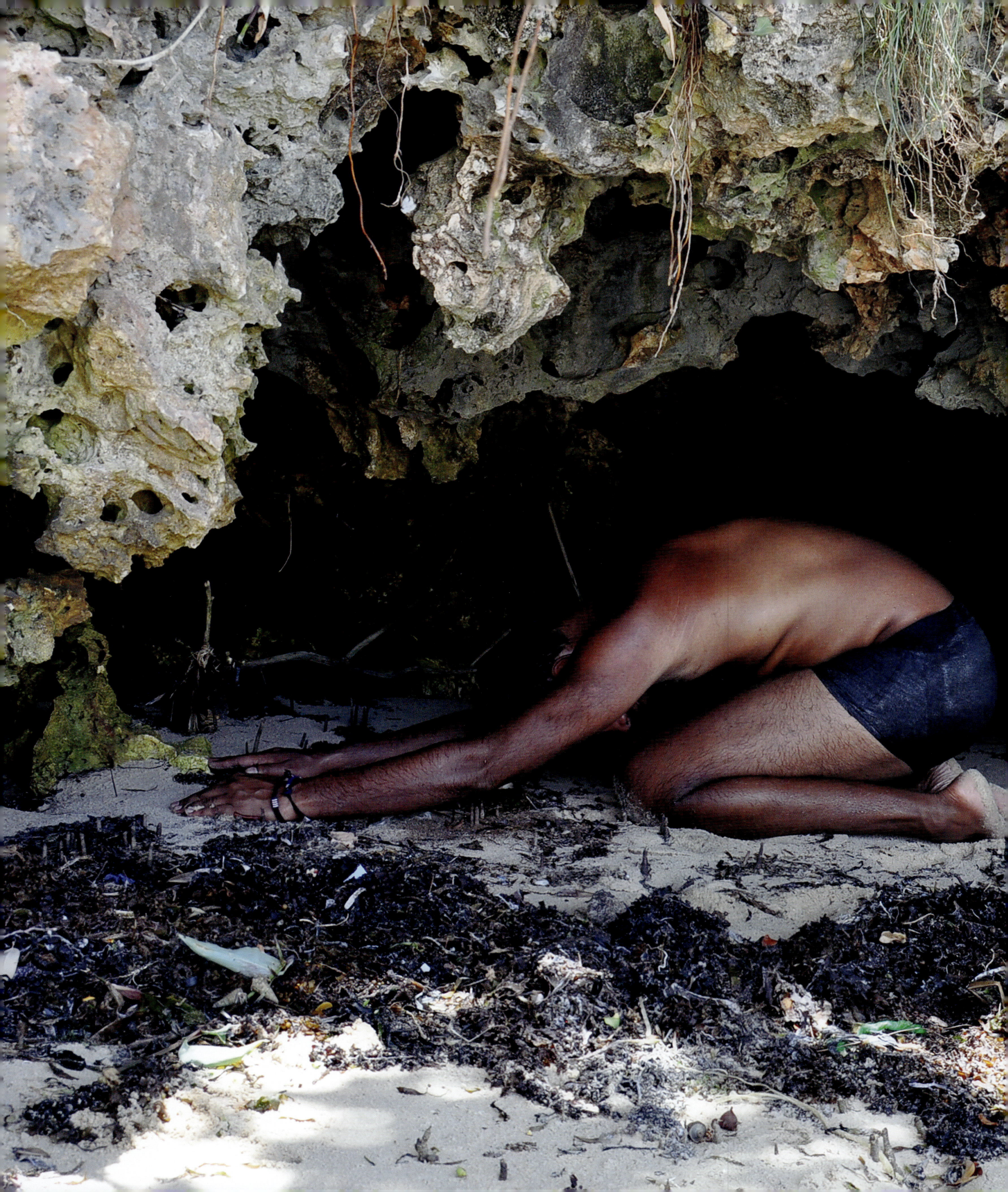

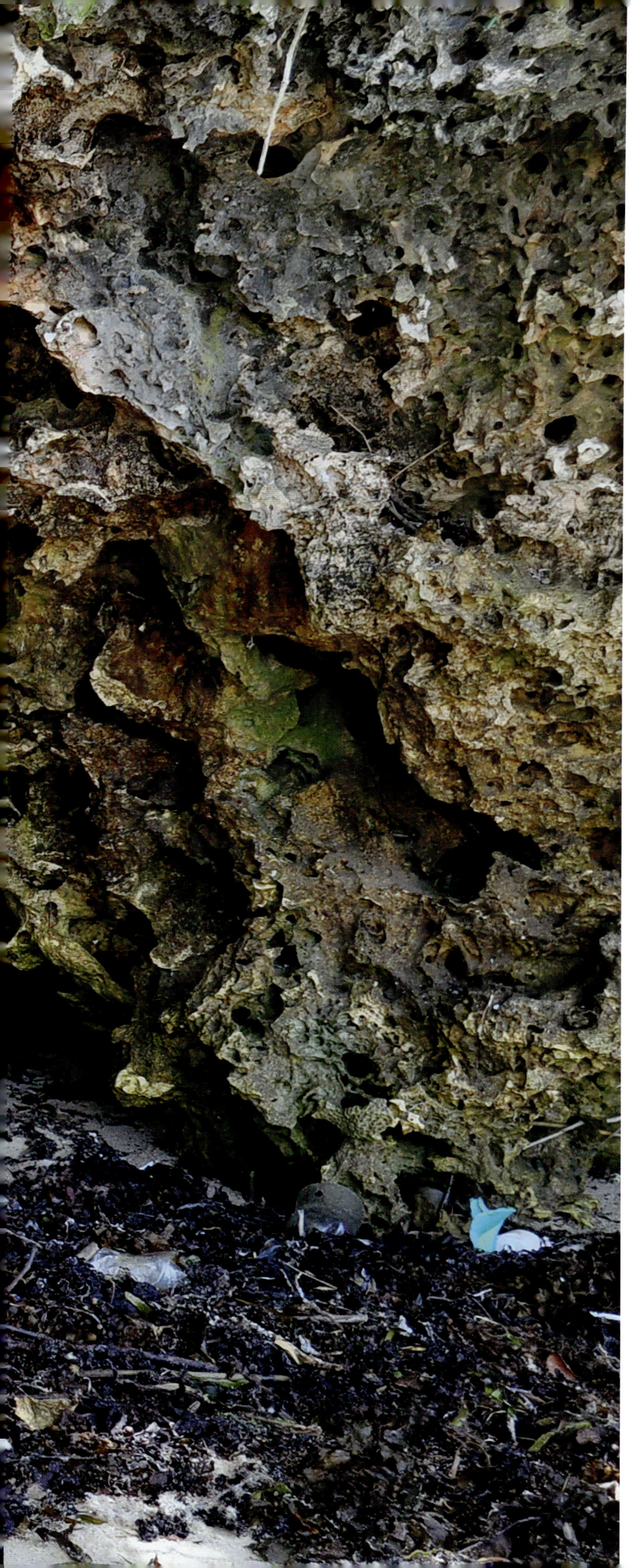

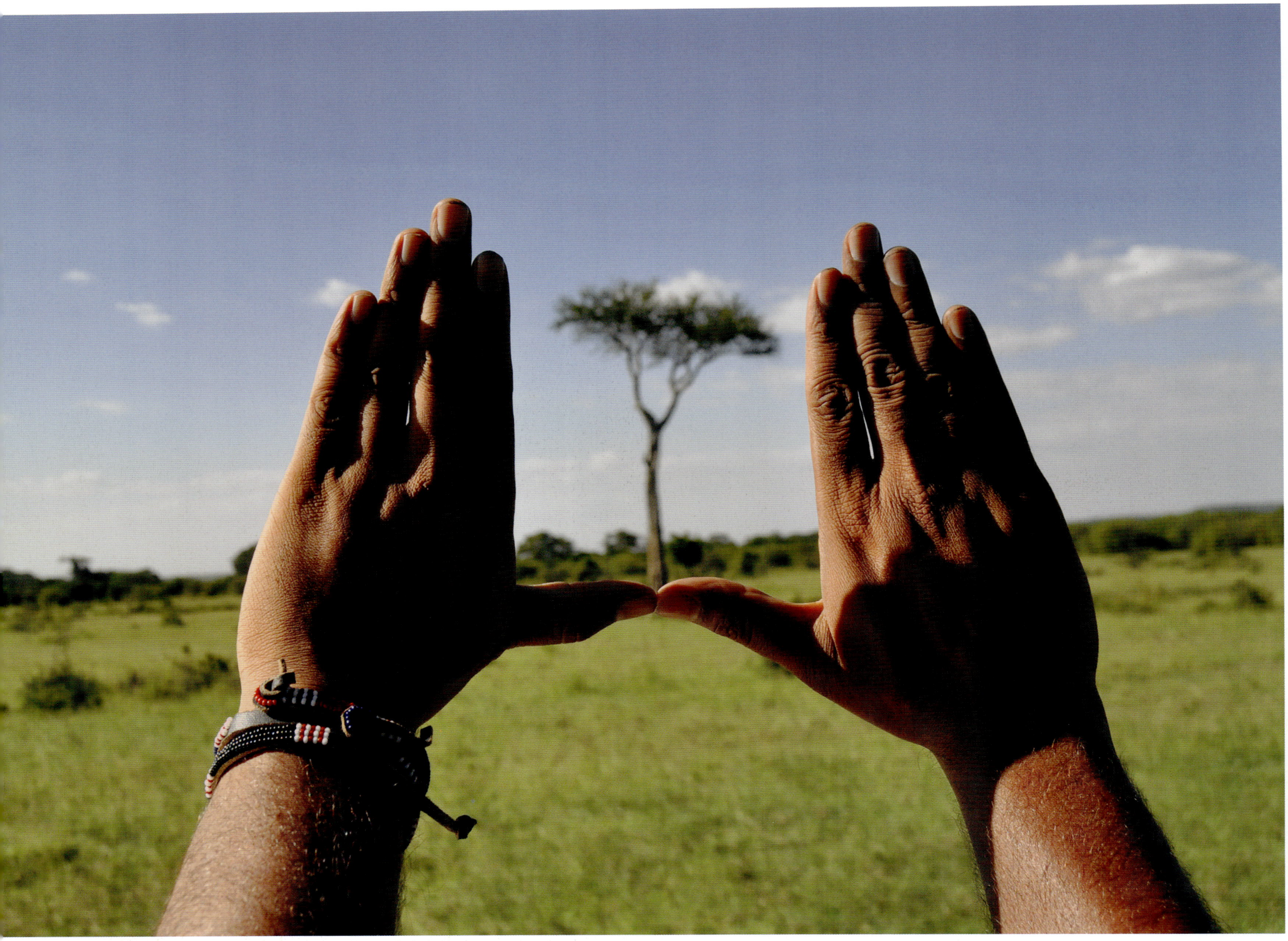

▲ **PRALAMBAMUDRA** · Kindness

DHOOPAGHADEEASANA · Sundial

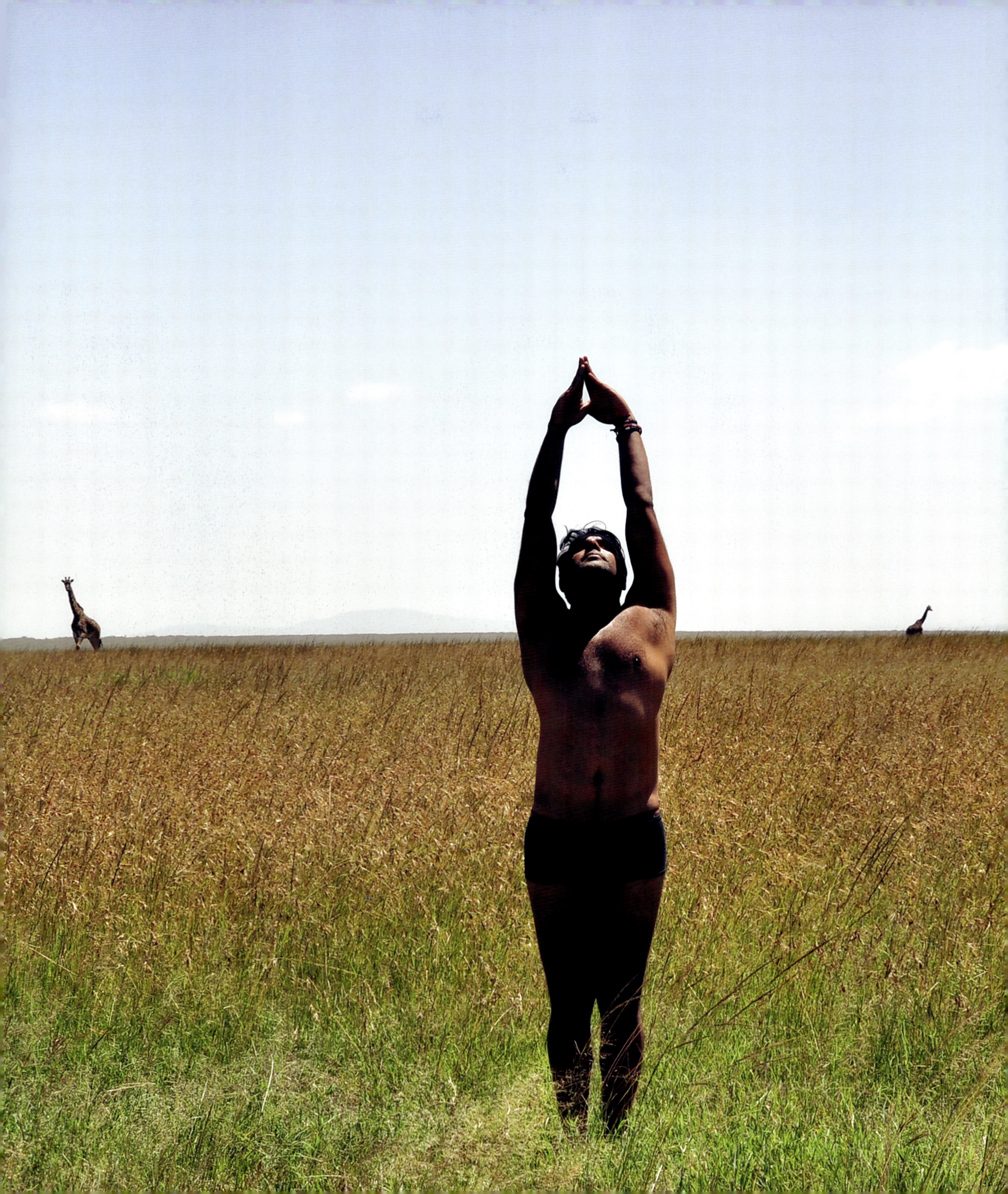

BRAHMA KUMBHA • Aquarius

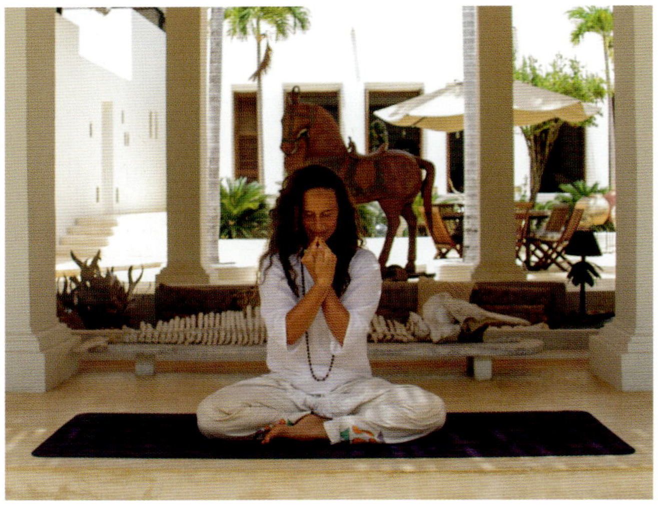

SIDDHASANA & NIRVANAMUDRA
Seated Accomplished & Awakening

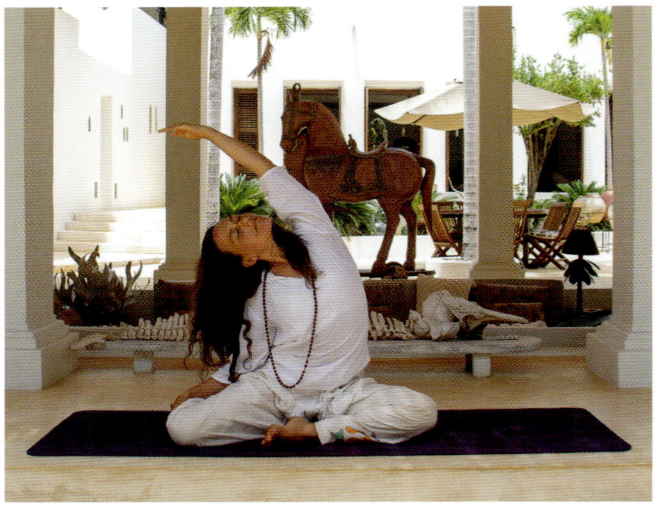

ARDHA HASTA SWASTIKASANA & HAMSIMUDRA
Side Reaching Auspicious & Illumination

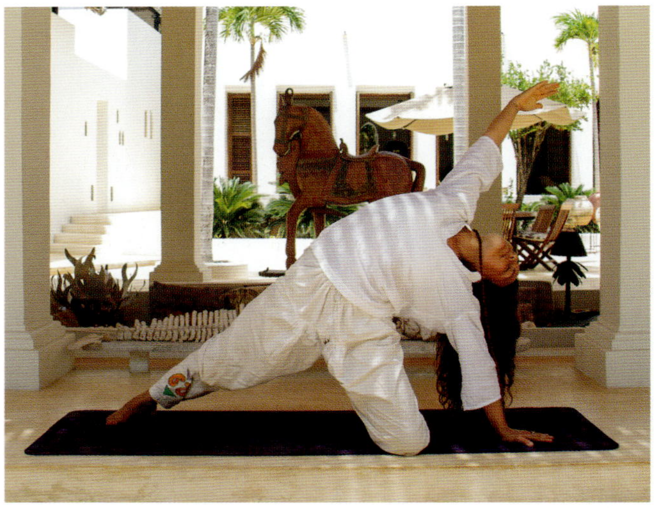

CAMATKARASANA
Enraptured Heart

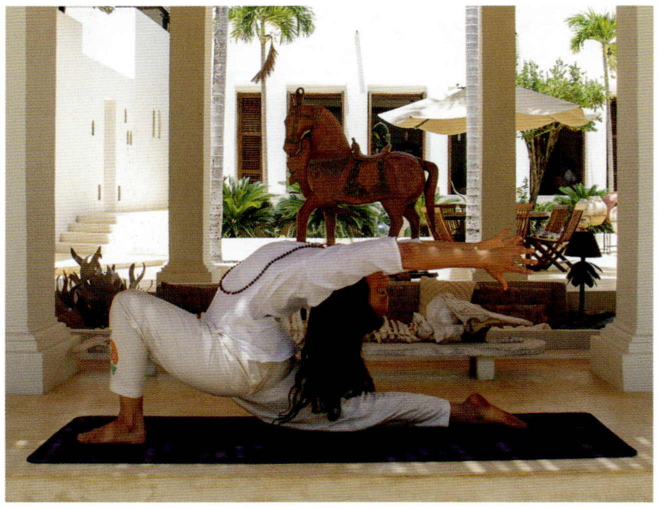

SAMDHI ANJANEYASANA
Horizon Crescent Lunge

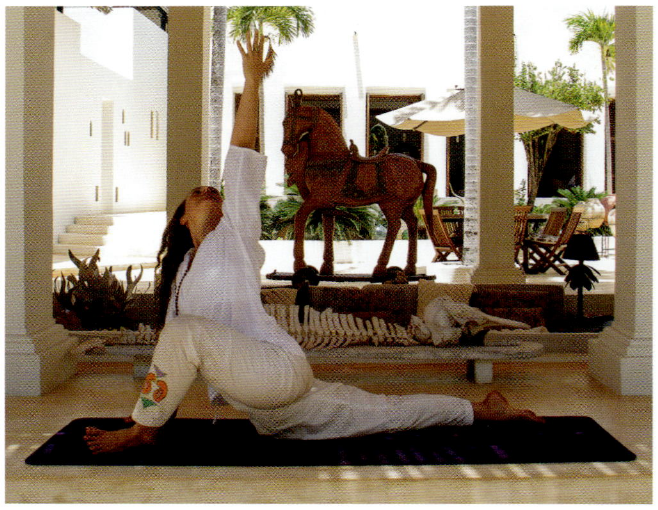

PARIVRTTA UTTHAN PRISTHASANA
Revolved Dragon Lizard

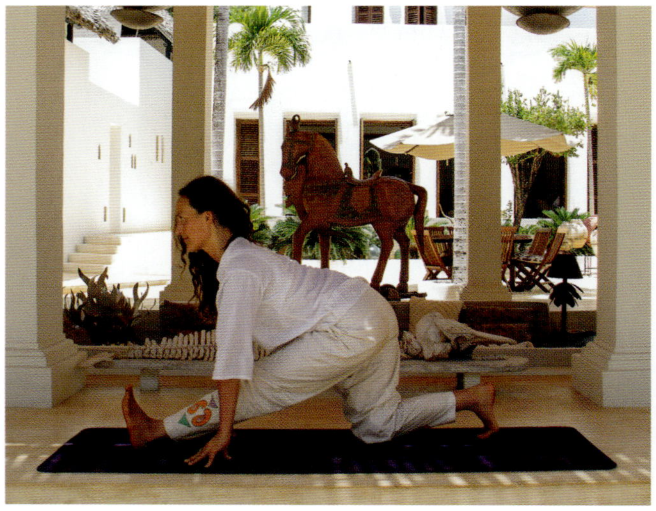

GAURAKHARASANA
Wild Donkey

In Brahma Kumbha, we are in the settled season of elemental air. This constellation of asanas provides an innovative way to unwrap the rebellious heart through graceful yet impressive poses. Through unconventional and original sequencing, the body acts as a framework and cosmic portal, a conduit for universal energy and prana to flow. The mudras create space for profound awakening and illumination. This prepares us for a humanistic existence based on kindness, selflessness, and the insights we find when we are fully in alignment with the cosmos.

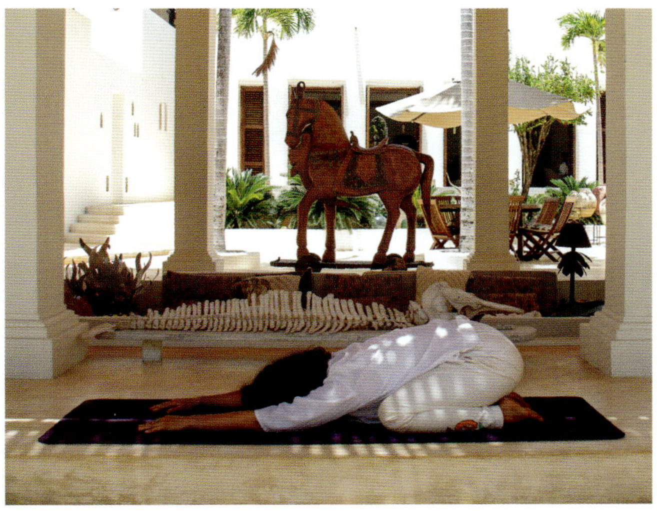

BALASANA
Child's

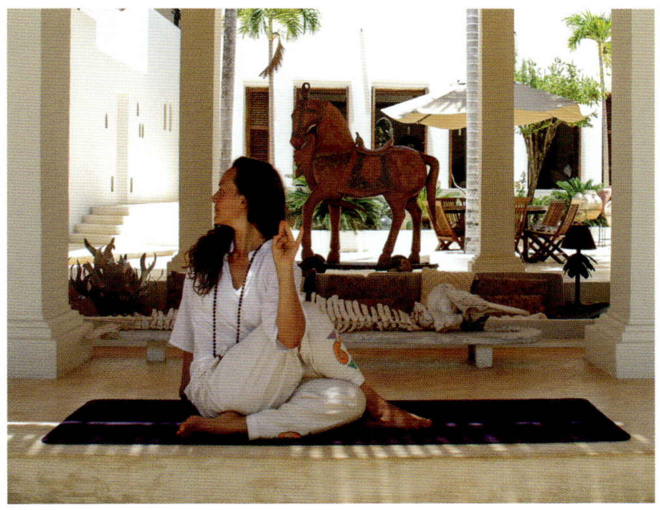

ARDHA MATSYENDRASANA & SHUNYAMUDRA
Half Lord of the Fish & Existence

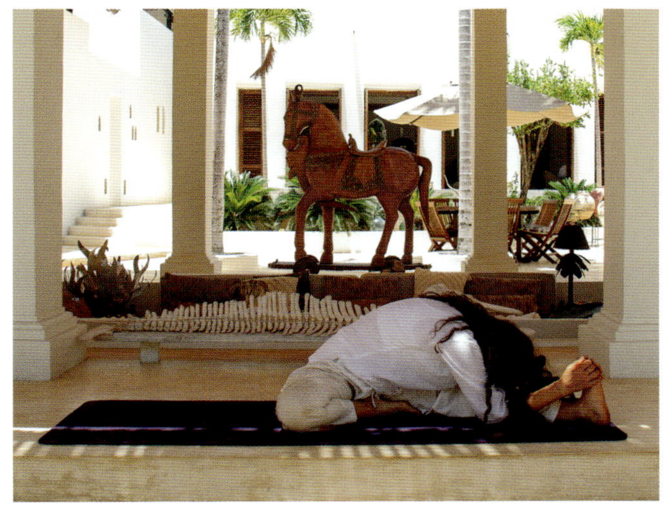

JANUSIRSASANA
Head-to-Knee Forward Bend

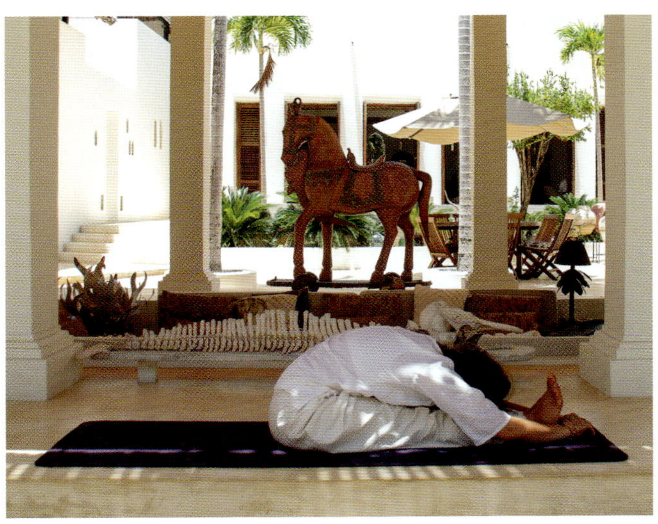

PASCHIMOTTANASANA
Forward Bend

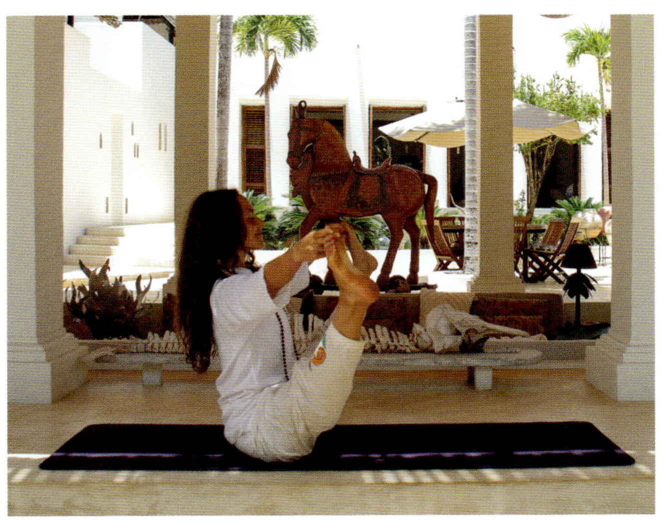

URDHVA UPAVISTHA KONASANA
Upward-Facing Wide-Angle Seated

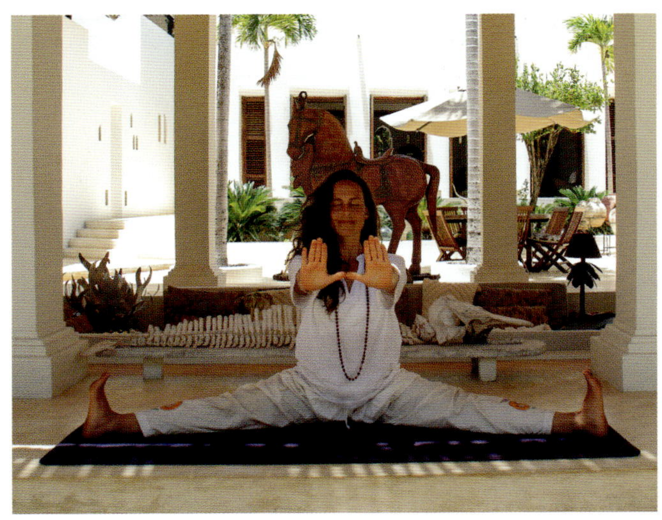

UTHITHA UPAVISTHA KONASANA & PRALAMBAMUDRA
Wide-Legged Seated & Kindness

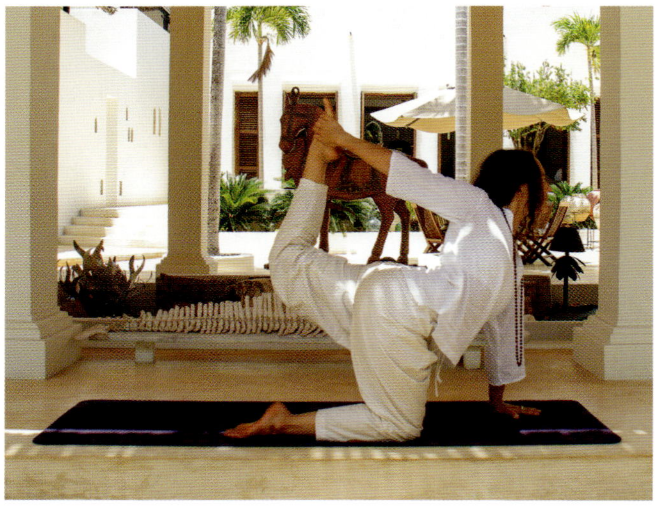

PARIVRTTA BHARMANASANA
Twisted Tabletop

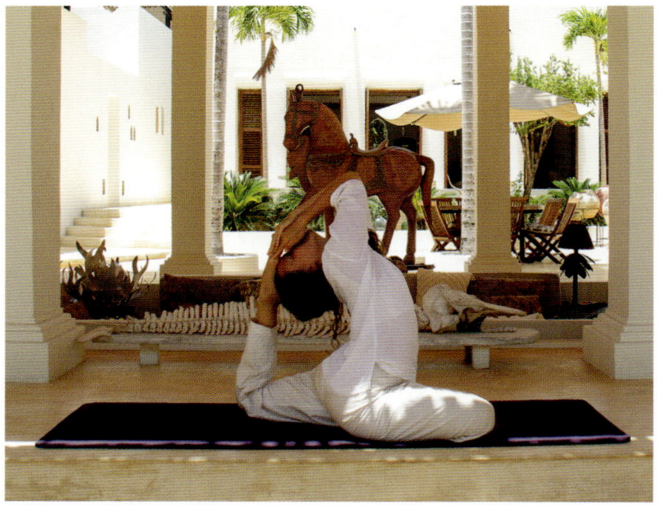

EKA PADA RAJAKAPOTASANA
King Pigeon

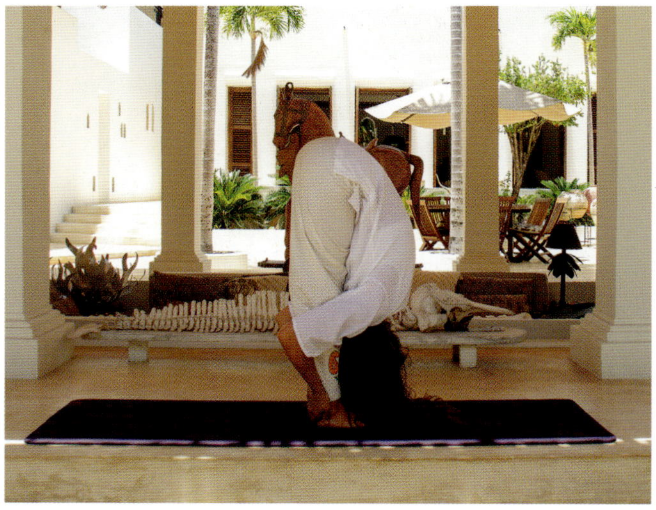

UTTANASANA
Standing Forward Fold

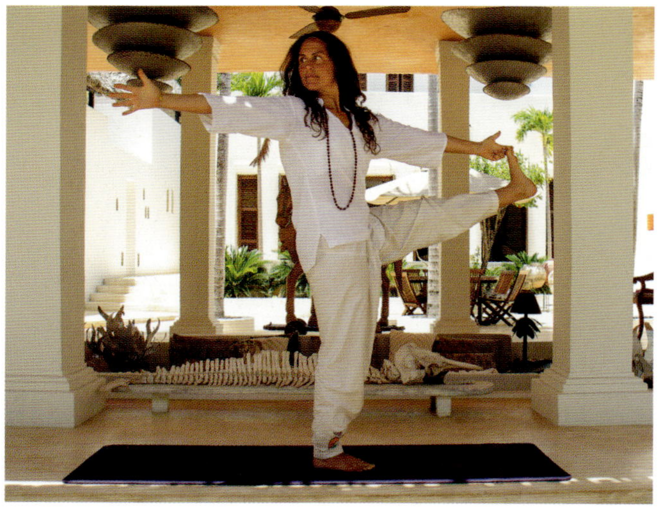

ANIMISA HASTA PADANGUSTHASANA
Blossoming Hand-to-Big Toe

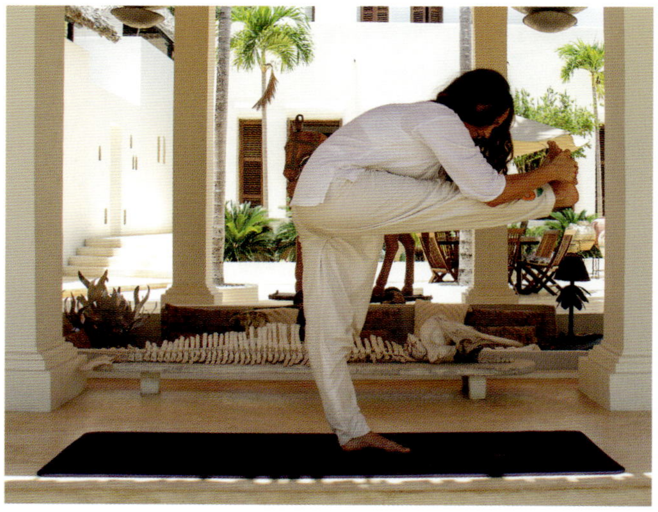

DANDAYAMANA JANUSIRSASANA
Standing Head-to-Knee

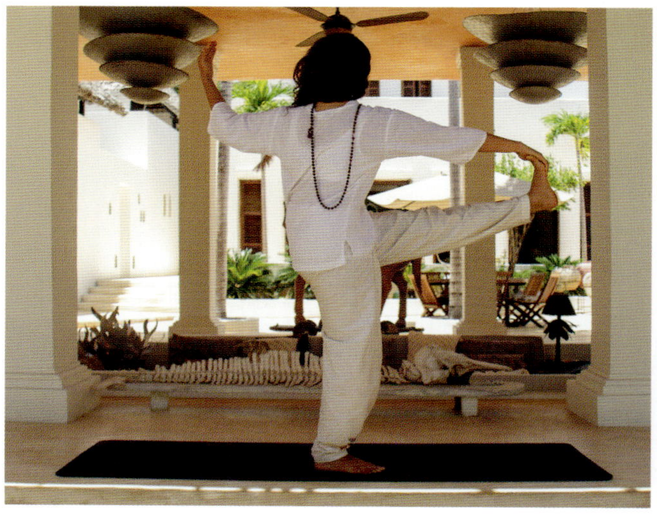

PARIVRTTA HASTA PADANGUSTHASANA
Revolved Hand-to-Big Toe

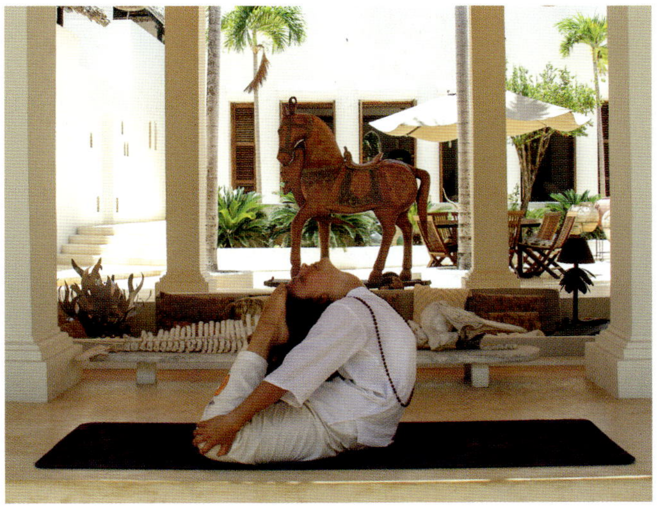

SALABHASANA PADA SIRSANA
Coiled Locust

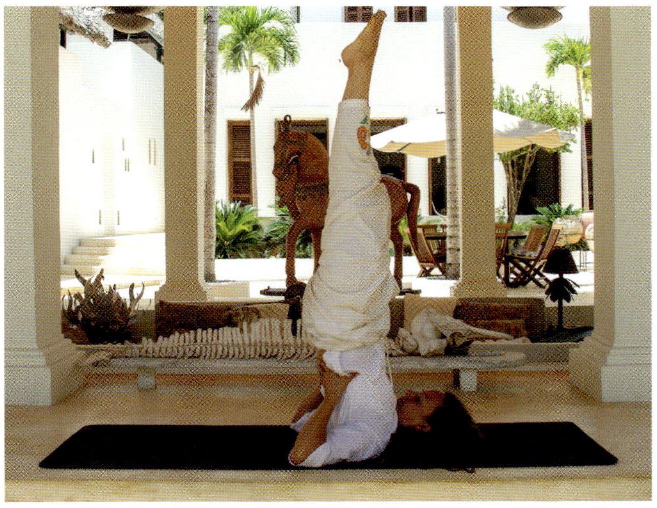

SARVANGASANA
Shoulder Stand

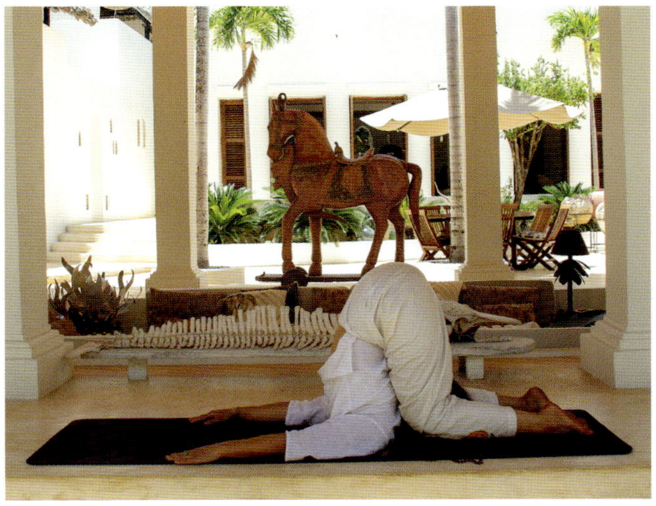

KARNAPIDASANA
Ear-to-Knee

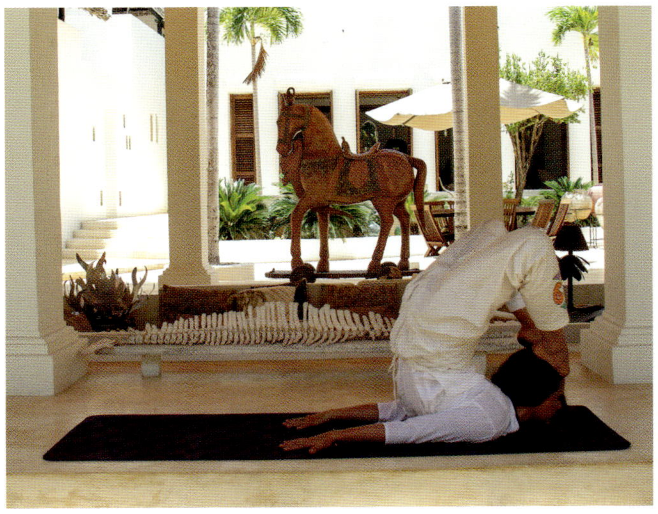

PURNA SALABHASANA
Locust

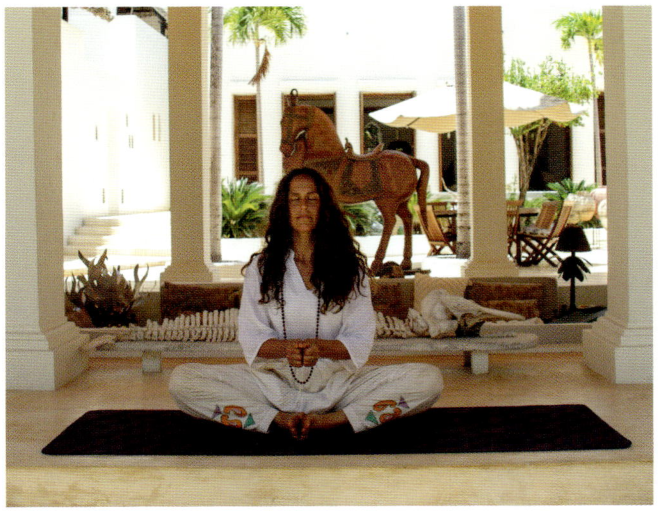

BADDHA KONASANA & MUSHTIKAMUDRA
Cobbler & Selflessness

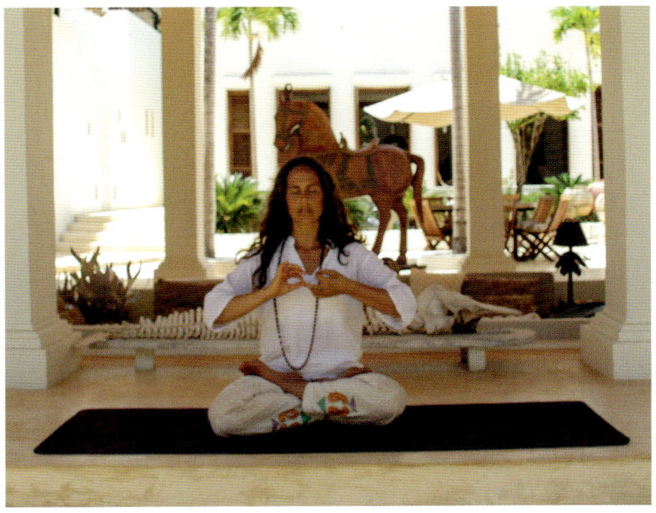

PADMASANA & DHARMACHAKRAMUDRA
Lotus & Alignment

BRAHMA MEENA • Pisces

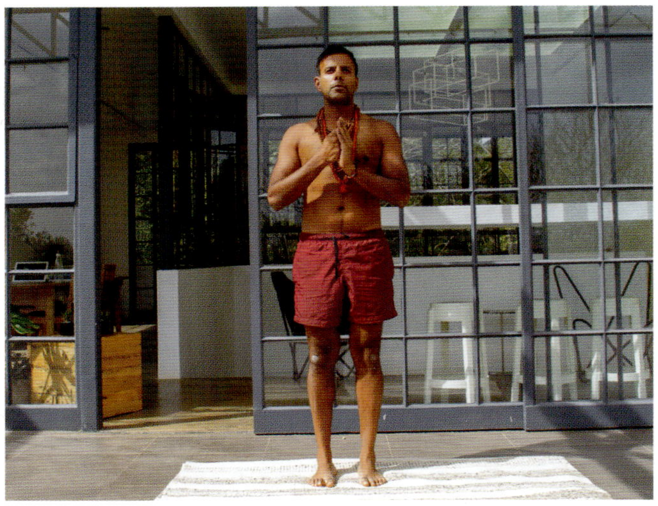

TADASANA, BHASTRIKA PRANAYAMA & SHANKHMUDRA
Mountain, Cleansing Breath & Mystery

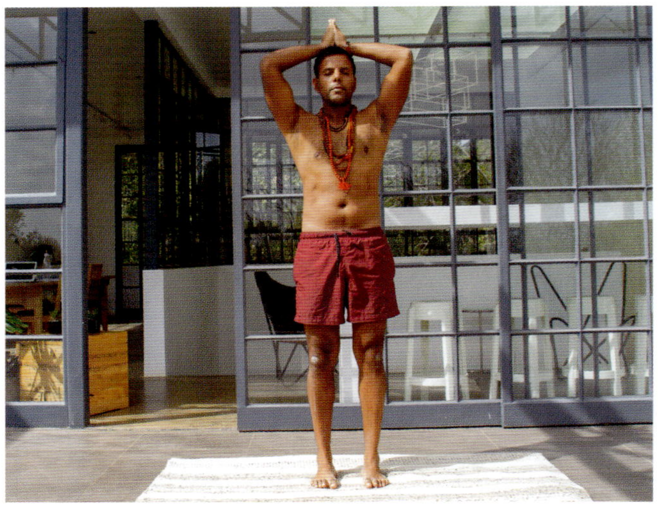

TADASANA, SAHASRARA & ANJALIMUDRA
Mountain, Crown Chakra & Love

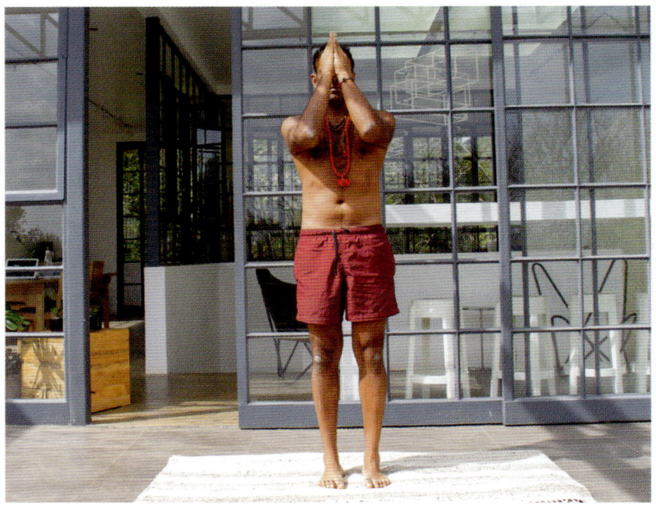

TADASANA, AJNA & ANJALIMUDRA
Mountain, Third Eye Chakra & Love

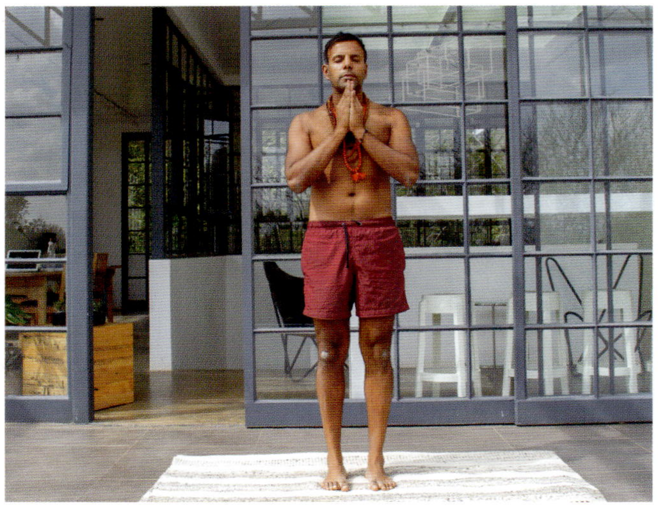

TADASANA, VISSHUDI & ANJALIMUDRA
Mountain, Throat Chakra & Love

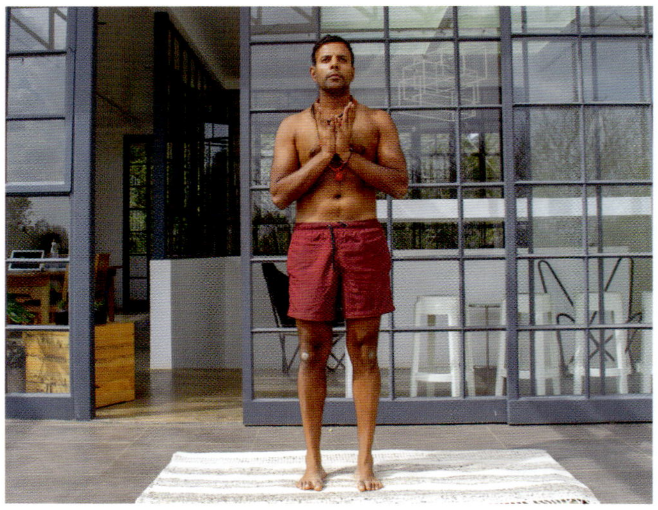

TADASANA, ANAHATA & PADMAMUDRA
Mountain, Heart Chakra & Enlightenment

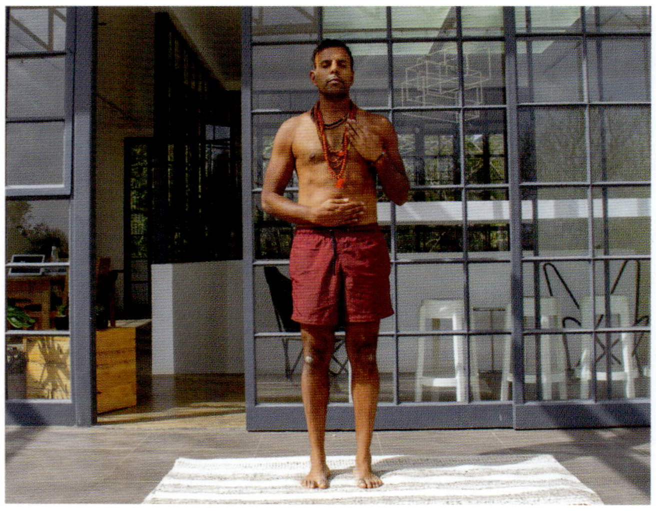

TADASANA & MANIPURA
Mountain & Solar Chakra

In Brahma Meena, we are in the shifting season of elemental water. This constellation of asanas invites us to reflect on the devotion and spirituality of our practice. The symbolic act of prostrating to the earth surrenders all experiences with nonattachment. The cooling breath is a sanctuary of calmness, and the fire breath releases our intuitive reservoir of imagination. The cleansing pranayama means we let go of any fear, and the artist within emerges. The mudras create awe and mystery, evoking the raptures of love and enlightenment. The sequence guides us through transcendence so we have freedom and are bonded with infinity.

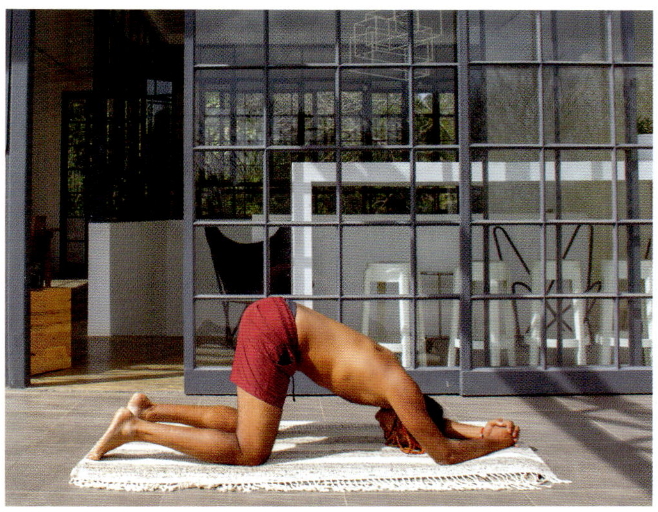

UTTANA SHISHOSANA & GRANTHITAMUDRA
Puppy Dog & Transcendence

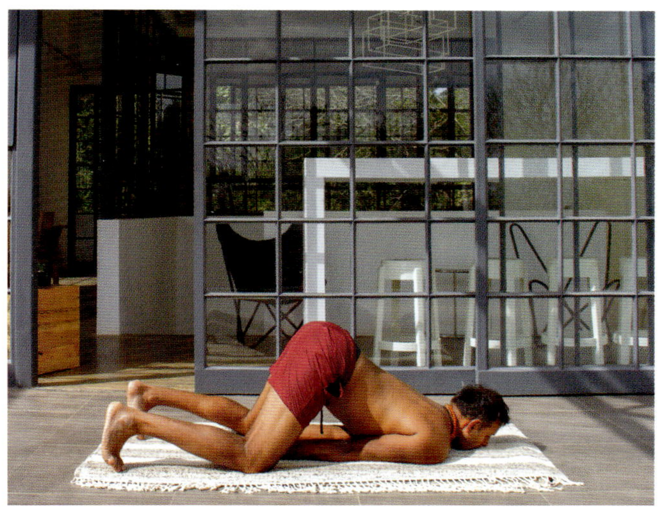

KUNDALINI SHAKTI ASHWINI MOOLA BANDHA
Merging with Sphincter and Perineum Seals

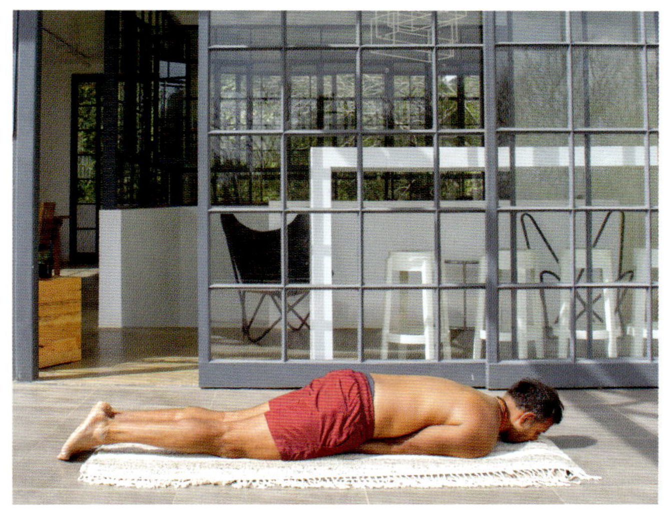

MAKARASANA
Crocodile

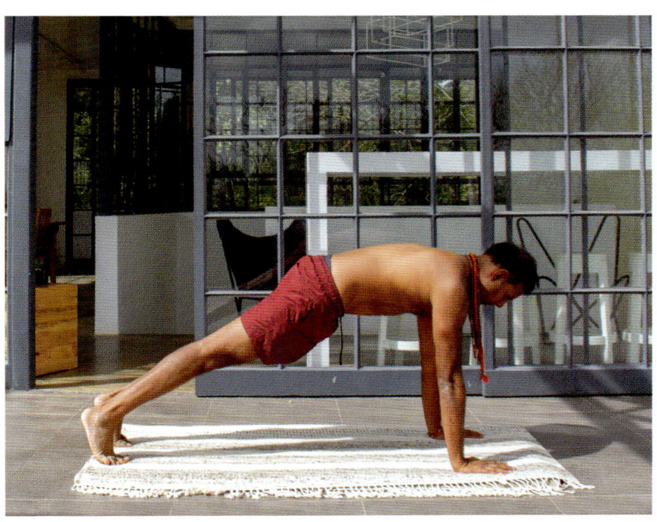

KUMBHAKASANA & 108 KAPALABHATI
Plank & 108 Fire Breath Pulsations

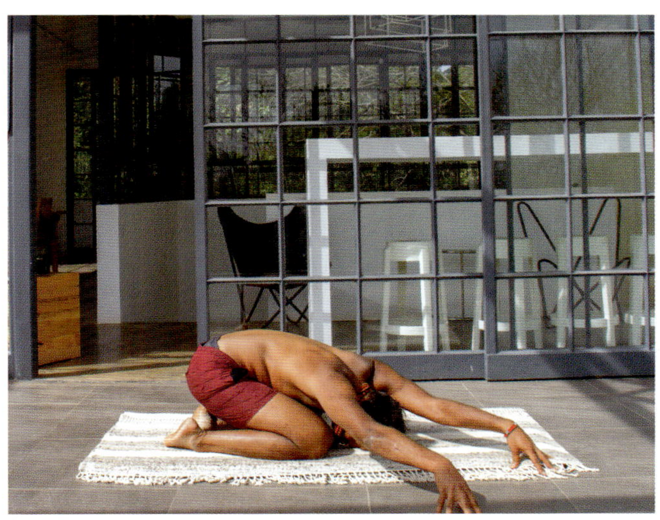

ARDHA BALASANA
Swaying Child

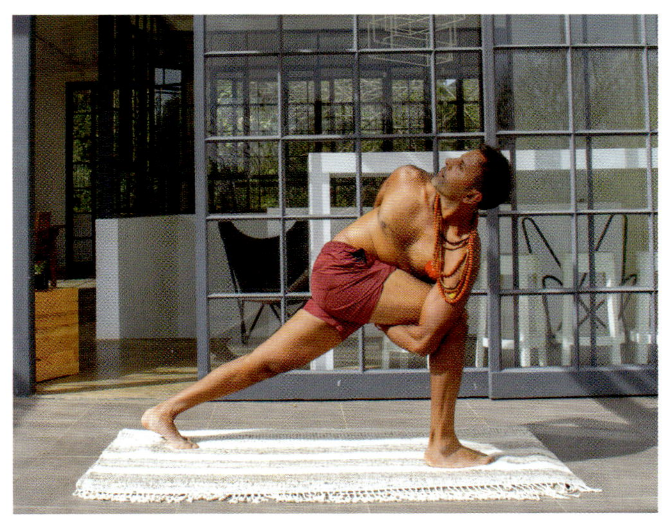

BADDHA UTTHITA PARSVAKONASANA
Bound Side Angle

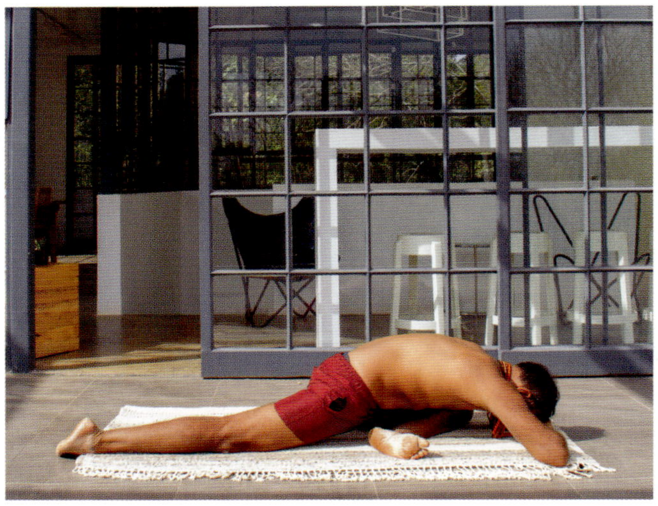

SONASVAINASANA
Sleeping Swan

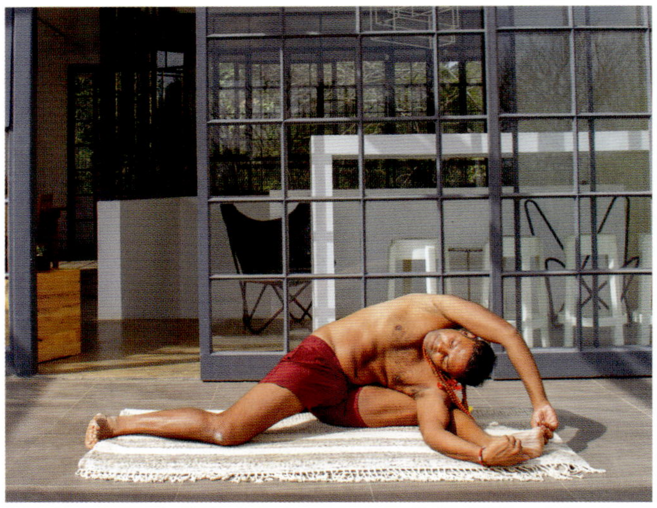

SUPTA ARDHA KAPOTASANA
Resting Half Pigeon

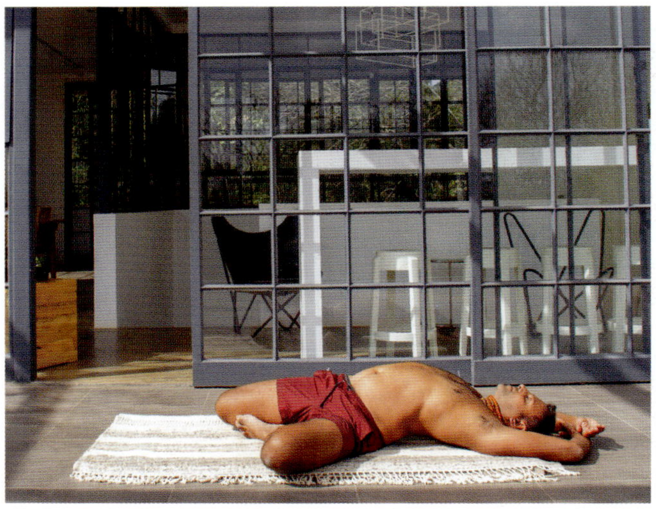

OKTOPASANA
Octopus

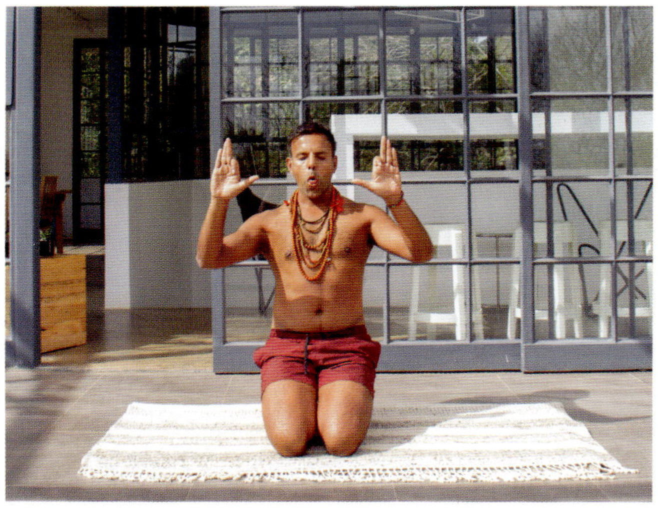

VAJRASANA SITALI PRANAYAMA & SHAKATAMUDRA
Thunderbolt Cooling Breath & Freedom

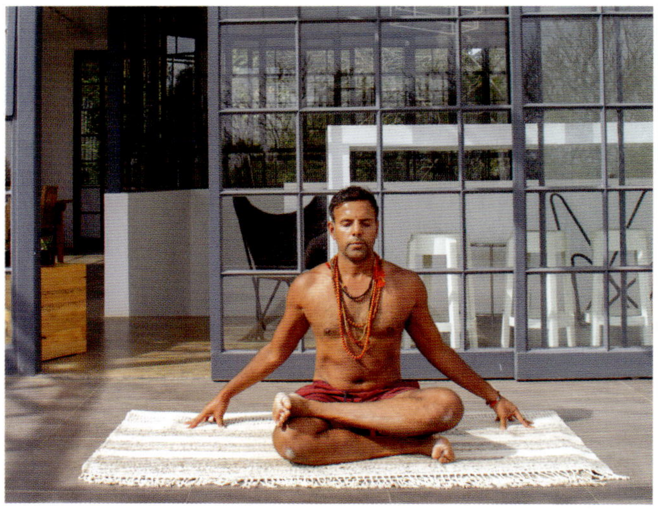

HASTA AGNISTAMBHASANA
Reaching Firelog

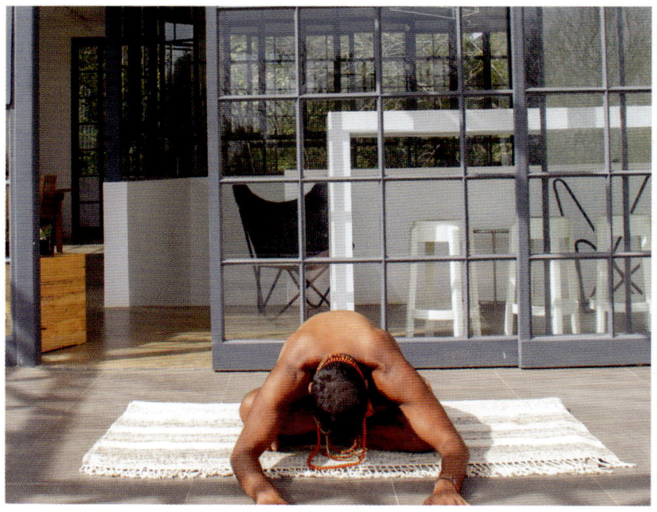

PASCHI AGNISTAMBHASANA
Folded Firelog

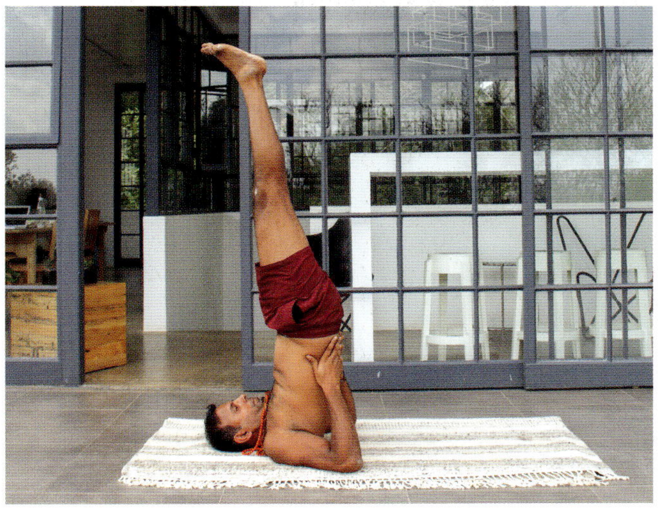

SARVANGASANA
Shoulder Stand

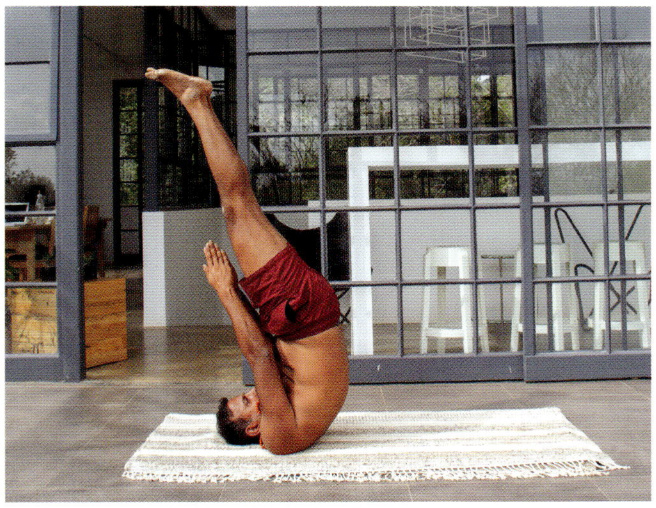

NIRALAMBASARVANGASANA
Candle Shoulder Stand

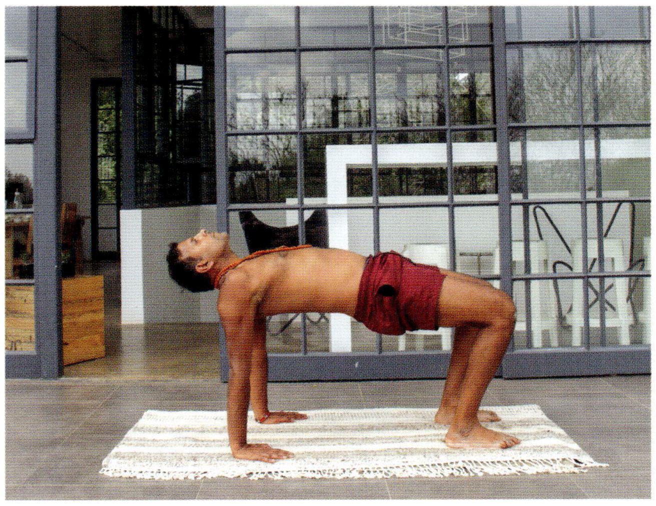

ARDHA PURVOTTANASANA
Half-Inclined Plane

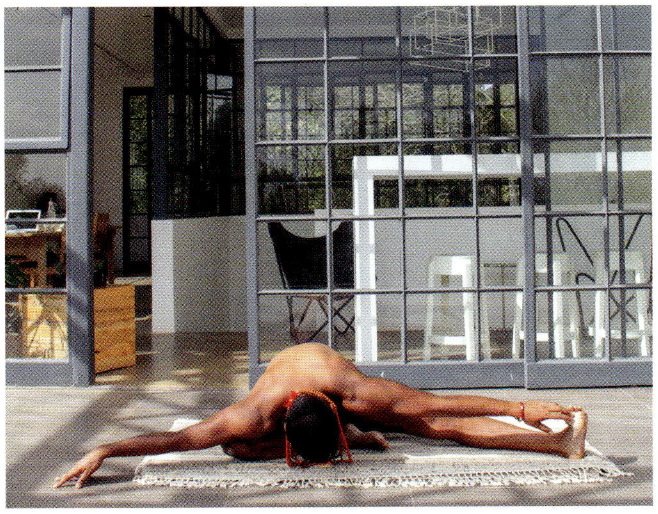

AMRAKUNAJASANA
Mangrove

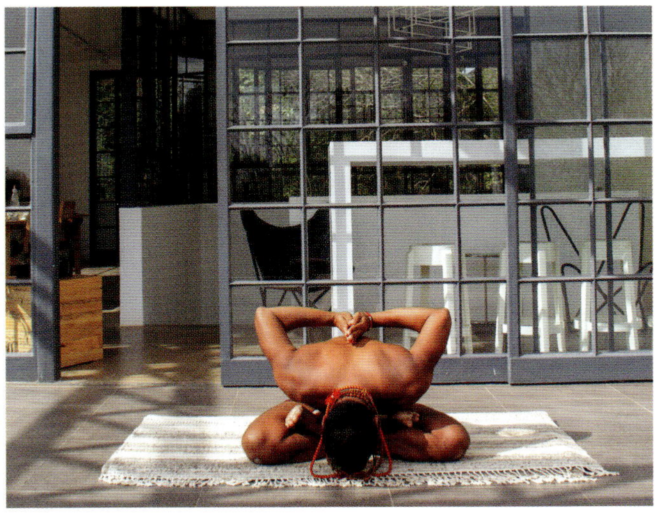

YOGA MUDRASANA
Deep-Seated Lotus Fold

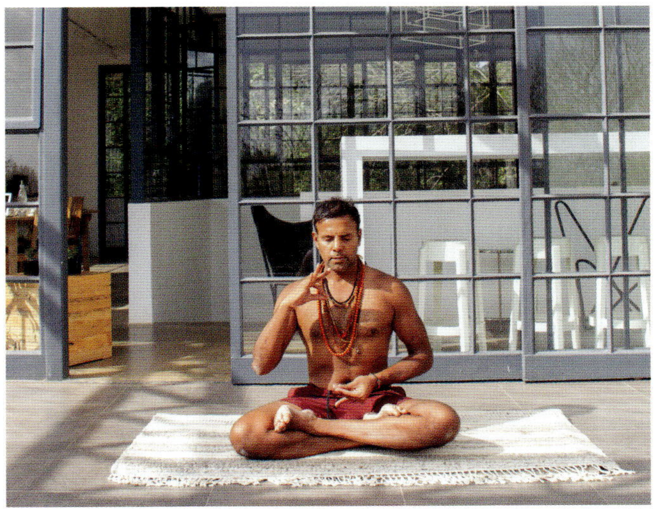

PADMASANA & BRAHMAMUDRA
Lotus & Infinity

THE TEMPLE

Ornate temple,
in this vast city,
with a thousand stories reverberating through civilizations
merging into the passage of time.
The silent threads binding to my dharma
through the allure, trappings, and misgivings of artha.
Time listens patiently to the drones and demands of destiny's desire
as we toil and curl, discard and batter our dreams
into fantastical hallucinations of meaning.
Suited not only for reason's sense,
nor fate's efficacy,
but in true denial of our spirit's nature.
The faded, jaded fabric of our lives naked,
uncovered, and banished from its source
as we replicate, rejuvenate, and replace our tender hearts.
The distraction of yet another other.
The hopeful wishes of mortals merely etched against these sacred walls.
Into its hollow crevices we dent our hopes
and we imagine the deities behold as our witness.
It's graceful to know, millennia along,
that we continue to search,
following the simmering scent of a flower,
hoping to find a field and not a pyre.

—Leo Lourdes

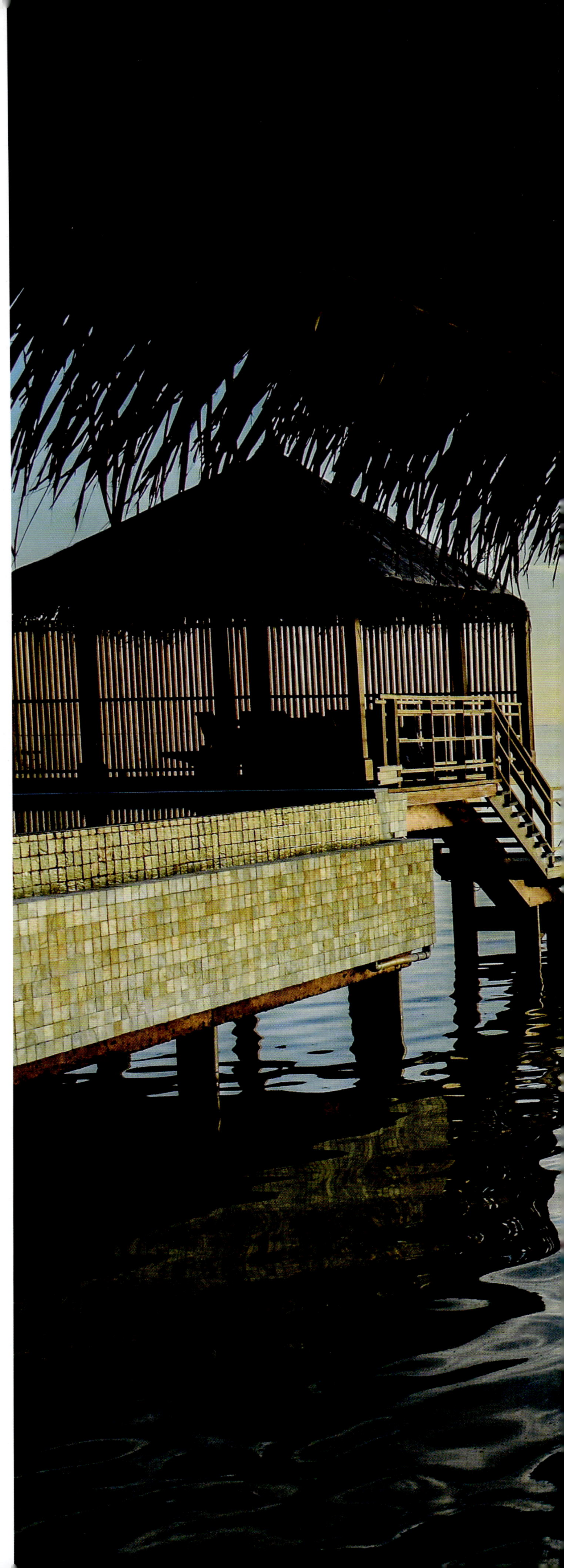

SANGA PARSVA URDHVA HASTASANA · Gathering Half Moon

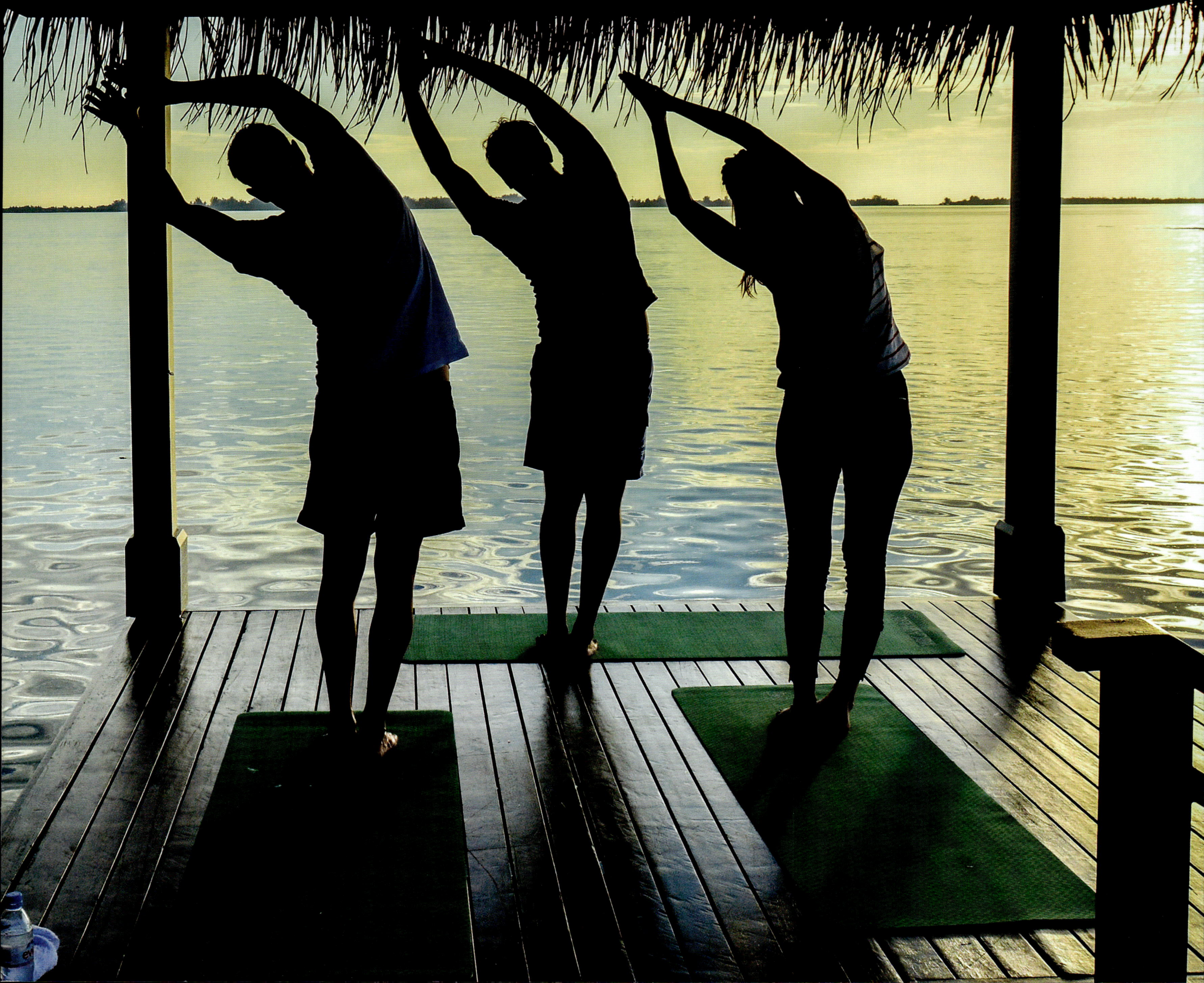

ACKNOWLEDGMENTS

First, I dedicate this book to my beloved beagle, Lamu, here on Earth, and my nephew, Kai Lourdes Wise, up in heaven. You both showed me the perfection of unconditional love that can exist in this world.

I am eternally grateful to my creative soul family who helped me realize this book, including African Ceremonies light bearers Carol Beckwith, Angela Fisher, Maria Alexander, and team; Big Life Foundation founder Tom Hill; Jimmy Nelson; Paya Ndiaye; Peter Adler of Pebble London; Deborah Coulson and David Coulson MBE, who discovered African rock art and taught me about humanity's origin in Africa; humanitarian photographer Alissa Everett; my best friend, conservationist and entrepreneur Peter Holmes à Court; the team at Afrika House; Nav Kumari; and photographers Anh Thai Bui, Jean Gabriel, Jodi Redhouse, and Carl Shanahan.

Additional thanks to the following: Katy Barker at Dhow House, Isabel Hansen at Mnarani House, the team at Honeymoon House, Monika Fauth at Banana House, and the Lamu Yoga festival crew; Robert Kuok and family for the beautiful home you blessed me with on Villingili Island in the Maldives; Qatari Diar and James Sellar for creating The Shard in London, which was home to my first yoga studio; Sir David Adjaye for designing the beautiful Lost House, which was a delightful home for Lamu and me; Tuuli Shipster, Rankin, and Damian Nixon; Tannah Matus, Nigel Kemp, and Elie Pippard-Kemp for their enduring belief in me; Christian Candy, Lance Uggla, Olly Olsen, and Charlie Green for being my role models in both design and business; team Blackstone, both in New York and London, for being the best clients ever—thanks for helping me feed people with the contributions we made to the Trussell Trust via my yoga classes during the global pandemic; the entire Smurfit family for our epic joyful yoga sessions; Maysa Salem and Rafel Bagot; Ken Lipper for your guidance; everyone at my publisher, Rizzoli—Charles Miers, James Muschett, Candice Fehrman, and Susi Oberhelman—for giving me a home as a first-time author; Juliette Cunliffe and the 42 children we look after at the Peace Pagoda in the Himalayas; Patrick Holford for your wisdom on nutrition; Mujassum Butt, Mark Anastasi, Mark Tyfield, and Evan Cramer, my soul brothers; Kavita Ramdya and Mansoor Sirinathsingh for your support, and Roopa Vyas and Ritchie Smith for your love; Merck Mercuriadis for believing in my dream of uniting my songs, music, and philanthropy; Dua Lipa for our enchanting conversations about the moon and for your radiant heart energy; Oprah Winfrey for your beautiful hugs, for listening to my vision after yoga in the Himalayas, and for initiating me by calling me "the singing yogi"; Eckhart Tolle for supporting me with my poem "The Temple"; and Khamis Abdullah for the tears we shared after a heart-wrenching visit to a former slave site in Zanzibar's Stone Town—I will always remember how you patiently waited while I sat on a rock at sunset and wrote the poem "Gems."

A big heartfelt wave of radiant love to all the teachers and yogis who agreed to model for me in this book, bringing the diversity and expression of the stunning asanas of my Brahma Yoga method to life: Awham Mohamed Al-Baidy, Alex Crockford, Madhvi Dalal, Samanta Duggal, Christel Flowers, Jawad Hamid, Samantha Howick, Mandy Jhamat, Vaida Kvedaraitė, Kieran Lowrie, Katariina Malkamäki, Natalie Cristal Morrison, David Mwashighadi Mwalugha, Robin Mydlak, Nalangu Naeku, Nkasiogi Nataana, Weronika Nowaczyńska, Mareen Pasedag, Salim Rollins, Lucrezia Romagnolo, Leila Sadeghee, Rebekah Sauder, Leboo Sironka, Alexandra Spyratos, Oriane Torode, Antoan Van, and Baghi Yemane.

Finally, I am eternally grateful to my birth family. I keep flying away from their nest to seek adventures, but they always receive me with love when I am wounded or need to rest. Thanks to my late grandmother, who brushed my teeth until I was five years old and told me my smile would bring many people happiness. Thank you to my mother, Caroline Alphonso, and my father, Louis Lourdes. Thanks to my in-laws, Michael Wise and Tony Heusner, who bring sanity to my eccentric family. And last, thanks to my siblings—Zita, Michelle, Veronica, and Rahul—and all my beautiful nieces and nephews—Shania, Tiana, Keira, Isaiah, Kai, Skye, and Aaliyah.

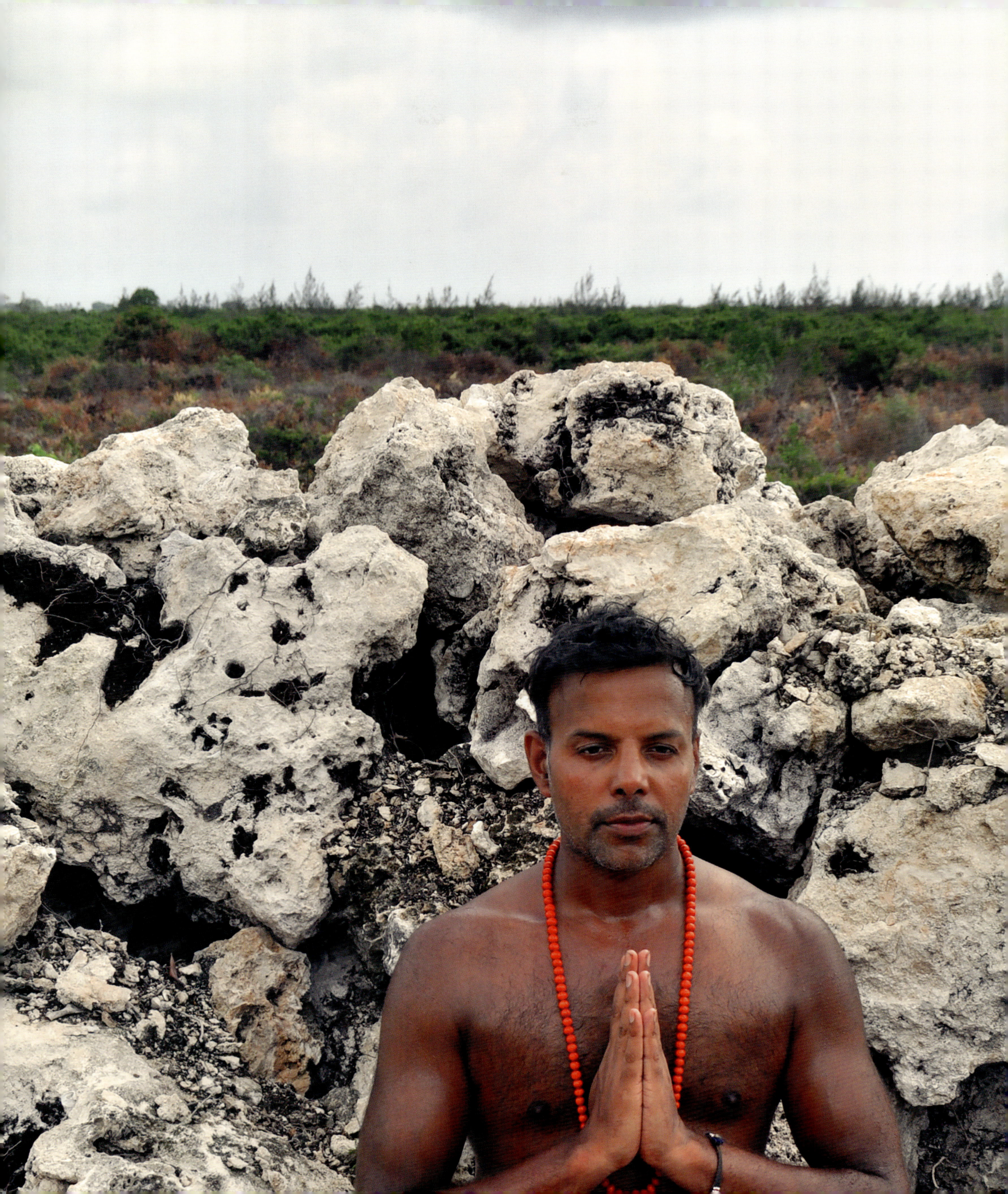

Yoga

Please visit www.ysyoga.co.uk to access the accompanying app with detailed instructions, class sequences, and guided visualizations available in multiple languages.

First published in the United States of America in 2023 by
Rizzoli International Publications, Inc.
300 Park Avenue South
New York, NY 10010
www.rizzoliusa.com

Publisher: Charles Miers
Associate Publisher: James Muschett
Managing Editor: Lynn Scrabis
Editor: Candice Fehrman
Design: Susi Oberhelman

Printed in China

2023 2024 2025 2026 / 10 9 8 7 6 5 4 3 2 1

ISBN: 978-0-8478-7235-0

Library of Congress Control Number: 2023933487

Visit us online:
Facebook.com/RizzoliNewYork
Twitter: @Rizzoli_Books
Instagram.com/RizzoliBooks
Pinterest.com/RizzoliBooks
Youtube.com/user/RizzoliNY
Issuu.com/Rizzoli

MIX
Paper from responsible sources
FSC® C104723